Essentials of
Immediate
Medical Care

Essentials of
Immediate
Medical Care

Dr C John Eaton MB BS Dip IMC RCS(Ed)

General Practitioner
Member of the British Association for Immediate Care
Saffron Walden
Essex, UK

SECOND EDITION

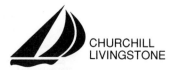
CHURCHILL
LIVINGSTONE

EDINBURGH LONDON NEW YORK PHILADELPHIA SYDNEY TORONTO 1999

CHURCHILL LIVINGSTONE
An imprint of Harcourt Brace & Company Limited

Robert Stevenson House,
1-3 Baxter's Place, Leith Walk,
Edinburgh, EH1 3AF, UK

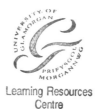
First edition 1992
Revised 1993
Second edition 1999

ISBN 0 443 05345 6

British Library Catologuing in Publication Data
A catalogue record for this book is available from the British Library

Library of Congress Cataloging in Publication Data
A catalog record for this book is available from the Library of Congress

Medical Knowledge is constantly changing. As new information
becomes available, changes in treatment, procedures, equipment
and the use of drugs become necessary. The author and the publishers
have, as far as it is possible, taken care to ensure that the information
given in this text is accurate and up to date. However, readers are
strongly advised to confirm that the information, especially with
regard to drug usage, complies with current legislation and standards
of practice.

Printed in China
NPCC/01

Preface

This book have been produced primarily for the doctor who is either practising, or considering practising Immediate Care, and in particular those preparing for the Diploma in Immediate Medical Care of the Royal College of Surgeons of Edinburgh (Dip IMC RCS Ed) and the new Fellowship in Immediate Medical Care of the Royal College of Surgeons of Edinburgh (FIMC RCS Ed). It should also be of interest to doctors and nurses involved in hospital mobile medical and surgical teams, doctors staffing minor casualty departments, which may have a triaging role in very rural areas, doctors in the armed forces on detached duty, doctors practising in remote areas, nurses involved in Immediate Care and both extended trained and non-extended trained ambulance personnel.

Immediate Care is a relatively new speciality, and at present there are few texts devoted to the subject. Most American texts are designed primarily for the paramedic, and with a few recent exceptions most British texts are either multiauthor, or have been written by experts who are primarily hospital orientated.

This book has been written in the form of a series of notes, each using the same format and style, so as to facilitate their use as revision material, and as a ready reference. The use of one author, albeit with input from many experts, hopefully has avoided the duplication and differing styles so often found in multiauthor books.

Although intended to be reasonably comprehensive, no attempt has been made to cover anything other than the Immediate Care aspects of most problems, and references are given at the end of the book for further reading should the reader wish to research any particular subject in greater depth. Anatomy and physiology have not been covered in depth as there are already many excellent textbooks which cover these subjects.

Guidelines where shown are those most universally agreed, and not necessarily the latest (but controversial) state of the art. I have deliberately included some procedures, which might more usually be carried out in hospital, for the benefit of those practising in remote areas or on detached duty, and for whom the travelling time to hospital may be many hours. Drug information is based on that in the current edition of the British National Formulary.

This book began life as a set of personal revision notes for the Diploma in Immediate Medical Care, which became the initial Course Notes on Immediate Care for the Cambridge Immediate Care Courses, organised by Dr John Scott. These were corrected and revised, and after a lot of help and constructive comments from many experts, became the second edition. Later a third edition was produced and that became the final proof for the first edition of this book.

This second edition has been very substantially revised, rewritten and enlarged with additional chapters on ECG recognition, mechanisms of injury, care of the elderly and psychiatric emergencies. There are over 350 new diagrams, with new sections dealing with some of the controversies in Immediate Care. This edition incorporates the revised guidelines developed by the British Thoracic Association for the management of acute asthma; the guidelines produced by Medical Commission on Accident Prevention for the out of hospital management of hypothermia; the revised Paediatric Resuscitation Chart produced by Dr Peter Oakley, the revised guidelines issued by the Meningitis Trust for the diagnosis and management of bacterial meningitis, and the new guidelines for Basic Life Support, Advanced Life Support, management of the Peri-arrest Arrhythmias, Paediatric Basic and Advanced Life Support, Resuscitation of Babies at Birth and Airway Management published by the European Resuscitation Council in 1996 and 1998.

C.J.E., 1999

Dedication

This book is dedicated to all of those involved in Immediate Care,
past, present, potential and future, and in particular to the father of
Immediate Care, Dr Kenneth Easton, and my personal mentor in
Immediate Care, Dr Robin Winch, without either of whom this book
would not exist, in the hope that it will enable the victims of trauma or
sudden serious illness to receive the best possible pre-hospital treatment.

Foreword for the Second Edition

Immediate Care by physicians in the UK is a largely unfunded specialty and almost totally depends on the goodwill, devotion and resourcefulness of the participants. Working in conjunction with the allied emergency services, they have proved their worth in providing medical knowledge and special expertise on countless occasions at accidents and medical emergencies.

Although it has taken years to achieve recognition. I believe it is now generally understood that a doctor, trained and versant in the techniques of Immediate Medical Care, is frequently required to amplify the work of the ambulance service. Paramedics have become skilled and adept in a large number of lifesaving procedures, including airway management, defibrillation and the administration of glucagon, salbutamol and intravenous fluids where appropriate. They are masters of extrication and splinting.

Medicine, however, moves on and it is now clear that there are an increasing number of prehospital and emergency situations which require clinical judgement by a doctor which only comes with medical education in depth. The interpretation of a 12-lead ECG and the decision to begin thrombolysis, the judgement of intravenous fluid requirements in patients with penetrating torsa injury and concomitant head trauma are instances which spring to mind.

John Eaton is a tyro in the field of Immediate Medical Care. He has devoted a substantial part of his medical career to the management of prehospital care and can write with an almost unique authority on the subject.

This book began from his personal notes in preparing for the diploma in Immediate Medical Care of the Royal College of Surgeons in Edinburgh. Through several improved and amplified versions of those notes he has now produced what is undoubtably the most comprehensive book on Immediate Care which is currently available. Though he has written the entire work himself, he has been painstakingly thorough in seeking help and criticism from experts in narrow fields and he can justifiably claim to have produced a book of authority and accuracy.

This work is to be recommended to all who deal with emergencies. This will include all family doctors, emergency physicians, anaesthetists and those who attend major incidents, sporting meetings and crowd events, not to mention medical students and paramedics, especially those preparing for degree courses.

Peter Baskett BA MB BCh BAO MRCP FRCA

Past Chairman, the British Association for Immediate Care

Foreword for the First Edition

Immediate Care has become a recognised and rewarding speciality within General Practice, Community and Hospital Practice. In the past, I believe some of the resistance to establishing new Immediate Care Schemes, was due to lack of experience and suitable reading material, rather than a lack of willingness on the part of the physician. Medical schools are now teaching more basic and advanced resuscitation skills, and they are being introduced into both qualifying and postgraduate examinations, providing further impetus and encouragement to doctors to carry appropriate resuscitation equipment at all times and to form BASICS schemes.

With the introduction of "The Diploma in Immediate Medical Care" by the Royal College of Surgeons of Edinburgh, we finally have a higher professional qualification, by which we can both evaluate and recognise a competent Immediate Care doctor. Appropriate literature to prepare for this examination has previously been scattered throughout many textbooks. Now that the practical skills can be refreshed at several Immediate Care courses throughout the United Kingdom, this timely volume provides an excellent, comprehensive and appropriate text, not only for use during the course, but for many years to come.

Judith M Fisher MB BS FRCGP

Past Chairman, the British Association for Immediate Care

Technical Note

The manuscript for this book was produced by the author on Acorn RISC PC, using Computer Concepts' Impression Publisher document processing software. A few diagrams were scanned in using a Computer Concepts' Scanlight Professional image scanner, but most were drawn by the author using Computer Concepts' Artworks professional graphics software. The entire book was then printed out onto paper plates using a Calligraph direct drive laser printer, which were then supplied to the printer.

Acknowledgements

I am very grateful to all those doctors and other experts, who have very kindly and so freely given me much constructive criticism and helpful advice, and I hope they will see that I have listened to them! It came as a very pleasant surprise to me, that without exception, they have all been so tremendously helpful. I hope that all those who use this book will also give me their comments, good and bad, so that future editions will be as comprehensive as possible.

I would like to acknowledge the help of the Resuscitation Council (UK) for their generous permission to use material and diagrams from *Resuscitation for the Citizen* and the *ABC of Resuscitation,* and the European Resuscitation Council for permission to use their diagrams for Advanced Life Support, management of the Peri-arrest Arrhythmias, Paediatric Basic and Advanced Life Support, Resuscitation of Babies at Birth and Airway Management. I am also grateful to Dr Brian Robertson, the editor of the *Basics Journal* for his permission to use line drawings from that journal; to the Officer Commanding HQ Search and Rescue Wing, RAF Finningley for his assistance in obtaining line drawings of the Wessex and Sea King helicopters; to the Controller of Her Majesty's Stationery Office and the Home Office (Fire Department) for permission to use various diagrams from the *Manual of Firemanship;* to Richard D Meyer M D to incorporate the diagrams on helmet removal; to Dr Peter Oakley and the *British Medical Journal* for permission to use his Paediatric Resuscitation Chart; and to Hoechst UK Ltd for permission to use ECG tracings from their *ECG Atlas.*

I am most grateful to Dr John Scott for using the precursors of this book as the manual for the BASICS Education five day courses on Immediate Care, held in Cambridge, to Clare Clenshaw, my secretary, for all her assistance, and to Peter Baskett (who has also kindly written the foreword for this edition), Nick Bateman, Mick Colquhoun, Anthony Handley, Ken Hines, David Humphriss, Brian Robertson, and David Zideman, for assistance with their specialist subjects and to Matthew Cooke, Peter Holden, Rod Mackenzie and Rachel Sutcliffe for proof reading the whole book. I would also like to thank Peter Richardson and Lucy Gardner of Churchill Livingstone for their invaluable help and advice with the first edition of this book and to Tim Horne and for his assistance and patience over the production of this new edition.

Finally I would like to thank my long suffering wife and partner Dr Catherine Brown who has provided me with much needed support and advice.

C John Eaton
Saffron Walden, 1999

Contents

Glossary of abbreviations

A&E	Accident and Emergency
ACCOLC	Access overload control
ACLS	Advanced Cardiac Life Support
AF	Atrial fibrillation
ALS	Advanced Life Support
AM	Amplitude modulation
AMI	Acute myocardial infarction
amp	ampoule
ARDS	Adult respiratory distress syndrome
ATLS	Advanced Trauma Life Support
AV	Atrio-ventricular
BA	Breathing apparatus
BLS	Basic Life Support
BP	Blood pressure
BP	British Pharmacopoeia
CNS	Central nervous system
CO	Carbon monoxide
CO_2	Carbon dioxide
COPD	Chronic obstructive pulmonary disease
CSF	Cerebrospinal fluid
CT	Computed tomography
CVA	Cerebrovascular accident
DC	Direct current
DGH	District General Hospital
DTs	Delirium tremens
ECG	Electrocardiogram
EMD	Electromechanical dissociation
ENT	Ear, nose and throat
ERC	Emergency reserve channel
FG	French gauge
FM	Frequency modulation
HACE	High altitude cerebral oedema
HANE	Hereditary angio-oedema
HAPE	High altitude pulmonary oedema
HAZCHEM	Hazardous chemical
HBIG	Hepatitis B immunoglobulin
HCO_3	Bicarbonate
Hg	Mercury
HIV	Human immunodeficiency virus
HPPF	Human plasma protein fraction
Hrs	Hours
GI	Gastrointestinal
ID	Identity
im	intramuscular
ITU	Intensive therapy unit
iv	intravenous
LED	Light emitting diode
LMA	Laryngeal mask airway
LSCS	Lower segment caesarian section
LTB	Laryngotracheobronchitis
MAOI	Monoamine oxidase inhibitor
MIO	Medical Incident Officer
mmHg	millimetres of mercury (pressure)
NAI	Non accidental injury
NATO	North Atlantic Treaty Organisation
N_2O	Nitrous oxide
NSAID	Non steroidal anti-inflammatory drug
O_2	Oxygen
PAC	Premature atrial contraction
PASG	Pneumatic anti-shock garment
PAT	Paroxysmal atrial tachycardia
pCO_2	Partial pressure of carbon dioxide
PEEP	Positive end expiratory pressure
PEFR	Peak expiratory flow rate
pO_2	Partial pressure of oxygen
PTLA	Pharyngeal tracheal lumen airway
PTSD	Post-traumatic stress disorder
PVC	Poly-vinyl chloride
PVCs	Premature ventricular contractions
RTA	Road traffic accident
RTS	Revised trauma score
SA	Sino-atrial
SpO_2	Arterial oxygen saturation
SCUBA	Self-contained underwater breathing apparatus
Sec	Seconds
SIDS	Sudden infant death syndrome
SOCO	Scenes of crimes officer
s/r	sustained release
SVT	Supraventricular tachycardia
SWG	Standard wire gauge
TIG	Tetanus human immunoglobulin
TREM	Transport emergency
TT	Tetanus toxoid
UHF	Ultra high frequency
UKHIS	UK hazard information system
VF	Ventricular fibrillation
VHF	Very high frequency
VSD	Ventricular septal defect
VT	Ventricular tachycardia

The concept and history of Immediate Care

> ## Definition of Immediate Care
>
> "Immediate (Medical) Care is the provision of skilled medical help at the scene of an accident, medical emergency, or during transport to hospital".

It consists of the recognition, resuscitation and stabilisation of the seriously injured and it extends beyond the preservation of life to the prevention of complications and the relief of suffering.

As such it may only be rendered by doctors and ambulance personnel who have received special training, using equipment specifically designed or adapted for use in the pre-hospital environment.

The chain of survival begins with self help and progresses to bystander First Aid, then with the arrival of an ambulance progresses to Ambulance Aid of varying sophistication depending on the training of those rendering it, and can vary from basic ambulance aid to that rendered by those with paramedic skills. Finally if an appropriately trained doctor arrives, he or she will practice Immediate Medical care.

Rationale

It has been realised increasingly over the last five decades, that if the seriously ill or injured patient receives effective immediate medical treatment, "Immediate Care", then the morbidity and the mortality are significantly reduced. In fact, it has recently been shown that in the critically injured, for every 20 minutes delay in instituting treatment, there is a threefold increase in mortality. This reduction in mortality and morbidity is due to a combination of the early performance of life saving procedures, and the prevention and treatment of life threatening pathophysiological events.

If the application of Immediate Care is to be effective, it must be rendered in a thoroughly disciplined, intelligent and rational manner, because time is of the essence; and once a procedure has been forgotten or not performed, there is seldom the opportunity for it to be done later, and for its full benefit to be experienced by the patient.

The history of BASICS

During the Second World War doctors became fully conversant with the requirements of emergency care, and were involved professionally with the rescue services and the public in the devastating effects of warfare waged upon the civilian population and armed forces alike. This expertise was a bonus to their patients during the post-war years of resettlement into general practice, the momentous commitment to a National Health Service in 1948, and the gradual evolution of the professional ambulance service. At the same time road traffic was increasing, although the roads were inadequate, and road traffic accidents accounted for more deaths and disabilities than had resulted from the previous armed conflict. Dr Kenneth Easton first became involved in this programme in 1949, when as Senior Medical Officer to the RAF Regiment Depot, Catterick, North Yorkshire, he was allowed to organise on-site medical care for the victims of road traffic accidents on the 15 mile stretch of the A1, a long way from the nearest hospital and where accidents occurred with monotonous regularity. He entered general practice at Catterick in 1950, retaining links with the RAF. After meeting several farseeing colleagues including Dr William Pickles, Dr Ekke Kuenssberg, Dr John Hunt, and Dr Ken Pickworth, who were later instrumental in forming the College of General Practitioners, he was invited to give lectures on "Immediate Care at road accidents" to groups of enthusiasts.

Deaths and injuries from road traffic accidents reached a peak in 1965, when it was obvious that these *ad hoc* rescue units needed improved co-ordination and co-operation between the statutory emergency services and general practitioners and hospital doctors, if unnecessary deaths and disabilities were to be prevented. Contact was made with Professor Eberhard Goegler of Heidelberg who had just published the results of a highly organised and funded scheme based on his University Surgical Clinic. By filling the "therapeutic vacuum" between the occurrence of the accident and hospital admission, Goegler had reduced the mortality and morbidity following serious injury by 20%, within a radius of 20 miles of his hospital. There seemed to be no reason why this "therapeutic vacuum" should not be filled in the United Kingdom by forming "Immediate Care Schemes", utilising the nearest general practitioners to provide this specialised medical care.

An approach made to Parliament asking both for the integration of the rescue services, and for better rescue equipment for the fire services, met with a surprising reply. Not only were fire services not obliged to attend persons trapped in road accidents, but any improvements in rescue procedures would necessarily depend upon local voluntary action. Thus the ground was prepared for the starting of the pilot Immediate Care scheme: "The Road Accident After Care Scheme (RAAC)" of the North Riding of Yorkshire, which covered 1,000 square miles and utilised the voluntary services of 34 doctors. The RAAC (Registered Charity No. 256843) went into operation in December 1967, and although its main concern was to be with road traffic accidents, all types of sudden illness and accidents were to be attended. Dr K.C. Easton and the late Dr E.L.R. McCallum addressed the BMA Annual Scientific Conference in July 1967, calling upon the profession to study the needs for establishing similar schemes in their own localities.

The Chairman of the BMA Scientific Conference of 1967, the late Mr Norman Capener, CBE, FRCS, was also Chairman of the Medical Commission on Accident Prevention, and he invited representation from the RAAC on that commission, their aims being mutual.

This avuncular relationship gave rise to the far ranging associations of the parent body, including the Royal Colleges, many eminent members of which joined in the First International Conference on Immediate Care held at Scotch Corner in May 1969. As new schemes came into existence, often as a result of lecture tours and enquiries, it was important to have national cohesion, a centre for information, and a source of help and encouragement to others. This role was fulfilled by the Immediate Care Subcommittee of the Medical Commission on Accident Prevention's Rescue and Resuscitation Committee. An evaluation of the efficiency of the schemes extant in 1977 was commissioned by the Department of Health and Social Security. This indicated a 20% improvement in the care expected and achieved.

The Medical Commission on Accident Prevention understood that the schemes would eventually become autonomous, and this came about in June 1977 with the formation of the British Association of Immediate Care Schemes (Registered Charity No. 276054). This title was later changed to the British Association for Immediate Care and the constitution altered so that individual doctors could become members as well. A room for a central office was made available to BASICS by The Royal College of General Practitioners in Princes Gate, until the needs of the College and BASICS occasioned a move out of London to Ipswich.

The aims of BASICS are to foster co-operation between existing Immediate Care Schemes, to encourage and aid the formation and extension of schemes in the United Kingdom and its surrounding waters; to strengthen and develop co-operation between all services in dealing with emergencies resulting in injury or risk to life; to encourage and assist research into all aspects of Immediate Care and accident prevention; and to raise the standards of Immediate Care and the training of all who undertake to practise the discipline.

Trauma and sudden illness have emerged as the pandemic of modern society. By the end of the 1980s, the annual accident toll in the United Kingdom had risen to 15,000 killed, 300,000 seriously injured, and some 5,000,000 hurt. One third of these arose from road traffic accidents. In 1996, the last year for which figures are available, the cost to society of one road traffic accident fatal casualty was nearly £984,000 and £118,030 for each seriously injured casualty. If these figures were related to some other disease they would shock both the medical profession and the general public into demanding urgent action.

By 1991 BASICS had a membership of nearly 2500 doctors in about 100 Immediate Care schemes. Schemes vary in size from one individual doctor working in close co-operation with the emergency services, to some with over 200 doctors. They cover between one third and one half of Scotland, England, Wales and Northern Ireland. The doctors involved give their time and expertise entirely without financial reward. BASICS has formed a valuable liaison with the statutory emergency services, especially the ambulance service, and with the Honorary Medical Advisers of the Royal National Lifeboat Institution; the latter forming one of BASICS schemes. Other organisations which have recently joined BASICS include the British Association of Aeromedical Practitioners (BAMPA), the British Association of Rally Doctors (BARD), the British Medical Equestrian Association, and the Mountain Rescue Committee.

Despite the recommendations of the House of Commons Expenditure and Social Services Committee in January 1974 that Immediate Care Schemes should have financial support and that "One Minister should have overall responsibility for the organisation of rescue services and for procedures for dealing with all types of accidents"; it was not until 1978, and then only through the good offices of the Parliamentary All Party Disablement Group under the chairmanship of Mr Jack Ashley, CH, MP, that Parliament asked the Department of Health and Social Security to provide financial assistance. A "pump priming" grant was made to BASICS for central administrative expenses only, for a limited period under Section 64. After several years this grant was reduced and eventually ceased altogether in 1988. Mr Ashley's group considered that moral and financial help should also be forthcoming from the Ministry of Transport and the Department of the Environment, thus reflecting the team effort required to provide effective Immediate Care on-site.

Although BASICS started as a national organisation, it has now become internationally recognised. In 1980 in association with the Association of Emergency Medical Technicians (AEMT, now Paramedic UK) and the Centre for Emergency Medicine, Pittsburgh, USA, it organised the First Brighton International Congress on Immediate Care. There is great value in the extension of these international links, which have continued to grow through BASICS representation on international bodies including the World Association of Emergency and Disaster Medicine.

It is the aim of BASICS to strengthen still further its ties with the Ambulance Service, and the British Association for Accident and Emergency Medicine. Through its various committees, working parties and publications, it is constantly seeking to extend its work in the fields of research and data collection and dissemination, radio-communications and emergency equipment, and in the education and training of the general public and medical profession in emergency medical procedures. It is hoped that there will be a concerted effort on the part of the Deans of Medical Schools and Postgraduate Deans of Universities to establish tuition in Immediate Care as a basic professional requirement. This aim was partially achieved in 1988, when after considerable input from leading members of BASICS, the Royal College of Surgeons of Edinburgh introduced a diploma examination in Immediate Medical Care. This was followed more recently by the introduction of a Pre-Hospital Emergency Care course, 'PHEC', and certification, as a baseline qualification for not only doctors, but also nurses and paramedics involved in pre-hospital emergency medicine. In 1992 BASICS Education was established, initially under the direction of Dr John Scott, and runs a variety of courses for all those involved in pre-hospital emergency medicine, and the Royal College of Surgeons of Edinburgh has established a Faculty of Pre-Hospital Care. Very recently BASICS has introduced accreditation for its members and schemes, and the Royal College of Surgeons of Edinburgh has agreed that that their diploma examination will be opened up to nurses and paramedics. and that a new fellowship examination for doctors, the Fellowship in Immediate Medical Care, 'FIMC', will be established, thus recognising the coming of age of the practice of Immediate Medical Care as a speciality in its own right.

BASICS members have played a full and active part in the recent series of major incidents including the King's Cross fire, the Lockerbie and Kegworth air crashes, the sinking of the Marchioness in the river Thames, and the train crashes at Purley and Clapham, following which an independent investigation under the chairmanship of Anthony Hidden QC into the Clapham Junction Railway Accident acknowledged the valuable part that BASICS members had played and in his recommendations advised the Department of Health to consider the role of BASICS in emergency planning and to review BASICS' funding arrangements. Similarly the Department of Health circular on major incidents, HC 90/25, recognised the value of Immediate Medical Care teams at major incidents and the role of the Medical Incident Officer. More recently, several prominent BASICS doctors have been appointed as Medical Director of their local ambulance service.

Thus after several decades, the value of Immediate Medical Care rendered by BASICS doctors and specially trained ambulance service personnel and nurses has eventually been recognised and given credence both by the medical profession and the Government. There is still however some way to go before this recognition is translated into active support, and this will only come about after all those practising Immediate Medical Care show themselves to be thoroughly professional in every aspect of their practice, even though most of them may be working in a voluntary capacity.

1

Guidelines for Immediate Medical Care

Guidelines for Immediate Medical Care

Introduction

- The aim of pre-hospital care is to reduce the mortality and morbidity in those seriously injured or taken dangerously ill out of hospital. This involves the rapid attendance of ambulance and medical personnel to perform advanced life and limb saving techniques, and to stabilise the patient's condition sufficiently to prevent deterioration, and maximise the chances of their receiving successful definitive hospital care
- Pre-hospital care should never be prolonged at the expense of evacuating the time-critical patient
- The aim of all treatment is to produce a neurologically intact survivor, with a reasonable quality of life
- Even for the experienced, it is advisable to use guidelines when dealing with life threatening problems, so that actions become automatic and rapid, rather than action interspersed with thought, which takes longer!
- These guidelines are based on recognised ALS, PHTLS, and PALS guidelines and should be used as the basis for all your actions. The pre-hospital situation may introduce many variables, and these guidelines should not be adhered to mindlessly, but used as a basis for action by the thinking person

Safety
- Protect yourself: wear appropriate protective identifying clothing
- Do not expose yourself unnecessarily to any hazards (present or potential):
    - Adverse weather
    - Overexertion
    - Infection, contamination
    - Falling masonry
    - Elecrocution
- Protect the scene, if necessary

Scene assessment
- Look for, identify and then neutralise or remove any life threatening hazards if possible, so as to avoid any potential injury to the rescuers and any further injury to the sick or injured. If necessary, remove the casualty to a place of relative safety
- Ascertain:
    - What has happened, how and why did it happen?
    - What injuries or problems might you expect?
- Assess the number and severity of casualties, and the resources needed for their management/evacuation

Triage (if there is more than one casualty)
- Rapidly sort (triage) the patients according to their priority for treatment and transportation

Primary survey and resuscitation

- This is the simultaneous assessment, identification and management of any immediate life threatening problems, followed by an assessment of the potential for developing other serious life threatening problems or complications. Remember: they may be suffering from more than one type of problem at the same time
- In the time critical patient, the identification and management of life threatening conditions is the first priority, and Immediate Care may not progress beyond the primary survey
- Assessment/examination of any patient follows the simple protocol: *look, listen and feel*

Guidelines for the primary survey

- Assessment: rapid assessment of the patient whilst approaching them and preparing for the examination
- **A**irway (with in-line cervical spine stabilisation, if trauma is involved)
- **B**reathing and the maintenance of adequate ventilation
- **C**irculation (with control of haemorrhage/fluid loss)
- **D**isability of the central nervous system (brief neurological examination)
- **E**xpose the whole patient to allow identification of any significant conditions not otherwise obvious

Note: If a life threatening problem is identified during the primary survey, manage it immediately, *not* later

Airway assessment and management with cervical spine control

- Initial assessment should be done without moving the neck (if possible):
    - It *must* be assumed that the casualty (especially if they are unconscious or has any significant injury above the clavicles) has a cervical spine injury, until this possibility can be reasonably excluded (*think spinal, do airway*)
- Check the casualty's responsiveness by gently shaking them by the shoulder or giving a command
- Is the airway clear or obstructed?
- Is there any risk of obstruction developing? e.g.:
    - In the unconscious/sedated patient (especially if he is lying on his back, trapped, sitting up, etc.)
    - In maxillo-facial and laryngotracheal injuries
    - From fractured dentures/teeth, bony fragments, foreign bodies (remove if present)
- Insert an airway if necessary:
    - Oropharyngeal airway (Guedel):
        - May provoke vomiting/retching resulting in airway compromise, neck movement and a rise in intracranial pressure
    - Nasopharyngeal airway:
        - May cause nasal haemorrhage, and should *not* be used if a basal skull fracture is suspected
- If the patient has resistant obstruction of the airway:
    - Consider cricothyrotomy
- If the patient has no gag reflex; protect the airway from pulmonary aspiration of gastric contents:
    - Intubate with a tracheal tube, maintaining in-line cervical stabilisation (intubation may be deferred until the secondary survey, if there is no immediate risk)
- Rapidly examine the neck for:
    - Tracheal deviation
    - Engorged neck veins
    - Swelling/deformity
    - Lacerations
    - Surgical emphysema
- Apply a rigid cervical collar and only remove it to examine the neck further whilst maintaining full spinal immobilisation

Breathing (ventilation) **with oxygen supplementation**
- Assess whether:
    - Respiration is spontaneous
    - Respiration is effective
    - There is any evidence of respiratory depression or distress, e.g. noisy breathing, wheeze
    - There is a pneumothorax
- Count the respiratory rate:
    - Is it normal? (12-20 respirations per minute)
    - If it is:
        - Under 12 or greater than 20 respirations per minute:
            - Consider high flow oxygen administration with a high concentration oxygen mask
        - Under 10 or greater than 30 respirations per minute:
            - Consider assisted ventilation
- If respiration is absent, impaired or inadequate:
    - Ventilate the patient
- If you suspect a chest problem, or if the patient has required ventilation:
    - Expose and examine the chest:
        - Look for chest movement:
            - Is it present and equal?
        - Consider percussing for dullness or hyper-resonance
        - Auscultate for breath sounds
            - Are they normal and present on both sides?
- Monitor the patient's arterial oxygen saturation (SpO_2) with a pulse oximeter
- If the patient is hypoxic, there is a risk of hypoxia or if they have suffered significant trauma:
    - Administer high flow (15 l/min) oxygen via a tight fitting non-rebreathing high % oxygen mask

Circulation care with control of haemorrhage
- Check the patient's:
    - Skin: colour, temperature (a warm pink patient is rarely suffering from hypotension, except in spinal or septic shock)
    - Pulse: presence or absence, rate, regularity (or irregularity), character
    - Blood pressure
- If necessary, perform basic and advanced cardiac life support, including defibrillation
- Is there any obvious major haemorrhage?:
    - If so, elevate and control with firm direct pressure (tourniquets should *only* be used when major haemorrhage can be controlled no other way or the limb is deemed to be non-viable)
- Assess whether there is any evidence of hypovolaemic shock *or* risk of hypovolaemic shock developing? e.g. from internal injuries or pelvic or long bone fractures, etc.
- If so:
    - Put up two intravenous infusions, using:
        - Peripheral veins (hand, forearm or antecubital fossa)
        - Large bore cannulae (14 or 16 gauge)
        - Colloid initially, followed by crystalloid
    - Splint any long bone fractures
    - Consider using a pneumatic anti-shock garment (PASG)
- If haemorrhage cannot be controlled adequately:
    - Convey to hospital immediately, and put up intravenous lines, etc. en route

PRACTICAL POINTS: Blood pressure measurement:
- *Many electronic blood pressure measuring devices can measure a patient's blood pressure through their clothing, even a leather jacket! The siting of the cuff on top of such clothing may be difficult, but flexing the elbow will allow identification of the antecubital fossa, and accurate placement of the cuff*

Disability (neurological state)
- Rapidly assess the patient's central (brain) and peripheral (spinal cord) neurological status:
    - Central nervous system:
        - AVPU scale:
            - **A** - Alert
            - **V** - Responds to verbal stimuli
            - **P** - Responds to pain
            - **U** - Unresponsive/unconscious
        - Assess the pupils: size, equality and reactivity
        - Ask the patient to put their tongue out
    - Peripheral nervous system:
        - Ask the patient if they can feel their:
            - Fingers
            - Toes
    - Ask the patient to:
        - Squeeze your hand with their fingers
        - Wriggle their toes

Exposure of the patient with control of the Environment
- Expose the whole patient if appropriate/necessary for the management of immediate life threatening problems (it is usually best to wait until the patient is in a place of relative safety, e.g. in the ambulance, if the incident has occurred outside, before removing all the clothing for a full examination)
- Only remove as much clothing as is necessary to determine the presence or absence of a suspected condition or injury
- Keep the patient warm and be aware of the risk of developing hypothermia, which can precipitate and may aggravate shock, which can be a major problem for the injured patient in the pre-hospital situation
- Cover any exposed area as soon as the examination (and treatment) is complete

Secondary survey and management

Subjective interview
- This is most useful in medical emergencies
- If possible try to obtain information from bystanders as well as the patient
- Try to ascertain:
    - What has happened?
    - What the patient is complaining of?
    - The patient's significant past medical history (see below)

Objective examination
- This must be omitted if it will cause undue delay in the evacuation of a time critical trauma patient
- The casualty should be completely undressed to enable a complete, comprehensive, head to toe examination, allowing identification and appropriate early management of the patient's injuries/illness

Guidelines for the secondary survey
- Systematic examination of the whole body in the following order:
    - **H**ead (including neurological status) and **N**eck
    - **C**hest
    - **A**bdomen and **P**elvis
    - **E**xtremities
    - **S**pine and **B**ack
- Obtain the **M**edical history (this should be considered first in the absence of a history of trauma)

- Reassess and re-evaluate the patient's response to treatment:
    - If there is any unexplained deterioration in the patient's condition, go back to the beginning of the primary survey and start again

General appearance
- Pale and/or sweating
- Cyanosed
- Pink

Examination of the head

Neurological state
- Monitor the patient's level of consciousness at regular intervals
- Note the patient's Glasgow Coma Scale (GCS) score, recording the three components separately

Scalp
- Perform a rapid visual inspection to reveal any obvious injuries
- Palpate the scalp from posterior to anterior checking for:
    - Lacerations
    - Swellings
    - Depression
    - Fractures at the base of lacerations
- Haemorrhage from the scalp should be stopped with :
    - Pressure dressing

Base of skull
- Look for mastoid staining/bruising
- Look for CSF:
    - Rhinorrhoea
    - Otorrhoea

Eyes
- If the patient is unconscious, test the:
    - Pupillary reflexes
- Look for:
    - Evidence of a penetrating injury
    - Foreign bodies under the eye lids
    - Haemorrhages

Face
- Palpate the face on both sides feeling for deformities and tenderness
- If there is a facial injury:
    - Check for loose or lost teeth
    - Grasp the upper incisors and check for instability of the maxilla (suggesting a middle third fracture)
    - Identify any fractures or injuries which may compromise the airway, and if necessary:
        - Pull the relevant fractured facial segment forward
        - Pull the tongue forward
- Does their breath smell: alcohol, ketones?
- Is there a nasal injury (deformity, bruising, swelling or epistaxis) and is the nasal airway patent?
- Is there evidence of haemoptysis or haematemesis?
- Look inside the mouth: lacerations, burns

Examination of the neck

- If trauma is involved and a cervical spine injury is suspected:
    - Leave the neck stabilised in a semi-rigid cervical collar and long board with full spinal immobilisation until the patient reaches hospital
    - Repeat the neurological examination to assess the patient's peripheral:
        - Motor power
        - Sensation
        - Reflexes

Examination of the chest

- Identify and treat any immediate or potential life threatening conditions, e.g. tension pneumothorax
- Inspect the anterior and posterior chest wall for:
    - Tracheal deviation (a late sign)
    - Signs of respiratory obstruction: stridor, intercostal recession, tracheal tug
    - Asymmetrical chest movement
    - Wounds
    - Bruising

Chest wall and lungs
- Examine the chest wall for:
    - Paradoxical chest movement (indicates flail chest):
        - If the patient shows signs of respiratory distress, consider:
            - Intubation and ventilation
    - Open chest wound:
        - Cover with an occlusive dressing and tape down on three sides (it will then act as a flutter valve)
        - Consider insertion of a chest drain
    - Tenderness and crepitus over the ribs and sternum:
        - If this is so painful that respiration is impaired, consider:
            - Analgesia
    - Surgical emphysema
    - Hyperresonance ⎤
- Auscultate for: ⎬ Indicates a pneumothorax: if tension, perform a needle decompression
    - Reduced air entry ⎦   and consider insertion of a chest drain
- Monitor the patient's:
    - Oxygen saturation (SpO_2)
    - Peak expiratory flow rate

Heart
- Suspect myocardial contusion/injury if the patient has suffered:
    - Massive deceleration
    - Penetrating thoracic injury
- Examine the neck for engorged neck veins
- Auscultate for:
    - Muffled heart sounds: and if associated with hypotension and engorged neck veins, perform:
        - Needle pericardiocentesis (pericardial aspiration)
- Perform an ECG if an acute myocardial infarction (AMI), cardiac dysrrhythmia or cardiac contusion is suspected

Examination of the abdomen/pelvis
- Examine the anterior abdominal wall, looking for:
    - Bruising
    - Movement
    - Open wounds; if present cover with saline soaked pads
- Palpate the abdomen for localised tenderness:
    - If there is bruising and tenderness over the lower ribs; suspect injury to the liver or spleen:
        - Monitor the haemodynamic state carefully
        - Put up two intravenous infusions with large bore cannulae and be prepared to infuse large volumes of fluid rapidly if there is any deterioration
    - Abdominal palpation may be unreliable, especially if the patient is head injured or intoxicated
- If there appears to be gastric distension: insert a naso-gastric tube
- Pelvic springing to elicit pain/movement/crepitus (may be unreliable as an indication of a pelvic fracture)

Examination of the extremities
- Inspect for:
    - Bruising
    - Wounds
    - Deformities
    - Burns
- If any injuries are found; check and record:
    - Distal pulses
    - Sensation
- Reduce and splint any fractures/subluxations:
    - Re-check the distal pulses and sensation after reduction
    - Record the position before and after reduction with polaroid photography
- Cover and seal (after first taking a polaroid photograph):
    - Compound fractures
    - Degloving injuries
- Collect any extruded fracture fragments and place in clean container for conveyance with the patient

Examination of the spine
- If spinal injury is suspected:
    - Do *not* move the patient unnecessarily:
        - If movement *is* necessary, move the patient with great care, in the horizontal axis only
    - Look for:
        - Motor deficit
        - Sensory deficit
        - Abnormal reflexes
        - Priapism

Examination of the back
- Log roll the patient, but with great care, if a spinal injury is suspected, and:
    - Examine the back for:
        - Bruising
        - Lacerations/open wounds
    - Auscultate the back of the chest
    - Examine the spine for:
        - Tenderness or muscular spasm
        - Boggyness
        - Irregularity (step deformity) of the contour of the spinous processes

Assessment and management of pain
- Assess whether the patient:
    - Is in pain or is likely to develop pain during the extrication process
- If the patient is in pain, remove the cause where possible:
    - If there is a fracture, splint it (after reducing it, if appropriate)
    - Remove any caustic substances
- If in pain administer adequate and appropriate analgesia:
    - Nitrous oxide/oxygen (Entonox) (but not for chest injuries where pneumothorax is a possibility)
    - Opiates
    - Non steroidal anti-inflammatory drugs
- Consider sedation if the patient is distressed, or hypoxic and violent:
    - Midazolam
    - Diazepam

Medical history
- Allergies
- Medicines
- Past medical history
- Last meal
- Events leading to the illness or injury

Unexplained deterioration
- If there is any sudden, severe or unexplained deterioration in the patient's condition:
    - Go back to the primary survey

Monitoring/reassessment of the patient
- This should be continuous, so as to detect any changes in the patient's condition and will allow modification of their management accordingly
- Is their condition:
    - Improving?
    - Deteriorating?: if so why? what can you do about it?
    - The same

Monitor
- Airway patency
- Breathing:
    - Appearance/colour
    - Respiratory rate
    - Chest expansion
    - SpO_2
    - Peak expiratory flow rate
    - End tidal CO_2
- Circulation:
    - Pulse rate
    - Blood pressure
    - Capillary refill
    - Peripheral pulses
- Disability/neurological status:
    - Glasgow Coma Scale score (record the three components)
- Pain severity
- Drug and fluid administration

Trending
- This allows early assessment of changes in the patient's condition, i.e. any improvement or deterioration, and gives a guide as to the efficacy of their management

Monitoring equipment/devices
- Sphygmomanometer: electronic/automatic
- Pulse oximeter
- ECG monitor/defibrillator
- End tidal CO_2 monitor
- Trauma scoring

Note: Always make certain that all your monitoring equipment is well maintained and regularly serviced. If you have a piece of equipment, make certain that you know how to use it, what its limitations are, and how to interpret the results. There is no point of using faulty or inaccurate equipment; if you use a device you must have confidence in it and believe what it is telling you!

Recording information
- Patient report form
- Photography
- Print out from monitor/defibrillator

Guidelines for patient assessment & management

Assess the Scene

Triage if there is more than one casualty per skilled rescuer

Primary Survey
- Airway with cervical spine stabilisation
- Breathing with oxygen supplementation
- Circulation with control of haemorrhage
- Disability
- Exposure with control of the environment

Secondary Survey
- Subjective interview
- Objective examination and management
    - Appearance
    - Head (including neurological status)
    - Neck
    - Chest
    - Abdomen
    - Pelvis
    - Extremities
    - Spine
    - Back
- Pain assessment and management
- Medical history (consider first, in the absence of a history of trauma)

Monitoring/reassessment

Figure 1-1 Guidelines for patient assessment and management

2

Basic life support

Basic life support

Introduction

Definition: Basic Life Support (BLS), is life support using no aids, to maintain the airway and support breathing and the circulation, to preserve cerebral function, (and when all three techniques are used together is called 'Cardiopulmonary resuscitation'). If an aid is used, e.g. a simple airway or face mask it may be called 'Basic Life Support with an airway adjunct'

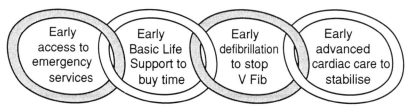

Figure 2-1: the Chain of Survival

- Basic Life Support is something in which every health care professional must be proficient, and many lives that are lost would be saved if a significant proportion of the population were trained in BLS, because no matter how good the emergency services are, it has to be the bystander who starts treatment
- Survival from cardiac arrest is greatest if the event is witnessed; if a bystander starts resuscitation; if the heart arrests in ventricular fibrillation; and when defibrillation is performed soon after the arrest: "the Chain of Survival", comprising early access, bystander BLS, rapid defibrillation, and early cardiac care
- These guidelines are those produced by the European Resuscitation Council in 1998, for use in the, and are primarily intended for use by the non-professional rescuer

---

Discussion point: cardiopulmonary resuscitation

- The commonest treatable cause of sudden cardiac arrest is ventricular fibrillation; the *only* effective management for which is early defibrillation, which may be up to to 85% successful if administered immediately, but the chances of success decline rapidly with increasing time
- Effective cardiopulmonary resuscitation helps to maintain some cerebral and cardiac circulation and may prolong the interval during which defibrillation is likely to be successful, i.e. it slows deterioration and buys time. If BLS is performed the chance of success declines by 10% per minute (20% if not)
- The aim of the Basic Life Support is to assess the patient rapidly, ask for help early if the patient is unresponsive, and only after that start resuscitation:
    - Clear any airway obstruction and ventilate the patient, if they are not breathing
    - If there are no signs of a circulation: maintain the patient's circulation, preserving the cerebral blood supply, until a defibrillator arrives and can be used

---

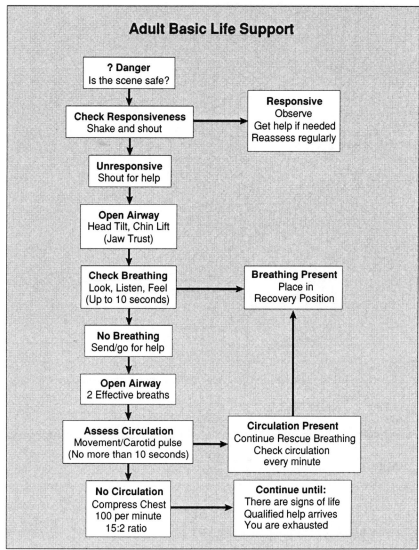

Figure 2-2 Algorithm for single rescuer Basic Life Support

Assessment

- Do not rush headlong into the situation, but quickly try to assess what has happened

The scene: ensure the safety of rescuer and casualty

- Look out for dangers to yourself and the casualty, e.g. electricity, gas, road traffic, dangerous chemicals and falling masonry

The casualty

Assess general appearance

- Rapidly assess the casualty:
    - Are they unconscious, pale or cyanosed?
- During the assessment look for other relevant signs which might indicate what is wrong with or has happened to the casualty. Is there:
    - Cyanosis, pallor, excessive salivation, gastric contents or foreign body present in the mouth/oropharynx
    - Unusual voice quality, abnormal breath sounds, wheeze/stridor indicates partial airway obstruction:
        - Stridor during inspiration indicates an obstruction above the larynx
        - Wheeze during expiration usually indicates an obstruction below the larynx

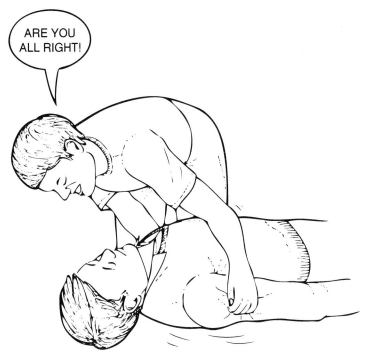

ARE YOU ALL RIGHT!

Figure 2-3 Assess the patient (if a cervical spine injury is a possibility put one hand on the forehead to stabilise the head/neck and shake a shoulder)

Check responsiveness
- Shake the patient gently by the shoulder (be careful not to exacerbate any injuries especially of the neck, chest or spine)
- Give a command such as "Open your eyes!" or ask loudly: "Are you all right?", "What's happened?" (the confused and disorientated patient will respond to a command better than to a question)
- In the unresponsive casualty, perform the assessment without moving them, if possible, especially if traumatic injury is suspected

- **If the patient responds by answering or moving:**
    - Leave the patient in the position in which you found them (provided they are not in further danger)
    - Check for any injuries
    - Reassess their condition at regular intervals and get further help if necessary

- **If the patient does not respond:**
    - Shout for a bystander to help

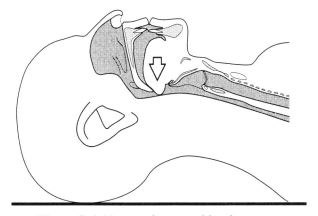

Figure 2-4 Airway obstructed by the tongue

Airway
- If the patient is not breathing, they may have an obstructed airway:
    - Airway obstruction may be caused by:
        - The tongue falling back onto the posterior pharyngeal wall, e.g. in unconsciousness
        - Vomit or blood
        - Foreign bodies, e.g. false teeth or food impacted in the oropharynx (sometimes both)
- Establishing and maintaining the airway is the single most useful manoeuvre that a rescuer can perform

Open the airway

Method
- Loosen any clothing around the patient's head or neck
- If possible, leave the patient in the position in which you found them, and open the airway
- If there is any possibility of a neck injury, perform a jaw thrust and *do not* tilt the head

Head tilt, chin lift (method of choice in most circumstances)
- Head tilt:
    - Lifts the tongue away from the posterior pharyngeal wall and lifts the epiglottis away from the pharyngeal opening by stretching the anterior tissues of the neck
- Chin Lift:
    - Used in conjunction with head tilt, this further assists anterior displacement of the tongue

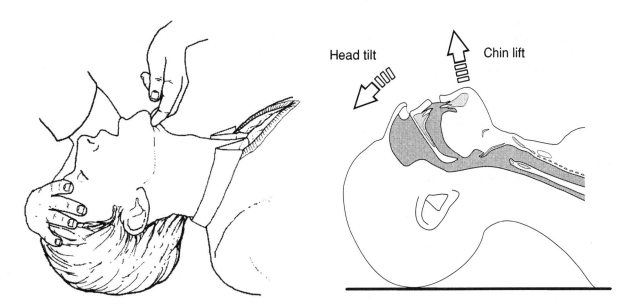

Figure 2-5 Head tilt, chin lift

Method
- Head tilt:
    - Place one hand on the forehead, and gently tilt the head, keeping the thumb and index finger free to close the nose, in case expired air ventilation is necessary
- Chin lift:
    - Simultaneously, lift the chin with the tips of the index and middle fingers of the other hand under the point of the chin to open the airway (this will often allow breathing to restart)

- If you have any difficulty, turn the patient onto their back (see below) and try again

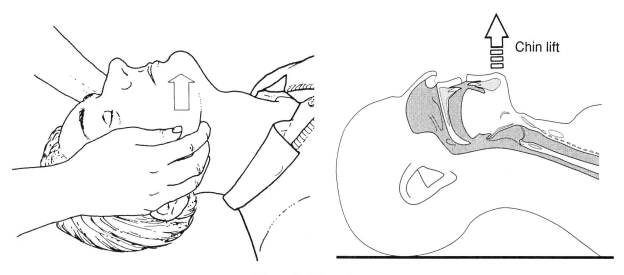

Figure 2-6 Jaw thrust

Jaw thrust (method of choice when cervical spine injury is a possibility, or when there are two rescuers)
  - Displaces the mandible, and with it the tongue, forwards

Method
  - Put one hand under each angle of the jaw, with the thumbs reaching forward to depress the point of the chin slightly to open the mouth, and lift it forwards and upwards

Note: This technique may be used in combination with head tilt to maximise displacement of the tongue away from the posterior pharyngeal wall, but is tiring and difficult to perform

Breathing
  - Once the patient has a clear airway, maintain the airway and check that they are breathing spontaneously, i.e. giving more than just an occasional gasp

Method
  - Put your cheek close to the patient's mouth looking along his chest and:
    - *LOOK* for chest movement ⎫ for up to 10 seconds
    - *LISTEN* at the patient's mouth for breath sounds ⎬ before deciding that
    - *FEEL* expired air on your cheek ⎭ breathing is absent

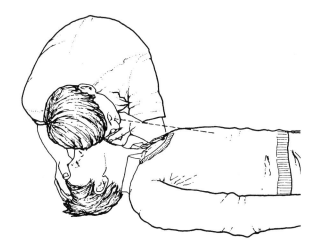

Figure 2-7 Look, listen and feel for signs of spontaneous respiration

- Causes of respiratory arrest include:
    - Airway obstruction by the tongue due to unconsciousness and an unprotected airway
    - Airway obstructed by vomit, or foreign body
    - Head injury
    - Chest injury
    - Poisoning from toxic gases or drug overdose
    - Near drowning

- If the patient is breathing spontaneously:
- Turn them into the *recovery position* (see below), unless this would exacerbate any injuries, supporting the chin to maintain the airway if necessary
- Send someone for help, if your initial call has not been answered, or if you are alone, leave the patient and go for help yourself
- Return and keep the patient under close observation, checking that they are breathing freely

- If the patient is not breathing:
- If you have not already done so, send someone for help, or, if you are on your own, leave the patient and go for help (see below), return and start expired air ventilations
- *Turn them onto their back*, if they are not already in that position (see below)
- Remove any visible obstruction from the patient's mouth, including dislodged dentures, but leave well fitting dentures in place (don't waste time trying to find hidden obstructions)
- Deliver 2 effective expired air ventilations (rescue breaths)

Expired air ventilation (rescue breathing)
- Expired air contains 16-17% oxygen (atmospheric air: 21% oxygen), which is more than sufficient to sustain life
- Expired air ventilation (rescue breathing) is most easily performed with the patient lying on his back, but can be done in almost any situation, e.g. swimming pool, when trapped, etc.

Mouth to mouth ventilation
- This is the most widely used method of expired air ventilation (rescue breathing)

Method
- Ensure that the patient's head is tilted and the chin is lifted
- Pinch the soft part of the nose with the index finger and thumb of one hand (which is already pressing on the forehead)
- Allow the patient's mouth to open a little, while still maintaining chin lift
- Take a deep breath and place your lips around their mouth, making sure that you have a good seal
- Blow out steadily into the patient's mouth for about 1½-2 seconds, until you can see the chest rise
- Lift your head away, maintaining head tilt and chin lift and allow the expired air to come out of the patient's mouth, while you take another breath in
- Allow the patient's chest to deflate fully (allowing a total of about 3 seconds for the inhalation/ exhalation cycle), before taking another breath and giving a second rescue breath

Note: 1. Only a small amount of resistance should be felt during mouth to mouth ventilation
2. The desired tidal volume in an adult is only about 400-500 mL in an adult, because carbon dioxide delivery during cardiac arrest is very low; this is the volume required to produce visible lifting of the chest. Higher tidal volumes are associated with gastric inflation

CAUTION
- If you try to inflate the lungs too rapidly, the resistance will be greater, less air will enter the lungs and gastric and oesophageal distension may occur, resulting in gastric inflation and pulmonary aspiration

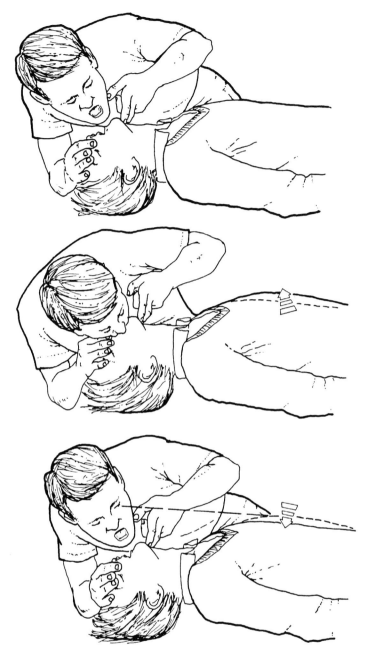

Figure 2-8 Mouth to mouth ventilation

Mouth to nose ventilation
- This may be aesthetically more acceptable than mouth to mouth ventilation especially if the patient has vomited
- May be indicated: if the patient has a clenched jaw, a mandibular injury, unusual/absent dentition or during water rescue, when one hand is required to support the body and cannot be used to close the nose
- May not be possible: if the patient has nasal obstruction or a nasal or maxillary injury

Method
- Open the airway with head tilt and chin lift, or jaw thrust
- Seal the patient's lips with the hand supporting the chin, but remember to open the mouth during the expiratory phase to allow expiration
- Take a deep breath, form a tight seal with your lips around the patient's nose and blow out
- Otherwise the method is similar to mouth to mouth ventilation

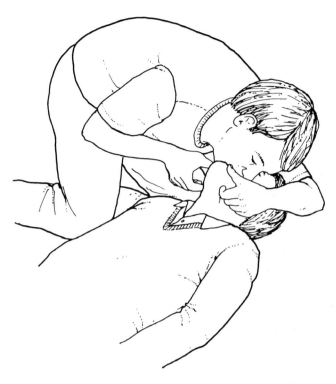

Figure 2-9 Mouth to nose ventilation using jaw thrust

Airway obstruction
- If you have difficulty achieving an effective breath (the chest does not rise with each ventilation), the airway is obstructed. Causes include:
    - Obstruction by vomit, blood or a foreign body: re-check the patient's mouth, and remove any obstruction (see Airway obstruction/Choking below)
    - Failure to extend the neck enough (extend the neck a bit further)
    - Failure to make an efficient seal around the mouth or nose (make a better seal)
- Make up to five attempts in all to achieve 2 effective ventilations
- Even if unsuccessful, move on to assessing the circulation

Note: **Patients with a laryngectomy and tracheotomy**
- Owing to earlier diagnosis and more effective treatment, there are more patients surviving carcinoma of the larynx with a laryngectomy and permanent tracheotomy
- Resuscitating these patients requires a slightly modified resuscitation technique, but most laryngectomees carry first aid instructions with them explaining this, for use in an emergency
- *Clearing the airway:*
    - Remove any clothing from around the neck (confirming that they are a laryngectomee), and make sure that their stoma is not obstructed
    - Clear mucus from around the stoma, being careful not to dislodge any tracheotomy tube
- *If the patient is not breathing and requires ventilating:*
    - Perform a head tilt and chin lift
    - Clear the airway as above
    - Pinch the nose between two fingers and place your thumb under the chin to keep the mouth tightly closed
    - Place your mouth over the tracheotomy stoma, forming a seal
    - Blow out slowly, watching the chest rise as you do so, as in mouth to mouth or mouth to nose ventilation (see above)
    - At the end of ventilation, take your mouth away from the stoma and let the chest fall completely, before ventilating the patient again

Circulation: assess the patient for signs of a circulation

- Look for any movement, including swallowing or breathing (more than an occasional gasp)
- Check for a central pulse (the best pulse to feel in any emergency is the carotid, but if the patient has a neck injury, the femoral pulse is a good alternative)
- Palpate for a pulse for no more than 10 seconds before deciding that it is absent (indicating a cardiac arrest)

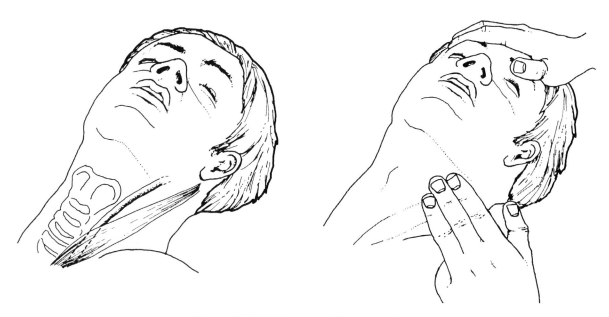

Figure 2-10 Palpation of the carotid pulse

- If you are certain that you can detect signs of a circulation within 10 seconds
- Continue rescue breathing (expired air ventilations), if necessary until the patient starts breathing on their own
- If a pulse is still present, continue doing ventilations alone, but re-check the pulse about every minute, taking no more than 10 seconds to do so each time
- If the patient starts to breathe spontaneously, but remains unconscious, put them onto their side in the recovery position. Check their condition regularly and be ready to turn the patient onto their back and start expired air ventilations if they stop breathing

Note: Research has shown that the carotid pulse can be very difficult to feel, especially for the inexperienced

- If the patient has no signs of a circulation or you are at all unsure:

- Start chest compressions

Method
- Locate the xiphisternal notch by running the index and middle fingers of one hand up the lower margins of the rib cage and find the point where the ribs join
- With your middle finger over the xiphisternum, place the tip of your index finger on the sternum above
- Place the heel of your other hand on the upper sternum, and slide it down towards the first hand until it touches the index finger. This should be the middle of the lower half of the sternum
- The heel of the first hand should then be placed on top of the other hand and the fingers interlocked, so that pressure is not applied over the ribs

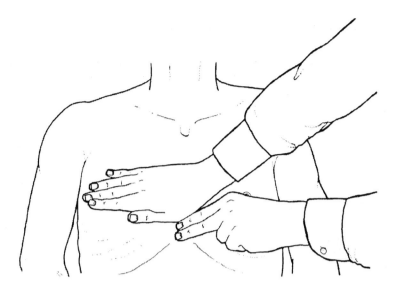

Figure 2-11 Positioning of the hand two fingers breadth above the xiphisternal notch

- Lean well over the patient, so that your shoulders are positioned directly above the hands, with the arms held straight at the elbows
- Press down firmly and vertically on the sternum using just enough force to depress it 1½-2 inches (4-5 centimetres) without allowing your elbows to flex. The movement should be well controlled. Erratic or violent action is dangerous and may cause unnecessary injury to the patient

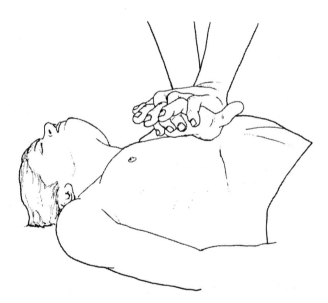

Figure 2-12 Intertwine the fingers and press down with the heel of the hand

- Release the pressure, still keeping your hand on the patient, and repeat the procedure at a rate of approximately 100 compressions per minute
- The compression phase should last at least 50% of the cycle
- Do not waste time checking for a pulse as it is unlikely that effective spontaneous cardiac function will return, without using advanced life support techniques, especially defibrillation
- If the patient makes a movement or takes a spontaneous breath, check the carotid pulse, to see if the patient has any productive cardiac output, taking no more than 10 seconds to do so. Otherwise *do NOT interrupt* resuscitation
- Combine ventilations and chest compressions

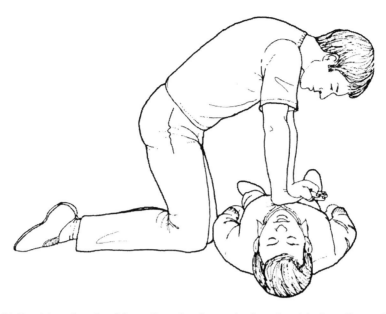

Figure 2-13 Position the shoulders directly above the hands with the elbows held straight

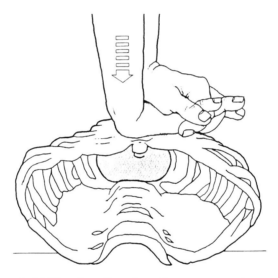

Figure 2-14 Showing direction of pressure on the sternum

Organisation

Single rescuer BLS (15:2)

Method
- The single rescuer should do two initial expired air ventilations, followed by 15 chest compressions, two expired air ventilations and then 15 chest compressions and so on
- If the patient moves or takes a spontaneous breath, check the carotid pulse to see if the patient has any effective cardiac output

Note: Pulse check:
- Do not stop basic life support to check for a pulse, unless the casualty starts breathing or regains consciousness
- A palpable pulse indicates a pressure wave and not necessarily the flow of blood

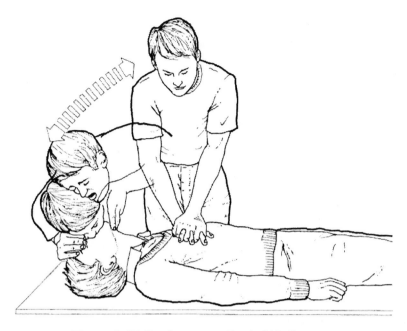

Figure 2-15 Single rescuer Basic Life Support

When to get help
- It is vital for rescuers to get help as quickly as possible
    - When more than one rescuer is available:
        - One rescuer should start resuscitation at 15:2 compressions/ventilations, while another rescuer goes for help
    - If there is only one rescuer:
        - They will have to decide whether to start resuscitation or to go for help first
        - If the casualty is an infant/child or if the likely cause of unconsciousness is trauma or drowning:
            - The rescuer should perform basic life support for about one minute before going for help
        - If the casualty is an adult, and the cause of unconsciousness is not trauma or drowning:
            - The rescuer should assume that the casualty has a heart problem, and go for help (a defibrillator) immediately it is clear that the casualty is not breathing

Two rescuer BLS (5:1)
- More effective than single rescuer BLS as it results in better ventilation and less interruption of chest compressions
- The first priority is to get help; one rescuer should start BLS, whilst the other goes for help and they should only change to two rescuer BLS once help has been summoned

Method
- The first rescuer (lung ventilator) should look after the airway, beginning with two inflations, following which the second rescuer (chest compressor) should do five chest compressions, counting out loud "1-2-3-4-5" between compressions, as they do so
- At the end of every five compressions, the second rescuer should pause just long enough for the first rescuer to do one lung inflation, but no longer. He should not remove his hands from the patient's chest
- Sellick's manoeuvre (cricoid pressure to compress the oesophagus) helps to reduce the risk of pulmonary aspiration of gastric contents and if indicated is usually performed by the lung ventilator
- When the second rescuer becomes tired, the rescuers should exchange positions
- If the pulse returns and spontaneous respiration begins, the patient should be put into the recovery position (see below), and their condition carefully monitored
- The usual convention is for the first rescuer to be in charge, and to give instructions to the second

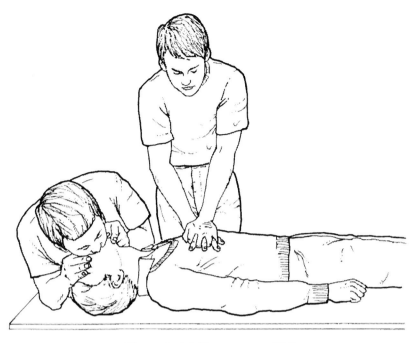

Figure 2-16 Two rescuer BLS

Continue resuscitation until:
- The victim shows signs of life
- Qualified help arrives
- You become exhausted

Active compression/decompression CPR (ACD CPR)
- A new device, the Ambu® *CardioPump*^{TM} has recently been introduced, which is used to actively decompress the thorax and heart during cardiopulmonary resuscitation (active decompression has been shown to increase the venous return and left ventricular filling, and increase cardiac output)
- Early studies are encouraging and show that the device is relatively easy to use, but so far its use has not been shown to improve outcome following cardiac arrest

Description
- The CardioPump is a hand held device, incorporating a soft silicone rubber vacuum cup which is designed to adhere to the anterior chest wall over the lower part of the sternum (even if it is hairy!); and a circular handle, incorporating a pressure gauge

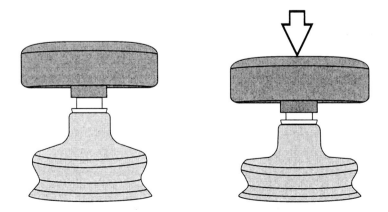

Figure 2-17 CardioPump

Method
- Grasp the device by the handle with both hands; apply it to the anterior chest wall over the lower sternum and exert downward pressure on the handle
- As soon as the pressure gauge indicates that chest compression is sufficient, pull the handle (and the anterior chest wall to which it is attached) upwards, actively decompressing the thorax

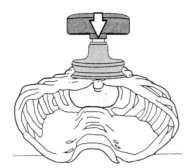

Figure 2-18 CardioPump compressing the thorax

Discussion point: mechanism of action of chest compression in standard and active compression/decompression cardiopulmonary resuscitation

Standard cardiopulmonary resuscitation
- The way in which chest compressions in standard CPR produce arterial blood flow has not been fully elucidated, but it is undoubtably effective and may achieve 10-30% of normal cardiac output
- There are two different models:
    - *Cardiac pump:*
        - External chest compression causes indirect compression of all chambers of the heart
        - Compression of the ventricles results in blood being forced out of the ventricles and into the pulmonary artery and aorta
    - *Thoracic pump:*
        - External chest compression causes a rise in intrathoracic pressure
        - This results in the pressure in the thorax being greater than that in the rest of the body, and causes blood to flow forward out of the thorax to the rest of the body
        - At the end of the external chest compression, the thorax decompresses due to its inherent elastic recoil, creating a fall in intrathoracic pressure, which becomes lower than that in the rest of the body
        - This results in blood flow from the rest of the body into the thorax because the veins at the thoracic inlet collapse, whilst the arteries remain patent
    Note: The valves of the peripheral venous system remain competent and aid the flow of venous blood towards the thorax and heart
- In practice, both mechanisms probably operate together
- Coronary artery flow usually only takes place during the passive decompressive phase

Active compression/decompression cardiopulmonary resuscitation
- In active compression/decompression (ACD) CPR:
    - The negative pressure in the thorax, during active decompression is much greater than with standard CPR, and results in more venous blood flowing into the thorax and more effective atrial filling. This in turn results in more efficient ventricular filling, greater cardiac output during compression, an increase in output (systolic) blood pressure and an increase in myocardial and cerebral blood flow
    - Coronary artery flow takes place during both compression and active decompressive phases

Recovery position

- There are many different positions in use throughout the world, but in general any position should:
    - Be in as near a true lateral position as possible, with the head dependant allowing the tongue to fall forward away from the posterior pharyngeal wall and any vomit or secretions to drain away from the corner of the patient's mouth by gravity
    - Be stable, i.e. not allow the patient to roll over
    - Avoid any pressure on the chest which might compromise breathing
    - Allow good access to and observation of the airway
    - Not by itself give rise to any injury to the patient
    - Be easily reversible, so that the casualty may be moved into the position and then back onto their back, if required, easily and safely, having due regard to the possibility of a cervical spine injury

Method
- Remove the patient's spectacles and any bulky or sharp objects from their pockets, e.g. keys, (explaining what you are doing to any onlookers, as you do so)
- Turn round (rotate) any rings, so that the stones are on the palmar aspect of the finger
- Kneel beside the patient and make certain that both their legs are straight
- Open the airway by tilting the head and lifting the chin

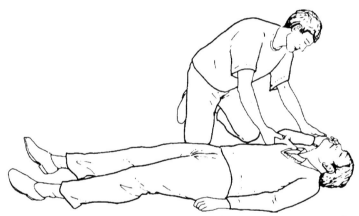

Figure 2-19 Moving a patient into the recovery position 1

- Take the arm nearest you, and place it at right angles to the body with the elbow bent and the palm of the hand uppermost
- Bring the furthest arm across the chest, and place the back of the hand against the patient's nearest cheek

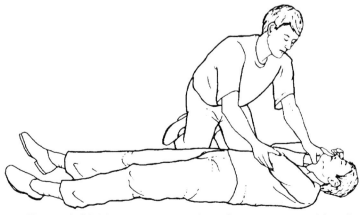

Figure 2-20 Moving a patient into the recovery position 2

- With your other hand grasp the far leg, just above the knee, and pull it up, bending the knee, but keeping the foot on the ground
- Keeping the patient's hand pressed against their cheek, pull on the leg to roll the patient towards you on their side
- Stabilise the patient's position, by adjusting the legs, as necessary

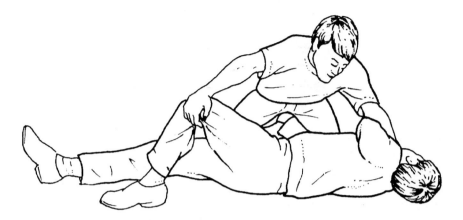

Figure 2-21 Moving a patient into the recovery position 3

- Adjust the upper leg so that both the hip and the knee are bent at right angles
- Adjust the lower arm so that the patient is not lying on it, and the palm is uppermost
- Tilt the head back so that the airway remains open
- Adjust the hand under the cheek, as necessary, so that the head stays tilted
- Check the breathing and pulse regularly, and monitor the peripheral circulation in the lower arm, ensuring that the length of time that there is pressure on the lower arm is kept to a minimum

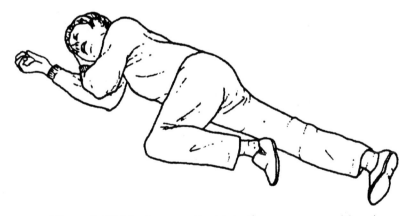

Figure 2-22 Moving a patient into the recovery position 4

Turning a patient onto their back

Method
- Kneel down beside the patient and place the arm nearest to you above their head
- Turn their face away from you
- Hold the far shoulder with one hand and the hip with the other, at the same time clamping their wrist to their hip
- With a steady pull, roll the patient over against your thighs
- Lower them gently to the ground on their back, supporting the head and shoulders as you do so, and place the extended arm by their side

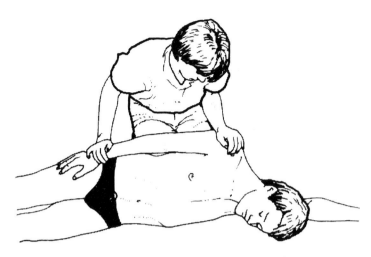

Figure 2-23 Turning a patient onto their back

Cervical spine injury
- Particular care should be exercised if there is any suspicion that the patient may have sustained a cervical spine injury with possible damage of the spinal cord, for example in:
  - Road traffic accidents
  - Falls from heights
  - Falls down stairs
  - Riding accidents
  - Rugby football accidents: scrum collapse
  - Diving accidents into shallow water
  - The unconscious head injured patient
- If cervical spine injury is suspected:
  - Avoid moving the neck any more than *absolutely* necessary
  - Use jaw thrust instead of head tilt, chin lift to maintain the airway, although limited head tilt with jaw thrust may be applied gently, until until the airway opens, in life threatening situations
  - If turning is necessary, log roll the patient (see chapter on Spinal Injuries)
  - Immobilise the neck with gentle manual in-line cervical stabilisation, followed by the application of a rigid cervical collar, and if available a spinal board and straps/spider harness and head blocks
  - Be careful to keep the immobilised patient horizontal, as spinal cord injury may result in significant hypotension

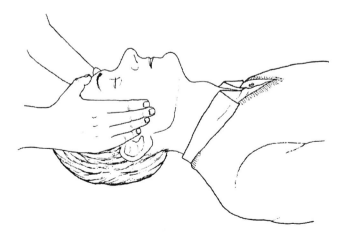

Figure 2-24 Immobilisation of the neck with manual in-line stabilisation

Airway obstruction by a foreign body/Choking

Incidence
- Airway obstruction by a foreign body is a relatively common problem

Aetiology
- Causes include:
    - Regurgitation of gastric contents associated with a depressed level of consciousness
    - Choking on large pieces of poorly chewed food

Symptoms/signs
- The patient will have difficulty with breathing, and may appeared cyanosed
- If conscious they may indicate that they are choking by grasping their neck with their hands or pointing to their throat

Conscious casualty

Management
- If the airway is only partially obstructed, the casualty may often able to dislodge the foreign body themselves by coughing
- If the airway obstruction is complete, urgent intervention is indicated to prevent asphyxia
- Obtain their confidence and encourage them to cough; this allows them to use their own muscles and so exert as much pressure as possible to expel the foreign body (this is successful in most patients)

- **If the airway obstruction appears to be complete, or the casualty shows signs of exhaustion with poor or absent air movement, or is cyanosed, administer:**

Back blows
- Firm blows to the back may dislodge the foreign body

Method
- Place the casualty either in the lateral position with a face down tilt or they may be standing (support the front of their chest with one hand) or sitting down (leaning over the back of a chair), preferably with the head below the chest to maximise the effects of gravity
- Lean the patient forwards, with the head down (preferably). This allows gravity to assist you
- Stand behind and to the side of the patient and give up to five firm blows smartly with the heel of the other hand to the middle of the back, between the scapulae

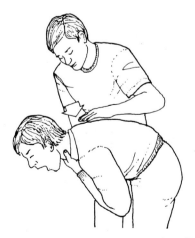

Figure 2-25 Back blows: patient bending over

- **If 5 back blows are unsuccessful, proceed to:**

Abdominal thrusts (Heimlich manoeuvre)
  - The sudden inward and upward movement of the upper abdomen against the diaphragm forces air up the oesophagus, and helps to expel the foreign body

Method
  - Stand or kneel behind the patient, and put both your arms round the patient's upper abdomen, above the umbilicus and well below the xiphisternum
  - Clench one fist and place it with the thumb inwards, immediately below the patient's xiphisternum.
  - Grasp the fist with your other hand, and pull both hands inwards and upwards towards you, with a quick thrust from the elbows
  - Continue to administer thrusts until the foreign material is expelled or the patient becomes unconscious

CAUTION
  - Excessive force may result in injury to the stomach, liver, diaphragm, spleen and aorta
  - Not recommended in pregnancy, gross obesity, or in infants and children under 5 years old

- **If neither method is successful, consider:** surgical airway management, if available

Back blows alternating with abdominal thrusts (or)

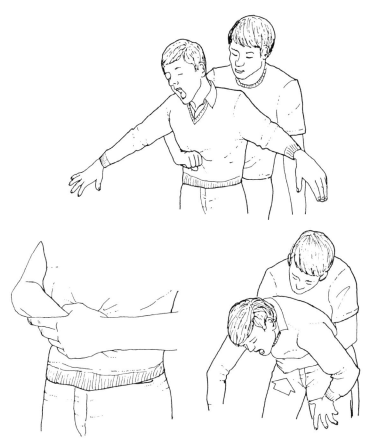

Figure 2-26 Abdominal thrusts: patient conscious

Unconscious casualty

- **If the casualty becomes, or is already unconscious, try:**

Finger sweeps

Method
- Place the casualty in the supine position for solid objects or lateral position for drainage of liquids
- Open the mouth by lifting the chin or prise the teeth apart manually
- Use an index finger to sweep inside the mouth and try to remove the foreign body digitally (well fitting dentures, however, may help to maintain a mouth seal during ventilation, so do not remove)

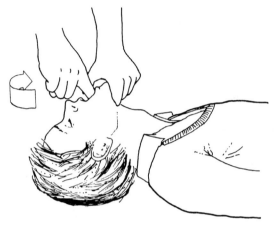

Figure 2-27 Finger sweeps

- **If this is not successful, administer:**

Five back blows

Method
- Turn the patient onto their side in the lateral position (see Recovery position above)
- Hold them with one hand, and with the other hand give up to five firm blows smartly with the heel of the hand to the middle of the back, between the scapulae

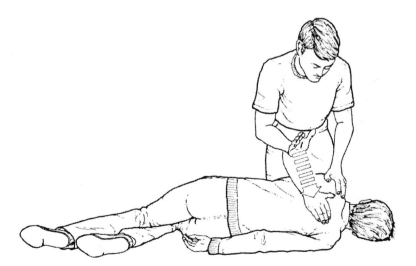

Figure 2-28 Back blows: patient unconscious

If this is not successful, administer:

Abdominal thrusts

Method
- Kneel astride, or if this is not possible, beside the patient
- Place the heel of one hand in the patient's epigastrium and cover it with the other hand, keeping the wrist dorsiflexed
- With both arms straight, give a quick inwards and upwards thrust aiming towards the patient's upper thoracic spine
- Repeat this up to four times as necessary (five in total)

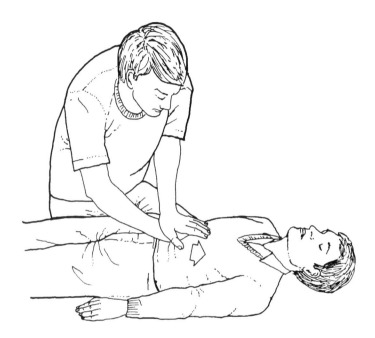

Figure 2-29 Abdominal thrusts: patient unconscious

Chest thrusts
- This may used as an alternative to abdominal thrusts (preferred method in children and when abdominal thrusts are contraindicated or ineffective

Method
- Use the same technique as for chest compressions during cardiac arrest (see above)

If the obstruction is not moved after 5 back blows and 5 abdominal thrusts and the casualty is not breathing, try expired air ventilations again. If this is still not successful, administer:

Further abdominal or chest thrusts (or consider direct laryngoscopy or surgical airway management, if available)

Note: If the casualty is found to be unconscious, with an obstructed airway on the initial assessment, start performing abdominal thrusts immediately, as the situation is desperate, and abdominal thrusts are more effective at removing inhaled objects than back blows

Resuscitation: when to stop

- When resuscitation attempts are obviously unsuccessful
- When the rescuers are exhausted
- Where there is evidence of irreversible brain damage
- Exceptions to this include:
    - Hypothermia
    - Drug overdosage
    - Drowning
    - Electrocution
    - In children

Note: The presence of *dilated pupils* is an unreliable sign of cardiac arrest, circulatory failure or established/ irreversible brain damage and should *not* be used to influence the management of a patient during or after cardiopulmonary resuscitation

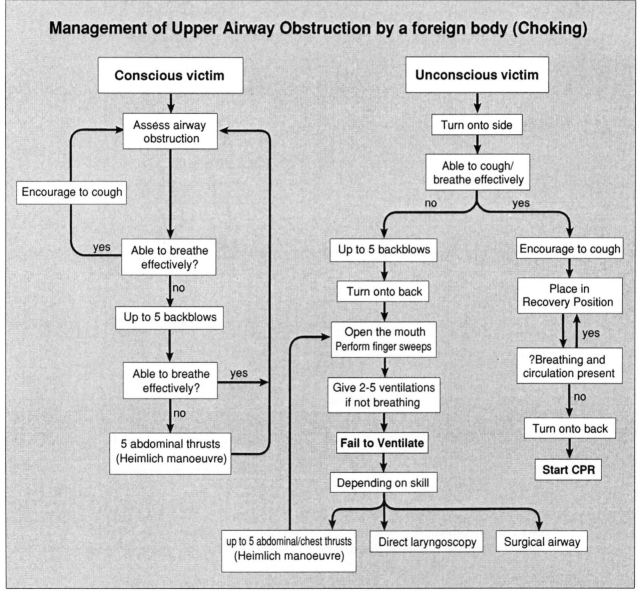

Figure 2-30 Algorithm for the management of choking
(copyright of the European Resuscitation Council, reproduced with permission)

Cross infection and expired air ventilation

- Hepatitis B and herpes viruses have been known to be transmitted by saliva and nasal discharge, and so it is advisable to avoid direct contact with these if possible, by using a simple and effective barrier device which does not hinder an adequate flow of air or significantly increase the dead space, e.g. a pocket mask (see chapter on Airway management)
- In human immunodeficiency virus (HIV) disease, contact with infected blood is the *only* risk, and even then the incidence of transmission is extremely low. Recent studies have shown that the HIV virus does not survive in human saliva
- About 70% of cardiac arrests occur in the home where the patient is known to the rescuer

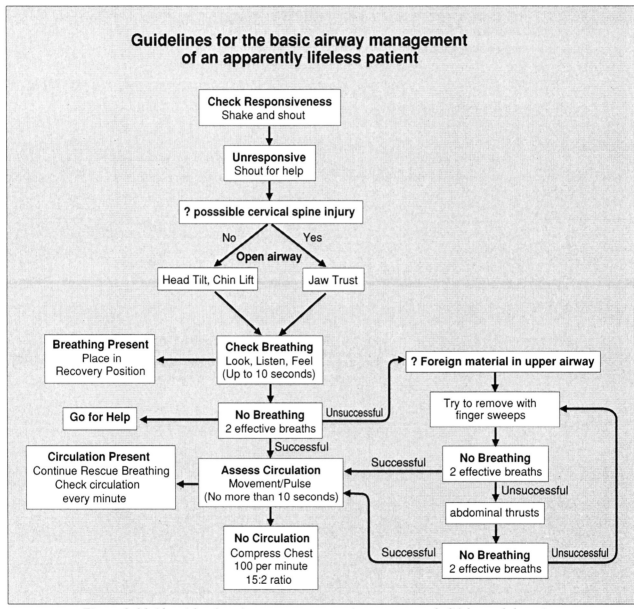

Figure 2-31 Algorithm for airway management in an apparently lifeless adult patient (adapted from the European Resuscitation Council, reproduced with permission)

3

Airway care

Airway care

Introduction

- Basic airway care is covered in the previous chapter on Basic Life Support
- Rapid assessment, and if appropriate, management of the airway must be the first potential problem to be addressed in every patient. The treatment is usually simple and may be lifesaving
- Bystander failure to recognise and treat airway obstruction is a common but preventable cause of death on all too many occasions: it is estimated that one in five of all preventable deaths following road traffic accidents occurs as a result of an obstructed airway

Respiratory failure
- Occurs when there is a failure of normal gas exchange in the lungs

Aetiology

Hypoxia

Unsuitable respirable atmosphere
- Carbon monoxide, smoke or other toxic constituents
- Hypoxic environment, e.g. high altitude hypoxia
- Drowning

Airway obstruction
- Above the larynx:
    - Excess mucus
    - Enlarged tonsils: severe quinsy
    - Enlarged adenoids
    - Foreign body: food, false teeth
    - Faciomaxillary injury
    - Angioneurotic oedema
- Laryngeal:
    - Tumours, acute epiglottitis, laryngeal trauma, burns
- Below the larynx:
    - Trauma, inhaled foreign body, tracheitis, burns
- In the lungs:
    - Asthma, bronchitis, bronchiolitis, pneumonia
    - Lung contusion, haemothorax, pneumothorax

Failure of oxygen transfer and utilisation
- Poisoning:
    - Carbon monoxide
    - Cyanide
- Profound anaemia and hypovolaemia

Ventilatory failure

Bellows failure
- Central depression:
    - Drugs: narcotics, hypnotics, tranquillizers, alcohol
    - Accidents: severe head injury, cerebrovascular accident
- Neuromuscular paralysis:
    - Cervical spine injury
    - Tetanus, polyneuritis, poliomyelitis
    - Myasthenia gravis
    - "Nerve" gases (organophosphates)
- Breach in the integrity of the thoracic cage:
    - Flail chest
    - Pneumothorax/stab wound
    - Ruptured diaphragm
- Rupture of trachea or bronchus

Pathophysiology
- Normal gas exchange fails, resulting in:
    - A reduction in the level of oxygenation of the blood (hypoxaemia)
    - An increase in the levels of deoxygenated haemoglobin in the blood (cyanosis)
    - A build up of carbon dioxide levels in the blood (hypercapnia)
    - A resultant respiratory acidosis

Symptoms/signs (depending on the underlying pathophysiology)

Respiratory distress
- Hypoxia/hypoxaemia (inadequate blood oxygenation):
    - Disturbance of cerebral function, restlessness
    - Pallor, sweating
    - Dyspnoea, tachypnoea, irregular respiratory effort, inability to cough, tracheal tug
    - Use of accessory muscles, intercostal recession, nasal flaring
    - Increase in heart rate, unless severe hypoxia, when heart rate starts to decrease
    - Oliguria: this is a relatively late development and therefore not usually relevant in Immediate Care
- Hypercapnia/hypercarbia (a build up of carbon dioxide in the blood due to inadequate ventilation):
    - Vasodilation: warm extremities
    - Tachycardia with a high volume pulse
    - Flapping tremor and drowsiness

Impending death
- Cyanosis:
    - Discolouration of tongue and lips: not usually seen until the PaO_2 is less than 60 mmHg.
    - Does not occur if the patient is very anaemic
- Drowsiness
- Irregular respiration, absence of wheeze (silent chest)
- Tachycardia >150 bpm, hypertension progressing finally to bradycardia and hypotension

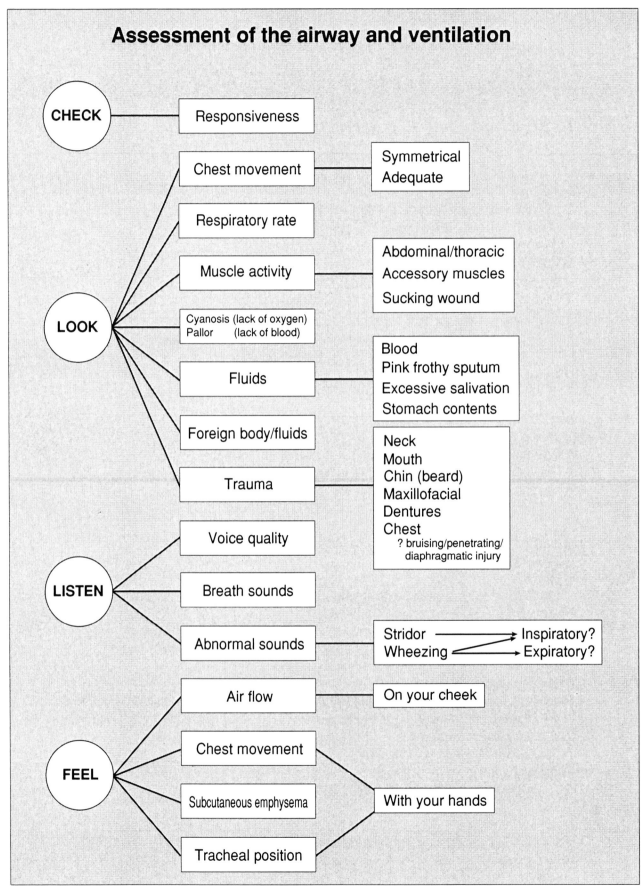

Figure 3-1 Algorithm for assessment of the airway and ventilation
(copyright of the European Resuscitation Council, reproduced with permission)

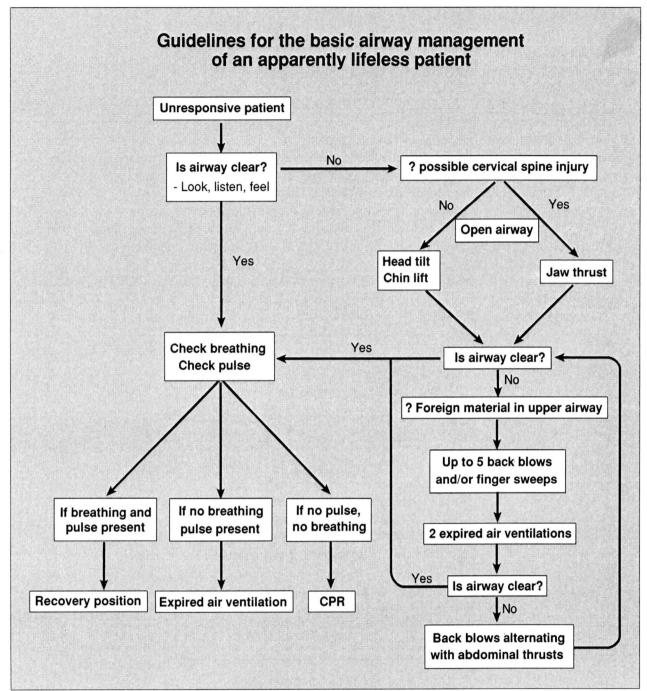

*Figure 3-2 Algorithm for basic airway management
(copyright of the European Resuscitation Council, reproduced with permission)*

Assessment/measurement of respiration

Oxygenation

Pulse oximetry
- This is a simple, reliable and accurate way of measuring the adequacy of arterial oxygenation, but it *does not* measure the adequacy of ventilation, or elimination of carbon dioxide (a pulse oximeter measures capillary blood oxygen saturation, not oxygen content)
- Has become established as the most convenient non-invasive method for the continuous monitoring of arterial oxygen saturation, and is now being used regularly in the pre-hospital situation to assess and monitor patients during entrapment and transportation to hospital
- It has several benefits as a monitoring tool, because of the difficulty of assessing oxygenation clinically:
    - Cyanosis is very difficult to detect with any accuracy, even for the experienced in good lighting conditions, and is particularly unreliable as a sign in the poor lighting conditions usually encountered out of hospital
    - Plethoric or polycythaemic patients may appear cyanosed despite adequate arterial oxygen tensions
- If pulse oximetry is used to assess or monitor the condition of a patient, the user *must* understand basic respiratory physiology, the way in which pulse oximetry works and its limitations as a diagnostic tool
- Under no circumstances must pulse oximetry be relied upon as the sole method of assessment to indicate such events as oesophageal intubation, cardiac arrest, breathing system disconnections, or failure of the oxygen supply

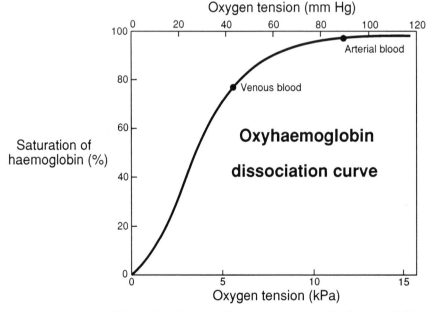

Figure 3-3 Oxygen dissociation curve for haemoglobin

Description
- A portable pulse oximeter is a solid state battery operated device which measures the oxygen saturation of arterial haemoglobin detected by a probe usually attached to a finger, toe, ear or the bridge of the nose
- Pulses of red and infrared light, produced by two adjacent light emitting diodes in the probe are transmitted through a pulsating arterial vascular bed, where the two different wavelengths of light are absorbed to a greater or lesser extent by the oxy- and total haemoglobin present, depending on the the amount of each haemoglobin present
- The remaining red/infrared light is then detected by a photodetector in the probe and an electronic signal sent via a screened cable to the processing unit, where it is then processed and displayed to give analogue digital readouts for the arterial waveform, oxygen saturation (SaO_2) and pulse rate

Pulse oximetry probe

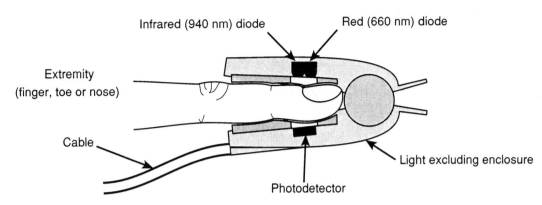

Figure 3-4 Pulse oximetry probe

- Oxy- and total (oxy- + deoxy-) haemoglobin absorb different wavelengths of red/infrared light (as do carboxy- and methaemoglobin, but these are not usually present in the circulation in any significant quantity, except in the patient who has suffered from smoke inhalation or crush injury)
- Bone, tissue and blood vessels containing venous blood absorb a constant amount of light over time, but the arterial vascular bed pulsates, and absorbs different amounts of light at different phases of the cardiac cycle, as the volume of blood in the arterial vascular bed increases in systole and decreases in diastole (the pulsatile component of the signal is only a small part of the total signal and is thus very susceptible to artefact, especially if there is poor peripheral circulation or movement)
- Oxygen saturation (SaO_2) as measured by pulse oximetry is commonly referred to as the "SpO_2"

- Oxygen saturation of arterial haemoglobin $= \dfrac{\text{haemoglobin sites occupied}}{\text{total haemoglobin sites available}}$

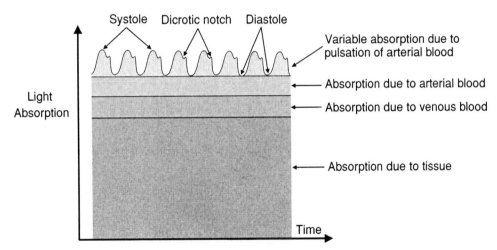

Figure 3-5 Photoplethysmography: absorption of light through various tissues

Normal values when breathing air
- Normal adult range: 97-100% (at sea level)
- Mild hypoxia: 90-96%
- Moderate hypoxia: 85-90%
- Severe hypoxia: <85%

Note: Some patients, especially those with chronic severe asthma and chronic obstructive pulmonary disease may tolerate relatively severe hypoxia surprisingly well

Limitations
- Pulse oximetry combines the inaccuracies of measuring oxygen saturation by this method, and the limitations of using arterial oxygen saturation as an indication of the cardiorespiratory status of a patient
- Accuracy (± 1-2%):
    - Becomes progressively less accurate, especially below 85%, because of the shape of the oxygen dissociation curve
- Supplemental oxygen:
    - If the patient is being administered supplemental oxygen, a pulse oximeter may show a normal oxygen saturation, *but will give no indication as to the adequacy of ventilation*
- Tracheal tube positioning:
    - An initially satisfactory pulse oximetry reading does *not* indicate satisfactory positioning of the tracheal tube following intubation, if the patient has been preoxygenated. This is because the lungs act as an oxygen reservoir, and it may take up to 8 minutes for the SpO$_2$ level to fall
- Anaemia/haemodilution:
    - Pulse oximetry will give no guide as to the adequacy of the total arterial oxygenation if the patient is anaemic. A severely anaemic patient with very few red blood corpuscles, all of which are carrying oxyhaemoglobin may have a normal oxygen saturation
- Peripheral circulation:
    - Pulse oximetry may not be accurate when there is poor peripheral perfusion, e.g. if the patient is hypovolaemic, and/or the ambient temperature is very low and there is peripheral vasoconstriction. There must be an effective arterial circulation in the part being monitored, and pulse oximetry only gives a crude indication as to the adequacy of the peripheral circulation. In fact the device is so sensitive that it may show a pulse signal even when the pulse pressure is so low that there is inadequate tissue perfusion and has even been observed to give a signal when the proximal artery has been occluded by a clamp! Thus the apparent presence of pulsation by itself does *not* give any indication as to the adequacy of cardiac output, arterial blood pressure or cardiac rhythm
- Carbon monoxide inhalation:
    - Pulse oximetry will give a false high reading in carbon monoxide poisoning (common when there has been smoke/car exhaust inhalation), as the photo-detector is unable to distinguish oxy- from carboxy-haemoglobin
- Methaemoglobinaemia:
    - This may be caused by the patient taking some drugs, e.g. nitrites, nitrates, chlorates, anti-malarials and amyl nitrate (used in the management of cyanide poisoning), and in the later stages of crush injury, and will bias any reading towards 85%, regardless of the actual oxygen saturation

Applications
- For measuring arterial oxygen saturation and detecting a reduced level (which indicates tissue hypoxia) and monitoring the pulse rate
- As an aid to diagnosis:
    - A low initial reading or a deteriorating reading gives an early warning that the patient has a respiratory problem, *but a normal reading does not indicate that there is no respiratory problem*
- Pulse oximetry has an important role in patient assessment in the following situations:
    - Trauma:
        - Head injury:
            - Obstructed airway, hypoventilation on air
        - Chest injury:
            - Flail chest, haemothorax or pneumothorax
        - Multiple injuries:
            - Hypovolaemic shock
        - Limb injuries:
            - Assessing the adequacy of the distal circulation (but always be aware of its limitations, and if possible compare any reading with that in the opposite uninjured limb)

- Medical emergencies:
    - Unconsciousness: upper airway obstruction
    - Asthma: degree of hypoxia
    - Respiratory depression: overdose, alcohol
    - Cardiogenic shock and arrest
    - Hypovolaemic and bacterial shock
- Assessing whether a patient's confusion is due to hypoxia, e.g. in silent pulmonary embolism
- Determining/monitoring trends:
    - Adequacy of oxygen therapy
    - Efficacy of analgesia in fractured ribs
    - Response to treatment
    - Effectiveness of the peripheral circulation (but always be aware of its limitations, and if possible compare any reading with that in the opposite uninjured limb)
- Checking the distal circulation in damaged limbs before and after movement, e.g. before and after extrication, splinting or reduction of a fracture

PRACTICAL POINTS

- *Choice of probe site:*
    - *A finger is the site of choice, although toes may be used instead, but poor perfusion is more likely, especially in hypothermia and in the older patient who may have peripheral vascular disease*
    - *The ear lobe or pinna may be considered for a clip probe after fingers and toes, but ear probes are not available for some devices; fixation can be more difficult and care must be taken to ensure that the clip does not exert so much pressure that it impairs the circulation*
    - *The bridge of the nose may be tried as an alternative when perfusion is poor, but there is no evidence that this is any better than the other sites*

- *Probe type:*
    - *Clip probes are the most expensive, but can be reused many times*
    - *Self adhesive probes are not generally reusable, but are the most useful when movement artefact is likely or when long term monitoring is necessary*

- *Pulse oximetry may produce artefacts and inaccurate results if:*
    - *The patient has painted finger and toe nails, as some nail varnish pigments (notably black, purple and blue) do not allow the light to pass through them*
    - *The probe is attached to skin which is covered in dirt, oil, grease (under-estimation)*
    - *The probe is uncovered in bright sunlight*
    - *The patient is shivering or is in a moving vehicle (movement artefact)*
    - *The probe is taped too tightly to the patient*
    - *The patient is peripherally shutdown: hypovolaemia, cold environment (try warming the skin or use a different site for the probe)*
    - *The patient is a heavy smoker (over-estimation due to carbon monoxide)*
    - *The probe or probe site is contaminated by dried blood (under-estimation)*

CONCLUSION
- Pulse oximetry is essential in Immediate Care for monitoring changes (*trends*) in the level of oxygenation in the severely ill or injured patient, but its limitations must be understood

Ventilation

Capnography
- This is the detection and measurement of carbon dioxide in a patient's expired gas (end tidal CO_2)
- The level of carbon dioxide produced at the end of expiration is almost identical to the level of carbon dioxide in alveolar gas, and as carbon dioxide passes easily across the alveolar membrane, the alveolar carbon dioxide level is a good representation of the arterial carbon dioxide level
- Its use in the pre-hospital situation is limited as it can only be used in patients who require some form of active airway or ventilation intervention

End tidal CO_2 detectors/monitors
- These are the devices used for measuring the levels of carbon dioxide in expired gas

Description
- The sampling part of the device is attached between the connector of the tracheal tube and the catheter mount, and is classified as a mainstream analyser (as it monitors carbon dioxide levels in the expired gas directly, unlike a sidestream analyser, which monitors the gas in a sidearm of the breathing apparatus attached to the patient)
- There are currently two types of device suitable for use in the pre-hospital environment:

Infrared end tidal CO_2 detector

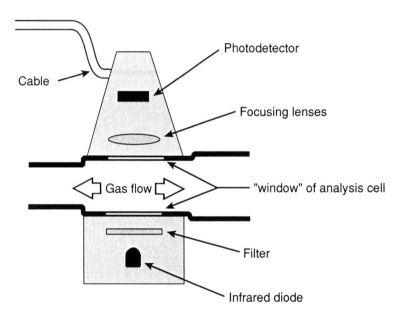

Figure 3-6 Infrared end tidal CO_2 detector

- This is a battery operated device which uses a solid state non-dispersive infrared carbon dioxide detector which clips over a disposable gas analysis cell/airway adaptor which fits between the airway and ventilating device, a cable and a processor unit
- In the detector, an infrared light emitting diode transmits a pulsed beam of infrared light through a filter (which prevents interference from other gases such as oxygen and nitrous oxide), across the gas in the analysis cell, after which it is focussed onto a photodetector. from which an electronic signal is sent via a screened cable to the processing unit
- The signal is then processed to give a visual (and in some devices an audible) indication of the amount of carbon dioxide present in each respiratory cycle

Disposable end tidal CO_2 detector
- This uses a rapidly acting chemical pH indicator to detect the presence of carbon dioxide.
- The colour varies from mauve, indicating a CO_2 level of <0.5% during inspiration, to yellow, indicating a CO_2 level of 2-5% during expiration, and responds sufficiently rapidly to detect changes in carbon dioxide levels breath by breath.

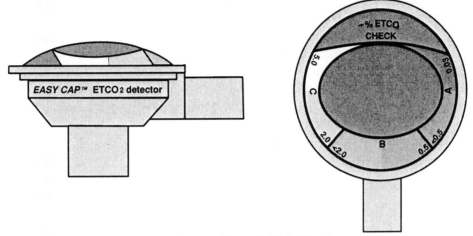

Figure 3-7 Disposable end tidal CO_2 detector

Applications
- Detection of hypo- or hypercapnia
    - Gives an early indication of:
        - Oesophageal intubation (is therefore very useful as an aid to confirm correct placement of the tracheal tube, especially useful for the infrequent or inexperienced intubator)
        - Adequacy of ventilation (hypoventilation)
        - Disconnection of the breathing system
- Provides a simple, rapid and non invasive method of measuring blood flow during resuscitation, and can indicate the return of spontaneous cardiac output or give warning of cardiorespiratory failure

Limitations
- Little or no CO_2 may be produced during cardiac arrest, so capnography may be of little use in this situation, except to indicate the adequacy of CPR and the return of respiration
- Sodium bicarbonate or carbonated drinks in the stomach can give significant CO_2 waveforms up to six breaths after oesophageal intubation (therefore ignore first six cycles of respiration)
- Electronic device:
    - Expensive
    - Relatively heavy and bulky
    - Delicate
- Disposable monitor:
    - Gastric acid contamination causes a permanent orange colour
    - Tracheal lidocaine or epinephrine will cause a permanent yellow colour
    - May not work when it is very cold

Advantages
- Capnography is less susceptible to error or artefact than pulse oximetry
- May give an earlier warning of imminent arterial desaturation than pulse oximetry

CONCLUSION
- Capnography is useful in Immediate Care as an aid for confirming tracheal intubation, and when used in conjunction with pulse oximetry is valuable for monitoring the respiratory state of intubated patients

Oxygen therapy

- This is the treatment of choice for hypoxia

Mode of action
- Increases the haemoglobin oxygen saturation
- Increases the amount of oxygen carried in solution in the blood

*Note:*1. Oxygen should be administered with caution in some patients, i.e. patients with chronic obstructive pulmonary disease (COPD), some of whom may depend on their hypoxic drive to maintain respiration, provided that there is no other cause for their hypoxia. If they do require oxygen this should be administered at a low flow rate using a relatively low oxygen concentration. This is not a problem if they are being artificially ventilated

2. Oxygen administration is contraindicated in paraquat poisoning

Administration

Oxygen masks
- Oxygen is often administered at inadequate flow rates, (e.g. 4-6 litres per minute); to be effective oxygen should be administered at flow rates of 8-15 litres per minute
- The oxygen concentration delivered varies with the type of mask used
- Oxygen may be in relatively short supply in the pre-hospital situation; use of the most appropriate mask and oxygen flow rate will help to avoid unnecessary waste of oxygen

Ventimask® medium flow oxygen mask

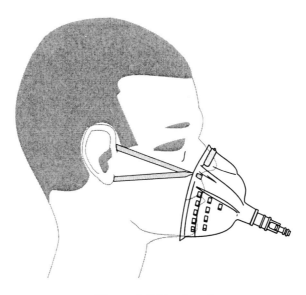

Figure 3-8 Ventimask

- The Ventimask is a fixed performance mask designed to provide a constant level of oxygen enrichment to inspired air, irrespective of the phase of respiration or the breathing pattern
- The inspired oxygen concentration is not dependent on the fit of the mask
- Only allows minimal rebreathing of expired air
- Delivers 24/28/35/40/60% oxygen via a range of interchangeable colour coded venturi adaptors

Note: The Edinburgh mask is similar to the Ventimask but has a variable flow venturi oxygen entrainment adaptor which allows adjustable oxygen concentration rates of 24-35%

Polymask, MC (Moderate Concentration) oxygen mask

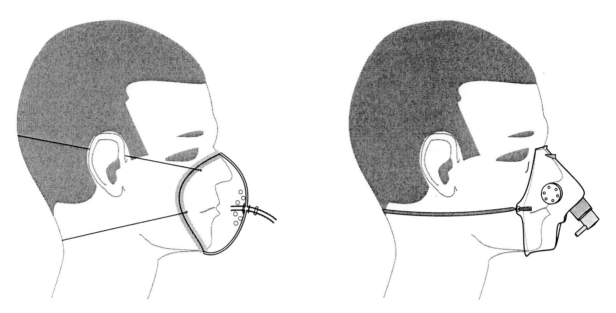

Figure 3-9 MC Masks from different manufacturers

- This is a range of masks designed to provide a moderate concentration of oxygen in inspired air, the oxygen concentration depending on the oxygen flow rate
- The air is drawn in by the wearer in an uncontrolled way, depending on the depth/rate of respiration
- The fit of the mask may also influence the inspired oxygen concentration
- Delivers approximately 60% oxygen at a flow rate of 8 litres/minute and 67% oxygen at a flow rate of 10 litres/minute

High concentration oxygen mask with oxygen reservoir

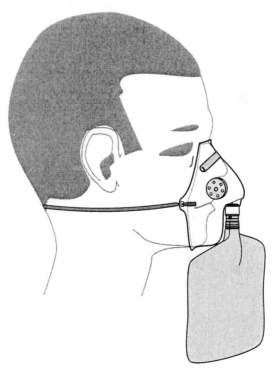

Figure 3-10 High concentration oxygen mask with oxygen reservoir

- Allows minimal re-breathing of expired air
- Delivers 98-100% oxygen at a flow rate of 8 litres per minute when tightly applied to the face
- Flow rates higher than 10 litres per minute may rarely result in gastric distension

CONCLUSION
- Should be used in patients who requires a high concentration of inspired oxygen (most trauma victims)

Oxygen cylinders

Identification
- Black cylinder with a white collar and neck

Sizes
- Size C is the most portable and may fit into a carrying case for use at the scene of an incident
- Size D is used in portable ventilators
- Sizes C and D have an integral contents gauge and can be recharged from larger cylinders using a charging valve (this is no longer recommended, but if necessary should be performed with appropriate precautions)
- Sizes E, F and G are not readily transportable, due to their weight and size
- Other sizes may be available, e.g.; 125, 230, and 370 litres
- Modern cylinders are made of aluminium and are lighter than older metal cylinders

Sizes and capacity of oxygen cylinders

Size	Capacity (litres)	Duration at 8 l/min (minutes)	Duration at 15 l/min (minutes)
C	170	21	11
D	340	42	22
E	680	85	45
F	1360	170	90
G	3400	420	225

Figure 3-11 Size and capacity of oxygen cylinders

Flow rates
- Fixed at 6, 8, 10 or 15 litres per minute
- Variable: 2, 4, 6, 8, 10 and 15 litres per minute

Duration
- Cylinder capacity in litres, divided by the flow setting

Maintenance
- All cylinders need to be pressure tested every 5 years after the date stamped on the neck of the cylinder

CAUTION: 1. NEVER lubricate any part of the oxygen regulator valve as an oil/oxygen mixture is explosive
*   2. Oxygen supports combustion, and so should be kept away from naked flames, cigarettes, and cutting equipment in use*

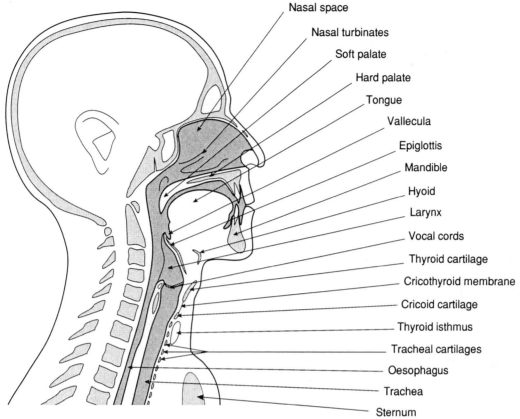

Nasal space
Nasal turbinates
Soft palate
Hard palate
Tongue
Vallecula
Epiglottis
Mandible
Hyoid
Larynx
Vocal cords
Thyroid cartilage
Cricothyroid membrane
Cricoid cartilage
Thyroid isthmus
Tracheal cartilages
Oesophagus
Trachea
Sternum

Figure 3-12 Anatomy of the upper airway: 1

Airway management

Introduction

- Effective airway assessment and management is the first priority in the care of the seriously ill or injured patient, for without a patent airway the patient will die in minutes
- The possibility of a cervical spine injury should always be borne in mind when managing the airway, especially if the patient is unconscious following an injury above the chest, and the neck handled with appropriate care (in-line cervical stabilisation)
- An understanding of the anatomy of the upper airway is essential for effective upper airway control

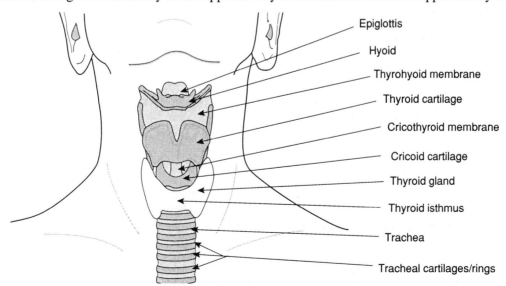

Epiglottis
Hyoid
Thyrohyoid membrane
Thyroid cartilage
Cricothyroid membrane
Cricoid cartilage
Thyroid gland
Thyroid isthmus
Trachea
Tracheal cartilages/rings

Figure 3-13 Anatomy of the upper airway: 2

Simple airways

Oropharyngeal airway (Guedel)

- The oropharyngeal airway improves airway patency in the unconscious patient by preventing the tongue falling backwards and obstructing the airway, and provides relief for the rescuer having to apply prolonged jaw thrust, although chin lift is frequently necessary

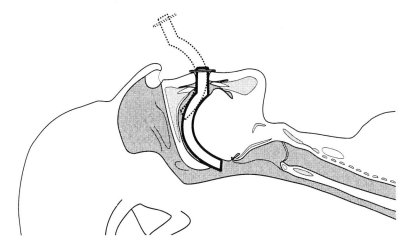

Figure 3-14 Oropharyngeal airway showing method of insertion

Indications
- Upper airway obstruction due to backward displacement of the tongue
- Can act as a protective 'bite block' when other airways are in place

Contraindications
- Clenched jaw (trismus), vulnerable dentition
- Imminent danger of the patient vomiting, active glossopharyngeal reflexes
- Haemorrhage from the oropharynx

Sizes
- 00 - infant   0 - small child   1 - child   2 - small adult   3 - medium adult   4 - large adult

PRACTICAL POINT: The correct length for an oropharyngeal airway is the same length as the distance from the corner of the mouth to the ear lobe

Method of insertion
- Invert the lubricated device and insert it into the mouth turning it through 180° as the end of it passes under the palate and into the oropharynx (except in infants/small children, when it should be inserted the right way up under direct vision)
- Check for unimpeded air entry (supplementary jaw support (chin lift) may be necessary)

Disadvantages
- May cause oropharyngeal stimulation and retching unless the patient is deeply unconscious
- If it is too long, the device may impinge on the epiglottis and bend it over the laryngeal opening
- If too short, it may not support the tongue
- The oropharyngeal airway does not protect the airway from gastric aspiration

CONCLUSION
- The standard simple airway

Nasopharyngeal airway

- The nasopharyngeal airway improves airway patency in the unconscious patient by preventing the tongue being displaced backwards and obstructing the airway

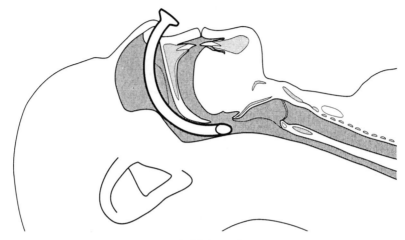

Figure 3-15 Nasal airway

Indications
- Patients who do not tolerate an oropharyngeal airway
- Severe faciomaxillary injury
- Trismus (clenched jaw)

Sizes
- Female: 6.0 mm   Male: 7.0 mm

Method of insertion
- Prepare the device by putting a safety pin through the proximal end to prevent it being lost inside the nose and lubricate it well.
- Carefully and gently insert the device into the right nostril, parallel to the palate.
- If resistance is experienced, withdraw the device and try the left nostril.
- Check for unimpeded air entry

PRACTICAL POINT: If no nasopharyngeal airway is available: a size 6.0 or 7.0 tracheal tube may be used instead. It should be cut to length and a safety pin inserted through the proximal end.

Advantages
- It is often better tolerated than the oropharyngeal airway, once it is in position

Disadvantages
- May cause severe haemorrhage from the nasopharynx ⎫ only a tube manufactured from
- May cause severe injury to the nasal mucosa, bone or cartilage ⎬ soft material should be used
- Should not be used in patients with a known or suspected anterior fractured base of skull (it may accidentally pass into the cranial cavity)
- Should be used with extreme caution in patients with a deformed or bilaterally obstructed nasal passage

CONCLUSION
- Nasal airways are useful simple airway devices and are often underused in Immediate Care.

Linder balloon® nasopharyngeal airway
- This is a development of the nasopharyngeal airway, but uses a soft deflatable introducer, which is less likely to cause nasopharyngeal trauma and resultant haemorrhage

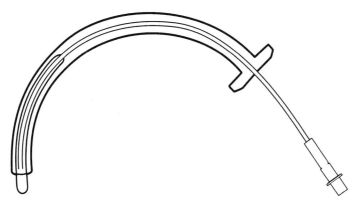

Figure 3-16 Linder balloon nasal airway: prior to inflation

Method of insertion
- Prepare the device by inserting the introducer until about one quarter of an inch of the balloon end protrudes from end of the airway tube
- Inflate the balloon with a 5 mL syringe to secure the introducer and airway together, until the protruding balloon is equal to the outside diameter of the airway
- Add some lubricant and insert the airway as described above
- After the airway has been full inserted, deflate the balloon completely with the syringe and gently withdraw the introducer

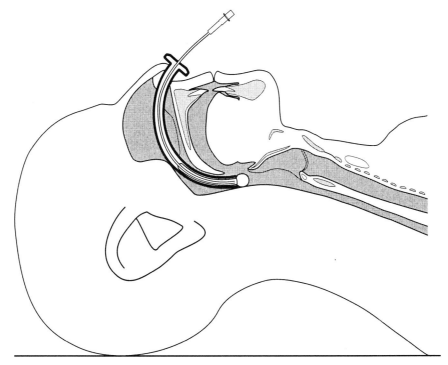

Figure 3-167 Linder balloon nasal airway: inserted with balloon inflated

CONCLUSION
- A useful modification to the standard nasal airway, but may be a bit more fiddly to use

Modified pharyngeal and laryngeal airways

Laryngeal mask® airway (LMA): Brain airway

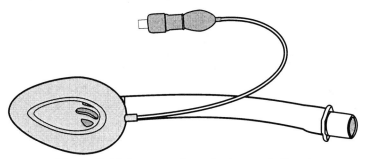

Figure 3-18 Laryngeal mask airway: inflated

Description
- The LMA consists of an oropharyngeal tube inserted into the upper end of a spoon shaped mask through a perforated window, with a standard connector at the proximal end
- The mask is surrounded by an inflatable cuff, which forms a laryngeal seal when adequately inflated
- Some versions have armoured tubes

Indications
- Requirement for ventilation in the presence of a cervical spine injury
- Facial injuries and supraglottic trauma, where use of a face mask is difficult
- When tracheal intubation is not possible due to the shape of the patient's neck/larynx
- When the operator is not trained/experienced in tracheal intubation
- As an aid to intubation (insert the LMA, pass down a gum elastic bougie, and then railroad down a small tracheal tube)

Sizes/cuff volume

-	1	- neonate/infant	up to 6.5 kg	2-4 mL
	2	- baby/child	6.5-15 kg	10 mL
	2½	- children	20-30 kg	14 mL
	3	- small adult	30-60 kg	20 mL
	4	- adult small male or female	50-75 kg	30 mL
	5	- Adult male	>75 kg	40 mL

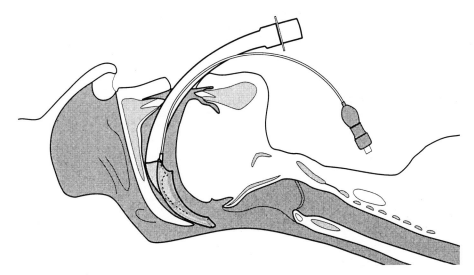

Figure 3-19 Laryngeal mask airway: correct insertion

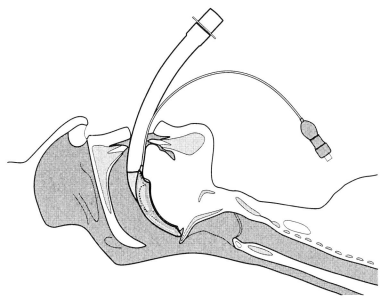

Figue 3-20 Laryngeal mask airway: impinging on the epiglottis

Method of application
- Prior to insertion, prepare the mask by deflating (sucking it completely flat with a syringe) and lubricating it
- Insert the mask behind the upper incisor teeth, with the solid line facing towards the nose, and carefully push it back along the roof of the mouth until it is deflected into the oropharynx by the soft palate (if it is pushed along the tongue, it may impinge on the epiglottis, folding it down and preventing correct insertion; if this happens, withdraw the device, and deflate it before attempting reinsertion)
- Push the device further down the oropharynx, until the tip comes to rest in the triangular shaped hypopharynx (further insertion is not possible unless excessive force is used). This signifies a definite end point which indicates correct placement of the mask around the laryngeal outlet
- Inflate the cuff with air, isolating the larynx from the rest of the pharyngeal space. The device moves upwards a little during inflation
- Confirm correct placement (may be accompanied by slight bulging of the soft tissues at the front of the neck) by attaching a bag, ventilating the patient and listening for breath sounds

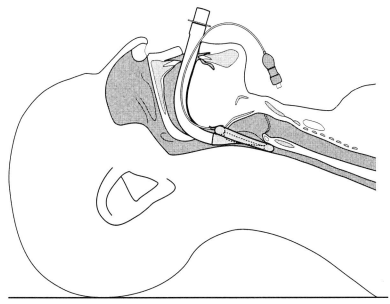

Figure 3-21 Laryngeal mask airway: correct position inflated

Advantages
- The device is easy to insert: the technique is simple and is easy to teach or learn
- Insertion:
    - Is much less traumatic than tracheal intubation, and does not require direct laryngoscopy
    - Requires minimum cervical movement
    - Can be performed with the operator sitting in front of the patient
    - Can be accomplished with less mouth opening than for tracheal intubation
- It is particularly useful in patients with "bull necks" in whom tracheal intubation is very difficult
- It reduces the risk of gastric aspiration (30% incidence with bag valve mask ventilation) and air leak compared to no airway, or a nasal/oropharyngeal airway
- It allows controlled ventilation, provided inflation pressures below 20 cm of water are sufficient for satisfactory lung expansion

Disadvantages
- Leak may occur around the cuff when using ventilatory pressures greater than 20 cm of water
- There is a small risk of pulmonary aspiration of gastric contents, especially in those patients in whom the mask does not seal the hypopharynx precisely (use a larger, rather than a smaller size)
- In theory it may be easily dislodged, e.g. during CPR, but in practice this doesn't appear to be a problem
- Only tolerated in patients in whom the gag reflex has been lost

CONCLUSION
- Particularly useful in the management of cardiac arrest as an alternative to bag-valve-mask ventilation with an oropharyngeal airway (*NOT* to tracheal intubation and ventilation)
- In trauma it may be useful; but the potential risk of aspiration has meant that it has been little used, except after failed tracheal intubation or for the sitting trapped patient in whom access does not allow intubation

Note: A modified LMA device, the intubating LMA which facilitates tracheal intubation is being evaluated

Pharyngeal tracheal lumen® airway (PTLA)
- The PTLA consists of two parallel tubes of differing length, held together by a length of moulded semi-rigid plastic, which conforms to the shape of the oropharynx
- The shorter tube has a large inflatable cuff proximal to its distal end, while the longer tube has a smaller inflatable cuff at its distal end. These cuffs are high volume, low pressure and are inflated via a single air entry port, with a one way valve and a universal connector. Air can be directed selectively to either cuff with the aid of a slide clamp on the air inlet to the longer tube

Indications
- Requirement for ventilation/airway protection in the presence of a cervical spine injury
- Patients who require ventilation and airway protection, in whom airway access is restricted, e.g. the unconscious patient, trapped sitting up in a vehicle
- Facial injury including unstable/fractured mandible, with requirement for airway protection/ventilation
- When the operator is not trained/experienced in tracheal intubation/failed intubation

Method of insertion
- The device is designed to be inserted blindly, and for the longer tube to enter the oesophagus, but if it is inserted into the trachea instead, the patient can still be ventilated and the airway protected
- Lift the jaw (there is no need to move the neck) and insert the device with its curvature following the natural curve of the oropharynx, until the tooth guard is reached (if resistance is met; withdraw the device and reinsert it)
- Inflate the cuffs by first blowing air into the cuff air entry port, and then into the short tube, following which check for breath sounds and chest expansion

- If ventilation is satisfactory; attach a bag or ventilator to the short tube
- If air does not enter the lungs:
    - Remove the stylet from the long tube, blow air down the long tube, and check for breath sounds/ chest expansion
- If ventilation is satisfactory; attach a bag or ventilator to the long tube
- If air still does not enter the lungs; look for airway obstruction
- Secure the device with the neck strap
- Once the device is in position; check for air leaks continually especially if the long tube is in the oesophagus
- If a leak does occur; clamp the long tube, and reinflate the oral cuff until the leak is controlled

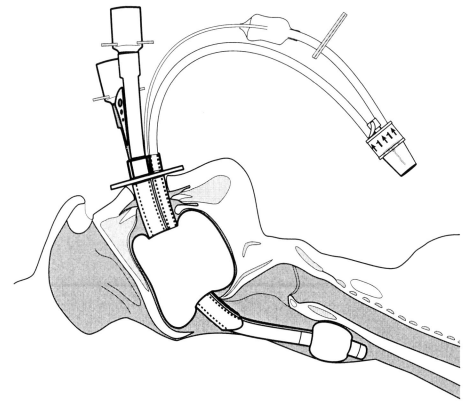

Figure 3-22 Pharyngeal tracheal lumen airway

Advantages
- Easy to use, although appears to be rather complicated initially
- Rapid insertion is possible, without the need for instrumentation
- Neck movement is unnecessary
- Controlled ventilation is possible

Disadvantages
- The tube is of fixed length, and care has to be taken using the device in very small or very large adults
- Airway obstruction may occur with the longer tube in the oesophagus
- The cuffs may be damaged by sharp teeth during insertion
- Requires wide mouth opening
- Unsuitable for use in patients with a high oesophageal stricture or severe oropharyngeal trauma

CONCLUSION
- Gaining acceptance for use in Immediate Care, but is a bit complicated to use initially, and may be superseded by the Combitube (see below)

Combitube®
- The Combitube consists of two parallel semi-rigid tubes (a longer blue tube labelled No.1 and a shorter white tube labelled No. 2), with two inflatable balloon cuffs, with pilot balloons labelled No.1 and No.2
- The smaller cuff is near the distal end of the tubes, and the larger (pharyngeal) cuff at their mid point
- The distal end of one tube is blind, but it has perforations between the two cuffs, and the other is open
- There are two ring marks near the proximal end of the tubes
- The device is supplied complete with a gastric suction tube, a 140 mL syringe for inflating the large cuff with 100 mL of air and a 20 mL syringe for inflating the smaller cuff with 15 mL of air
- There are two sizes; the smaller size being suitable for the majority of patients

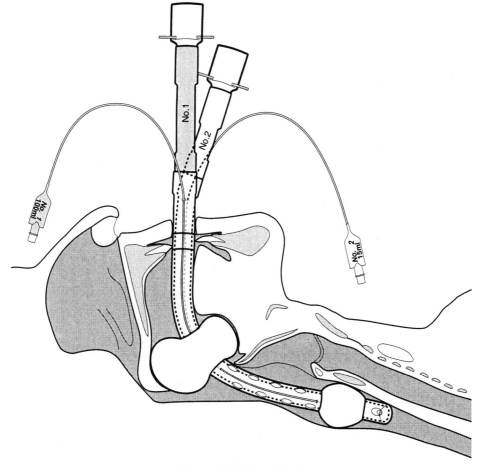

Figure 3-23 Combitube

Indications
- Similar to the PTLA

Method of insertion
- The device is designed to be inserted into the oesophagus, but if it is inserted into the trachea (2-4%), the patient can still be ventilated and the airway protected from gastric aspiration
- Insert the device blind (there is no need to move the neck of the patient) until that part of the tubes between the ring marks is aligned with the patient's teeth
- Inflate the cuffs with the syringes provided, starting with the pharyngeal cuff (blue pilot balloon No.1)
- Blow air into the longer blue (No.1) tube and check for breath sounds and chest expansion
- If ventilation is satisfactory:
    - Attach a bag or ventilation device to the long tube (the shorter tube can be used for gastric suction)
- If breath sounds are absent and there is no chest expansion, the device has entered the trachea:
    - Attach a bag or ventilation device to the shorter white (No.2) tube, and ventilate the patient

Advantages
- Similar to the PTLA, but simpler to use
- The distal cuff may be damaged by sharp teeth during insertion
- Allows gastric suctioning to empty the stomach (when correctly inserted)

Disadvantages
- Rather bulky and difficult to fit into equipment containers
- Designed for single use, and is rather costly
- May be associated with local trauma and may stimulate vomiting

CONCLUSION
- *A useful device* for protecting the airway in Immediate Care, when intubation is not possible

Tracheal tube
- A tube with an inflatable cuff near its distal end, which is inserted through the vocal cords and into the trachea
- The distal cuff prevents pulmonary aspiration of gastric contents and gas leakage during ventilation
- It provides a secure and clear airway through which ventilation and oxygenation can be administered

Indications
- Apnoea
- Upper airway obstruction
- Respiratory insufficiency necessitating positive pressure ventilation
- Risk of gastric regurgitation or blood entering the lungs, especially in the unconscious and/or head injured patient
- Risk of airway compromise, e.g. after facial burns, continuous fitting in spite of administration of intravenous diazepam or midazolam

Tube sizes (external diameter: approximately the size of the patient's little finger)
- Adults: Male 8.0 - 9.0 mm
           Female 7.0 - 8.0 mm

Tube length
- Twice the length from the corner of the mouth to the tip of the ear lobe
- Adults: Males: approximately 23 cm
           Females: approximately 21 cm

Advantages
- Provides a patent and secure airway, through which effective positive pressure ventilation can be applied
- Protects the airway from aspiration of foreign material, especially gastric contents
- Allows access for tracheal suction
- Allows release of skilled staff for other tasks

Disadvantages
- Correct insertion is very difficult for the inexperienced to perform; regular practice is required
- It cannot be performed in a conscious patient without anaesthesia, e.g. in severe facial burns
- There is a danger of:
    - Accidental intubation of the oesophagus or right main bronchus
    - Causing local trauma during insertion
    - Gastric aspiration during insertion
- If the patient is not anaesthetised insertion may cause a rise in intracranial pressure and bradycardia

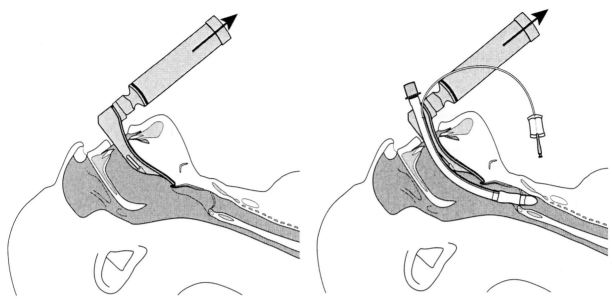

Figure 3-24 Tracheal intubation using a curved blade

Tracheal intubation: equipment

Suction equipment (see below)

Lubricant
- For lubricating the tube during insertion

Laryngoscopes
- Usually have detachable blades:
    - Curved blade: better for intubation of adults
    - Straight blade: probably better for the intubation of infants and small children
- Illumination may be:
    - Bulb in the blade
    - Fibre optic lighting system: better as the light source is brighter (for use in daylight) and less bulky

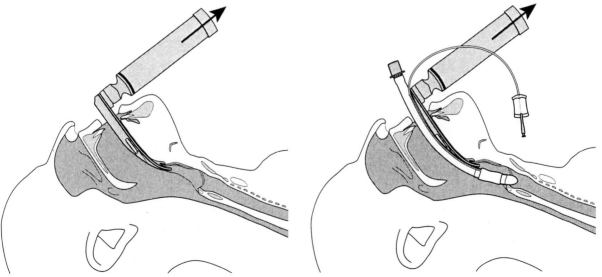

Figure 3-25 Tracheal intubation using a straight blade

Gum elastic bougie
- This is inserted through the cords before passing the tracheal tube, which is then passed down over it
- Essential equipment for pre-hospital airway care, especially for inexperienced intubators and if laryngeal oedema is present

Magill's forceps (not often used in Immediate Care, but should be!)
- Used for manipulating the tracheal tube through the cords/removing objects obstructing the airway
- The distal shaft is bent at an angle of 45°

Light wand
- A stylet with a light source at its tip used as an aid to tracheal intubation

Capnography
- This is the direct measurement of carbon dioxide (CO_2) in expired air, and can be used to confirm tracheal placement (except when the patient has no cardiac output)

Syringe 1 (5-10 mL)
- For inflating the cuff

Syringe 2 (50-60 mL)
- Attached directly to the tube connector and used as an oesophageal detector (an excellent alternative to capnography)

Tracheal intubation: method
- Assemble the equipment and make certain there is an appropriately sized tube cut to the correct length
- Always pre-oxygenate the patient before attempting insertion, with a bag-valve-mask device
- Position the patient correctly: with cervical flexion and head extension (sniffing the morning air), unless the patient has a possible cervical spine injury, when all neck movement should be avoided.
- Take and hold a deep breath yourself
- Holding the laryngoscope in the left hand, insert the blade into the right side of the mouth, making sure that the lower lip is not trapped between the blade and lower teeth

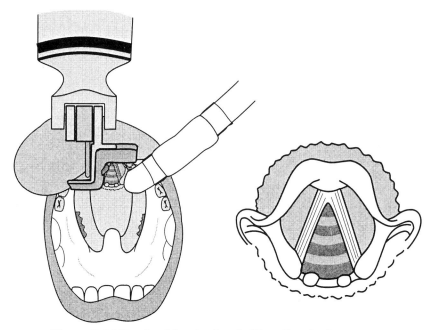

Figure 3-26 Tracheal intubation 1: Visualise the larynx

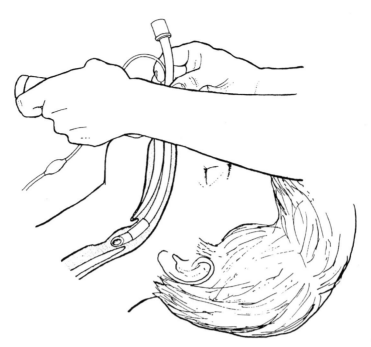

Figure 3-27 Tracheal intubation 2: Insertion of the tube

- Advance the tip of the blade, aiming it towards the posterior pharyngeal wall, displacing the body of the tongue to the left as you do so
- Lift the laryngoscope handle upwards and forwards, and slide the tip of the curved blade laryngoscope into the space between the base of the tongue and the root of the epiglottis, maintaining the position of the patient's head with your right hand as you do so (if you are using a straight bladed laryngoscope, the tip of the blade should be placed below the epiglottis)
- Be careful not to press the laryngoscope blade against the patient's upper teeth, as this can damage them
- Visualise the larynx, adjusting the position of the blade, so as to obtain the best view. Cricoid pressure (Sellick's manoeuvre) may make the larynx easier to see, especially if neck movement is contraindicated, and helps to reduce the danger of pulmonary aspiration of gastric contents
- Insert a lubricated tracheal tube into the right hand corner of the patient's mouth, and pass it down through the vocal cords under direct vision (if necessary rotate the tube anti-clockwise through 90° to ease its passage through the glottic opening)
- Continue inserting the tube until the cuff has completely passed through the vocal cords
- If you can only visualise the epiglottis or arytenoids, use a gum elastic bougie:
    - Pass it down behind the epiglottis and it will usually pass through the vocal cords and into the trachea. Tracheal placement is confirmed by feeling it 'click' across the tracheal rings, or when it is held up in the bronchial tree
- Inflate the cuff with air using a syringe attached to the cuff port, and apply positive pressure ventilation, checking for air leaks as you do so. Cease inflating the cuff when the sound of leaking air disappears. If this does not happen after fully inflating the cuff, check under direct vision, that the tube has not been misplaced in the oesophagus.
- Correct placement of the tube should be confirmed by:
    - Seeing the tip of the tube going through the vocal cords by direct laryngoscopy
    - Using a 50 mL syringe as an oesophageal detector:
        - Depress the plunger to expel the air, attach the syringe to the proximal end of the tube, and attempt to aspirate air, by withdrawing the plunger:
            - Easy air aspiration signifies tracheal placement
            - Difficulty in air aspiration and the presence of negative pressure indicates oesophageal placement

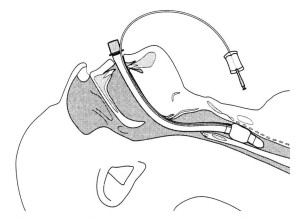

Fig3-28 Correct placement of the tracheal tube (cuff inflated)

- Ventilating the patient with the cuff of the tube fully inflated and confirming:
    - Absence of air leak around the cuff
    - Chest expansion and air entry into both sides of the lungs on auscultation of both axillae
    - Absence of sounds in the epigastric area on inflation
    - Changes in carbon dioxide levels in the inspired and expired gases using capnography
- Secure the tube with tape and re-check placement

Note: Intubation should take no longer than 30 seconds in the apnoeic patient (when you need to take your next breath, so does the patient!). If you have not been successful within this time, ventilate the patient for a few minutes with oxygen, before trying again

PRACTICAL POINT: 1. It saves time to pre-cut and pre-assemble the tubes for immediate use
2. If tracheal intubation is difficult: pass a laryngeal mask airway. Ensure that there is lung inflation and then pass a bougie, following which remove the LMA, and pass tracheal tube down over the bougie. Check satisfactory placement (see above). A modified LMA, the intubating LMA, is being developed, which may make this easier

Sellick's manoeuvre
- Cricoid pressure to compress the upper oesophagus and protect the airway from gastric regurgitation (and brings the vocal cords into view during intubation)

Method
- Apply continual downward pressure to the cricoid cartilage with the thumb and index finger of one hand, whilst exerting counter pressure to the back of the neck with the other

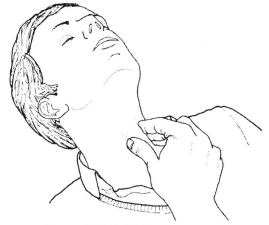

Figure 3-29 Sellick's manoeuvre

CONCLUSION
- Tracheal intubation provides a reliable, clear and secure airway by means of which effective positive pressure ventilation of the lungs can be achieved, and is the *method of choice*. However, the technique required for insertion is difficult to learn, and once learnt difficult to perform without practice
- Tracheal intubation is rarely required in the pre-hospital situation; but it may be lifesaving. Unfortunately it may also be especially difficult to perform, and those required to do so may lack recent experience of intubation. As a result various alternative methods of intubating the patient in difficult circumstances and different devices to provide the patient with a secure airway, which are easier to use and require less training, have been developed

Tracheal intubation: alternative methods

Blind digital intubation

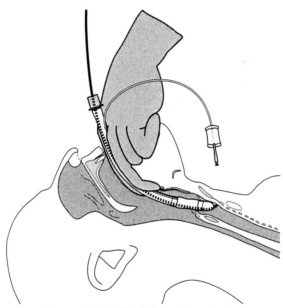

Figure 3-30 Blind digital intubation

Indications
- When intubation using a laryngoscope is not possible because of the patient's position, e.g. trapped, sitting upright in a vehicle

Method of insertion from the front
- May only be used in the deeply unconscious patient
- Lubricate the tracheal tube with gel, insert a malleable stylet into it, and form it into a "J" shape.
- Place yourself on the patient's right side, facing towards their right shoulder. Hold the tracheal tube in the right hand and put the left index and middle fingers into the patient's mouth, opening it as you do so and hold back the tongue
- Move your fingers along the lower border of the teeth until they reach the back of the tongue, and come into contact with the epiglottis
- Insert the tube and stylet, guiding it down between your fingers, and manoeuvre it just behind the epiglottis before slipping the tip of the stylet and the tube into the larynx
- Push the tube down over the stylet and further into the trachea
- Once the tube is in place, withdraw the stylet, inflate the cuff and secure the tube
- Confirm correct placement

CONCLUSION
- Requires practice (and long fingers) and is *rarely used* in Immediate Care

Nasotracheal intubation

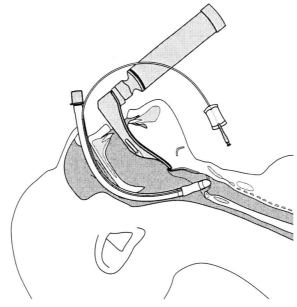

Figure 3-31 Nasotracheal intubation

Indications
- When intubation is indicated but orotracheal intubation is not possible
- It should *not* be used if there is a possible basal skull fracture

Tube size
- 1 mm smaller than that used for normal intubation, cut to 23-27 cm long

Method of application
- Lubricate the tube with gel
- If possible try to position the head and neck in the clear airway position, by applying gentle pressure to the occiput
- Insert the tube through the right nostril and gently push it backwards in a straight line. If resistance is met, withdraw and try the left nostril
- Continue inserting the tube, until it enters the nasopharynx, try to manipulate it through the glottis and into the trachea, if necessary using a laryngoscope to obtain direct vision
- If difficulty is experienced with insertion of the tube into the larynx, tracheal displacement and direct manipulation using Magill's forceps may help
- Once the tube is in place, inflate the cuff
- If the patient is breathing spontaneously, correct placement is indicated by the presence of breath sounds

Disadvantages
- Relatively difficult to perform, with a high risk of unrecognised oesophageal placement
- Risk of causing nasal haemorrhage
- Possibility of introducing infection from the upper (nasal) to the lower respiratory tract

Note: The *Endotrol*® is a modified nasotracheal tube with a flexible tip, which allows the end of the tube to be bent to different angles by traction on a pull ring

CONCLUSION
- *Not often used* in Immediate Care

Airway obstruction: surgical management

Aetiology
- Trauma:
    - Severe faciomaxillary injury resulting in:
        - Tongue displacement
        - Gross retroposition of the middle third of the maxilla
        - Actual or potential oedema of the pharynx or glottis
        - Uncontrollable oronasopharyngeal haemorrhage, e.g. from the lingual artery
    - Laryngeal injury
    - Blast, burn or missile injury to the face
- Infection:
    - Larynx (laryngotracheobronchitis) or epiglottis (epiglottitis)
- Physical obstruction:
    - Foreign body: Incompletely chewed food, children's toy, soft tissue swelling of neck, etc.
- Allergy:
    - Acute laryngeal oedema, e.g. insect stings, drug anaphylaxis

Management

Cricothyrotomy
- Minimum lumen for prolonged effective spontaneous ventilation: 6.0 mm.
- Assisted ventilation by a bag or ventilator is unlikely to be effective with a lumen under 4.0 mm

Advantages
- It is a rapid and safe procedure in trained hands
- The anatomical landmarks in the adult are usually easy to identify
- There is little danger of causing oesophageal damage
- There are rarely any overlying veins, thyroid tissue, muscles, or calcification to cause problems

Disadvantages
- It may cause haemorrhage within the airway
- It may result in trauma to the posterior laryngeal wall (especially in infants and young children)
- There is a risk of faulty placement of the tube in the subcutaneous tissues
- The procedure should not be performed in infants unless the situation is desperate, because the larynx/tracheal cartilages are immature and soft
- Carbon dioxide retention occurs as time passes

Complications
- Asphyxia
- Aspiration
- Cellulitis
- Oesophageal perforation
- Haemorrhage
- Perforation of the posterior tracheal wall
- Tissue emphysema

Cricothyrotomy devices/techniques

*Devices inserted using the "***Blind stab technique***"*

Needle cricothyrotomy (using a 12 or 14 gauge intravenous cannula).
- Can give temporary oxygenation and ventilation if placed through the cricothyroid membrane, using a flow rate of 15 litres of oxygen per minute

Method
- With the patient in the supine position (if possible), extend the neck, palpate the larynx and identify the cricothyroid membrane
- Attach the cannula to a 10-20 mL syringe, and pierce the skin directly over the cricothyroid membrane in the midline
- Direct the needle caudally (towards the feet) at an angle of 45°, to avoid damage to the vocal cords
- Carefully insert the needle through the lower part of the cricothyroid membrane, withdrawing the plunger on the syringe as you do so
- Aspiration of air indicates entry into the trachea
- Continue to insert the needle, being careful not to perforate the posterior laryngeal wall, withdrawing the stylet as you do so
- Attach the tube to an adaptor and "Y" piece (or 3-way tap), and oxygen tubing for jet ventilation
- Ventilate the patient using the device to ensure its correct placement
- Secure the needle with tape and adjust the oxygen flow rate to 15 l/min

Ventilation (jet ventilation)
- The patient may be ventilated by placing a thumb over the open end of the "Y" piece, using a rhythm of about 1 second on to 4 seconds off:
    - Each chest inflation should be observed carefully and the inflation pressure released as soon as some chest expansion occurs, to prevent pulmonary barotrauma (overinflation)
    - Ample time should be allowed after each inflation for lung deflation

Note: 1. Using this method, a patient can be adequately ventilated for only 10-15 minutes
2. It is essential that the larynx and upper airway are patent, so exhalation can occur through the mouth or nose

CONCLUSION
- Considered by some to be *the method of choice for obtaining a surgical airway in infants and young children*: others prefer the Mini Trach

Mini Trach II® cricothyrotomy device
- This device was originally developed for the treatment of post-operative sputum retention
- The standard device has a 4 mm lumen, but a new device with a 6.5 mm lumen which may be inserted after serial dilations has recently been produced

Method
- Place yourself at the patient's head, preferably with the patient in the supine position and extend the neck
- Palpate the larynx and identify the cricothyroid membrane
- Stretch the skin over the cricothyroid membrane with the thumb and index finger of the left hand and, holding the guarded scalpel in the right hand with the blade pointing towards the patient's feet, incise the skin and cricothyroid membrane vertically in the midline up to the guard
- Withdraw and discard the scalpel, and without moving the fingers of the left hand, take the introducer and insert it through the stab incision and into the trachea
- With the end of the introducer well inserted into the trachea, pass the cannula over the introducer and into the trachea
- Hold the flange in place against the skin and withdraw the introducer
- Ventilate the patient via the device to check that it is correctly positioned and secure it with the neck tapes

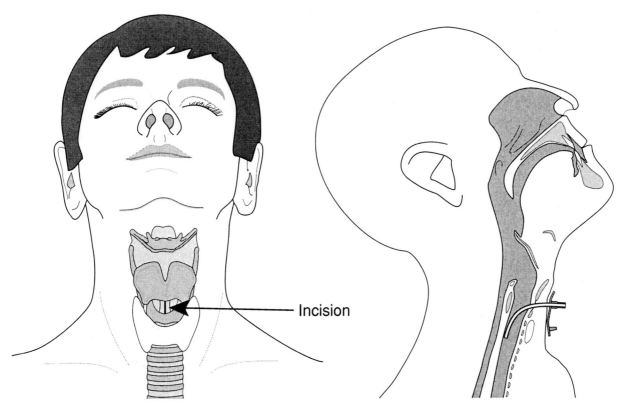

Figure 3-32 Mini Trach II

Complications
- As for needle cricothyrotomy, but there is less risk of damaging the posterior pharyngeal wall, as the scalpel has a guard which prevents the blade being inserted too far
- Malpositioning in the tissues of the neck, especially if the left hand is released and tissue alignment lost

CONCLUSION:
- Possibly the *device of choice*, but the 4 mm tube usually gives *only temporary relief*
- Not designed for use in children

Quicktrach®
- A curved cricothyrotomy device, incorporating a syringe and a large bore needle
- Available in two sizes:
    - Adult: 4 mm
    - Paediatric: 2 mm

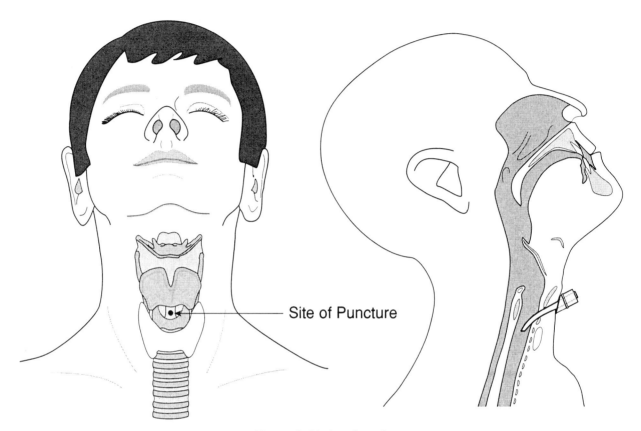

Site of Puncture

Figure 3-33 Quicktrach

Method
- Assemble the device by attaching the syringe to the Quicktrach, making certain that the depth gauge and the red markers are adjacent to each other
- Position the patient in the supine position (if possible) and extend the neck slightly.
- Palpate the larynx and identify the cricothyroid membrane
- Hold the device vertically by the syringe
- Puncture the skin overlying the cricothyroid membrane in the midline with the Quicktrach, gently withdrawing the plunger as you do so
- Move the syringe so that it makes an angle of 45° to the horizontal and continue insertion
- The device is in the trachea when air enters the syringe freely
- Continue inserting the device until the depth gauge is reached
- Remove the depth gauge, holding the the needle firmLy by the syringe, and slide the cannula down over the needle until the hub of the cannula is reached
- Withdraw the syringe and attached needle, and ventilate the patient via the device to confirm that it is correctly positioned
- Secure the device with the neck tape provided

Complications
- As needle cricothyrotomy

CONCLUSION
- A relatively new device, which has *not yet been evaluated* in Immediate Care
- Not suitable for long term ventilation as the lumen is narrow (4 mm)

Nutrach®
- A new device similar to the Quicktrach, but it also incorporates a set of trochar dilators, of increasing diameter. These are used to dilate the opening in the cricothyroid membrane, until finally a tube of 6.0-6.5 mm diameter can be placed in the trachea

Complications
- As needle cricothyrotomy

CONCLUSION
- A *useful* device for use in Immediate Care, as it *allows satisfactory relatively long term ventilation*
- Less likely to cause tissue damage than the Mini Trach

Percutaneous dilational cricothyroidotomy
- This is when the airway is inserted through the cricothyroid membrane using the Seldinger needle and wire technique

Method
- A stab incision is made through the middle of the cricothyroid membrane with a hollow needle, as in needle cricothyrotomy (see above)
- A guidewire is then passed down through the needle, and the needle withdrawn, keeping the guidewire in place
- A series of increasingly large dilators are then passed down over the wire, until the hole in the cricothyroid membrane is large enough to allow placement of a 6.0-6.5 mm tracheal tube through it

Complications
- As needle cricothyrotomy

CONCLUSION
- As Nutrach.
- Takes a relatively long time and is fiddly to use in the pre-hospital situation

Surgical cricothyrotomy (using a small tracheotomy or tracheal tube)

Method
- With the patient in the supine position, palpate the larynx and identify the cricothyroid membrane
- Stabilise the thyroid cartilage with the left hand, and with a scalpel in the right hand, incise the skin and underlying membrane horizontally, over the lower half of the membrane
- Insert the scalpel handle (or ideally tracheal dilators if available) through the incision and rotate it through 90º to enlarge the opening
- Insert a small tracheotomy or cut down tracheal tube through the opening, inflate the cuff and ventilate the patient
- If tube location problems are experienced; a gum elastic bougie may be placed in the trachea first, and the tube slid down over it, and into the trachea (as when inserting a *Mini Trach*)
- Auscultate the chest to confirm correct placement of the tube
- Secure the device in place with neck tapes

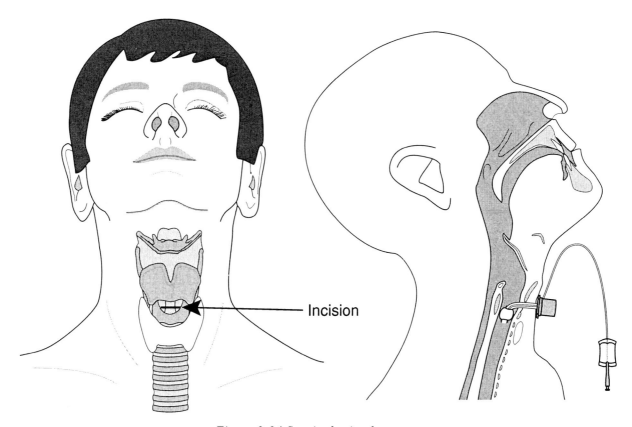

Figure 3-34 Surgical cricothyrotomy

Complications
- As needle cricothyrotomy, with the addition of:
    - Creation of a false passage in the tissues
    - Subglottic/laryngeal stenosis
    - Mediastinal emphysema
    - Vocal cord damage: hoarseness, paralysis

CONCLUSION
- Can give adequate ventilation and oxygenation, and is *probably the best method* in Immediate Care

Tracheotomy devices/techniques

Indications (for experts)
- When cricothyrotomy is not appropriate
- Laryngeal trauma

Surgical tracheotomy

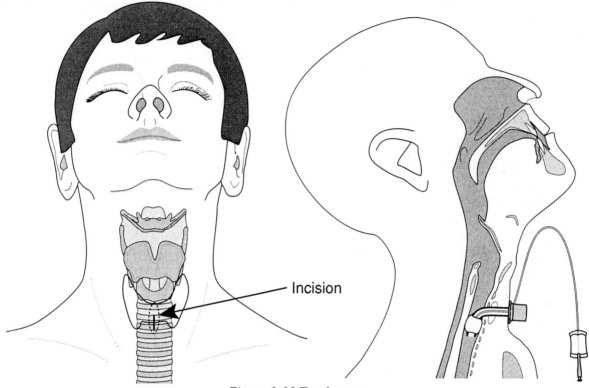

Incision

Figure 3-35 Tracheotomy

Method
- Make a vertical incision from the cricoid cartilage to just below the thyroid isthmus
- Divide the second to fourth tracheal rings and insert tracheal dilators
- Insert the tube, inflate the cuff and ventilate the patient
- Auscultate the chest to confirm correct placement and secure the device in place with neck tapes

Complications
- Haemorrhage
- Creation of a false passage in the tissues
- Mediastinal emphysema
- Laryngeal stenosis

CONCLUSION
- Should not really be considered as an emergency procedure; cricothyrotomy is preferable

Percutaneous tracheotomy
- This is when the airway is inserted using the Seldinger technique (see percutaneous dilational cricothyrotomy above)
- Very difficult to perform in the pre-hospital situation, but less likely to cause complications

:es

quipment for resuscitation which is used to clear the oropharynx of: blood,
etions

- .ld have:
    - exert an adequate vacuum and flow rate to enable the effective and rapid removal of both liq and semisolid material
    - A container of adequate size or an overflow for aspirated matter
    - The facility for the easy attachment of a suction catheter or Yankauer sucker
    - An integral power source
- It should be:
    - Lightweight, portable and easy to use
    - Easy to dismantle for cleaning and maintenance and reassemble without error
    - Reliable and robust
- In the prehospital situation, the equipment may be:
    - Hand powered:
        Advantage
        - Lightweight
        Disadvantages
        - Requires the operator both to power the device and manipulate the suction tip with the same hand, and may therefore be difficult to control accurately
        - When full, may overflow over the operator's hands
    - Foot powered:
        Advantage
        - Allows hands free operation
        Disadvantages
        - May be difficult to operate on uneven ground or in a moving vehicle
        - Fairly heavy
    - Electrically (battery) powered:
        Advantage
        - Allows hands free operation
        Disadvantages
        - Relatively heavy and bulky
        - The battery has a limited useful life
    - Gas powered: Usually powered by the oxygen cylinder connected to a ventilator
        Advantage
        - Very effective.
        Disadvantage
        - Uses up a considerable amount of oxygen

Suction ends
- There are two basic types:
    - Yankauer:
        - Rigid, only used for sucking out the upper airway
    - Soft:
        - Flexible (not recommended for use in Immediate Care)
        - Only used for aspiration down a tracheal tube/nasal or oral airway

Breathing (ventilation care)

Introduction

- Once the airway has been secured, attention should be paid to the patient's breathing, and the chest examined
- The maintenance of adequate ventilatory support is essential for the successful resuscitation of the severely ill and injured

Symptoms/signs

- Expose the chest completely and evaluate the patient's breathing by:
    - Observing their respiratory movement and quality of respiration
    - Palpating the chest wall
    - Auscultation
- In particular look for:
    - Intercostal and supraclavicular muscle retraction
    - The signs of chest injury
    - Evidence of impending hypoxia (often subtle and difficult to detect):
        - An increase in respiratory rate
        - A change in the breathing pattern, with respiration usually becoming more shallow
- Measure the SpO_2

Management

Severe spontaneous pneumothorax
- Needle decompression

Tension pneumothorax
Open pneumothorax
Massive Haemothorax

See chapter on
Chest Injuries

Flail chest
- Controlled ventilation

Controlled ventilation

Indications
- Hypoxia
- Apnoea
- Excessive respiratory work
- Ventilatory insufficiency
- In severely head injured patients to prevent hypoxia/hypercarbia

Expired air ventilation
- May be:
    - Mouth to mouth   see chapter on Basic Life Support
    - Mouth to nose
    - Mouth to mask, e.g. Pocket Mask
    - Mouth to tube

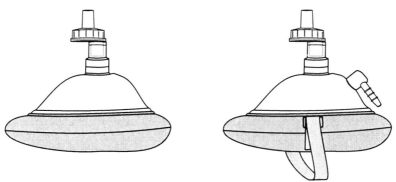

Figure 3-36 Pocket masks: standard model and oxygen model with oxygen inlet and head strap

Air ventilation
- Resuscitation bag/valve pocket mask (an oropharyngeal airway may be inserted first)
- Resuscitation bag/valve cricothyrotomy device

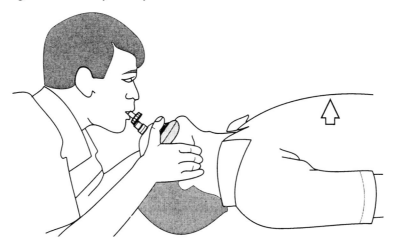

Figure 3-37 Pocket mask in use showing positioning of hands

Bag/valve/mask ventilation
- A self inflating bag with two one-way valves, one which is connected to a mask or airway, and the other to an oxygen reservoir with air inlet

Advantage
- When connected to an oxygen supply, it provides a higher inspired oxygen concentration than expired air ventilation

Disadvantage
- Can be a difficult technique to perform singlehandedly because of difficulty in aligning the airway and achieving an airtight seal between the mask and face. Those with small hands may have difficulty producing an adequate tidal volume with one hand. The result is usually not effective if performed unassisted, unless by a very experienced operator

Supplemental oxygen

Pocket Mask with oxygen inlet *(Laerdal®)*
- Probably the best device available at present to supplement the inspired oxygen concentration with expired air ventilation, although there is a risk of causing an excessive rise in airway pressure with subsequent gastric inflation
- Delivers up to 55% oxygen with flow rates of 8-10 litres per minute

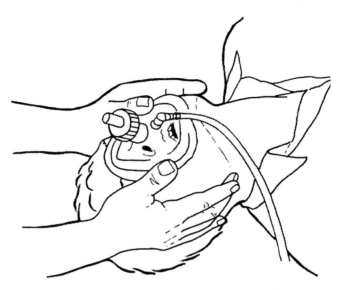

Figure 3-38 Pocket mask with supplemental oxygen

Bag/valve/mask *(Laerdal®/Ambu®)*
- Use of a bag/valve/mask with an oxygen reservoir can increase the concentration of inspired oxygen up to 90%, with oxygen flow rates of 8-10 litres per minute

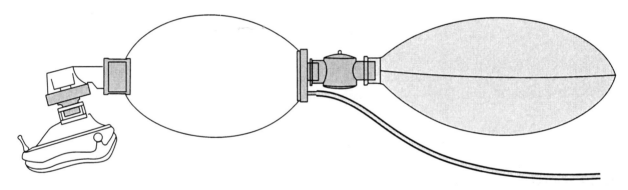

Figure 3-39 Bag and mask with oxygen reservoir

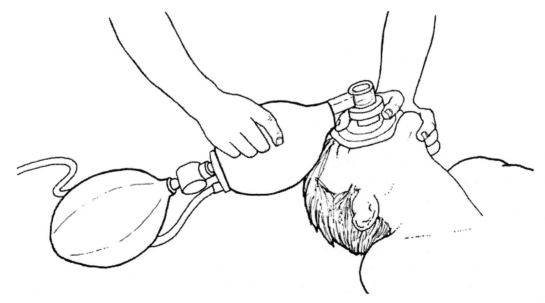

Figure 3-40 Bag and mask, showing hand positions

Mechanical ventilation

Manually triggered oxygen powered ventilators
- These devices have a high pressure oxygen supply attached to a manually triggered valve which, when opened, inflates the lungs via a face mask or ventilation tube
- Most devices incorporate a demand valve which allows the patient to breathe spontaneously when able to do so

Advantage
- Both hands can be used to provide jaw support and apply the mask to the face, whilst lung inflation is triggered by a thumb

Disadvantage
- They lack the "feel" that allows the trained operator to judge when lung inflation is complete or gastric inflation is occurring

Automatic oxygen powered ventilators
- Most modern automatic ventilators used in Immediate Care can be used for controlled ventilation or in patient triggered mode, and have a straight oxygen therapy facility
- They usually function best when connected to a ventilation tube, i.e. tracheal tube, LMA, Combitube, etc., but can be effective with a face mask with good airway alignment and seal

Requirements
- They should be:
  - Robust, reliable and require little maintenance
  - Lightweight, portable and easy to use
  - Self powered: usually by oxygen, ideally with air entrainment to conserve oxygen
- They should:
  - Enable the patient to trigger their own respirations, and recommence controlled ventilation, if spontaneous breathing ceases
  - Give an audible warning of high inflation pressures
  - Provide a range of tidal volumes, and rates of ventilation depending on patient size
  - Not generate flow rates greater than 40 L/min
  - Be volume controlled and time cycled

Advantage
- As with manually triggered models, when connected to a ventilation tube, it permits hands free operation
- Consistent ventilation rate and pattern

Disadvantages
- As the manually triggered models: prone to cause gastric distension if airway not correctly aligned
- Limited life of oxygen cylinders

Anaesthesia: rapid sequence induction
- This is the preferred method of administering anaesthesia in all trauma patients, especially in the pre-hospital situation, because of the reduced risk of aspiration of gastric contents

Indications
- Head injury with a Glasgow Coma Scale Score of <12
- Agitated and combative patients, for whatever reason, who are compromising their own management
- Patients with compromised ventilation, e.g. due to multiple rib fractures, flail chest or high cord injury
- Pain from injuries, e.g. multiple limb fractures or pelvic injury, likely to result in significant hypovolaemia and hypoxia

Method
- Attach equipment for monitoring pulse rate, blood pressure and oxygen saturation
- Apply manual in line cervical stabilisation
- Open the patient's rigid cervical collar if one has been applied (if an appropriately sized collar has been fitted; the patient's mouth should hardly open, so it will not be possible to insert a laryngoscope)
- Pre-oxygenate the patient:
    - If the patient is breathing spontaneously, ensure that an oxygen mask with reservoir bag has been fitted and is functioning correctly:
        - Ensure that the oxygen reservoir is unfolded, full and emptying with inspiration
        - In cold conditions the plastic of the reservoir may be stiff, so rub it to enhance compliance
    - If ventilation is poor it should be augmented with a bag valve mask (make certain that the oxygen reservoir and oxygen line are attached to the ventilation bag)
- Apply cricoid pressure, using the two handed method (to prevent movement of the cervical spine)
- Secure vascular access. Make certain that injuries do not compromise the venous flow to the heart, e.g. vascular access below the pelvis in an obvious pelvic fracture, or penetrating chest wound on the same side as an antecubital fossa cannula
- Administer etomidate/propofol followed by suxamethonium (if the patient is severely hypotensive or unresponsive, consider reducing or even omitting the etomidate, as a catastrophic fall in blood pressure due to vasodilation can accompany sedation and positive pressure ventilation in these patients, in whom effective management of hypovolaemia is vital)
- If the patient's position or condition make it likely that intubation will be difficult or impossible, it is advisable to check that *before* administering the muscle relaxant (suxamethonium). Once the patient has stopped breathing, manual ventilation is possible, but should be performed gently to avoid distending the stomach with the attendant risk of pulmonary aspiration
- After fasciculations have occurred, the patient should be intubated
- Confirm successful intubation:
    - Observe the tracheal tube pass through the vocal cords
    - Look for chest and abdominal wall movement
    - Listen for air entry in both axillae and over the stomach
    - Attach capnography or oesophageal detector
- After successful intubation:
    - Secure the tube with tape
    - Close the cervical collar
- Maintain anaesthesia/sedation with bolus doses or infusion of propofol or midazolam:
    - Avoid episodes of hypertension; try to administer the bolus doses smoothly; rather like a continuous infusion, without allowing the blood pressure to drop

Drugs used in anaesthesia
- The ideal pre-hospital anaesthetic should:
    - Have a quick onset of action resulting in the rapid loss of consciousness
    - Have analgesic properties
    - Not have any respiratory depressant action
    - Not impair the laryngeal reflexes and thus not interfere with the reflex protection of the upper airway
    - Have no effect on the patient's cardiovascular status (and doesn't increase intracranial pressure)
    - Not induce a histamine response
    - Have a short duration of action, allowing a rapid recovery
- Such an agent does not yet exist, a compromise must be used

Intravenous anaesthetics/induction agents

Etomidate (*Hypnomidate*®)

Description
- Etomidate is an intravenous induction agent, associated with a rapid recovery

Presentation
- 10 mL ampoules of 2 mg/mL in propylene glycol 35%

Dosage
- For induction: 0.3 mg/kg

Onset of action
- 30-45 seconds (this will be delayed if there is a reduction in cardiac output)

Duration of action
- Approximately 2-3 minutes

Advantages
- Is relatively cardiostable, and causes less hypotension than other induction agents
- Convenient preparation for use in Immediate Care as it does not need reconstituting

Disadvantages
- Should not be used for the maintenance of anaesthesia
- High incidence of extraneous muscle movement and pain on injection (especially with small veins)
- May cause excitatory and emergence phenomena (and suppression of adrenal cortisol synthesis with long term administration)
- Contra-indications include porphyria and adrenal insufficiency

CONCLUSION: Etomidate is the most commonly used induction agent

Ketamine (*Ketalar*®)
- See chapter on Pain management

Propofol (*Diprivan*®)

Description
- Propofol is an intravenous induction agent, associated with a rapid recovery without hangover

Presentation
- 20 mL ampoules of 10 mg/mL

Dosage
- For induction:
    - 2 mg/kg (if the patient is hypovolaemic or elderly, administer slowly in a titrated dose)
- For maintenance:
    - 20-30 mg every 2-3 minutes

Onset of action
- 30-45 seconds (this will be delayed if there is a reduction in cardiac output)

Duration of action
- Approximately 2-3 minutes

Advantages
- Significant extraneous muscle movements do not occur

Disadvantages
- Contraindicated in those with egg protein allergy, and possibly in the pregnant patient
- May cause hypotension and bradycardia, and (rarely) an allergic reaction and convulsions

CONCLUSION: Propofol is the preferred agent for maintaining anaesthesia in the pre-hospital situation; it may also be used as an induction agent, but its hypotensive effects are greater than etomidate

Muscle relaxants
- Muscle relaxants specifically block the neuromuscular junction, enabling light levels of anaesthesia to be used. They relax the vocal cords to permit tracheal intubation
- Patients who have received a muscle relaxant should always have assisted ventilation until the drug has been deactivated or antagonised
- Always try to avoid administering a second dose of suxamethonium
- Assess the adequacy of ventilation before administering a muscle relaxant
- Never administer a long acting muscle relaxant before you are absolutely certain that the tracheal tube is correctly positioned
- Wait until there is movement before administering a long acting muscle relaxant after suxamethonium
- Remember: muscle relaxants *never* sedate the patient, so administer an anaesthetic as well in all but the profoundly comatose

Suxamethonium (*Anectine®*)

Description
- A short acting depolarising muscle relaxant with a rapid onset of action

Presentation
- 2 mL ampoules of 50 mg/mL

Dosage
- 1 mg/kg, if necessary the second dose should be approximately ¼ of the first dose (+ atropine)

Onset of action
- 30-40 seconds

Duration of action
- 2-5 minutes

Advantages
- Rapid onset and short duration of action

Disadvantages
- May cause:
    - Hypotension
    - Potassium release
    - Bradycardia/asystole, especially after the second dose and in children (usually responds to atropine)
- Contra-indications:
    - Renal failure and burns
    - Scoline apnoea (rare)

Pancuronium (*Pavulon®*)

Description
- An aminosteroid which is a long acting non-depolarising muscle relaxant with a relatively rapid onset of action

Presentation
- 2 mL ampoules of 2 mg/mL

Dosage
- 0.1 mg/kg

Onset of action
- 2-3 minutes

Duration of action
- 30-40 minutes

Advantages
- Does not require reconstituting, and has a vagolytic effect so is therefore cardiovascularly stable

Disadvantages
- May cause tachycardia and hypertension due to vagal blockade
- Contra-indications:
    - Known allergy (very rare)

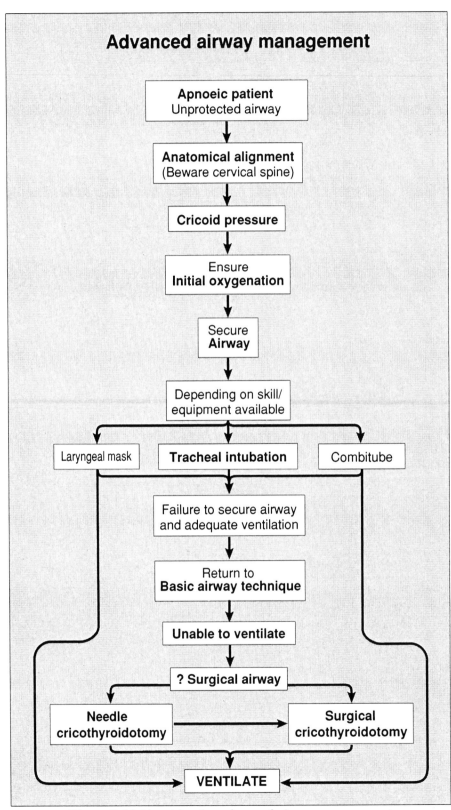

Figure 3-41 Algorithm for advanced airway management
(copyright of the European Resuscitation Council, reproduced with permission)

Circulation care: shock

4

Circulation care: shock

Introduction

Definition: Shock is a condition characterised by impaired cellular function as a result of a reduction in the effective circulating blood volume, resulting in an inadequate supply of oxygen and nutrients to cells, tissues and organs, inadequate oxygen utilisation and inadequate removal of waste products. It may arise from a variety of causes. Shock is the start of the dying process

Hypovolaemic shock
- Occurs as a result of a reduction in the circulating blood volume, e.g. as a result of haemorrhage, dehydration (prolonged vomiting, diarrhoea or heatstroke) and burns

Cardiogenic shock
- This is caused by pump (cardiac) failure, e.g. as a result of acute myocardial infarction, electrocution, tension pneumothorax, myocardial contusion, cardiac tamponade, or air embolism

Neurogenic shock
- This is caused by stimulation of the autonomic nervous system, resulting in vasodilation and the sudden enlargement of the vascular bed, e.g. as a result of head injury, fainting or spinal cord injury

Bacteriological shock (rarely encountered in Immediate Care)
- This is due to cellular poisoning followed by circulatory failure, e.g. septicaemia, peritonitis
    - **Septic shock**: Caused by Gram negative or other organisms
    - **Toxic shock**: Caused by toxins from *Staph. aureus* or rarely by endotoxins from *Haemolytic strep*

Anaphylactic shock
- This is an acute allergic response resulting in respiratory failure, pump failure, vasodilation, capillary leakage and tissue damage

Pathophysiology
- The body responds to shock by attempting to maintain tissue oxygen delivery by increasing oxygen extraction
- Oxygen delivery varies with cardiac output and vascular dynamics
- Oxygen consumption depends on the cardiac output and the arterio-venous oxygen saturation difference
- Tissue hypoxia results in anaerobic metabolism causing an initial metabolic acidosis, which together with continuing hypoxia causes a reduction in cardiac output, multi-organ failure and so a vicious cycle develops
- The secondary effects of shock, which can take up to an hour to develop, include the release of various substances as a result of cellular damage; including enzymes, kinins, hormones and complement

Symptoms/signs
- Pallor
- Tachycardia
- Reduction in pulse pressure
- Peripheral vasoconstriction
- Hypotension
- Sweating
- Hyperventilation/tachypnoea
- Anxiety/confusion
- Unconsciousness

Assessment
- Patient's appearance (peripheral perfusion)
    - Colour (may be difficult in the pre-hospital situation, due to poor lighting conditions)
    - Temperature
- Measurement of:
    - Pulse rate
    - Capillary refill time
    - Pulse oximetry: see chapter on Airway Care
    - Blood pressure: systolic and diastolic (to estimate pulse pressure)
    - Respiratory rate
    - Temperature

Capillary refill test
- Press on the skin for five seconds. As you remove the pressure say "capillary refill" to yourself
- If the skin is still pale at the end of this time, the capillary refill time is prolonged (>2 seconds)

Note: This test is best done at the nail bed and requires adequate lighting for its correct interpretation

---

Hypovolaemic shock

Incidence
- This is a very common avoidable cause of death and morbidity

Aetiology
- Hypovolaemic shock may be caused by:
    - Fluid loss:
        - Haemorrhage
        - Severe vomiting, diarrhoea or evaporation (heatstroke)
    - An increase in capillary permeability due to mediator release and prolonged hypoxaemia:
        - Oedema due to severe soft tissue injury, including burns and anaphylaxis

Pathophysiology
- In haemorrhage:
    - The initial fluid loss is from the intravascular compartments
- In oedema:
    - The initial fluid loss is from the interstitial compartment
- Haemorrhage is often associated with tissue injury

Hypovolaemia

Cardiac response
  - The initial cardiac response to hypovolaemia is a compensatory increase in the cardiac output to maintain the arterial oxygen saturation
  - If hypovolaemia and hypoxaemia continue, cardiac output and oxygen saturation will fall resulting in a further reduction in tissue oxygenation

Pulmonary response
  - The initial pulmonary response is:
    - Hyperventilation to increase blood oxygenation
    - Pulmonary vasoconstriction in hypoxic areas:
      - This helps divert the pulmonary blood flow to areas where the alveolar oxygen concentration is higher, and so improves blood oxygenation
      - This increases the pulmonary resistance and the force needed to pump blood to the lungs, and hence the cardiac work load

Fluid compartments
  - The intravascular and interstitial fluid compartments are normally in equilibrium with each other
  - Loss of fluid from one compartment will normally result in donation to that compartment of fluid from the other compartment
  - Intravascular fluid loss will result in depletion of the interstitial compartment by approximately 25% of the overt blood loss

Vascular changes
  - Initially:
    - There is a reduction in the circulating blood volume, which causes initially a reduction in pulse pressure and later a fall in the systolic blood pressure
    - The sympathetic response to blood loss is catecholamine release causing:
      - Peripheral vasoconstriction which results in an increase in the peripheral vascular resistance (excluding the cerebral and myocardial vessels, thus diverting blood to these vital organs) and:
        - A contribution from the vascular pool of up to 1 litre
        - An increase in heart and pulse rate
        - An increase in myocardial contractility and cardiac output
      - The increase in pulse rate and myocardial contractility results in an increase in myocardial oxygen demand
    - A reduction in the venous return to the heart, causing a drop in arterial pressure and hypotension
    - This arterial hypotension together with the peripheral vasoconstriction results in a reduction in tissue perfusion which together with the increase in myocardial oxygen demand results in myocardial ischaemia eventually leading to cardiac failure
    - The reduction in tissue perfusion results in anaerobic metabolism and a metabolic acidosis
  - Later, if haemorrhage or intravascular fluid loss continues until 20% or more of the circulating blood volume has been lost:
    - There is multisystem failure as sympathetic vasoconstriction ceases and the heart rate, peripheral resistance and arterial pressure fall

Tissue injury
- Local tissue injury may result in a systemic (generalised) response, which varies depending on the amount of tissue damaged and the location of the injury, e.g. pulmonary tissue damage will have an adverse effect on respiration

Pathophysiology
- Tissue injury results in the release of various mediators including:
  - Endotoxin
  - Histamine
  - 5-Hydroxytriptamine
  - Bradykinin
  - Leukotrienes
- These cause vasodilation, increased microvascular permeability and activation of macrophages and neutrophils, which in turn release further mediators including elastase, platelet-activation factor, tumour-necrosis factor and toxic oxygen metabolites
- The overall effect may be to maintain the amount of oxygen available for tissue utilisation, by increasing oxygen extraction, if oxygen delivery begins to fail

Signs/symptoms
- Erythema
- Swelling
- Pain
- Local heat
- Loss of function

Symptoms/signs

Circulation
- Tachycardia (catecholamine release)
  - Tachycardia is present when the heart (pulse) rate is more than:
    - 160 beats per minute in an infant
    - 140 beats per minute in a pre-school child
    - 120 beats per minute from school age to puberty
    - 110 beats per minute in an adult
- Reduced pulse pressure
- Reduced systolic and diastolic pressures
- Reduced central venous pressure (hypovolaemia and possibly myocardial insufficiency)
- Pulse oximetry plethysmograph will show flattening of the waveform, unless automatic compensation is incorporated in the device

Normal blood volumes
- The total blood volume of an individual is approximately 8% of their total body weight, i.e. 80 mL/kg.

Children	12 months	10 kg	800 mL
	10 years	30 kg	2400 mL
Adults	Female	55 kg	4400 mL
	Male	70 kg	5600 mL

Blood loss estimation
- In acute trauma the cause of blood loss may be obvious, but one must be aware of the potential for covert blood loss from thoracoabdominal injuries, and also from pelvic and long bone fractures
- Relatively minor injuries, which can bleed a lot, e.g. scalp lacerations, may cause significant blood loss, especially in infants and children

Approximate blood loss from untreated fractures in first 4 hours (*double this,* if the fracture is compound)

Humerus:	500-1000 mL
Radius/ulna:	250-1000 mL
Thorax(ribs):	150-2000 mL
Pelvis:	500-3000 mL
Shaft of femur:	1000-2000 mL
Tibia/fibula:	500-1000 mL

Approximate blood loss from other organs

Scalp:	250-1000 mL
Liver/spleen	1000-4000 mL

Blood pressure estimation
- As a rough guide:
    - If the brachial (radial) pulse is palpable: systolic BP >90 mmHg
    - If the femoral pulse is palpable: systolic BP >80 mmHg
    - If the carotid or femoral pulse is palpable: the systolic BP >70 mmHg

Mental state
- This changes progressively from anxious, restless, and talkative, to aggressive, confused, drowsy and eventually unconscious (cerebral hypoxia)

Symptoms
- Thirst (hypovolaemia)
- Feeling cold (vasoconstriction)
- Blurring of vision, weakness, faintness and giddiness (hypoxia and acidosis)

Skin appearance
- Pale, cold and clammy (vasoconstriction secondary to catecholamine release)

Respiration
- Shallow rapid respirations (hypoxia and acidosis)

Urine output (not usually measured in Immediate Care)
- Reduced (reduced renal perfusion)
- Should normally exceed 30 mL/hour

Modifying factors
- The patient's symptoms and signs may be modified by various factors:

Age
- Modest blood loss will have a greater effect in the very young (small blood volume) and the old (myocardial insufficiency)

Fitness
- The young and fit compensate for hypovolaemia very effectively initially (efficient catecholamine response), but may suddenly and rapidly decompensate
- Athletes will have a larger than normal blood volume, and a slower than normal pulse rate

Pregnancy
- A pregnant patient's blood volume increases by 50% in the third trimester, without a similar increase in oxygen carrying capacity. They may tolerate fluid loss better initially than the non pregnant female, before suddenly decompensating

Injury severity
- Extensive tissue damage may result in an increase in the severity of the shock

Previous medication
- e.g. β-blockers may prevent tachycardia, masking the early signs of hypovolaemic shock

Hypothermia
- The severity of shock will be greater if the patient is hypothermic, and will make shock more difficult to manage due to peripheral vasoconstriction

Pre-existing medical conditions
- These may modify the patient's response to hypovolaemia:
    - Anaemia will reduce the blood's oxygen carrying ability and the patient will tolerate less blood loss
    - Patients with coronary artery disease may become hypotensive due to myocardial insufficiency after only modest blood loss
    - A pacemaker will maintain a constant pulse rate, regardless of the patient's haemodynamic state

Classification of hypovolaemic shock in adults

Class I haemorrhage: up to 15% (up to 750 mL)

Pathophysiology
- Blood loss of up to 750 mL is usually well tolerated and results in minimal symptoms or signs

Symptoms/signs
- A slight tachycardia
- Normal blood pressure

Class II haemorrhage: 15-30% (750-1500 mL)

Pathophysiology
- The body responds with catecholamine release

Symptoms/signs
- Anxiety or aggression
- A normal systolic pressure with a slightly raised diastolic pressure and a narrow pulse pressure (systolic pressure does not consistently fall until >30% blood volume is lost), with absent/reduced jugular venous pulses when the patient is lying flat
- A tachycardia with a slow capillary refill (>2 seconds)
- A normal SpO_2

Class III haemorrhage: 30-40% (1500-2000 mL)

Pathophysiology
- The patient's compensatory mechanisms begin to fail

Symptoms/signs
- Pallor of the face and extremities
- Anxiousness, aggression or drowsiness
- Shallow respiration with a marked tachypnoea
- A marked tachycardia, with a reduction in both systolic and diastolic pressures and a weak pulse
- A slightly reduced SpO_2

Class IV haemorrhage: >40% (>2000 mL)

Pathophysiology
- This is life threatening fluid loss

Symptoms/signs
- Ashen complexion with cold clammy sweaty skin, especially in the extremities
- Confusion, impaired consciousness and eventually unconsciousness, coma and death
- A marked tachycardia, with a profound fall in systolic and diastolic blood pressure
- A reduced SpO_2

Classification of hypovolaemic shock according to blood loss

Class of shock		I	II	III	IV
Blood loss	(%)	<15	15-30	30-40	>40
	Volume (mL)	<750	750-1500	1500-2000	>2000
Pulse rate	(beats per minute)	normal or <100	100-120	>120	>140
		slight tachycardia	tachycardia	thready	very thready
Blood pressure	Systolic	unchanged	normal	reduced	very low
	Diastolic	unchanged	raised	reduced	very low or unrecordable
Pulse pressure		normal or increased	decreased	decreased	decreased
Capillary refill		normal	>2 sec	>2 sec	undetectable
Respiratory rate	(per min)	normal (14-20)	normal (20-30)	tachypnoea (30-40)	tachypnoea (>35)
Oxygen saturation		normal	normal	slightly low	low
Urine output	(mL/hr)	>30	20-30	5-15	0-10
Extremities		normal colour	pale	pale	pale & cold
Complexion		normal	pale	pale	ashen
Mental state		alert	anxious or aggressive	anxious, aggressive or drowsy	drowsy, confused lethargic or unconscious

Figure 4-1 Classification of hypovolaemic shock in adults based on a 70 kg male

Management

Aim
- Control/prevent further blood loss if possible (see below)
- The aim of effective management of hypovolaemia is to:
    - Maintain tissue oxygenation and restore it to normal
    - Prevent irreversible hypoxic damage to vital organs; the brain, heart, and kidneys
- The maintenance of an adequate oxygen carrying capacity requires:
    - A packed cell volume of more than 30%
    - Normal electrolyte levels
    - Normal clotting factors
    - A normal colloid osmotic pressure

Airway
- Ensure that the patient has an adequate airway with cervical spine control if indicated
- Administer oxygen:
    - All shocked patients, especially the elderly and those with ischaemic heart disease, tolerate hypoxia badly and should be given high flow oxygen, at a high inspired concentration
    - In severe shock: use 100% oxygen

Breathing
- Ensure that the patient's ventilation is adequate
- Intubate and ventilate unconscious patients. This optimises oxygenation and avoids gastric distension, which impairs effective ventilation and exacerbates shock

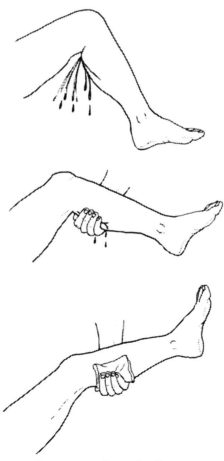

Figure 4-2 Haemorrhage control: apply direct pressure and elevate

Circulation

- Assess the amount of blood lost, the cause of the blood loss and the potential further blood loss
- Control/prevent the blood loss, where this is possible:
    - Limb elevation
    - Application of firm direct pressure with a dressing
    - Application of pressure on appropriate pressure points, e.g. femoral, popliteal, brachial
    - Application of a tourniquet to prevent life threatening exsanguination
- Treat the cause of the blood loss, e.g. reduction of the fracture with appropriate splinting
- Establish intravenous access with large bore cannulae and provide adequate fluid replacement
- Consider application of a pneumatic anti-shock garment (PASG) for life-threatening exsanguination

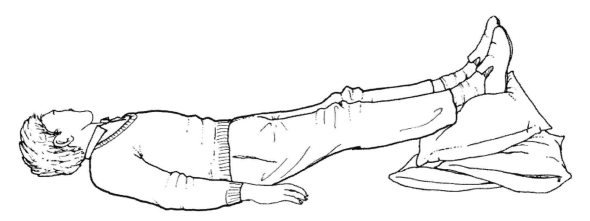

Figure 4-3 Leg elevation

Position

- Elevate the patient's legs to aid the venous return
- Make the patient comfortable and warm, and minimise/reduce heat loss

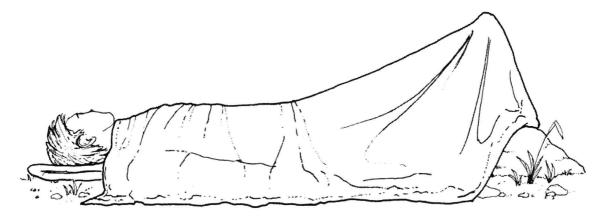

Figure 4-4 Keeping the patient warm

Pain Relief

- Provide adequate pain relief (see chapter on Pain management)

Circulation

Control of blood loss

Tourniquets
- Should only be used in: appropriate acute life threatening emergencies, e.g. sudden traumatic amputation
- In severe crush injury application of a tourniquet may protect the rest of the body from the toxins produced by the non-viable tissue, i.e. potassium, myoglobin and lactic acid
- If a tourniquet is applied, the time and date of application and the name of the person applying it should be recorded
- It is most important that when a tourniquet is applied, the pressure exerted is sufficient to prevent arterial flow, not only when it is applied, but also when the patient's blood pressure rises to normal after resuscitation (*if too low a pressure is applied, the tourniquet may act as a venous tourniquet and will make bleeding worse*)
- Should be broad (narrow tourniquets may cause permanent damage to the underlying tissues, e.g. nerves. If only a narrow tourniquet is available, apply it over padding
- May be removed after an effective pressure bandage has been applied

Note: The use of artery forceps/haemostats is *not* recommended

Pneumatic anti-shock garment (PASG)
- PASGs have been widely used in the USA and several other countries, but are becoming less popular
- Their use has not been generally accepted in the UK or Europe, and they are not commonly available
- Current evidence suggests that their only use is for the management of unstable pelvic fractures in the pre-hospital situation, together with appropriate fluid replacement

Description
　　A PASG is:
- An inflatable pair of trousers, separated into different compartments:
    - One for the patient's abdomen and one for each leg
- Usually made from radiolucent double layered polyurethane coated fabrics
- Inflated up to 100 mmHg by a foot pump, the pressure in each compartment is indicated by a pressure gauge
　　In addition:
- There is an opening in the groin to allow catheterisation, and rectal and vaginal examination without deflation
- Each compartment is colour coded, as are the securing Velcro strips
- Each trouser leg can be shortened if necessary

Mode of action
- An inflated PASG effectively transfers up to one and a half to two units of blood (or up to 25% of the patient's available blood volume) from the lower extremities to the upper, protecting the vital organs from the initial effects of shock
- The exact mode of action is not fully understood but may include:
    - Reduction in the total peripheral vascular capacitance/increase in the peripheral vascular resistance
    - Tamponade of bleeding vessels
    - Autotransfusion
- In addition it may splint lower limb and pelvic fractures reducing further blood loss and pain

Advantages
- Reduces the initial amount of blood/fluid required to replace blood loss
- Facilitates venepuncture in the hypovolaemic patient: makes the upper limb veins more prominent
- Other advantages: splinting of fractures

Disadvantages
- Impaired ventilation and dyspnoea may be caused by use of a PASG, which should therefore *not* be used in the patient with a chest injury or cardiac failure:
    - Management: oxygen and a reduction in the PASG pressure
- Defecation, urination and vomiting may rarely occur as a result of the raised intra-abdominal pressure
- Metabolic acidosis and compartmental syndromes have been recorded
- There is a potential risk of puncture of the PASG from sharp objects, e.g. compound fractures, glass

Application
- If possible/practical lay out the PASG on the ambulance trolley, before lowering the patient onto it
- Inflate the leg compartments first and then the abdominal compartment noting the time
- Use inflation pressures of 40-50 mmHg initially, increasing to 80 mmHg, if the systolic pressure fails to improve

Deflation
- This should only be performed where there are facilities for rapid blood transfusion, e.g. in an operating theatre, with at least two wide bore intravenous lines in place and with careful monitoring of the patient's haemodynamic state
- The garment must be deflated slowly; compartment by compartment starting with the abdominal compartment (this may take up to 30 minutes; if the staff at the hospital are unfamiliar with the PASG, you should stay and supervise deflation)

Indications
- Stabilisation of severe unstable pelvic fractures associated with major blood loss
- Possible indications include:
    - Ruptured aortic aneurism
    - Ruptured ectopic pregnancy
    - Neurogenic shock, e.g. spinal cord injury
    - Infective or anaphylactic shock

Contraindications
- Absolute:
    - Chest injuries (a recent study has demonstrated an increased mortality rate when PASGs are used in patients with a chest injury)
- Relative:
    - Injuries causing blood loss outside the area covered by the PASG (may cause an increase in blood pressure and a resultant increase in blood loss)
    - Head injury with a risk of raised intracranial pressure
    - Respiratory distress, cardiac failure, pulmonary oedema
    - Suspected or actual diaphragmatic rupture

CAUTION: Inflation of the leg compartments *only*, is advised for:
    - Pregnancy: more than 26 weeks
    - Abdominal evisceration or impalement

Intravenous fluid replacement

Introduction
- It is vital to obtain adequate venous access early in severely injured patients, as once hypovolaemic shock (and venoconstriction) has developed, achieving venous access becomes increasingly difficult
- Two large bore cannulae (12 to 14 gauge), should be inserted into the peripheral veins of different, preferably uninjured limbs, to provide an adequate rate of flow for rapid fluid replacement
- In the severely hypovolaemic patient, obtaining venous access and providing fluid replacement must not delay their access to surgical management of their haemorrhage
- Assess the patient's injuries and vital signs so that blood loss and iv fluid requirement can be estimated

Intravenous fluid flow rates
- The rate of flow of a fluid in a cannula depends on:
    - The diameter of the cannula (radius^4, and therefore the most important factor)
    - The length of the cannula (inversely proportional)
    - The viscosity of the fluid
    - The pressure at which the fluid is infused (pressure differential):
        - Elevation of the fluid container increases the pressure differential and hence the rate of flow
    - To achieve a high rate of flow use a large bore cannula and elevate and compress the fluid container
- Rates of flow for different gauges of intravenous cannulae in ideal circumstances:
    - 14 gauge: 1 litre in 3 minutes
    - 16 gauge: 1 litre in 6 minutes
    - 18 gauge: 1 litre in 20 minutes

Discussion point: Controlled hypotension/permissive hypotension

Concerns
- Recent studies have shown a poorer outcome for patients with severe penetrating trauma who have received aggressive fluid replacement in the pre-hospital phase of their management, when compared to those who have had no pre-hospital fluid replacement

Evidence
- After significant blood loss, blood pressure drops, and this together with clot formation and spasm in many severed arterial blood vessels, results in reduction and sometimes cessation of arterial blood loss
- If the blood pressure is then restored to normal because of intravenous fluid replacement, haemorrhage from these damaged arterial vessels may begin again
- If, as usually occurs, the fluid used for blood replacement is not blood (and contains no clotting factors), dilution of the patient's blood occurs and clotting is impaired, thus increasing the tendency to bleed
- The young compensate for hypovolaemia very effectively, but may eventually decompensate rapidly
- Patients with some injuries, e.g. splenic injury, partial major vessel injury, may suddenly bleed profusely and their condition deteriorate precipitously and fatally, if they are not managed rapidly and aggressively by surgical intervention

Conclusions
- The definitive management of hypovolaemia due to trauma is surgery
- The aim of pre-hospital fluid replacement is to prevent severe hypotension and vital organ injury
- It is suggested that the desired blood pressure for a patient with hypovolaemia is probably 20-30 mmHg below the normal blood pressure for that patient (and *not* their normal blood pressure), with the exception of serious head injuries in whom an *increase* in blood pressure may be important to maintain cerebral perfusion in the presence of brain swelling and the resultant increase in intracerebral pressure
- Two large bore cannulae should be inserted without causing any delay in evacuation, in the patient with severe or potentially severe injuries, and they should be infused cautiously, with continuous monitoring of their haemodynamic state, using the blood pressure or the radial pulse as a guide, so that if their condition deteriorates suddenly, appropriate action can be taken
- Restoration of blood flow is the aim of treatment, not normalisation of blood pressure

Intravenous cannulation sites
- The usual route for fluid replacement in the pre-hospital situation is intravenous, although the intraosseous and rectal routes may be used in special circumstances, e.g. in children under the age of seven or when intravenous cannulation is not possible
- Some protocols suggest than one intravenous line be inserted above and one below the diaphragm, to avoid any of the problems associated with mediastinal or cervical injury which might compromise the delivery of intravenous fluid from the the limbs to the central venous circulation. In practice this is seldom a problem
- Central venous cannulation is not advised in the pre-hospital situation, unless there is no alternative

Peripheral venous cannulation
- In hypovolaemic shock the peripheral veins should be used in preference to the central veins for venous access and fluid replacement:
    - Fewer risks
    - Easier technique for the non-anaesthetist
    - Faster flow rates
- The usual sites are:
    - Cephalic, median cubital, and basilic veins in the antecubital fossa
    - Cephalic vein in the wrist
    - Long saphenous vein at the ankle

Note: It is best, especially for the inexperienced, to start with the easy veins in the antecubital fossa

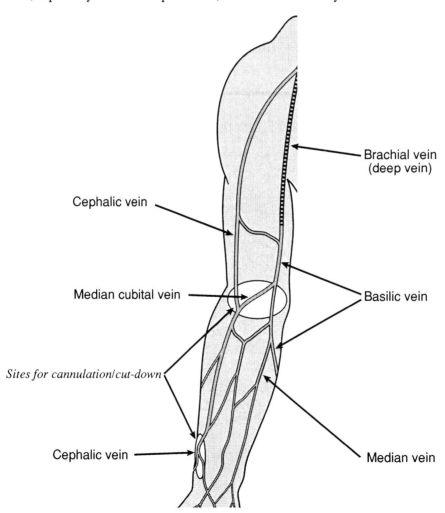

Figure 4-5 Veins of the upper limb showing sites for cannulation/cut down

Venous cut down
- A cut down is rarely if ever necessary in Immediate Care, unless there is very considerable delay in initiating fluid replacement
- The best sites are:
    - The long saphenous vein in the ankle
    - The sapheno-femoral vein in the groin
    - The cephalic vein near the wrist

Long saphenous vein cut down

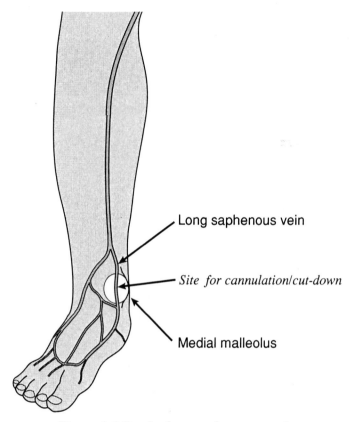

Figure 4-6 Site for long saphenous cut down

Method
- Identify the long saphenous vein, which lies just anterior (about one inch superior and one inch anterior) to the medial malleolus at the ankle (it is not always visible)
- Cleanse the skin (if circumstances permit)
- Make a transverse incision through the skin, and using artery forceps spread the skin to display the vein which should be visible lying at right angles to the line of the incision
- Mobilise the vein by using the forceps for blunt dissection
- Grasp a suture with the forceps, pull it back under the vein and cut the top of the loop, so that there are two sutures, each one having one end each side of the vein. Separate these sutures so that there is approximately half to one inch between them
- Tie off the distal part of the vein with the distal suture
- Elevate and stabilise the vein using the proximal suture
- Nick the vein transversely with sharp-pointed scissors (use the scalpel, if these are not available)
- Insert the wide bore intravenous cannula and secure it by tying the proximal suture
- Suture the skin (if circumstances permit) and tape the giving set and cannula firmLy in place

Note: Always secure an intravenous line with a loop of tubing, to prevent it being pulled out accidentally

Central venous cannulation

- A central vein may be used for administration of cardiac drugs, and will reduce circulatory transit time
- With the exception of femoral vein cannulation, central venous cannulation should not be performed by the inexperienced (when the risk of complications is doubled) out of hospital, except in the shocked and severely hypovolaemic patient when there is no alternative, because:
  - There is a relatively high risk of complications (up to 10% failure rate even for the experienced), including:
    - Pleural puncture resulting in pneumothorax
    - Subclavian artery puncture resulting in haemothorax
    - Carotid artery puncture with the approach to the internal jugular vein
    - Local haematoma formation
    - Air embolism
    - Myocardial injury: perforation or penetration
    - Local or systemic infections
  - The central venous route is unsuitable for rapid high volume fluid replacement if a long catheter is used, because of the cannula length. A short cannula should be used in patients with trauma
- The usual sites used are:
  - The femoral vein at the saphenofemoral junction
  - The internal jugular vein
  - The subclavian vein

Femoral vein cannulation (proximal saphenous vein cannulation)

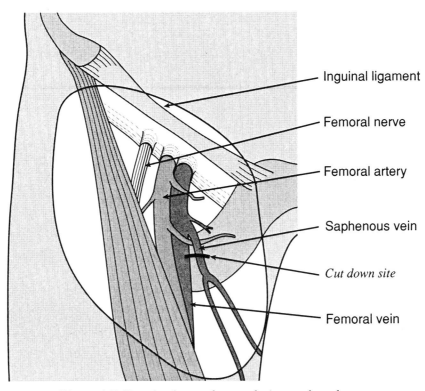

Figure 4-7 Sites for femoral cannulation and cutdown

Method
- Enter the skin over the femoral vein, with the point of the cannula pointed towards the head and at an angle of about 45º to the skin
- Advance the tip of the cannula, until there is a flashback of blood, following which reduce the angle of the cannula to the skin to about 15-20º and advance it further up to the hilt
- Connect the giving set and secure both in position with tape or a suture

Femoral vein cut down (proximal saphenous vein cut down)

Method
- Position yourself on the same side of the patient as the vein that you are going to use
- Identify the femoral artery about two finger-breadths below the mid-point of the inguinal ligament, and using two fingers over the artery pull the artery slightly laterally to tighten the skin
- Make an incision approximately 5 cm long just medial to the pulsations of the femoral artery
- Clear the subcutaneous fat and tissue with artery forceps using blunt dissection
- Dissect the vein free (it lies just below Scarpa's fascia)
- Using the same technique as for long saphenous vein cut down, elevate the vein, insert the cannula and secure it and the giving set. Do *not* tie off the vein peripherally

Note: In patients requiring immediate high volume fluid replacement, the end of a sterile giving set may be cut off obliquely and then inserted directly into the vein instead of a cannula. Infusion rates of up to 1 litre per minute may be obtained using this method (the fluids should be warmed first)

Internal jugular vein cannulation

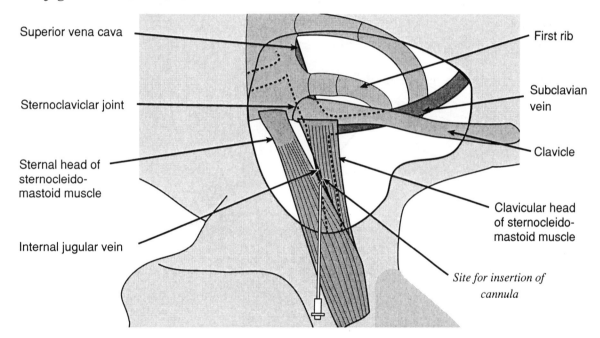

Superior vena cava

First rib

Sternoclaviclar joint

Subclavian vein

Sternal head of sternocleido-mastoid muscle

Clavicle

Internal jugular vein

Clavicular head of sternocleido-mastoid muscle

Site for insertion of cannula

Figure 4-8 Cannulation of the internal jugular vein viewed from the patient's head

Method
- Lie the patient down, head down and turned to one side with the legs elevated (if possible), to reduce the risk of air embolism and help distend the neck veins
- Approach the patient by standing at the head, facing towards the legs
- Identify the sternal and clavicular heads of the sternocleidomastoid muscle and the apex of the triangle that they form
- Using a 10 mL syringe and a 12-14G cannula, insert the needle at the apex of the triangle (or at the middle of the anterior border of the sternal band of sternocleidomastoid) at an angle of 30° aiming towards the right nipple
- Withdraw the syringe plunger as soon as the needle is under the skin, and continue insertion and aspiration until there is a flashback of blood. *CAUTION:* The carotid artery is situated just medial and anterior to the vein
- Advance the cannula into the vein, withdrawing the syringe and needle as you do so
- Attach the giving set to the cannula

Complications
-   Arterial puncture:
    -   This is usually obvious. If it occurs, leave the cannula in situ and seal it, as withdrawal may result in an extensive haematoma

Subclavian vein cannulation

Infraclavicular approach

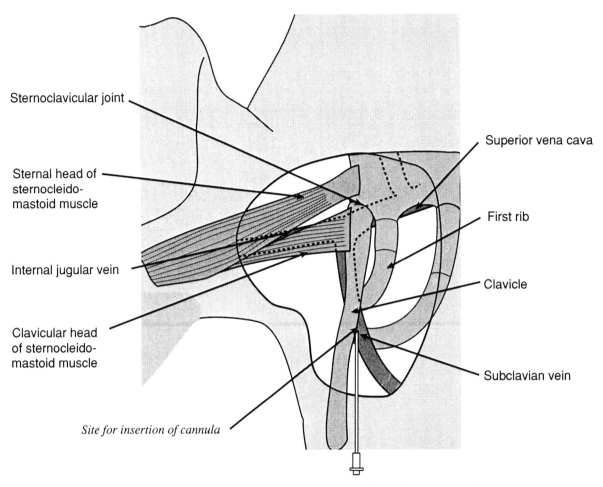

Sternoclavicular joint

Sternal head of sternocleido-mastoid muscle

Internal jugular vein

Clavicular head of sternocleido-mastoid muscle

Site for insertion of cannula

Superior vena cava

First rib

Clavicle

Subclavian vein

Figure 4-9 Subclavian cannulation: infraclavicular approach

Advantages
-   Avoids moving the neck
-   Leaves both arms free

Method
-   With the patient supine, identify the clavicle, and find its mid point
-   Insert the cannula horizontally one finger's breadth below the clavicle, along the inferior border of the clavicle aiming for the opposite sternoclavicular joint
-   Gently withdraw the plunger of the syringe until there is a flashback of blood
-   Then proceed as for cannulation of the internal jugular vein

Complications
-   Arterial puncture (may be undetected)
-   Pleural puncture

Supraclavicular approach

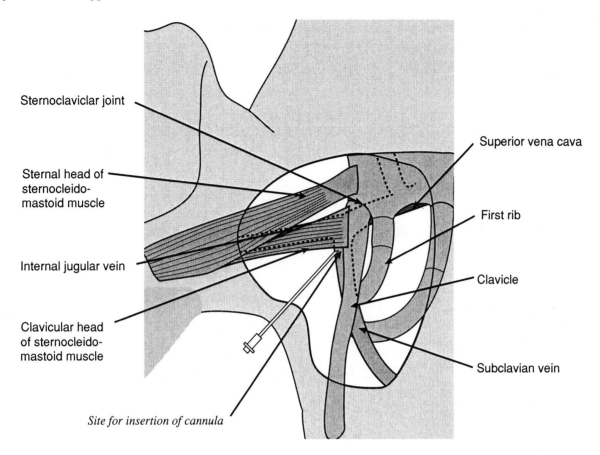

Figure 4-10 Subclavian cannulation: supraclavicular approach

Advantage
- Less likely than the infraclavicular approach to cause problems

Method
- With the patient supine and the head down, elevate the legs to prevent the risk of air embolism, and to help distend the neck veins
- Position yourself by the patient's right shoulder and turn the patient's head to the left
- Identify the clavicle, the clavicular head of the sternocleidomastoid muscle, and the angle that they form
- Insert the needle horizontally above the clavicle, bisecting the angle, and pass it directly behind the clavicle
- Gently withdraw the plunger of the syringe until there is a flashback of blood
- Proceed as for cannulation of the internal jugular vein

Complications
- Arterial puncture (may be undetected)
- Pleural puncture

PRACTICAL POINTS: 1. In cold weather local application of a "Warm Pak®" may help dilate the peripheral veins
2. Application of a PASG may aid venous cannulation of the central and upper limb veins in the very shocked hypovolaemic patient

Intraosseous infusion
-   This is a relatively simple and useful technique for emergency vascular access particularly in children, especially those under seven years old, in whom it is now considered to be the method of choice
-   In older children it should be used in preference to a venous cut down or central venous cannulation, when peripheral venous cannulation is difficult or unsuccessful

Advantages
-   Much quicker and easier to perform than establishing difficult intravenous access
-   Provides rapid access to the central circulation for fluid and/or drug administration (except bretylium)

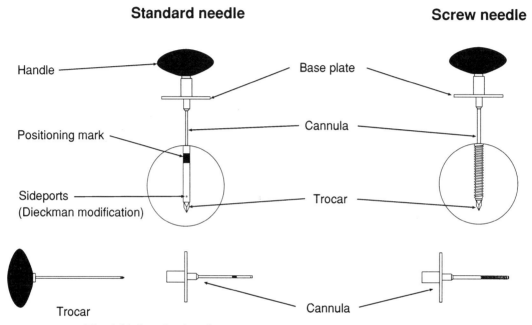

Fig 4-11 Standard and screw intraosseous cannulae and trochars

Sites
-   Proximal tibia:
    -   1-3 cm below the mid point between the tibial tuberosity and the medial edge of the tibia over the antero-medial (broad flat) surface of the tibia
    -   Suitable for children up to the age of 5 years old (it may be difficult to penetrate bone after this)
-   Distal tibia:
    -   Just proximal to the medial malleolus over the medial surface of the tibia
    -   Suitable for all ages
-   Distal femur:
    -   2-3 cm above the lateral femoral condyle

Contraindications
-   *Never* insert an intraosseous needle distal to a fracture site
-   Proximal fracture
-   Bleeding diathesis
-   Local sepsis

Method
-   Identify the relevant anatomical landmarks, and prepare the insertion site with antiseptic solution
-   If the patient is awake or alert, administer local anaesthetic
-   Incise the skin over the intended insertion site

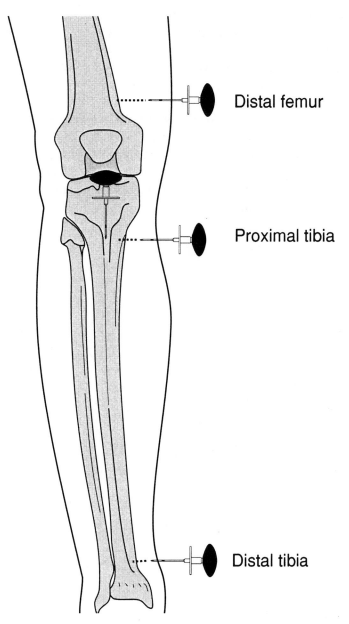

Figure 4-12 Sites for intraosseous infusion

- Grasp the intraosseous needle (if this is not available, a 16 gauge intravenous cannulation needle (18 gauge for babies under 8 months old) may suffice), and insert it perpendicularly into the bone to a depth of about 1.5-2.0 cm, rotating the device, and if appropriate aiming away from the growth plate

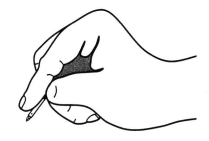

Figure 4-13 Hold for intraosseous needle

- Needle entry into the marrow cavity is shown by:
  - A loss of resistance
  - Sustained positioning of the needle without support (in infants and small children, there may be very little support, and the device has to be held in place by hand or secured using the Molynar Disc (included with some devices)
  - Free flow of marrow aspirate or infusion fluid
- Remove the stylet and attach a syringe. Withdraw the plunger and aspirate a little marrow to confirm correct placement (save marrow for grouping and cross-matching later)
- Administer blood replacement fluid by giving syringe boluses using minimal pressure, attach a giving set (although the rate of flow may be rather slow), or preferably attach a giving set, syringe and a three-way tap to the intraosseous needle, which will make fluid administration easier and faster
- Be careful not to over infuse children/infants!

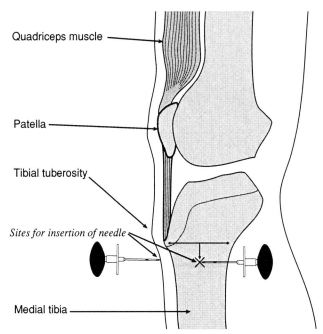

Figure 4-14 Intraosseous infusion: locating site for proximal tibia

Rate of infusion
- Gravity: 100 mL per hour (at best)

Complications
- Osteomyelitis: 0.6%
- Skin infection: 0.7%
- Growth plate injury
- Subcutaneous infusion/oedema
- Subperiosteal infusion
- Over penetration through to the other side of the bone

PRACTICAL POINTS
- *In hypovolaemic and cold patients, especially females, the peripheral veins may collapse, making intravenous cannulation of the large antecubital fossa veins difficult. To bring up these veins:*
  - *Apply a tourniquet at the mid humeral level and ask the patient to clench and unclench their hand*
  - *Place a warm pack on the back of the patients hand for a few minutes, remove it and insert a butterfly cannula into one of the veins*
  - *Syringe or run in 100-200 mL of intravenous fluid, until the antecubital fossa veins stand out*
  - *Cannulate the antecubital fossa veins in the usual way*

Types of intravenous infusion fluid

Introduction
- The ideal infusion fluid/blood substitute should be:
    - Cheap, with a long storage life at any temperature
    - Inert:
        - No risk of allergic, toxic, or incompatibility reaction
        - Does not interfere with grouping and cross matching
        - Has no effect on haemostasis or coagulation
        - No risk of electrolyte disturbance
    - Isotonic with blood: low risk of fluid overload; both intravascular and interstitial
- It should have:
    - A pH of 7.4 (similar to blood), but with a buffering effect
    - A relatively short half life, and be rapidly excreted
    - Good oxygen carrying capacity and oxygen release
    - No effect on renal function
    - No risk of disease transmission
- The container should be:
    - Robust
    - A convenient shape
    - Squeezable
    - Fitted with a good integral hanging loop
    - Easy to connect to a giving set

Crystalloids

Sodium chloride intravenous infusion 0.9%

Action
- Provides short term fluid replacement (30-60 minutes blood volume replacement) as rapid diffusion into the interstitial space occurs
- At least three times the blood loss must be infused to achieve full fluid replacement

Advantages
- Low cost
- Long shelf life of five years or more
- Low risk of infection or allergy
- Availability in convenient soft plastic containers, e.g. *Viaflex*®

Disadvantages
- The large volumes required to provide blood replacement
- If large volumes are infused, the risk of causing:
    - Tissue oedema, especially cerebral and pulmonary oedema
    - Hypernatraemia

CONCLUSION: Only useful for short term fluid replacement and when fluid lost has been mostly sodium chloride, e.g. in vomiting, dehydration, etc.

Hartmann's/Ringer Lactate solution: sodium lactate intravenous compound

Description
- A buffered solution, similar to saline, but containing sodium and chloride ions in physiologically more normal quantities, and also containing potassium, calcium and bicarbonate (as lactate) ions

Advantages
- Lower sodium and chloride content than saline
- Has some buffering action

Disadvantage
- In the hypovolaemic patient, who already has a lactic acidosis due to hypoperfusion, addition of lactate ions may result in an increased accumulation of lactate, and a metabolic acidosis. Although this is theoretically a problem, it has not been found to be so in practice

CONCLUSION: Probably the *crystalloid of choice* in pre-hospital care

Dextrose 5%: Glucose intravenous infusion 5%

Description
- 5% dextrose in 0.18% saline

Action
- Dextrose is a readily utilizable energy source

Disadvantages
- Prone to cause local venous thrombophlebitis
- Low pH: 3.5-5.0

CONCLUSION: Preferred by some for low volume intravenous infusions following myocardial infarction, and in paediatric resuscitation; it has no role in the management of hypovolaemia

Colloids

Action
- Provide long term volume replacement

Advantages
- There is a low risk of tissue oedema
- Generally iso-oncotic with blood, which they replace on an equal volume basis
- Rapidly restore circulating fluid volume

Disadvantage
- Do not replace interstitial fluid loss
- Are more viscous than crystalloid, resulting in a slower infusion rate with some cannulae
- Recent meta-analysis has shown that they may confer no advantage in the blood loss situation

Plasma substitutes
- Macromolecular substances, which are only slowly metabolised

Gelatins/Bovine albumins

Haemaccel®

Description
- A modified fluid gelatin, average molecular weight 30,000, 4% in sodium chloride 0.9%

Action
- Promotes an osmotic diuresis and has a half life of several hours

Advantages
- Relatively cheap
- Is generally non toxic and does not affect the clotting mechanisms, except when large volumes are infused, which may result in dilution of clotting factors
- Presented in convenient plastic containers
- Is not affected by changes in storage temperature
- Has a long shelf life of 5-8 years according to the storage conditions

Disadvantages
- Liable to freeze in cold weather
- There is a (low) risk of anaphylactic reactions: minor histamine release effect
- Should not be mixed with citrated blood as the calcium ions may cause blood to clot in the giving set
- Increased risk of pulmonary and cerebral oedema in the first hour

Gelofusine®

Description
- Similar to Haemaccel (Polygelene: degraded/modified gelatin), average molecular weight 35,000, but has a lower potassium and calcium content, a higher sodium content and a slightly longer half life

Disadvantages
- Hyperoncotic with blood and there is a greater risk of fluid overload, due to its fluid expanding effect
- Gels below 3°C

CONCLUSION: Recent meta-analysis has suggested that these fluids are no better than crystalloid

Modified starches

Hydroxyethyl starch: Hetastarch 6%: *Hespan®/Elohes®*

Description
- Hetastarch 6%, in sodium chloride 0.9%
- Similar to Dextran 70 physiologically

Advantages
- Relatively cheap, compared to plasma, but is much more expensive than either gelatins or crystalloid
- Half life: long (12-14 hours)
- The shelf life is 2 years; it should be stored below 25°C and above freezing
- There is little risk of histamine release or anaphylactic reaction.

Disadvantages
- Tends to coat platelets and therefore has an anticoagulant effect; by prolonging the clotting time
- Should be used with caution in renal impairment
- There is a small risk of allergic reactions; the mechanism is not known
- Can fill the intravascular space for some time and cause problems with getting an adequate volume of blood infused with the possibility of fluid overload

CONCLUSION: Gaining increasing acceptance in hospital practice. Not used in pre-hospital care at present

Dextrans

- Hydrolytic starch products, fractionated to produce solutions with molecules of a consistent size
- Molecule sizes available are 40,000 (40) and 70,000 (70)
- Coat the red cell membrane which may interfere with blood grouping and cross matching
- Increase coagulation times by impairing platelet function and fibrin formation
- Stored in glass bottles, which are heavy, bulky, fragile and impractical for pre-hospital use

Dextran 40: *Gentran 40®, Lomodex 40®, Rheomacrodex 40®*

Description
- 10% dextrans of average molecular weight 40,000 in 5% glucose or 0.9% sodium chloride solution

Advantages
- Promotes the microcirculation in small volumes

Disadvantages
- May cause irreversible renal damage if it is used for resuscitation in acute hypovolaemic shock

CONCLUSION: Not recommended for the treatment of hypovolaemic shock

Dextran 70: *Gentran 70®, Lomodex 70®, Macrodex®*

Description
- 6% dextrans of average molecular weight 70,000 in 5% glucose or 0.9% sodium chloride solution

Advantages
- An effective blood substitute
- Long shelf life: 5 years

Disadvantages
- Can interfere with coagulation (and hence with cross matching)
- Has a long half life of several days, which means that no more than 1 litre should be infused
- There is a small risk of allergic reactions due to histamine release and other mechanisms
- Should be stored at a steady room temperature; temperature variation may result in flaking

Contraindications
- Congestive cardiac failure
- Bleeding diatheses due to: thrombocytopenia, hypofibrinogenaemia

CONCLUSION: No longer used in pre-hospital care in the UK

Plasma

Albumin 5%

Description
- Freeze dried plasma; it is stored as a dry powder and has to be reconstituted

Disadvantages
- It is expensive and in short supply
- May cause serum homologous jaundice and has a high potassium content which can be dangerous in rapid transfusion
- The shelf life is relatively short: 6 months
- Recent research has indicated an increased mortality when albumin is used in the treatment of burns

CONCLUSION: Has now been *replaced by HPPF*

HPPF (Human plasma protein fraction)

Description
- A 5% solution of protein, containing 88% albumin

Advantages
- Does not carry the risk of producing either a serum homologous reaction or hyperkalaemia
- Has a long shelf life of up to 5 years if stored between 2-25ºC
- The risk of disease transmission is very low

Disadvantages
- It is in short supply, and is very expensive
- Comes in a glass bottle and needs an air vent

CONCLUSION: Theoretically physiologically perhaps the ideal blood replacement fluid, but due to its cost, it has been reserved for replacement of plasma albumin in burns. However recent analysis has suggested that survival rates in burns patients is reduced when HPPF is used. *Not used* in pre-hospital care

Whole blood

Disadvantages
- It needs careful storage between 3-6 ºC
- The shelf life is very short: between 21 and 35 days depending on the the preservative used
- Allergic and incompatibility "transfusion" reactions. There is a significant risk of this, even with unmatched O Rh NEG blood; therefore type specific blood should be requested at least
- Contamination with pathogenic organisms, e.g. hepatitis, HIV. This risk is very low in the UK, as all blood is heat treated irrespective of screening
- Hypothermia, and cardiac arrest may occur if the blood is not warmed sufficiently prior to infusion
- It has a high viscosity (the microcirculation in shock may be improved by a reduction in the packed cell volume)
- If stored for more than a few days, platelets and white cells tend to fragment rapidly and lose their normal function, and there is a rise in the serum potassium
- Overtransfusion with a consequent increase in viscosity, and pulmonary oedema may occur due to the difficulty of estimating blood loss accurately
- There may be coagulation problems if more four units are infused (clotting factors, especially factor VIII, rapidly degrade in stored blood)

CONCLUSION: Because of its short shelf life and special storage requirements, whole blood is not readily available and *not usually necessary* in Immediate Care, except for the patient with major blood loss who is trapped for some time

Guidelines for provision of blood out of hospital

Introduction
- Doctors in Immediate Care Schemes (and doctors in Hospital Flying Squads, or Hospital Surgical Teams) may on rare occasions need to administer blood products at the roadside
- In each area guidelines should be agreed with the consultant in charge of the Accident and Emergency Department and the relevant hospital Transfusion Service for the provision of blood outside hospital
- Because of the dangers of mismatched blood, the most important factor is accurate patient identification. To achieve this it is necessary to register the patient with a hospital, which will issue the patient with a unique patient identification number to reduce the risk to the absolute minimum
- For trauma patients blood banks usually supply packed red cells of the casualty's ABO and Rh D group

- In ideal circumstances cross-matched packed red cells can be issued in about 20 minutes of the blood bank receiving a correctly labelled blood sample. However, especially at night and at weekends, when on-call haematology staff may have to be called in, it may take considerably longer. A realistic minimum time span between requesting blood from the scene and receiving it, is one hour. In view of this fact, requests for blood should be made early, especially out of hours
- Once the decision has been made that blood is required, it will be necessary to involve Police or Ambulance Officers for transporting specimens from the scene, and to bring blood products back

Patient registration
- Once the decision has been made that blood is required, the casualty should be accurately and uniquely identified by registering the patient with the A&E Department, which should be contacted by cellphone or radio telephone on the Ambulance Service radio frequency
- The Accident and Emergency Department should be provided with as much information about the patient as possible, including the following details:
    - First name, surname, actual or approximate age and date of birth if available
    - The sex and ethnic origin of patient
    - The location of accident
    - The name, status and call-sign of the person requesting blood
- The Accident and Emergency Department may ask for additional information and will then allocate a unique A&E identity number to the patient. This should be written on an identity band, which is then placed around the casualty's wrist or ankle
- At least one company can supply an armband with a unique patient number and a strip of numbered stickers for blood sample and other specimen containers for patients of unknown name or identity

Taking and labelling blood samples
- For adults a 10 mL blood sample bottle without coagulant is usually used for the blood sample
- The blood sample bottle should be labelled with a label taken from the identity band at the same time that the blood sample is taken
- It is vital that the casualty's correct name is used, if in doubt the casualty should be referred to as 'Unidentified male/female', and this together with the casualty's unique A&E number, the name and call-sign of the doctor requesting blood, the location of the incident, and the date and time of taking the specimen *must* be put on the blood sample bottle label

Transport
- The full blood sample bottle should the be put in a polythene bag and given to the Police or Ambulance Officer, who will transport this to the Accident & Emergency Department (in the interim the Medical Records staff can, if details are known, identify whether the patient is known to the hospital and release a pre-existing hospital number, if appropriate)
- On arrival at the hospital the specimen should be given to a doctor in the Accident & Emergency Department (who will have been alerted in advance), who will then check the details and complete the appropriate blood transfusion request form (it is normal practice to order 6 units of red cells for critical trauma)
- The blood specimen and associated paperwork is then taken to the blood bank
- Type O Rhesus negative blood is often available immediately to most Accident & Emergency Departments. If the patient's condition is such that O Rh negative blood is required immediately, the Accident & Emergency Department should be informed as soon as possible, so that the person delivering the blood sample can return to the accident scene with two units of O Rh negative blood, whilst cross-matched blood is being prepared

Administration
- When blood products arrive on scene, they must be checked to ensure that it is the correct blood for the correct casualty

- Blood components carry a label applied to them by the blood transfusion centre that produced them, and a label from the hospital blood bank (usually called the Compatibility Label), which contains information that uniquely identifies the patient for whom the blood is intended
- With the exception of unmatched O Rh negative blood from A&E, this information includes the casualty's name and date of birth, their unique A&E number, the ABO, Rhesus group and unique donation number of the unit, and the date and time that the blood was requested
- The blood bank will also provide a compatibility report on a slip of paper which states the patient's full identity (as far as it is known), the patient's ABO and Rhesus group and the unique donation number of each unit supplied, which should be recorded by the doctor in the patient's notes together with the time it was used
- It is the responsibility of the Immediate Care doctor to check that all the details on the compatibility report and the labels, including the expiry date, on each unit of blood exactly match the identity of the patient, **If in any doubt do not transfuse**
- Blood must be administered through an infusion set with an integral filter, and not a fluid infusion set
- Never add any other infusion solution/drugs to any blood component, and do not try to warm the blood

Temperature
- Transfusion of cold blood at rates of more than 100 mL/minute has been associated with cardiac arrest
- Blood warmers are not usually available in the pre-hospital situation, thus keeping the patient warm and controlling the infusion rate is especially important (do *not* try to warm the blood without a blood warmer)

Adverse reactions
- If the casualty develops any unexplained adverse symptoms/signs/evidence of allergy, stop the infusion
- Over transfusion may be indicated by the signs of systemic venous engorgement (a raised JVP) and pulmonary oedema (basal crackles)

Intravenous fluids: composition

Crystalloids	Na+	K+	Ca++	Cl-	Albumin	Globulin	pH	Osmolality
	(millimoles/litre)				(g/l)	(g/l)		(mmol/kg)
NaCl. 0.9%	150			150			5.5-6.5	Normal
Hartmann's	131	5.0	2.0	111 (lactate)			5.0-7.0	Normal
Dextrose 5%							3.5-5.5	Normal
Colloids								
Haemaccel®	145	5.1	6.26	145	35 (polygeline)		7.3	300-306
Gelofusine®	154	<0.4	<0.4	125	40 (gelatin)		7.4	279
Albumin 5%	140	5	2.0		43	7	7.0	300
HPPF	136-160	2		112	45 (95% Albumin)		7.3	Normal
Blood	136-145	3.5-5.0	2.0-2.5	100-106	34-45	20-30	7.4	285-295

Figure 4-15 Composition of intravenous fluids

Class of shock and fluid replacement

Class I (blood loss <15%): oral fluids are usually sufficient
Class II (blood loss 15-30%): Fluid replacement with a combination of intravenous crystalloid and colloid
Class III (blood loss 30-40%): Rapid fluid replacement with colloid and crystalloid followed by blood
Class IV (blood loss >40%): Rapid aggressive fluid replacement with colloid, crystalloid and blood

---

Discussion point: Choice of intravenous fluid

Concerns
- For many years there has been debate as to which type of fluid is best for the initial restoration of blood volume following traumatic hypovolaemia, with crystalloid being generally favoured in North America and colloid being generally favoured in Europe
- Any tendency of the fluid to cause an increase in interstitial pulmonary fluid, which may predispose the patient to the adult respiratory distress syndrome (ARDS), is a disadvantage
- The application of the Starling principle (which states that the maintenance of colloid osmotic pressure in the intravascular space by the infusion of albumin or a similar colloid reduces fluid extravasation into the interstial space) is inappropriate in traumatic hypovolaemic shock and septic shock, because in these conditions the situation is not one of just intravascular fluid loss, but also of local tissue injury. As a result of this injury, and also as part of the body's general response to injury or infection, capillary permeability increases considerably, and albumin and other colloids which would normally stay in the intravascular space diffuse into the interstitial space. This is particularly a problem in the lungs where the albumin may become trapped in the irregular latticework of collagen and elastin fibres in the interstitial space, increasing the osmotic pressure and drawing in fluid, resulting in pulmonary oedema

Evidence
- In hypovolaemia, the first priority is to restore the circulating blood volume rapidly, thus ensuring the adequate delivery of oxygen to the tissues by the blood. A modest reduction in the number of blood cells available in the blood for oxygen transportation does not impair delivery of oxygen to the tissues significantly, and may in fact improve it by reducing the viscosity of the blood. However a further reduction in the number of red blood cells may result in impaired oxygen transportation and delivery
- When crystalloid alone is used to replace traumatic blood loss, much greater volumes have to be used to restore the patient to the same haemodynamic state than when colloid is used
- Theoretically, if large volumes of crystalloid are infused, there will be dilution of the colloid in the blood and a reduction in the intravascular colloid osmotic pressure, resulting in the transfer of fluid from the intravascular space to the interstitial space, reducing the intravascular fluid volume
- In the few studies that have been performed (involving fit individuals), it has been found that falls in intravascular osmotic pressure have not resulted in impaired pulmonary function or an increase in pulmonary fluid retention. It is thought that any undesirable increase in pulmonary fluid is prevented by an increase in lymphatic drainage

Conclusion
- Recent research has shown that colloid is no more effective than crystalloid (volume for volume), for restoring blood volume rapidly, in view of which it is suggested that:
    - Blood loss of up to 15% blood volume can safely be replaced by colloid or crystalloid alone
    - If the blood loss is greater than 15%, then one unit (500 mL) of colloid may be used followed by 2 units (1000 mL) of crystalloid
    - In the pre-hospital situation, when treatment may be started shortly after the initial blood loss, colloid is probably the fluid of first choice, as it replaces the blood lost the most efficiently. If there is more than 30 minutes delay in starting the infusion, there may be significant interstitial fluid loss. In this case the initial infusion fluid should be crystalloid, followed by colloid

Complications of large volume fluid replacement
- Large volume transfusion of colloid/crystalloid followed by blood may result in:
  - Hypothermia
  - Acid/base disturbance
  - Hyperkalaemia
  - Hypocalcaemia
  - Clotting problems
  - ARDS
- Rouleaux formation, if blood is administered through the same giving set as colloid

PRACTICAL POINTS
- *At low temperatures intravenous fluids, especially colloids, may increase in viscosity, freeze or form crystals, which can cause difficulty with infusion, patient cooling and cardiac arrhythmias*
- *Storage of intravenous fluids:*
  - *Ideally intravenous fluids for immediate use should be kept in an insulated container at body temperature, e.g. the Transwarm® intravenous fluid warming system*
  - *Alternatively:*
    - *At least one unit of each type of transfusion fluid should be kept in the passenger compartment of the vehicle, so as to keep it relatively warm*
    - *The first bottles of fluid used should probably be those carried on the ambulance, as most ambulances are kept in centrally heated garages. Check with your local ambulance service!*
- *Warming intravenous fluids:*
  - *Fluids can be kept warm during infusion by wrapping the infusion bottle and drip chamber in a "Hot pack®", or using an Infupak® which is a purpose designed intravenous fluid warming device, consisting of an insulated bag into which a reusable Hot pack® and a bottle of infusion fluid can be inserted. An insulated sleeve for the giving set and line is also provided to reduce fluid cooling due to wind chill*
  - *Fluid warming is not only important for warming up cold infusion fluids, but also for administering warm fluids to warm up hypothermic and hypovolaemic patients*
- *Administration of intravenous fluids*
  - *In very cold or windy situations the fluid container, giving set and line should be insulated*

Pain relief
- Pain relief is important, as severe pain alone may raise the blood pressure and heart rate (see chapter on Pain management)

Monitoring
- Measurement/assessment:
  - Pulse rate
  - Pulse pressure
  - Oxygen saturation and pulse oximetry plethysmography
  - Arterial pressure
  - Respiratory rate
  - Temperature
  - Mental state
  - Jugular venous pressure; if raised together with a low arterial pressure and tachycardia, it indicates:
    - Tension pneumothorax
    - Cardiac tamponade
    - Cardiogenic shock

Cardiogenic shock

Incidence
- May occur following acute myocardial infarction (see chapter on Cardiac care: acute myocardial infarction)
- Occurs relatively rarely following trauma

Aetiology
- Following acute myocardial infarction
- May occur in trauma as a result of:
    - Cardiac contusion caused by blunt chest injury
    - Cardiac tamponade due to penetrating injury
    - Tension pneumothorax
    - Air embolism (rare)

Pathophysiology
- A severe reduction in cardiac output which is caused by:
    - Loss of sufficient active myocardium as a result of:
        - Acute myocardial infarction
        - Cardiac contusion
    - Reduced cardiac filling (reduced preload) as a result of;
        - Cardiac tamponade
        - Tension pneumothorax
        - Air embolism

Symptoms/signs
- These are similar to, but not identical, to those for hypovolaemic shock
- The differences are:
    - Skin appearance:
        - Slightly pale in cardiogenic shock, very pale in hypovolaemic shock
    - Jugular venous pressure:
        - Raised in cardiogenic shock, low in hypovolaemic shock
    - ECG pattern: Injury pattern in cardiogenic shock, normal in hypovolaemic shock

Management

- *Airway*
    - Airway maintenance, with cervical spine stabilisation if there is a history of recent trauma

- *Breathing*
    - Tracheal intubation and ventilation if the patient is unconscious, oxygen

- *Circulation*
    - Treatment of the cause:
        - Thrombolysis
        - Pericardiocentesis
        - Thoracocentesis
    - Establish a slow intravenous infusion with crystalloid, if there is no associated hypovolaemic shock. This may also be used for intravenous drug administration if required
    - Administration of:
        - Opiates
        - Nitrates

Neurogenic shock

Incidence
- Commonly encountered, often in combination with other types of shock
- More common in the young female and elderly

Aetiology
- Head or spinal cord injury
- Sudden severe anxiety

Pathophysiology
- Autonomic stimulation or disruption of the sympathetic pathways descending in the cervical and upper thoracic spine, results in loss of vasomotor tone and arteriolar tone with sudden venous dilation and vascular pooling without any reflex cardiac stimulation

Symptoms/signs
- Hypotension
- Bradycardia
- Syncope

Management
- Leg elevation is usually sufficient in severe anxiety
- In very persistent cases consider:
    - Cautious intravenous fluid administration with very careful monitoring of the patient's haemodynamic state
    - Atropine:
        - Incremental doses of 0.5-0.6 mg, administered intravenously over 5 minutes, up to a maximum of 3 mg

Septic shock

Definition: Septic shock is a more severe form of the sepsis syndrome; which includes those conditions previously described as septicaemia, bacteraemia and fungaemia, and is the clinical situation that results from the presence of micro-organisms in the bloodstream
Septic shock results in severe tissue hypoperfusion, and is usually associated with profound hypotension and organ failure

Introduction
- Septic shock is a rare, but potentially lethal condition, with a high mortality which may present to the General Practitioner or Accident and Emergency department, but may also be encountered by Ambulance crews and Immediate Care doctors

Incidence
- Septic shock occurs in about 20% of patients with bacteraemia, and increases the mortality to about 60%
- Streptococcal shock syndrome (*Strep. pyogenes*):
    - 600 cases per year in the UK
    - 30% are fatal
    - 5% are associated with chickenpox
- Toxic shock syndrome (*Staph. aureus*):
    - 18 cases per year in the UK
- Waterhouse-Friderichsen syndrome/meningococcal septicaemia (*Neisseria meningitides*):
    - Over 400 cases per year in the UK with a mortality of over 20%

Aetiology
- Septic shock may occur if:
    - There is a penetrating injury with contamination of the abdominal cavity by intestinal contents
    - The patient cannot be conveyed from the scene of their accident for many hours, e.g. in prolonged or complicated entrapment
    - The travelling time to hospital is very long, e.g. in remote areas or at sea
- Toxic shock may occur as a result of infection associated with the following:
    - Childbirth:
        - Due to abortion or the retained products of conception
    - Inappropriate vaginal tampon use in menstruating women
    - Any injury (accidental or iatrogenic) or illness, e.g. minor wounds, burns, abscesses and sinusitis and areas affected by postinfluenzal bronchopneumonia, tracheitis and empyema

Bacteriology
- Septic shock is commonly considered to be a complication of Gram-negative rod bacteraemia, but the causative organism may also be:
    - Gram-positive organisms including the toxin producing *Staph. aureus*
    - β-haemolytic streptococci group A, which produces an endotoxin such as lipopolysaccharide A
    - Fungi and other similar organisms
- In the majority of patients, the prime initiator is an *endotoxin,* which is a lipopolysaccharide component of the bacterial cell wall of Gram-negative bacteria
- In some patients septic shock may be caused by *exotoxins* released by bacteria (Toxic shock)

Pathophysiology
- Infection with a wide range of different organisms results in a similar clinical picture because they cause tissue injury by a common final pathway:
    - Lipopolysaccharide (*endotoxin*) stimulates the release of cytokines, including tumour necrosis factor, from monocytes

- Lipopolysaccharide and Gram-positive cell wall compounds stimulate :
    - The activation of neutrophils, which adhere to each other and to vascular endothelium and may cause vascular and tissue injury, resulting in impaired ability to absorb oxygen, and capillary wall damage at the site of the infection, resulting in a leak of albumin and water
    - Factor XII which promotes intrinsic and extrinsic coagulation pathways causing disseminated intravascular coagulation leading to consumptive coagulopathy, generalised bleeding and hypovolaemia. It may also influence the release of bradykinin
  - Cytokines and endotoxin stimulate inductible nitric oxide synthase to produce nitric oxide, which activates cyclic GMP in vascular smooth muscle, causing peripheral vasodilation
- There is a compensatory rise in cardiac output, and the systemic vascular resistance falls because of peripheral vasodilation secondary to pyrexia, and also because of the release of vasoactive mediators, such as kinins and tumour necrosis factor
- The cardiac output may later fall due to hypovolaemia, and vascular resistance rises as a result of the sympathetic response
- The cardiac preload falls as hypovolaemia develops
- A vicious cycle may then develop with a further reduction in blood pressure and myocardial performance, resulting in general organ failure and eventually death

Symptoms/signs
- The typical symptoms of septic shock include:
    - Dizziness/postural syncope due to hypotension:
        - Systolic BP <90 mmHg
        - A *wide pulse pressure* with a postural drop in diastolic pressure of at least 15 mmHg
    - A modest tachycardia and tachypnoea
    - Hypoxia resulting in confusion, drowsiness, without focal neurological signs when the fever and hypotension have been corrected
    - A pyrexia with warm pink skin, or hypothermia
    - Blotchy macular erythema: which may be patchy, localised or generalised
    - Myalgia
    - Diarrhoea and vomiting
- Septic shock may be associated with:
    - Acute renal failure
    - Adult respiratory distress syndrome
    - Disseminated intravascular coagulation
- None of the typical features are essential for the diagnosis to be made, and it is unusual for them to all be present at once
- In the young, the elderly and the immunocompromised, the physical signs/symptoms may be very subtle
- There are no signs which help to distinguish Gram-positive from Gram-negative infections reliably, except the rash of meningococcal infection
- Patients with a combination of septic shock and hypovolaemia are difficult to distinguish clinically from those who have hypovolaemia alone

Management
- Oxygen
- Intravenous fluid administration with crystalloid/colloid
- Treatment of the cause/prevention of further production or absorption of toxin:
    - Removal of tampon, etc.
    - Drainage of abscess
- Intravenous antibiotics:
    - Flucloxacillin and/or benzylpenicillin (or erythromycin), depending on the likely causative agent
- Steroids

Anaphylactic shock

Definition: Anaphylactic shock is a state of immediate generalised hypersensitivity (a severe acute allergic reaction), following exposure to a foreign substance in a previously sensitised individual

Introduction
- This is one of the most acute medical emergencies, and requires immediate recognition and aggressive management as the patient may die in minutes

Note: Anaphylactic shock is the most extreme/severe type of allergic response. Many patients suffer from much less severe allergic reactions/symptoms and do not require such aggressive management

Incidence
- Relatively uncommon, but increasing

Aetiology
- Exposure to a diverse range of specific allergens, by inhalation, ingestion, injection or bite:
    - Protein drugs (hormones):
        - Insulin, ACTH and vasopressin
    - Non protein drugs (haptens)
        - Antibiotics:
            - Penicillin, sulphonamides and cephalosporins
        - Vitamins:
            - Thiamine and folic acid
    - Allergen extracts:
        - Pollens, mould and animal dander
    - Foods:
        - Nuts and seeds: peanuts, tree nuts (hazelnut, brazil, almond, walnut, pecan, pistachio)
        - Cow's milk and dairy products, (rare except in young children), chocolate
        - Fruit: strawberries, citrus fruit, apples (with tree pollen allergy), tomatoes, bananas, avocado
        - Fish, shellfish, chicken, eggs, cereals (wheat, corn, rice)
        - Vegetables: potatoes, celery, peas and soya
    - "Foreign" protein:
        - Tetanus antitoxin, gamma globulin, venom antitoxin and semen
    - Vaccines:
        - Pertussis, typhoid and hyposensitising (allergen) preparations
    - Therapeutic agents:
        - Iron injections, anti-inflammatory analgesics, heparin, and neuromuscular blocking agents
    - Enzymes:
        - Trypsin, chymotrypsin and penicillinase
    - Diagnostic agents:
        - Radio-opaque dyes
    - Venoms:
        - Bee, wasp, fire ant and snake
    - Parasites:
        - Hydatid cyst rupture
    - Chemicals:
        - Formaldehyde and ethylene oxide gas
    - Latex:
        - Surgical gloves and catheters
- Commonest causes are parenteral antibiotics and other substances, insect stings and food, especially nuts
- More likely to occur after parenteral administration, in atopic individuals and those on β-blockers

Pathophysiology
- Anaphylaxis is an acute generalised type I hypersensitivity reaction in previously sensitised individuals, caused by antigens binding with IgE antibody, or the shorter term sensitivity antibody IgG, attached to the cell membranes of interstitial mast cells and circulating basophils, and releasing histamine and other potent mediators, resulting in:
    - An urticarial rash, with peripheral vasodilation
    - Laryngeal oedema
    - Bronchial constriction with mucus secretion, similar to acute severe asthma
    - Severe hypotension:
        - This usually occurs after the appearance of the urticarial rash and is secondary to the peripheral vasodilation, resulting in a drop in cardiac preload, an increase in heart rate and a fall in systemic vascular resistance
        - Later there may be bradycardia, followed by cardiac arrest
- The onset may be extremely rapid, especially in the presensitised patient, e.g. insect stings, or relatively slow, e.g. when there has been no prior exposure and the route of administration is the alimentary canal

Note: An *anaphylactoid* reaction describes a similar clinical syndrome to anaphylaxis, involving similar mediators, including histamine, but not IgE or IgG, and there may be no history of previous exposure

History
- There is usually, but not always a history of atopy with similar, but milder attacks

Symptoms/signs
- There may be considerable variation in the severity of an acute allergic reaction, from relatively mild with a gradual onset to the sudden onset of life threatening anaphylaxis, or the pattern may be biphasic, with the reoccurrence of symptoms in 5% of patients 1-72 hours after the initial reaction
- The severity of a reaction can vary from one individual to another, and from one allergen to another
- Anaphylaxis will be more severe, if there has been recent, repeated exposure to the allergen
- There may be a feeling of impending doom with nausea, vomiting, abdominal cramps and diarrhoea
- *Pruritis* which may develop rapidly, usually beginning with the palms of the hands and soles of the feet
- An *urticarial rash*, which may become confluent later, rhinitis and conjunctivitis
- *Angio-oedema* with swelling of the face, especially the lips and eyelids
- Pallor, limpness and apnoea (the commonest signs in children)
- *Laryngeal oedema* with stridor and hoarseness, and later cyanosis
- *Bronchospasm*, retrosternal tightness, dyspnoea, an audible expiratory wheeze, and pulmonary oedema
- An initial sinus tachycardia and peripheral vascular vasodilation progressing to profound shock with *hypotension* and a marked tachycardia, and finally to severe bradycardia, coma and cardiac arrest. Circulatory collapse may occur rapidly and without any skin or respiratory symptoms or signs

Note: The differential diagnosis of anaphylactic shock is a panic attack with hyperventilation and syncope

Management
- Rapidly assess the extent and severity of the symptoms
- Treat the patient according to the symptoms and their severity, and monitor the haemodynamic state
- Be prepared to treat aggressively if there are signs of laryngeal oedema, bronchospasm or shock

Reduce further absorption of the agent causing anaphylaxis
- For injections and stings apply a tourniquet proximal to the site
- Remove bee stings
- Stop administering injections
- Remove food allergens from the mouth, and if the patient is conscious rinse out the mouth with water
- Induce emesis of recently ingested food

Position
- Lay the patient flat with the legs elevated (to aid venous return and reduce hypotension due to dependent venous pooling), but not if the patient has breathing difficulties, when sitting them up may be best
- If the patient is unconscious, but their condition is otherwise satisfactory:
  - Put them into the recovery position

Epinephrine (adrenaline)
- Reverses all the effects of anaphylaxis; if the first dose is ineffective, administration may be repeated:
  - α-receptor antagonist:
    - Reverses peripheral dilation and reduces oedema
  - β- receptor antagonist:
    - Dilates the airways, increases the force of myocardial contraction, suppresses histamine and leukotriene release
- Most effective if administered soon after the onset of symptoms, so it should be administered immediately to all patients with anaphylaxis or a severe allergic reaction, unless there is a strong central pulse, their symptoms are only mild and their general condition is satisfactory
- Should be administered with caution intravenously as it may cause severe hypertension (headache), myocardial ischaemia and infarction, a profound tachycardia with dysrhythmias and severe vasospasm if administered intra-arterially
- Epinephrine may be less effective for late reactions or if the patient is on β-blockers
- Anaphylaxis is almost unknown in children under 2 years old, for whom epinephrine is rarely indicated
- The roles of all other drugs in the management of anaphylaxis are subsidiary to epinephrine

Epinephrine 1:1000 (one in a thousand)

Presentation:
- 1 mL 1/1000 solution in a preloaded syringe *(IMS)*

Administration:
- By deep intramuscular or subcutaneous injection
- In the case of a reaction due to injections or stings, the injection should be given close to the site

Dosage:

Age (yrs)	Dose (mg)	mL
<2	0.0625	0.0625 (dilute further)
2-5	0.125	0.125
6-11	0.25	0.25
>12	0.5	0.5 (use a smaller dose for elderly/those of slight build)

Epinephrine 1:10,000 (one in ten thousand)

Presentation:
- 10 mL 1/10,000 preloaded syringe *(IMS)*

Administration:
- By *slow* intravenous (or intraosseous in young children) injection over several minutes, titrated against the patient's response, and with careful monitoring of the patient's haemodynamic state
- The dose may be repeated at 5-15 minute intervals up to three times, depending on the response

Dosage:

Age (yrs)	Dose (mg)	mL
>2	0.0625	0.625
2-5	0.125	1.25
6-11	0.25	2..5
>12	0.5	5.0

Epinephrine 300 µg auto-injector (self administration device) (*Epipen®, Ana-Guard®*)
- Carried by many individuals who have a risk of anaphylaxis, e.g. previous anaphylactic reaction, nut allergy, food allergy and asthma

Descriptions:
- *Epipen®:*
    - This consists of a fully assembled syringe and needle delivering a dose of epinephrine 300 µg by intramuscular injection
    - A 150 µg version is available for use in children
- *Ana-Guard®:*
    - This consists of a pre-filled syringe capable of delivering two 300 µg doses of epinephrine by intramuscular or subcutaneous injection
    - The syringe can supply smaller doses for children

Discussion point: Administration of epinephrine: method and dosage
- There has been considerable debate about the correct dose and best way of administering epinephrine

Evidence

Subcutaneous/intramuscular routes
- In the past the subcutaneous/intramuscular routes of administration have been advised as the routes of choice (there is little difference between them, although some prefer the intramuscular route)
- It is easy to administer drugs by either route, and in the early stages of anaphylaxis, when there is urticaria with peripheral vasodilation, epinephrine administered by either route should enter the central circulation rapidly
- If the patient has become shocked with peripheral circulatory failure, epinephrine will not be absorbed satisfactorily if administered by either route

Intravenous route
- This is the ideal route for administering epinephrine in anaphylaxis, but it may be difficult for the inexperienced to find a vein, when the patient has generalised urticaria, or if the patient is shocked

Dosage
- There has been little scientific research into the optimal management of anaphyalaxis
- Intravenous epinephrine may cause:
    - Cardiac arrhythmias (tachyarrhythmias) with myocardial ischaemia and infarction
    - Severe hypertension
- These side effects will be minimised if the epinephrine is diluted

Conclusion
- Satisfactory absorption of epinephrine may be obtained by the subcutaneous/intramuscular routes before the patient becomes shocked, and should be used in most circumstances
- If the patient has severe anaphylaxis with circulatory collapse, the intravenous route is the most effective, and should be utilised with care
- It is suggested that for intravenous administration, epinephrine be diluted to 1:100000, and be administered slowly with constant monitoring of the patient's ECG and haemodynamic state

Antihistamines (H$_1$ blockers)
- Histamines should be administered routinely in all anaphylactic reactions to counter histamine mediated vasodilation

Chlorpheniramine *(Piriton®)*

Indications:
- Antihistamines are a useful adjunct to epinephrine, and oral administration of chlorpheniramine 4 mg 6 hourly may be continued for 24-48 hours after the initial intravenous dose, to prevent relapse
- Should be administered after epinephrine

Presentation:
- 1 mL ampoules 10 mg/mL.

Dosage:

Age (yrs)	Dose (mg)
1-5	2.5-5
6-11	5-10
>11	10-20

Administration:
- Intravenously, diluted in the syringe with 5-10 mL of blood and injected slowly over 1 minute (any side effects, e.g. drowsiness, giddiness and hypotension, should then be transient)

Airway

Oxygen
- Administer high-flow (10-15 litres/minute) oxygen, using a high concentration oxygen mask

Airway maintenance
- If the patient is unconscious, insert an oropharyngeal airway or pass a tracheal tube
- If there is stridor due to laryngeal oedema, consider:
    - Administration of nebulised epinephrine, preferably by oxygen driven nebuliser
    - Tracheal intubation using a gum elastic bougie (but this should *only* be attempted by the experienced intubator, as a clumsy or failed intubation will only increase laryngeal oedema and may precipitate complete airway obstruction)
- If there is severe airway obstruction due to laryngeal oedema, perform a cricothyrotomy *immediately*

Breathing: bronchospasm

Ventilation
- Ventilate the patient if there is no spontaneous respiration

Bronchospasm

Nebulised β$_2$ adrenergic stimulants } see under Medical emergencies: Asthma
Intravenous aminophylline

Steroids
- The role of steroids in the acute management of anaphylaxis is being increasingly questioned in pre-hospital care, unless travelling time to definitive care is very long, or the patient is asthmatic
- Steroids are slow to take effect (up to several hours) and have a short duration of action, but may reduce the incidence of delayed/recurrent symptoms, especially if there is bronchospasm
- If used, these should be administered as soon as possible after epinephrine (tablets are as effective as the intravenous route)

Hydrocortisone succinate/sodium phosphate

- *Presentation:*
  - Ampoules of:
    - Dry powder which has to be mixed with water (*Solu-Cortef®*) *or*
    - Solution: 100 mg/mL in 1, 5 mL ampoules (*Efcortisol®*)
- *Dosage:* (4 mg/kg)

Age (yrs)	Dose (mg)
1-5	50
6-11	100
>11	100-500

- *Administration:*
  - By slow intravenous injection over 0.5-1 minute

Prednisolone

- *Presentation:*
  - Tablets: 5, 25 mg
- *Dosage:*
  - 30-60 mg

Glucagon
- Administer glucagon 10 mg immediately if the patient is on β-blockers

Circulation

Circulatory support
- Basic life support if appropriate
- If the patient is shocked:
  - Secure intravenous access with two wide bore cannulae and infuse rapidly with colloid
- Consider the application of a pneumatic anti-shock garment (PASG)

Local allergic reaction

Infiltration with epinephrine
- This may be useful in cases of acute localised reactions to injections or insect bites
- Acts by causing local vasoconstriction, and hence reduces further systemic absorption
- Great care has to be taken not to administer epinephrine intra-arterially into the peripheral circulation, i.e. limbs, and fingers or toes, as peripheral gangrene due to arterial spasm may result

Monitoring
- All patients who have had a significant anaphylactic reaction, and in particular all patients who have shock necessitating the administration of epinephrine should be monitored for 8-24 hours following the resolution of symptoms, as there is the risk of both prolonged and biphasic anaphylactic reactions
- Monitoring should include:
  - SpO_2
  - Respiratory rate
  - Peak expiratory flow
  - Pulse volume and rate
  - Blood pressure
  - ECG

Guidelines for the management of anaphylactic shock

Primary survey/management

Remove the allergen

Position
- Lie the patient down, with their legs elevated

Airway
- Administer high-flow **oxygen** using a high concentration oxygen mask
- Check that the patient has a clear airway:
    - If the airway is clear:
        - Insert an oropharyngeal airway or tracheal tube (unless the patient is fully conscious)
    - If the airway is obstructed (due to laryngeal oedema):
        - Perform a cricothyrotomy *immediately*

Note: If there is stridor do *not* attempt tracheal intubation, unless you are very experienced

Breathing
- Check that the patient is breathing:
    - If there is no spontaneous breathing:
        - Ventilate the patient

Circulation
- Check for a pulse (radial or carotid)
    - If there is no pulse:
        - Administer external chest compressions
- **Administer Epinephrine 1:1,000**
    - By intramuscular injection, unless the patient is severely shocked, when it should be epinephrine 1:10,000, which should be administered slowly intravenous/intraosseously
    - This should be repeated at 5 minute intervals if there is no improvement
- If there is any evidence of hypotension:
    - Set up two **intravenous infusions** (of colloid or crystalloid), using wide bore cannulae
    - Consider application of a PASG

Disability (neurological)
- If the patient is unconscious:
    - Place in the recovery position

Secondary survey/management
- Consider the administration of:
    - Antihistamines (chlorpheniramine 10-20 mg) by slow intravenous injection
    - Steroids by slow intravenous injection, especially if there is bronchospasm
- If there is stridor, consider the administration of nebulised:
    - Epinephrine or budesonide
- If there is wheeze, respiratory distress or a reduced peak expiratory flow (indicating bronchospasm), administer:
    - Nebulised salbutamol and/or intravenous aminophylline

Figure 4-16 Guidelines for the management of anaphylaxis

5

Pain management

Pain management

Introduction

Definition: Pain is an unpleasant sensory and emotional experience associated with actual or potential
tissue damage, or described in terms of such damage

- Apart from any humanitarian reasons, effective pain management has a high priority in Immediate Care
following the preservation of life and the treatment of major injuries, as pain alone can cause significant
deterioration in the patient's condition, e.g.
    - The pain from an abdominal or chest injury, e.g. fractured ribs may prevent adequate chest expansion,
    reducing the tidal volume and and hence impairing ventilation and exacerbating any hypoxia
    - The severe pain from acute myocardial infarction and trauma may increase catecholamine release
    resulting in an increase in cardiac work, oxygen demand and blood pressure, at a time when cardiac
    activity and oxygen delivery are compromised and may result in an increase in haemorrhage
- The complete abolition of pain, however, may not always be desirable, as the onset of increased pain can
indicate further tissue injury, knowledge of which may be important during extrication, especially when
there is restricted or poor access to the patient
- Effective analgesia may allow accelerated evacuation and facilitate early transportation to definitive care
- The requirement for analgesia may vary from one individual to another

Anatomy/physiology
- Knowledge of the anatomy, physiology and psychology of pain is necessary, to achieve an understanding
of the different ways in which pain perception can be prevented or modified

Peripheral nerves
- Pain receptors (nociceptors):
    - Are present in the skin and most other tissues, including muscle, parietal pleura and periosteum,
    but not the lung, liver, spleen, or most of the brain
    - Respond to mechanical, thermal or chemical stimulation
- Pain sensation is transmitted to the spinal cord by either:
    - 'Fast' or 'C' fibres: small unmyelinated fibres conveying sharp, localised and short-lived pain
    - 'Slow' or 'A' fibres, which usually convey signals of touch, pressure and proprioception, but
    some of which ('Aδ') fibres may convey signals of diffuse, on-going pain

Neurotransmission
- Pain sensation is transmitted up the spinal cord via the opposite spinothalamic tract to the thalamus and
cerebral cortex, where it is interpreted
- In the spinal cord the transmission of pain impulses to the brain may be modified by input from other
sensory nerve fibres, and by descending inhibitory fibres

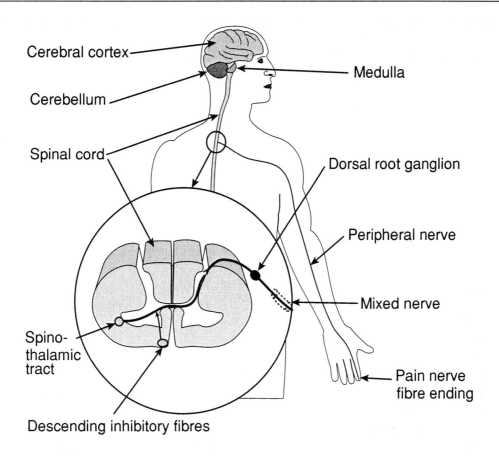

Figure 5-1 Nervous pain mediating pathways

Descending inhibition
- There is a system of descending nerve fibres which go back to the posterior grey column/dorsal horn cells, which have the effect of inhibiting or damping down incoming pain impulses

Wind up
- This is the process whereby both peripheral and central neurones becomes sensitised, resulting in amplification of the pain signal

Gate theory
- This is a theory which explains the processing of pain in the posterior grey column/dorsal horn of the spinal cord
- The wider open the gate, the more signals than can pass through it. The most significant control of the gate comes from the brain via the descending inhibitory nerve fibres, but the state of the gate may also be influenced by impulses from the periphery, e.g. touch (rubbing, massage, transcutaneous nerve stimulation) may reduce pain perception, or in some situations, e.g. if the patient is particularly anxious touch may actually intensify the perception of pain

Psychology
- Pain perception/interpretation may depend on a complex mixture of arousal, perception, emotion, interpretation and memory
- The soldier in battle or the driver of the vehicle anticipating an accident may produce a surge of epinephrine and other catecholamines which stimulate endorphins release, and modifies (reduces) pain perception
    - A notable historical example of this was the Marquis of Anglesey who had a leg shot off during the battle of Waterloo, but didn't realise it until the battle was over

Pathophysiology
- Pain causes an increase in circulating catecholamines resulting in vasoconstriction, tachycardia and hypertension
- This may cause reduced tissue perfusion and cellular damage, an increase in intracranial pressure, and myocardial ischaemia
- Pain may also cause an increase in muscle tone and metabolism, and can precipitate or exacerbate shock.
- In the hypovolaemic trauma patient pain may cause further impairment of the peripheral circulation, and increase tissue hypoxia
- In the patient with an acute myocardial infarction, pain will increase and the resulting tachycardia and increase in myocardial oxygen demand will aggravate myocardial ischaemia and infarction, and predispose the myocardium to arrhythmias

Symptoms/signs
- The nature and severity of pain may vary depending on its cause and the patient's state of mind
- Pain alone may cause:
    - Pallor with cold extremities, sweating and nausea
    - Tachycardia and hypertension

Assessment/measurement
- Pain assessment is important in Immediate Care, as severe pain by itself may be harmful
- It is important to detect changes in pain perception:
    - Increased pain may be caused by further injury, or ineffective analgesia
    - Decreased pain may result from reduced injury, e.g. effective splinting, effective analgesia or impairment of the nerve supply
- Pain can be very difficult to measure, as different patients may perceive pain in different ways, and different causes of pain may cause different types of pain. In Immediate Care, it is probably the severity of the pain that is the most important, rather than its character (although this may be important in making a diagnosis, especially in medical emergencies), as the more severe the pain the greater the physiological response,
- The quickest and most effective way to measure pain severity is by the Visual Analogue Scale. This consists of a 10 cm scale, one end of which is marked 'No pain' and the other 'Worst pain ever', with a numerical scale on the back. The patient is asked to mark their pain on the scale, with a slider. The scale can then be turned over to give them a precise score. In the pre-hospital situation, it may not be possible or practical to show them the scale, in which case the patient should be asked to score their pain out of 10 or 100
- The patient's pain perception should be assessed at regular intervals as is done with the vital signs

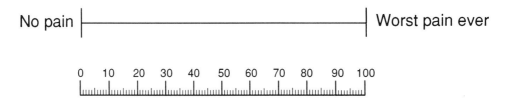

Figure 5-2 Visual analogue scale for measuring the severity of pain

Management

Airway care with cervical spine stabilisation in the case of trauma

Breathing with the maintenance of adequate ventilation and oxygen supplementation

Circulation care with control of haemorrhage

Disability

Exposure (if appropriate)

Pain management

- Treatment of the cause of the pain should be attempted where appropriate:
    - Splinting and reduction of fractures (which may itself require analgesia)
    - Reduction of dislocations
    - Removal of caustic substances
    - Surface dressing of burns
    - Surface cooling
- Analgesia (relief of pain):
    - Inhalational
    - Intravenous/intramuscular drugs
        - Opiates
        - NSAIDs
        - Sedatives
- Anaesthesia (loss of all sensation):
    - General
    - Local or regional

Note: Do not forget that simple reassurance, a calm voice, a held hand, and information about what is happening or going to happen (which may have to be repeated many times!) will help to minimise the patient's natural anxiety

---

Sites of action of different techniques for pain relief

Site	Technique
Pain nerve fibre ending	Local anaesthetic Simple analgesic NSAIDs
Peripheral nerve	Peripheral nerve block
Cerebral cortex	Opiate analgesics Sedatives Anaesthetic agents

Figure 5-3 Sites of action of different methods of pain relief

---

The ideal pre-hospital analgesic

- Effective
- Rapid onset
- Easily administered
- Packaging: small, tough, easily portable, easy to see
- Short duration of action: maximally 1-2 hours
- Cause minimal respiratory depression
- Have no negative inotropic effects
- Cause some sedation, without psychomimetic effects

Inhalational analgesic

Nitrous oxide/oxygen (*Entonox®/Nitronox®*)
Description
- A 50% mixture of nitrous oxide and oxygen
- Nitrous oxide is a gas, which liquefies at temperatures below -7°C, and is a strong analgesic at concentrations of 50%
- The analgesic effect of 50% nitrous oxide is equivalent to that obtained with 10 mg intravenous morphine
- Causes little sedation

Presentation
- Blue cylinders (usually size D for pre-hospital use) with a white and blue quartered collar

Administration
- The gas is usually self administered by mask or mouthpiece (which can be easier to use for the fully conscious patient or for children)
- Gas flow can only be triggered by the patient inspiring deeply whilst applying the face mask tightly to the face to ensure an airtight seal (unless the over-ride valve is depressed). This requires the patient to be conscious, able to co-ordinate and co-operative, and ensures that the patient doesn't continue to inhale the gas, if they become drowsy or unconscious due to the effects of the gas or for other reasons
- Some of the more recent giving sets are more compact than the original British Oxygen Company set, and have the demand valve connected to the mouthpiece enabling greater separation of cylinder and patient, and require a lower triggering pressure

Advantages
- It is rapidly effective (2-5 minutes) due to a combination of the low solubility of nitrous oxide in blood, which allows rapid equilibration with alveolar gas concentrations, and its low lipid solubility, which means that it is not redistributed in fat
- Its effect is rapidly reversible, due to its low fat solubility, and because it is excreted unchanged by the lungs
- The 50% oxygen content of the mixture is of benefit to the shocked or hypoxic patient

Disadvantages
- The two gases separate out at very low temperatures (below -7 °C), with oxygen which is less dense than nitrous oxide going to the top of the cylinder, which may result in the patient initially receiving pure oxygen (and no analgesia), followed by pure nitrous oxide, which is potentially dangerous:
    - Cylinders should therefore be stored horizontally and inverted several times before use in cold weather
    - If available, cylinders from a relatively warm ambulance interior should be used in preference to those from a cold car boot
- The apparatus is relatively heavy (6 kg), cumbersome, and expensive
- Portable cylinders only last about 20 minutes
- There is some danger of further depressing left ventricular function resulting in hypotension and heart failure, if it is combined with high doses of morphine in patients with impaired cardiac function However, it may be used in addition to morphine if heart failure can be excluded or is minimal

Contraindications
- Chest injuries, where there is a risk of pneumothorax (nitrous oxide is more soluble than nitrogen and diffuses into air filled body cavities faster than nitrogen can diffuse out, resulting in a build up of pressure causing a pneumothorax to become a tension pneumothorax)
- Use at high or low altitudes or after diving
- After major head injury, due to the possibility of an aerocele developing secondary to a skull fracture
- In cardiac failure

Precautions
- Due to its oxygen component, it should be used with care where there is a risk of combustion, e.g. where cutting equipment is being used

CONCLUSION: It is still the *analgesic of choice* for relief of mild to moderate pain in the pre-hospital situation, including cardiac pain

Systemic analgesics

Introduction
- As a general rule, the best drugs are those with which the user is familiar, and is confident to use

Administration
- Most analgesic drugs should *only* be given *intravenously, sublingually or by inhalation* in the Immediate Care situation, and *not intramuscularly or subcutaneously*
    - In the shocked and hypoperfused patient, drugs which have been administered intramuscularly may be poorly absorbed initially and thus be ineffective, but later as the patient's tissue perfusion improves, they may enter the circulation as a bolus, causing relative overdosage, e.g. opiates may cause respiratory depression and hypotension
- If drugs are administered intramuscularly following acute myocardial infarction, they may cause a spurious rise in muscle enzymes, which may cause diagnostic problems, and bruising if the patient is subsequently given thrombolytics
- The oral route is not recommended because:
    - Drugs administered by that route are slowly absorbed (1-1½ hours)
    - The increased risk of gastric aspiration if taken with a substantial amount of fluid (especially in trauma patients who may need a general anaesthetic once they reach hospital)
- It should be borne in mind when administering analgesics, that many patients suffering trauma may also have consumed alcohol, which may increase the side effects of the analgesic, and that the elderly and those who are not medically fit will require a smaller dosage
- Some analgesics, e.g. opiates and buprenorphine may cause hypotension and should therefore not be given to patients who are sitting, but only to those who are supine
- After analgesic administration, the patient's cardio-respiratory status should be monitored carefully at regular intervals with measurement of the:
    - Respiratory rate
    - SpO_2
    - Capnography
    - Pulse
    - Blood pressure

Opiates/opiate analogues

Description
- Opiates are very effective and are widely used, being the analgesics of choice for the relief of cardiac pain
- Opiate analgesics are thought to act at three principal receptor sites (other receptor sites do exist, but their clinical importance in Immediate Care is unclear):
    - *Mu* (µ) receptor stimulation results in:
        - Analgesia
        - Euphoria
        - Respiratory depression
    - *Kappa* (κ) receptor stimulation results in:
        - Central sedation without respiratory depression
        - Spinal level analgesia
    - *Sigma* (σ) receptor stimulation results in:
        - Psychomimetic effects including delirium

- Their overall effects include:
    - A strong centrally acting analgesic effect
    - Relief of anxiety and fear
    - Peripheral vasodilation

Administration
- By slow intravenous injection. The elderly require a reduced dose

Major problems
- They are 'Controlled Drugs', which means that they have to be kept securely, and there are special regulations regarding their prescribing, storage and stock control (see page 143)

Disadvantages
- They may cause:
    - Nausea and vomiting, especially during transport, and although these symptoms are rarely seen in the patient with very severe pain, opiates should be administered with an antiemetic such as metoclopramide
    - Respiratory depression
    - Hypotension (due to peripheral vasodilation), which may aggravate or precipitate shock
    - Drowsiness
    - Constricted pupils
- They should be *used with caution*, and are not contraindicated *in the head injured patient*. They should be used with caution when there is respiratory embarrassment, shock, or where there is a history of chest disease or asthma

Note: Naloxone, a competitive opiate antagonist should always be available when opiates or their analogues are administered, in case of overdosage (see below)

Morphine sulphate injection

Description
- A potent and effective analgesic, with anxiolytic properties
- It has a rapid onset and a duration of action of about two hours, which may cause prolonged masking of the vital signs

Presentation
- 10, 15, 30 mg/mL in 1 and 2 mL ampoules

Dosage
- Best given in small incremental doses, titrated to the patient's requirements
- Adults:
    - 5-10 mg initially followed by aliquots of 1-2 mg every few minutes up to a maximum of 20-25 mg or until satisfactory pain relief is achieved. Peak effect occurs at around 15 minutes
- Children:
    - 0.1-0.2 mg/kg

Disadvantages
- Prone to cause:
    - Nausea and vomiting
    - Respiratory depression
    - Hypotension

Morphine sulphate/cyclizine (*Cyclimorph®*)

Presentation
- Cyclimorph 10: 10 mg morphine tartrate, cyclizine 50 mg in 1 mL ampoule
- Cyclimorph 15: 15 mg morphine tartrate, cyclizine 50 mg in 1 mL ampoule

Advantages
- Cyclizine is an anti-histamine which is most effective for the treatment of nausea and vomiting due to motion sickness and labyrinthine disorders

Disadvantages
- Cyclizine has been shown to cause coronary artery spasm and an increase in pulmonary artery pressure which may aggravate severe heart failure, and counteract the beneficial haemodynamic effects of opiates if administered following an acute myocardial infarction

Dosage
- Adults: 10-15 mg initially

CONCLUSION: A convenient combination preparation that is *widely used* in Immediate Care, but should be administered with caution to the patient who has just had an acute myocardial infarction

Diamorphine

Description
- About twice as potent as morphine with a more rapid onset (due to its greater lipid solubility when compared to morphine) and shorter duration of action (2 hours)
- Possibly more sedative and less likely to cause nausea/vomiting and hypotension than morphine, but has a greater euphoric effect

Presentation
- 5 mg or 10 mg as a dry powder

Dosage
- Adults: 2.5-7.5 mg initially followed by aliquots of 0.5-1 mg every few minutes up to a maximum of 10 mg or until satisfactory pain relief is achieved

Disadvantages
- Presented as a powder and has to be reconstituted, just prior to administration
- May cause profound respiratory depression

CONCLUSION: The opiate of choice for the relief of cardiac pain (in combination with an anti-emetic)

Pethidine hydrochloride

Description
- A less potent analgesic than morphine/diamorphine, and is more likely to increase the heart rate
- Rapid onset of action (5 minutes) and relatively short acting (2-3+ hours)
- It has anti-spasmodic properties (useful in renal and biliary colic)

Presentation
- 50 mg/mL in 1 and 2 mL ampoules

Dosage
- Adults: 50-100 mg intravenously administered as an initial dose of 25-50 mg followed by aliquots of 10 mg up to a maximum of 100 mg or until satisfactory pain relief is achieved

Disadvantages
- May cause respiratory depression, nausea/vomiting and marked hypotension
- Contraindicated in patients taking a MAOI, e.g. tranylcypromine (*Parnate®*), phenelzine *(Nardil®)*

CONCLUSION: A popular alternative to morphine but is *not widely used* in Immediate Care

Synthetic opiate analogues

Pentazocine (*Fortral®*)

Description
- A mixed opiate agonist/antagonist (therefore only partially reversed by naloxone)
- It is much less effective as an analgesic than morphine

Presentation
- 30 mg/mL in 1 and 2 mL ampoules

Dosage
- Adults: 30-60 mg
- Children: 0.5-1 mg/kg

Disadvantages
- Hallucinogenic and should not be used in the patient with respiratory depression or a head injury
- Can cause an increase in heart rate, blood pressure and cardiac work and should not be used in acute myocardial infarction

CONCLUSION: Not widely used in Immediate Care, and *not particularly effective*

Alfentanil hydrochloride (*Rapifen®*)

Description
- A new potent narcotic analgesic, with a rapid onset of action and a very short half life
- Opiate agonist reversible by naloxone

Presentation
- 500 µg in 2 and 10 mL ampoules
- It is also available as:
    - Rapifen dilute: 100 µg/mL in 5 mL ampoules (500 µg)
    - Rapifen concentrate: 5 mg/mL in 1 mL ampoules

Dosage
- Adults:
    - 500 µg initial bolus given over 30 seconds
- Children:
    - 30-50 µg/kg initially followed by increments of 15 µg/kg (children metabolise alfentanil more rapidly than adults)
- The peak effect takes about 90 seconds, giving profound analgesia for 5-10 minutes. Further increments of 250 µg may be given as required

Disadvantages
- Causes profound respiratory depression, and is contra-indicated where there are respiratory problems
- May cause:
    - Transient hypotension, and bradycardia leading to asystole reversible by atropine (so the pulse must be carefully monitored)
    - Muscle spasms (rigidity), so ideally a muscle relaxant should be given first (not often practical in Immediate Care)
- Concomitant medication with erythromycin may result in impaired alfentanil metabolism

CONCLUSION: Not recommended for use in Immediate Care at present

Buprenorphine (*Temgesic®*)

Description
- Long acting (6-8 hours) synthetic mixed opiate agonist/antagonist, approximately thirty times as potent as morphine
- Only partially reversible by naloxone, this may cause problems if:
    - The patient requires stronger (opiate) analgesia, as it competes with conventional opiates and may block them from receptor sites, resulting in a reduced analgesic effect
    - Administered to an opiate abuser; it may result in opiate withdrawal symptoms

Presentation
- 200/400 µg: small sublingual tablet
- 300 µg/mL in 1 and 2 mL ampoules

Dosage
- Sublingually: 200-400 µg initially
- Intravenously: 300-600 µg

Disadvantages
- Can cause:
    - Nausea/vomiting (in 15-20% of patients, more marked in the elderly)
    - Drowsiness, dizziness, confusion and psychomimetic symptoms
    - Severe respiratory depression (rarely)
- In the UK it is a 'Controlled Drug' and subject to the same legal restrictions as conventional opiates

CONCLUSION: Not recommended for use in Immediate Care

Nalbuphine hydrochloride (*Nubain®*)

Description
- A long acting semi-synthetic opioid analgesic, with mixed opiate agonist/antagonist properties, fully or partially reversible by naloxone, indicated for moderate to severe pain, including cardiac pain
- It has somewhat less efficacy, but fewer side effects than morphine, especially nausea, vomiting and cardiovascular side effects. It has also been suggested that it causes less respiratory depression, but this should be treated with caution and the patient's respiratory status monitored after nalbuphine administration
- Rapid onset of action after iv administration (2-3 minutes), with a long duration of action (3-6 hours)
- Because of its mixed opiate agonist/antagonist properties, morphine may be less effective if administered after nalbuphine has already been used

Presentation
- 10 mg/mL: 1 and 2 mL ampoules

Dosage
- 10-20 mg administered slowly intravenously until analgesia is achieved (a further 20 mg may be administered after 30 minutes if necessary; further increments rarely produce any greater analgesia)

Advantages
- A reasonably effective analgesic which causes less nausea and vomiting than other opioids
- It does not have any cardiovascular effects in patients with a healthy cardiovascular system
- It is not a controlled drug (at present)

Disadvantages
- It may cause some respiratory depression
- It may also cause sedation and less frequently, sweating, nausea, vomiting, dizziness, dry mouth, vertigo and headache
- Use of nalbuphine will affect the effectiveness of subsequent opiate analgesic administration

CONCLUSION: Considered to be *the best synthetic opioid, and is used by many ambulance services*

Naloxone (*Narcan®* and *Narcan Neonatal®*)

Description
- A specific opiate antagonist used to treat opiate overdosage, especially respiratory depression induced by natural/synthetic opioids, and the mixed opiate agonists/antagonists pentazocine and buprenorphine

Presentation
- Naloxone hydrochloride 400 µg/mL: 1 and 2 mL ampoules
- Narcan Neonatal: 20 µg/mL: 2 mL ampoule

Dosage
- Adults:
    - 200-400 µg as an intravenous bolus, repeated at 2-3 minute intervals if there is no improvement in respiratory function up to a maximum of 10 mg
    - Larger doses are required for the treatment of overdosage with mixed opiate agonists/antagonists than for pure agonists, when it may be better to administer naloxone intramuscularly and assist ventilation in order to prevent acute opiate withdrawal
    - It has a short duration of action (half life: 1 hour), and further increments may be necessary
- Children:
    - 10 µg/kg intravenously initially up to a maximum of 100 µg

CONCLUSION: An *essential* drug for the Immediate Care practitioner to carry

Non steroidal anti-inflammatory drugs (NSAIDs)
- Although these drugs may appear superficially to be suitable for pre-hospital emergency use, they do have several important disadvantages:
    - In hypovolaemia:
        - They may cause a reduction in renal prostaglandins synthesis resulting in renal failure
        - They may inhibit platelet aggregation and increase the tendency to bleed
    - They may precipitate bronchospasm in asthmatics, and peptic ulceration and bleeding
    - They should not be used to provide analgesia in labour

Diclofenac (*Voltarol®*)

Description
- An NSAID with marked analgesic and anti-inflammatory properties, which has been shown to be as effective as pethidine when used for pain relief in renal and biliary colic. It may potentiate the analgesic effects of opiates when used in musculoskeletal injuries
- It has a relatively slow onset of action and lasts for 6-10 hours

Presentation
- 25 mg/mL: 3 mL ampoule

Dosage
- 75 mg.
- In renal colic the dose may be repeated after 30 minutes depending on response

Administration
- By deep *intramuscular* (intragluteal) injection, which can cause induration and local pain. In the shocked patient, it may only be poorly absorbed
- By slow intravenous injection, but not if the patient is hypovolaemic

Advantages
- Causes little sedation or respiratory depression

Disadvantages
- Can cause gastrointestinal haemorrhage and ulceration

CONCLUSION: *Useful for providing pre-hospital analgesia for renal/biliary colic*; diclofenac *may also have a role* in providing additional analgesia for patients with fractures, but should be used with caution if the patient is hypovolaemic

Ketoprofen (*Oruvail®*)

Description
- An NSAID with marked analgesic properties, which has been shown to be as effective as pethidine, morphine and pentazocine when used for the relief of pain from musculoskeletal injuries
- It has a rapid onset of action and lasts for approximately four hours

Presentation
- 50 mg/mL: 2 mL ampoule

Dosage
- 50-200 mg

Administration
- By deep *intramuscular* (intragluteal) injection

Advantages
- Causes little sedation or respiratory depression

Disadvantages
- Can cause gastrointestinal problems including ulceration
- Contraindicated in patients with renal problems

CONCLUSION: *May have a role* as an analgesic in Immediate Care, especially for providing additional analgesia for patients with fractures, but should be used with caution if the patient is hypovolaemic

Ketorolac (*Toradol®*)

Description
- A NSAID with marked analgesic properties, which has been shown to be almost as effective as intramuscular pethidine and morphine, when used for the relief of pain from musculoskeletal injuries
- It has a rapid onset of action resulting in significant analgesia within 30 minutes and maximum analgesia within 1-2 hours and lasts for approximately six hours

Presentation
- 30 mg/mL:1 mL ampoule

Dosage
- 30 mg, initially then 10-30 mg every 4-6 hours as required. Not recommended for those under 12 yrs
- The dose should be reduced in the elderly as ketorolac is excreted mainly by the kidneys and excretion may be delayed in the elderly and those with impaired renal function

Administration
- By deep *intramuscular* (intragluteal) injection. In the shocked patient, it may only be poorly absorbed and should be given intravenously

Advantages
- Causes little sedation or respiratory depression

Disadvantages
- Can cause gastrointestinal problems including ulceration, but is associated with significantly less gastric or rectal mucosa injury than many other NSAIDs
- Contraindicated in patients with renal problems

CONCLUSION: *May have a role* as an analgesic in Immediate Care, especially for providing additional pain relief for patients with fractures, but should be used with caution in the young or elderly, or if the patient is hypovolaemic

Other non opiate analgesics
- There has been little experience in Immediate Care of the use of many of the newer analgesics, and what little use there has been has failed to show that they offer any significant advantages over opiates

Tramadol (*Zydol®*)

Description
- A new centrally acting analgesic with a dual mode of action; it:
    - Is a weak selective pure agonist at μ, δ, or κ opioid receptors
    - Inhibits neuronal uptake of norepinephrine and serotonin, thus enhancing spinal inhibitory systems

Presentation
- 50 mg/mL: 2 mL ampoule.

Dosage
- 50-100 mg, administered slowly intravenously over 2-3 minutes
- Precipitation may occur if tramadol is mixed in the same syringe with injections of diazepam, diclofenac or midazolam

Administration
- Given *intravenously or intramuscularly* when 15-20 minutes is required for the onset of action but it lasts up to 6 hours

Advantages
- Causes little sedation or respiratory depression compared to opiates
- It is not a 'Controlled Drug'

Disadvantages
- Not recommended for patients suffering from acute intoxication with hypnotics, centrally acting analgesics, or psychotrophic drugs

CONCLUSION: A new drug that is *gaining some acceptance* in the pre-hospital situation

Nefopam (*Acupan®*)

Description
- A new analgesic unrelated to either opiates or NSAIDs, which does not affect the vital signs, and is less likely than narcotics to cause sedation

Presentation
- 20 mg/mL: 1 mL ampoule

Dosage
- 20 mg

Administration
- Given *intramuscularly*, it takes 15-20 minutes to act and lasts for up to 6 hours

Disadvantages
- Contraindicated in patients with a history of epilepsy, and those taking monoamine-oxidase inhibitors (MAOIs)

CONCLUSION: Should not be used for analgesia in myocardial infarction, as there is no clinical experience of its use in this situation
It is best used for musculoskeletal pain and can be used in the head injured patient
Its value in Immediate Care is *unproven*

Sedating agents

Benzodiazepines
- These have anxiolytic and anti-convulsant properties, and can potentiate the effect of analgesics
- Retrograde amnesia may occur
- At high doses they have an anaesthetic effect
- Should be administered with caution if administered concurrently with opiates as increased respiratory and cardiovascular depression may occur

Diazepam

Description
- Relatively long acting, and fat soluble

Presentation
- Intravenous injection:
    - *Valium*® (aqueous solution, which is highly irritant, causes local pain, inflammation and phlebitis)
    - *Diazemuls*® (an emulsion which causes no inflammation or pain on injection):
        - 5 mg/mL: 2 mL ampoules
- Rectal infusion (*Stesolid*®):
    - 2 mg/mL, 4 mg/mL: tubes of 2.5 mL (5, 10 mg)

Dosage
- Intravenously:
    - 10-30 mg:
        - Initially give a 5-10 mg bolus then administer the next 10 mg in 2 mg boluses over 30 minutes, titrated to the patient's response, e.g. ptosis
- Rectally:
    - Adults: 10 mg
    - Children (1-3 yrs): 5 mg, over 3 yrs: 10 mg
    - The elderly: 5 mg

Disadvantages
- *Valium*® is highly irritant and should only be given into a large vein (or rectally in children)
- May cause apnoea and more rarely hypotension

CONCLUSION: There are better benzodiazepines for use in Immediate Care (see below)

Midazolam (*Hypnovel*®)

Description
- A short acting water soluble benzodiazepine, which at body pH becomes lipid soluble and hence centrally acting
- In pre-hospital care, it is used mainly as a sedating agent, but can be used as an anaesthetic

Presentation
- Ampoules of: 10 mg/2 mL, 10 mg/5 mL (probably best for pre-hospital use)

Dosage
- 10 µg/kg initially, i.e. 7 mg for a 70 kg man

Administration
- It is given intravenously with the dose carefully titrated against the patient's response, as apnoea may occur even at very small doses

Half life
- Midazolam has a half life of about 2 hours

Advantages
  - Speed of onset of action, short half-life, anti-convulsant properties, excellent antegrade amnesic properties, an antiemetic effect, and minimal overall side effects
  - May be used concurrently with opiates, provided that the respiratory status of the patient is monitored
  - If it causes any problems, its effect may be rapidly reversed by flumazenil (see below)

Disadvantages
  - May (rarely) cause respiratory depression associated with severe hypotension, and should be administered with caution, especially to the elderly and those with cardiorespiratory disease
  - Once midazolam is administered, it will impair the patient's conscious level for some time, (and make monitoring difficult)

Note: Midazolam is often used with ketamine

CONCLUSION: In Immediate Care it can be *very useful* for sedating the head injured patient who is hypoxic and violent, and for tranquillising the very anxious, however as always, care of the airway and ventilation to ensure adequate oxygenation must remain paramount

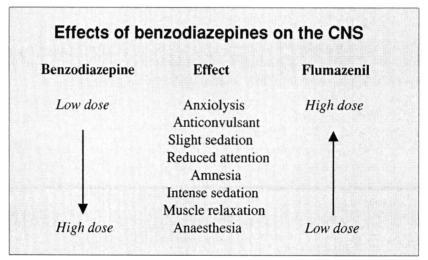

Effects of benzodiazepines on the CNS

Benzodiazepine	**Effect**	**Flumazenil**
Low dose	Anxiolysis	*High dose*
	Anticonvulsant	
	Slight sedation	
	Reduced attention	
	Amnesia	
	Intense sedation	
	Muscle relaxation	
High dose	Anaesthesia	*Low dose*

Figure 5-4 Effects of benzodiazepines on the central nervous system

Flumazenil (*Anexate*®)

Description
  - The first specific benzodiazepine antagonist

Action
  - A benzodiazepine itself, it acts by competing for, and then blocking benzodiazepine receptors

Indications
  - Reversal of benzodiazepine induced central sedative and respiratory effects

Presentation
  - 100 µg/mL: 5 mL ampoule

Dosage
  - Administer by slow intravenous infusion, titrated against patient response
  - Initially 200 µg should be given over 15 seconds, with a further 100 µg every 60 seconds as necessary. Usual dose 300-600 µg, the maximum dose is 1 mg
  - It has a rapid onset of action, and a short duration of action, which can result in re-emergence of the effects of the original benzodiazepine after as little as 70 minutes
  - Should be administered with care as cardiac arrhythmias may be precipitated

CONCLUSION: An *essential drug* if benzodiazepines are carried for pre-hospital use

Anaesthetic agent

Ketamine (*Ketalar®*)

Description
- Ketamine is an anaesthetic agent unrelated to other anaesthetic agents, with analgesic properties in sub-anaesthetic doses
- Ketamine increases pulse rate, cardiac output, blood pressure and muscle tone by direct CNS stimulation
- Ketamine does *not* cause:
    - Significant depression of the pharyngeal reflexes (but protection of the airway cannot be guaranteed, so airway care must be meticulous in the patient anaesthetised with ketamine)
    - Respiratory depression in analgesic doses
- Ketamine has a mild bronchodilator effect and is safe for use with asthmatics

Presentation
- 10 mg/mL: 20 mL vials, 50 mg/mL: 10 mL vials, 100 mg/mL: 5 mL vials

Dosage
- Analgesia:
    - Intravenously: 0.25- 0.5 mg/kg by slow injection
    - Intramuscularly: 0.5-1.0 mg/kg
- Anaesthesia:
    - Intravenously:
        - 1-2 mg/kg administered over at least 60 seconds usually gives good anaesthesia which is effective in 30-60 seconds and lasts for 5-10 minutes
    - Intramuscularly:
        - 8-10 mg/kg gives surgical anaesthesia in 3-4 minutes lasting 15-25 minutes (but absorption may be unreliable, especially in the hypovolaemic)

Contraindications
- Hypertension
- Head injury

Advantages
- Has a hypertensive action and is particularly useful in field amputations (but it may exacerbate pre-existing hypotension in the already hypovolaemic and shocked trauma patient, in whom no further cardiac stimulation is possible and the peripheral vasodilating effect is unmasked)

Disadvantages
- May induce unpleasant dose related nightmares with or without psychomotor activity manifested by confusion and irrational behaviour, 'emergence delirium' (these can be minimised by concurrent administration of diazepam or midazolam)
- May not be effective in the alcoholic
- May cause respiratory depression if administered too rapidly intravenously

CONCLUSION: Its value in immediate care is *underrated*, but it should *not* be used by the inexperienced

Local anaesthesia

- The advantages of local anaesthesia in the pre-hospital situation include:
    - Almost complete analgesia in an injured limb with relief of muscle spasm allows free movement of the limb for manipulation and reduction of fractures, application of splintage and during extrication
    - Rapid onset and short duration of action
    - Relative lack of systemic effects, e.g. respiratory depression, impairment of consciousness or protective airway reflexes which is a particular advantage if the patient is medically unfit
- In the pre-hospital situation, there may however, be problems due to lack of operator expertise, access to the injection site, difficulty in obtaining sterile conditions and local complications due to problems with distorted local anatomy due to trauma and an enhanced risk of inadvertent intravascular injection and toxicity

Local anaesthetic agents

Lidocaine/lignocaine hydrochloride (*Xylocaine®/Lidocaine®*)

Presentation
- 0.5, 1, 1.5 or 2% solutions with or without epinephrine, in a large variety of sizes, and containers:
    - Ampoules, vials and pre-filled syringes

Dosage
- Adults:
    - 3 mg/kg maximum equivalent to 0.3 mL/kg of a 1% solution (21 mL for a 70 Kg adult).
- 'Lidocaine with epinephrine' is best avoided in Immediate Care as intra-arterial injection or injection into digits results in severe vasoconstriction and may lead to peripheral gangrene and loss of the digit or limb

Advantages
- Rapid onset of action with good tissue penetration
- Stable over a wide range of temperatures

Side effects
- Restlessness, tremors and convulsions
- Cardiac and respiratory depression

CONCLUSION: The *most widely used* local anaesthetic

Bupivacaine *(Marcaine®)*

Description
- A newer more potent and longer acting local anaesthetic than lidocaine

Presentation
- 0.25, 0.5% solutions with or without epinephrine and 0.75% plain solution, in 10 mL ampoules.

Dosage
- Adults:
    - 0.5% up to 30 mL for a peripheral block
    - 0.25% up to 60 mL for local infiltration

Disadvantages
- Prolonged period of onset of action
- Accidental intravenous injection may cause severe toxic reactions including refractory ventricular fibrillation

CONCLUSION: It is a useful local anaesthetic where prolonged action is required, but its use is *best avoided in the patient who is shocked*

Nerve blocks
- Nerve blocks are excellent for providing short duration, but very effective analgesia with abolition of muscle spasm in limbs (especially useful for facilitating free movement of injured limbs for extrication or splintage)
- Require skill, but with practice has a small failure rate

Femoral nerve block
- Probably the most useful block in Immediate Care, as it is relatively easy to give
- It produces deep anaesthesia over the medial part of the thigh and lower leg, including the periosteum
- The nerve lies just lateral to and slightly deeper than the femoral artery

Indications
- Fractured shaft of femur
- Severe quadriceps muscle spasm

Method:
- Identify the anterior superior iliac crest, the pubic tubercle, and the inguinal ligament
- The injection is given 1-2 cm lateral to the femoral pulse, just below the inguinal ligament at a depth of about 3-4 cm, while withdrawing gently on the plunger of the syringe, to indicate penetration of the femoral fascia
- Re-aspirate to make certain that the femoral artery has not been punctured and inject about 10-15 mL of 1% lidocaine, *without epinephrine*, or 10 mL of 0.5% plain bupivacaine, moving the needle fanwise
- Aspirate regularly to make sure the needle is not in the femoral artery

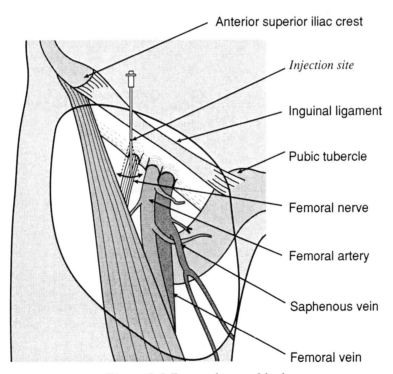

Figure 5-5 Femoral nerve block

Complications
- Femoral artery puncture
- Acute local anaesthetic toxicity
- Neuropathy (nerve damage)
- Infection

Brachial plexus nerve block
- May be very difficult to perform and is best left to the expert!

Wrist nerve block
- Blocks of the radial, ulnar or median nerves are possible, but are of limited use in Immediate Care

Digital nerve block
- Blocks of fingers and toes may be useful where these are trapped in machinery

Method:
- Insert the needle at the base of the finger on the extensor surface on one side of the finger and push the needle in down the side of the phalanx and inject 1-2 mL of lidocaine alongside the digital nerve.
- Repeat the process on the other side of the finger, and wait for anaesthesia (up to 10 minutes)

Ankle nerve block
- Similar to the wrist

Intercostal nerve block
- May be use in the patient with a flail chest, in whom pain is impairing their respiratory effort, but there is a risk of pneumothorax

Indications
- Multiple rib fractures causing pain severe enough to impair respiration

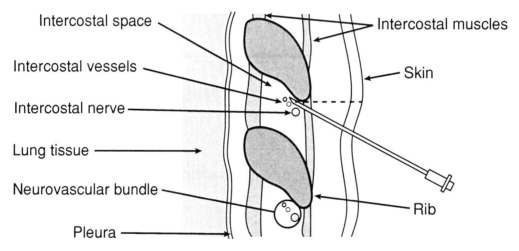

Fig 5-6 Intercostal nerve block

Method:
- Pull down the skin over the rib and insert the needle just beneath the rib, perpendicular to the skin, about 6-7 cm lateral to the spinous process of the vertebra (if accessible), until it comes into contact with the lower border of the rib
- Withdraw the needle a little and then advance it aiming towards the head at an angle of 10-20° to the skin sliding it over the lower border of the rib, as you do so
- Aspirate to make certain that the pleura or a blood vessel has not been punctured, and inject 5 mL of lidocaine 1%, or bupivicaine

Complications
- Pneumothorax
- Acute local anaesthetic toxicity

Controlled drugs regulations

The law

Misuse of Drugs Act 1971
- The basic law governing the supply and use of controlled drugs is the Misuse of Drugs Act 1971, which prohibits the manufacture, supply or possession of 'Controlled drugs'
- The penalties applied to offences involving these drugs are graded broadly according to the harmfulness of the drug when misused

Class A
- Alfentanyl, cocaine, diamorphine, opium, LSD, methadone, morphine, opium, pethidine and class B substances in injectable form

Class B
- Oral amphetamines, barbiturates, cannabis, cannabis resin, codeine, pentazocine and pholcodeine

Class C
- Some amphetamine related compounds, buprenorphine, most benzodiazepines, androgenic and anabolic steroids and human and non-human chorionic gonadotrophins

Misuse of Drugs Regulations 1985
- In 1985 the drugs were reclassified into schedules 1 to 5 by the Misuse of Drugs Regulations 1985, each of which specifies the requirements such as import, export, production, supply, possession, prescribing and record keeping which applies
- It also defines the classes of person authorised to supply/possess controlled drugs whist acting in their professional capacities, and lays down the conditions under which these activities may be carried out

Schedule 1 drugs
- Drugs such as LSD and cannabis, which are not used medicinally
- Possession and supply are prohibited, except in accordance with Home Office authority

Schedule 2 drugs
- Opiates and some opiate analogues (controlled drugs) including: morphine, diamorphine, pethidine, and amphetamines in medical use
- Subject to the full controlled drugs regulations relating to prescriptions, safe custody, registers, etc., unless exempted in Schedule 5

Schedule 3 drugs
- Barbiturates, pentazocine, diethylpropion, temazepam and buprenorphine
- Subject to the special prescription requirements (except phenobarbitone and temazepam), but not to the safe custody requirements (except buprenorphine, diethylpropion and temazepam) nor the need to keep registers, although there are requirements to keep receipts for 2 years

Schedule 4 drugs
- Benzodiazepines, androgenic and anabolic steroids and human/non-human chorionic gonadotrophins
- Subject to control regulations; but not subject to control drug prescriptions or safe custody regulations

Schedule 5 drugs
- This exempts those medicines which contain small quantities of the drugs mentioned in schedule 4, from control, e.g. those containing codeine, dihydrocodeine, pholcodeine and dextropropoxyphene

Possession and supply of controlled drugs
- Doctors, acting in their professional capacity, have authority to possess and supply these drugs
- They may administer or direct any other qualified person to administer such drugs

Safe custody of controlled drugs
- Doctors must keep Schedule 2 controlled drugs and buprenorphine in a locked receptacle that can only be opened by them or somebody authorised by them

Note: 1. A locked car is not considered to be a locked receptacle, but a locked case inside a locked car is acceptable. A locked glove compartment in a locked car is not acceptable
2. This can present a considerable problem especially for doctors involved in Immediate Care, as they need to keep their emergency drugs including opiates ready for instant use. It is suggested that they carry the minimum quantity of controlled drugs, and should keep them in a locked car safe

Controlled drug registers
- Doctors must keep a register of Schedule 2 drugs and buprenorphine, which must be bound, rather than loose leaf, for recording all transactions relating to these drugs. There should be an 'in' and 'out' page for each separate drug, and for each strength of each drug
- All entries must be in chronological order, made within 24 hrs of supplying or obtaining a drug. The 'in' page must show the date of purchase, the supplier, the name, quantity and strength of the drug supplied The 'out' page must state the date of supply of the drug together with the name and address of the patient to whom the drug was supplied, and the strength and quantity of the drug
- Entries must be in ink and no entries may be cancelled, obliterated or altered. Any correction must be made with an explanatory marginal note or footnote, which must be dated
- Registers must be preserved for 2 years since the last entry, and should be available for Home Office inspectors (who have the right of entry) to examine them without warning (they may also inspect a doctor's stock of controlled drugs)

Destruction of controlled drugs
- Doctors may not destroy opiates in their stock, except in the presence of someone authorised by the Secretary of State. Such persons include Home Office Inspectors, Regional Medical Officers, Health Authority Medical Advisors and all police officers
- A record must be made of the quantity destroyed, and the date on which they were destroyed, and must be signed by the authorised person

Prescriptions for controlled drugs: Drugs in schedules 2 and 3
- These must be hand written in indelible ink by the prescriber in full, including their usual signature and the date (which alone may be stamped), and must contain:
    - The name and address of the patient
    - The form of the preparation: tablets, capsules and description if appropriate, e.g. s/r (slow release)
    - The strength and the dose to be taken
    - The total number of tablets, capsules or ampoules (or total volume of a liquid) in words and figures

Importation/exportation of controlled drugs
- Patients may only carry 15 days' supply of any Schedule 2 or 3 controlled drugs for their own use
- If high doses are prescribed/the treatment is for 15 days or more, a Home Office licence may be required

Licence for importation of controlled drugs
- Doctors importing schedule 2 and 3 drugs into the UK must have a personal valid Home Office licence, which is renewable annually
- This is of particular importance for doctors doing aeromedical work, who may wish to carry these drugs with them on flights to treat patients and bring them back into the country if not used

6

Cardiac care: anatomy, physiology and the ECG

Cardiac anatomy, physiology and the ECG

Introduction

- An understanding of the anatomy and physiology of the heart together with the ability to interpret an ECG (electrocardiogram) accurately is essential for the informed, proficient practice of pre-hospital cardiac care

Anatomy
- The heart is a powerful cone shaped hollow muscular organ, about the same size as its owner's fist
- It is situated in the mediastinum between the lungs, lying obliquely more to the left than the right with its base lying towards the patient's head and its apex pointing down and to the left
- The heart lies within a fibrous sac, the outer or parietal pericardium, and is covered by a serous membrane, the visceral pericardium

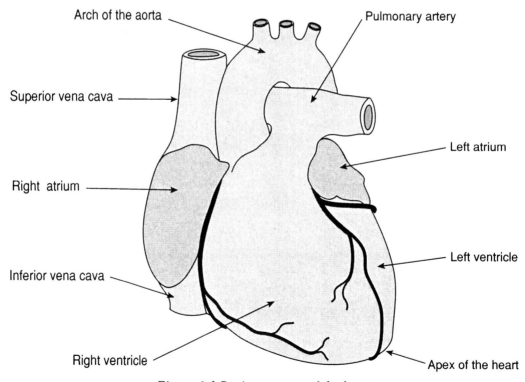

Figure 6-1 Basic anatomy of the heart

- The heart itself is composed of specialised cardiac muscle, the myocardium, together with its arteries and veins, and is lined on the inside by endocardium
- The heart is divided into right and left sides by a septum; the inter ventricular septum, and each side is further divided by a fibrous atrioventricular ring, into thin walled upper chambers, the atria, and lower thick walled chambers, the ventricles. The left ventricle is larger than the right ventricle
- The chambers of each side of the heart are connected by an atrioventricular valve:
    - The right atrioventricular valve has three cusps and is known as the tricuspid valve
    - The left atrioventricular valve has two valves and is called the mitral valve
- The valves are prevented from everting (opening upwards) into the atria by fibrous strands; the chordae tendinae which are attached to the inferior surface of the valve and run down to projections on the inner surface of the myocardium called the papillary muscles
- Each ventricle empties into to a major artery by a three cusped valve; the pulmonary artery and pulmonary valve on the right side of the heart, and the aorta and aortic valve on the left side of the heart
- The myocardium has its own blood supply, the right and left coronary arteries, which take their blood supply from near the beginning of the arch of the aorta, just distal to the aortic valve. The coronary veins drain into the coronary sinus, which in turn empties into the right atrium

Physiology

Right side of the heart
- The right atrium collects venous blood from the two main veins of the body, the superior vena cava from the top of the body and the inferior vena cava from the lower half of the body
- When the right atrium contracts (atrial systole), it pumps venous blood through the tricuspid valve into the relaxed right ventricle. It then relaxes (atrial diastole), allowing more venous blood to flow in and fill its chamber
- Immediately the right atrium has finished contracting and begun to relax, the right ventricle contracts (ventricular systole), causing the tricuspid valve to close and forcing open the pulmonary valve, through which venous blood is pumped into the pulmonary artery, and from there to the lungs

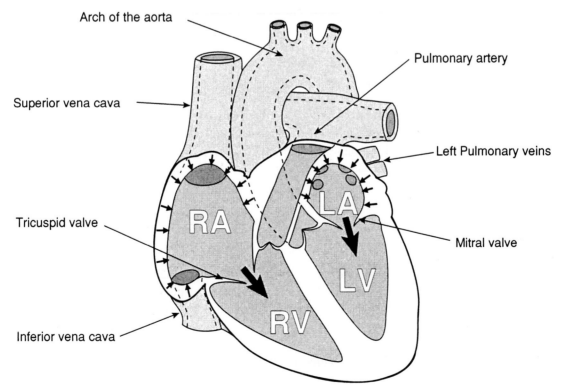

Figure 6-2 Atrial systole, ventricular diastole

- After it has contracted, the right ventricle then relaxes (ventricular diastole), allowing the tricuspid valve to open. As it does so, the right atrium contracts again pumping blood into the right ventricle, The pressure difference between the pulmonary artery and the relaxed ventricle forces the pulmonary valve to close and prevents blood flowing back into the ventricle from the pulmonary artery
- Venous (deoxygenated) blood is thus pumped into the lungs via the pulmonary arteries, where it gives off carbon dioxide, becomes oxygenated, and returns to the left side of the heart via the pulmonary veins

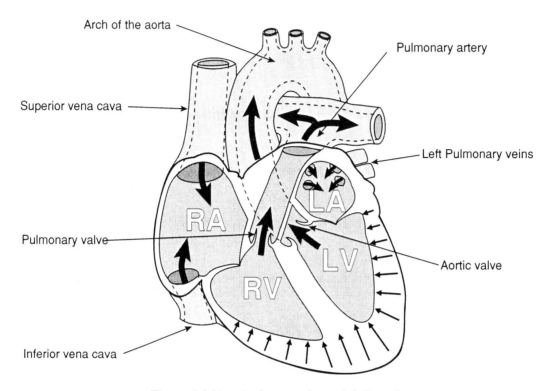

Figure 6-3 Ventricular systole, atrial diastole

Left side of the heart
- The left atrium collects oxygenated blood from the four pulmonary veins, which empty directly into it
- At the same time the right atrium contracts, the left atrium contracts, pumping blood into the left ventricle via the mitral valve (atrial systole); it then relaxes to allow atrial filling
- The left ventricle then contracts (at the same time as the right ventricle), forcing the mitral valve closed, and pumps its oxygenated blood through the aortic valve, which is forced open in the process
- After contracting, the left ventricle relaxes (ventricular diastole), the aortic valve closes to prevent retrograde blood flow, and the mitral valve reopens to allow ventricular filling during atrial systole

Conducting system
- The heart has its own specialised muscle stimulating system

Sinoatrial (SA) node
- The SA node is a small clump of muscle cells situated in the wall of the right atrium near the opening of the superior vena cava. From it runs a system of fibres, the inter-nodal pathways for conveying impulses to the AV node, and Bachmann's bundle for conveying impulses to the left atrium

Atrioventricular (AV) node
- The AV node is a small clump of muscle cells situated in the wall of the atrial septum near the atrioventricular valves

Bundle of His
- This is a group of specialised fibres originating from the AV node which cross the fibrous ring separating the atria and ventricles
- At the upper end of the interventricular septum the bundle of His divides into right and left bundle branches, which run down either side of the septum before entering the myocardium of the ventricular walls. The left bundle branch subdivides into anterior and posterior fascicles
- In the ventricular myocardium the branches become progressively smaller until they become single small fibres, the Purkinje fibres, which end in the muscle fibres of the myocardium

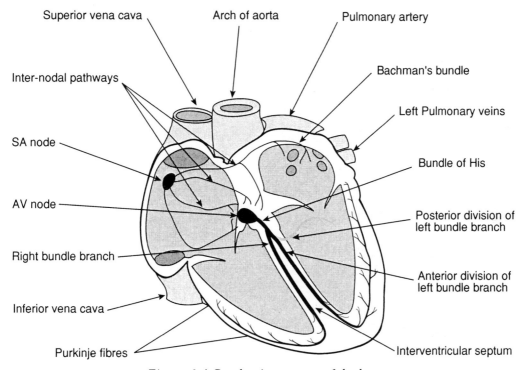

Figure 6-4 Conducting system of the heart

Nerve supply
- The heart is controlled from the higher centres of the brain by the parasympathetic and sympathetic nervous systems, and by the release of catecholamines and other hormones

Parasympathetic (vagus) nerves
- The vagus nerves (parasympathetic) supply the SA and AV nodes, and atrial muscle
- Stimulation slows the heart rate and reduces the force of contraction

Sympathetic nerves
- These run from the medulla oblongata via the spinal cord to the SA and AV nodes and the myocardium of both atria and ventricles
- Stimulation increases the heart rate and the force of myocardial contraction

Catecholamines
- These are the principal adrenergic transmitter substances in the sympathetic nervous system and are produced by the adrenal medulla:
    - Epinephrine and norepinephrine both increase the heart rate and force of myocardial contraction

Electrocardiogram (ECG) and cardiac events

Introduction
- The electrocardiogram is a very important diagnostic tool; its principal use in Immediate Care is in the diagnosis of acute myocardial infarction and life threatening arrhythmias

Electrophysiology
- All cardiac cells exhibit excitability, whereby an electrical stimulus of sufficient strength will result in a rapid membrane depolarisation, followed by a slower repolarisation
- Depolarisation in myocardial cells results in their contraction
- Only specialised cardiac conducting tissue normally depolarises spontaneously (i.e. exhibits 'automaticity'), although other cardiac cells will discharge spontaneously in some situations, if they are not stimulated frequently enough

Iso-electric line
- When there is no electrical activity taking place in the heart, no deflection is seen on the ECG tracing, this is described as the iso-electric line

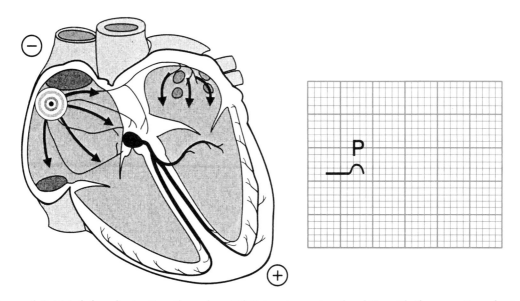

Figure 6-5 Atrial depolarisation (based on ECG tracing using lead II, with the negative electrode attached to the right arm/shoulder, and the positive electrode attached to the left leg/ lower abdomen)

P wave
- An electrical impulse is generated within the SA node and a results in a wave of depolarisation which spreads out through the right atrium to the AV node (and via 'Bachmann's bundle' to the left atrium), causing atrial muscle contraction (atrial systole)
- The P wave represents this depolarisation and is relatively small (the muscle mass of the atria is relatively small, compared to that of the ventricles)
- The deflection seen on the ECG tracing is positive initially, as the wave of depolarisation spreads towards the positive ECG lead, but when atrial depolarisation is complete, the ECG tracing returns to the iso-electric line

PR interval
- The wave of electrical depolarisation then enters the AV node, where it is delayed
- As there is no muscle depolarisation during this time, the ECG tracing returns to the iso-electric line
- The PR interval represents the time taken for excitation to spread from the SA node down to the AV node, and down through the bundle branches to the ventricles

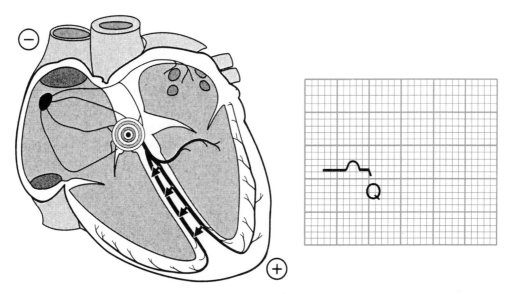

Figure 6-6 Depolarisation of the AV septum (based on ECG tracing using lead II)

QRS complex

- After a short delay in the AV node, the wave of depolarisation spreads rapidly down the Bundle of His to the right and left bundle branches and from these to the Purkinje fibres, from where it spreads to the ventricular muscle, resulting in ventricular contraction (ventricular systole)
- The ECG deflection is large as the muscle mass of the ventricles is relatively large
- The QRS complex represents the time taken for depolarisation to spread from the Bundle of His to the right and left bundle branches and from these to the Purkinje fibres and through to the ventricles

Q wave

- The first part of the ventricles to respond to the wave of depolarisation is the inter-ventricular septum which depolarises from left to right as seen in lead II
- This causes a small negative ECG deflection, as the wave of depolarisation is away from the positive ECG lead (it should *not* be confused with the pathological Q waves seen after an acute myocardial infarction, which indicate an area of non-conducting myocardium)

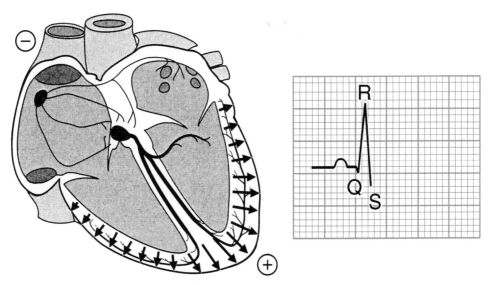

Figure 6-7 Ventricular depolarisation (based on ECG tracing using lead II)

R and S waves
- The R and S waves represent ventricular depolarisation which spreads from the bundle branches to the myocardium nearest the interventricular septum first, from there to the cardiac apex and finally up the walls of the ventricles
- Depolarisation spreads from the inside wall of the myocardium (endocardium) to the outside wall (epicardium)
- The ECG tracing shows an initial large upwards deflection as the wave of depolarisation spreads to the apex and left ventricle (and towards the positive ECG electrode), and is then followed by a smaller downwards deflection as the wave of depolarisation spreads up the walls of the less muscular right ventricle (and away from the positive ECG electrode)

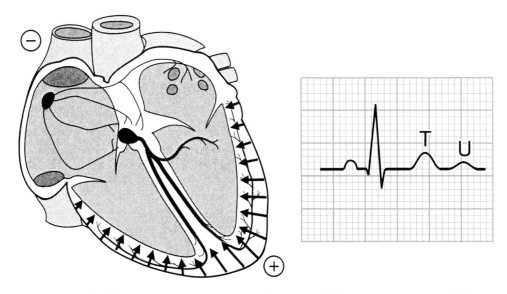

Figure 6-8 Ventricular repolarisation (based on ECG tracing using lead II)

ST segment
- After ventricular depolarisation, there is a short interval during which the myocardium remains at rest in a depolarised state (ventricular diastole/relaxation), during which the ECG tracing should be iso-electric

T waves
- After a short period of rest, the ventricles repolarise during ventricular relaxation/diastole
- This takes place in the opposite direction to depolarisation, with the outside walls of the ventricles repolarising first, resulting in a positive deflection on the ECG tracing, and usually takes more time than depolarisation

U waves
- Occasionally a late wave of ventricular repolarisation, occurring just after the T wave, can be seen on the tracing. These are usually shallower and broader than P waves with which they should not be confused

Note: Deflections showing atrial repolarisation may not be seen on the ECG tracing, as they are low energy, and may be hidden by the QRS complex

Conduction abnormalities and ectopic cardiac pacemakers

Ectopic pacemakers
- All cardiac cells exhibit excitability, and if they are not stimulated frequently enough they will discharge spontaneously; those higher up the conduction chain having the highest intrinsic firing/discharge rate
- The SA node has the highest intrinsic firing/discharge rate, but if it fails, the AV node/junction may discharge spontaneously, usually providing a junctional escape rhythm at a slower rate
- If the firing rate of the SA node is too slow, i.e. <30-50 per minute, or if conduction through the Bundle of His fails (complete heart block), then a focus further down the conduction chain or in the ventricular myocardium may take over as the pacemaker for the ventricles, resulting in a ventricular escape rhythm (idioventricular rhythm).
- Sometimes part of the ventricular myocardium may become 'irritable' and discharge spontaneously

Heart rate
- Conduction through the AV node is relatively slow and as a rule does not exceed 220 impulses per minute. This ensures that there is usually an adequate delay between atrial and ventricular contraction for optimum cardiac function and that the ventricles are protected from excessively rapid atrial rhythms
- If the heart rate exceeds 120-140 beats per minute, then there may not be enough time for the ventricles to fill adequately, and the cardiac output may be reduced
- Very rapid heart rates increase oxygen demand, reduce the strength of heart contractions and aggravate myocardial ischaemia, especially after a myocardial infarction, and may result in further infarction

Calculation of the heart rate

- ECG machines in the UK run at the standard speed of 25 mm/second

Time: Each small square = 40 milliseconds
Each large square = 5 small squares = 200 milliseconds

Heart rate:
- Divide 300 by the number of big squares between two QRS complexes
or - Count the number of QRS complexes in 6 secs (30 large squares) and multiply by 10 (best method if the rhythm is irregular)

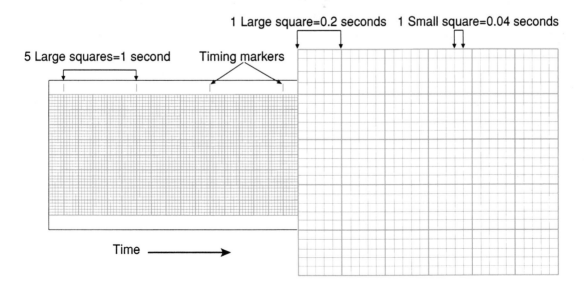

Figure 6-9 Standard ECG graph paper with a paper speed of 25 mm/sec

Regular QRS rhythm

$RR_1 = RR_2 = RR_3$

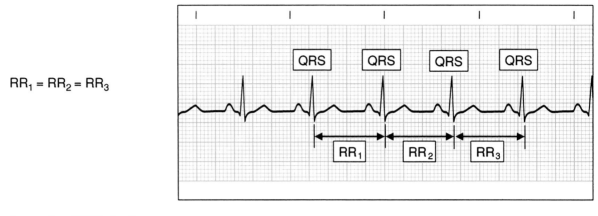

Irregular QRS rhythm

$RR_1 \neq RR_2 \neq RR_3$

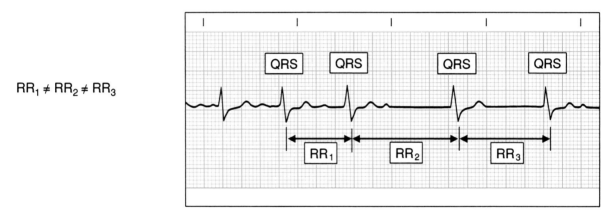

Figure 6-10 QRS rhythms: regular and irregular complexes

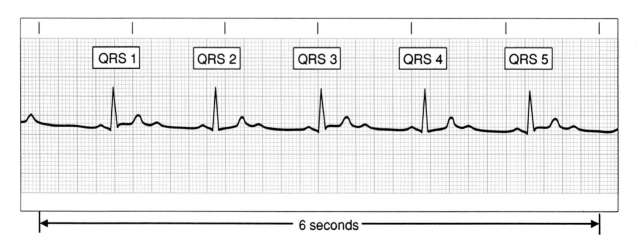

Figure 6-11 Calculation of heart rate: counting QRS complexes

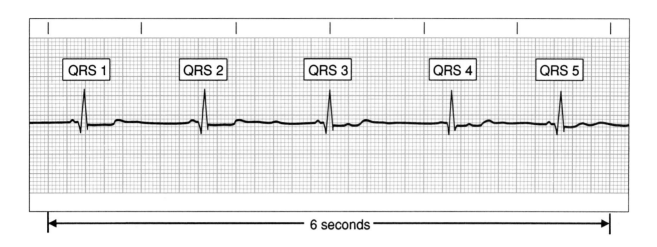

Figure 6-12 Calculation of heart rate: bradycardia

Heart rates

Normal heart rate:
- 60-110 beats per minute (may be slower in athletes, faster in children)

Bradycardia:
- <60 beats per minute

Sinus tachycardia:
- 120-160 beats per minute

Supraventricular tachycardia:
- 140-220 beats per minute

Ventricular tachycardia:
- 100-250 beats per minute

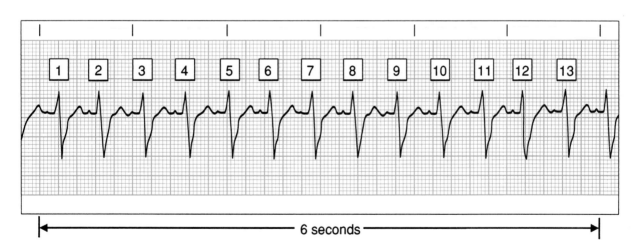

Figure 6-13 Calculation of heart rate: tachycardia

The ECG leads

-   The standard ECG tracings are obtained from pairs of electrodes attached either to the limbs or the anterior chest wall, each of which looks at the electrical activity of the heart from a different angle
-   The standard diagnostic ECG uses 12 leads, and although obtaining a full 12 lead ECG is not always possible or indeed desirable in the pre-hospital emergency situation (except for diagnosing acute myocardial infarction, when a 12 lead ECG tracing is nearly always desirable), an understanding of the electrophysiology will help the pre-hospital practitioner practise pre-hospital cardiac care rationally and more effectively
-   Each lead is firmLy attached to the body using conducting jelly to ensure a good electrical contact with the skin, and is held in place by either a rubber band, clips, suction cup or skin adhesive

The groups of ECG leads

-   There are three groups of leads which look at the heart from different directions:
    -   Bipolar limb leads: I, II, and III (plus a non-recording stabilising lead)
    -   Unipolar limb leads: aVR, aVL, and aVF
    -   Unipolar chest leads: V_{1-6}

Bipolar limb leads

-   The signal is recorded from two positions at once
-   There are four leads, one attached to the surface of each wrist and one to each ankle
-   Only the two arm electrodes and the left ankle electrode are used for recording purposes; the right ankle electrode is used to stabilise the ECG tracing

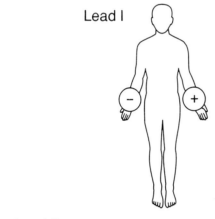

Lead	Positive	Negative
I	Left arm	Right arm
II	Left leg	Right arm
III	Left leg	Left arm

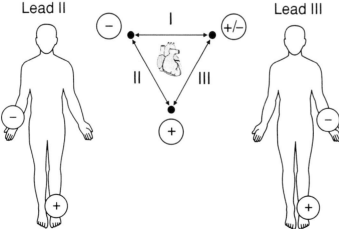

Figure 6-14 Positions for recording the bipolar limb leads

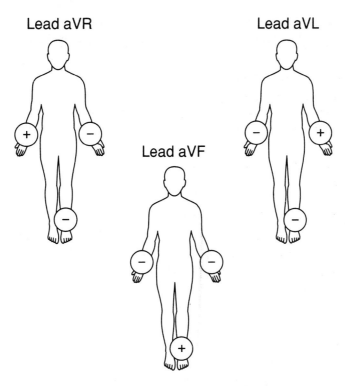

Lead aVR   Lead aVL

Lead aVF

Figure 6-15 Unipolar limb leads

Unipolar limb leads
- This uses the same three electrodes as the bipolar limb leads
- The signal is recorded from only one position; the right or left wrist or the left ankle, and compared with the mean of the negative electrodes

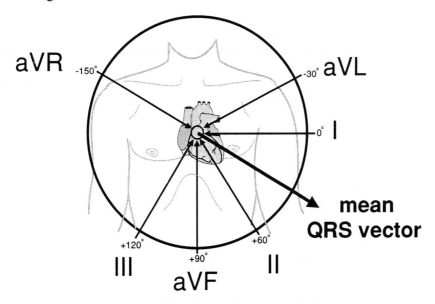

Figure 6-16 Electrical views of the heart

Cardiac axis
- The instantaneous electrical vectors generated during ventricular depolarisation can be combined to produce the mean QRS vector in the frontal plane (cardiac axis) which is usually in about the same direction as shown in the diagram above
- An independent vector for atrial depolarisation can also be calculated, and normally points in roughly the same direction as the mean ventricular QRS vector

- Although the cardiac axis will usually be as shown in the diagram, it may vary (axis deviation) from one individual to another, as its direction also depends on the position of the heart, and the relative size of the ventricles:
    - Short, broad people tend to have horizontal hearts in which the cardiac axis is rotated upwards to the left
    - Tall thin people tend to have vertical hearts in which the cardiac axis is rotated downwards
- The cardiac axis may also be rotated if there is an abnormality of cardiac conduction, e.g. bundle branch or fascicular block

Estimating the cardiac axis
- The cardiac axis will be nearest the lead with the tallest QRS complex (usually lead II)
- Deep S waves will be found in leads facing in the opposite direction to the cardiac axis
- An equiphasic QRS complex, i.e. one that has positive (up) and negative (down) components of equal size, indicates that the lead being used is positioned at right angles (90°) to the cardiac axis
- Normal cardiac axis: QRS predominantly upwards in I, II and III (still normal if downwards in III)
- Right axis deviation: QRS predominantly downwards in I
- Left axis deviation: QRS predominantly downwards in II and III

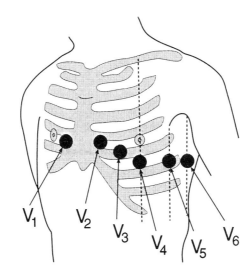

Figure 6-17 Positions of the unipolar chest leads

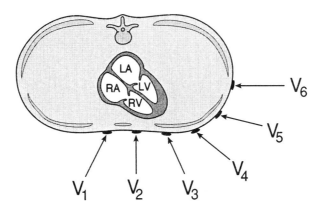

Figure 6-18 Electrical views of the front of the heart from the V leads

Unipolar chest leads
- These use a series of positive electrodes which are positioned across the anterior chest wall.
- The chest leads may all be attached at once, or there may be a movable electrode with a suction cup for attaching it to the chest wall which may be positioned in each location in turn

Chest lead positions
- V_1 4th intercostal space, just to the right of the sternum
- V_2 4th intercostal space, just to the left of the sternum
- V_3 Midway between V_2 and V_4
- V_4 5th intercostal space, in the mid clavicular line
- V_5 In the left anterior axillary line, at the same horizontal level as V_4
- V_6 In the left mid axillary line, at the same horizontal level as V_5

Electrical views of the heart
- The different chest leads enable the electrical activity of the heart to be examined from different angles in the horizontal plane:
  - Leads: V_1 and V_2 Wall of the right ventricle
            V_3 and V_4 Inter-ventricular septum and anterior wall of the left ventricle
            V_5 and V_6 Anterior and lateral walls of the left ventricle
- A combination of limb leads and chest leads as used in the 12-lead ECG give a three dimensional electrical picture of the heart, which with careful analysis enables the position of many localised cardiac abnormalities to be worked out:
  - Leads: II, III, aVF   Inferior surface
            I, aVL, V_{5-6} Lateral border
            V_{2-3}, sometimes V_1 and V_4 Depolarisation of the interventricular septum
- Lead II is usually the lead closest to the mean QRS vector (cardiac axis) and also the mean P wave vector, and as a result will show the tallest R and P waves. It is thus the best single lead for showing P waves and QRS complexes

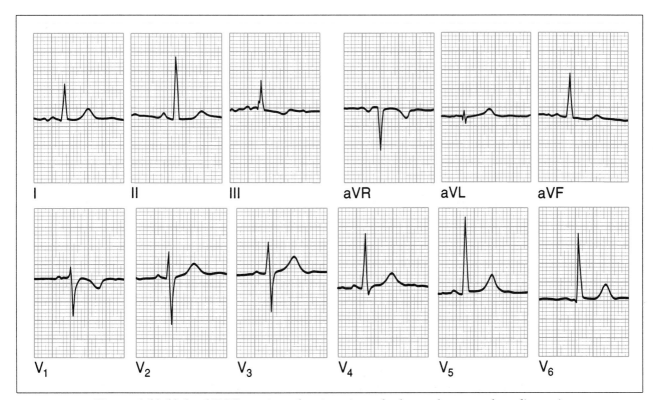

Figure 6-19 12-lead ECG tracing, showing sinus rhythm and a normal cardiac axis

Naming the different parts of the ECG tracing

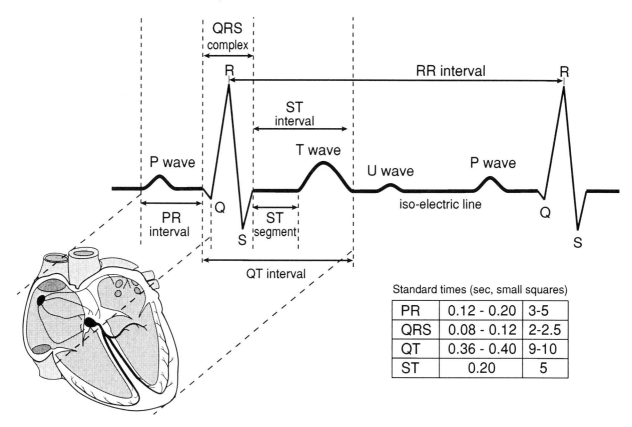

Fig 6-20 Naming the different parts of the ECG tracing and normal values

	Standard times (sec, small squares)	
PR	0.12 - 0.20	3-5
QRS	0.08 - 0.12	2-2.5
QT	0.36 - 0.40	9-10
ST	0.20	5

Labelling the QRS complex
- The different parts of the QRS complex are arbitrarily labelled as follows (regardless of the lead used):
    - The first downward (negative) deflection is called a Q wave. If there is only a downward deflection (and no upward/positive deflection), it is called a QS wave
    - Any upwards (positive) deflection is called an R wave (whether or not it is preceded by a Q wave. If there is a second upwards deflection it is called an R'
    - Any downwards (negative) deflection below the baseline occurring after an R wave is called an S wave. If there is a second downward deflection it is called an S' wave

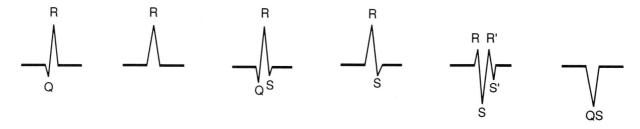

Figure 6-21 QRS complex labelling

ECG interpretation

Determine the heart rhythm (is the QRS rhythm regular or irregular?)
- Identify the QRS complexes
- Do they occur regularly or irregularly?
- If they are irregular:
    - Is there a regular irregularity?
    - Are they totally irregular?

Determine the heart rate (what is the ventricular rate?)
- Calculate the heart rate:
    - If the QRS complexes occur regularly:
        - Count the number of large squares between the R waves of two adjacent QRS complexes, and divide 300 by that number
    - If the QRS complexes occur irregularly, calculate the approximate heart rate:
        - Count the number of QRS complexes occurring over 6 seconds (30 large squares) and multiply by ten

Analyse the P waves (is atrial activity present?)
- Are P waves present?
- If P waves are present, do they have a normal shape? or do they look abnormal?
- If they look abnormal, are they:
    - Peaked (>3 small squares tall) in right atrial hypertrophy (caused by tricuspid valve stenosis or pulmonary hypertension) in leads II and III
    - Bifid and broad (>3 small squares wide) in left atrial hypertrophy in leads II or III
    - Lost or inverted in ectopic rhythms and tachycardias
    - **f waves**
        - Representing atrial depolarisation in atrial fibrillation:
            - Atrial rate: 350-600 per minute
        - May be fine or coarse
    - **F waves**
        - Representing atrial depolarisation in atrial flutter:
            - Atrial rate: 240-360 (usually about 300) per minute
        - Usually coarse: saw tooth pattern
- What is the relationship of the P waves to a QRS complex? Are they:
    - Followed by a QRS complex? Always? Sometimes?
    - Lost in or dissociated from the QRS complex
- If there are no visible P waves:
    - They may be obscured by, e.g. a QRS complex
    - An ectopic focus below the atria may be acting as pacemaker

PR interval (how is atrial activity related to ventricular activity?)
- The PR interval represents the time taken for excitation to spread from the SA node down over the atria to the AV node, down through the bundle of His, and to the ventricular muscle
- Normally: >120 milliseconds (>3 small squares), but <210 milliseconds (<5 small squares)
- The PR interval may be shorter:
    - If electrical conduction from the atria to the ventricles has occurred via an abnormal conduction pathway, e.g. in the Wolff Parkinson White and other pre-excitation syndromes
- The PR interval may be prolonged:
    - If there is delayed conduction through the AV node, e.g. in First (and sometimes Second) Degree Heart Block

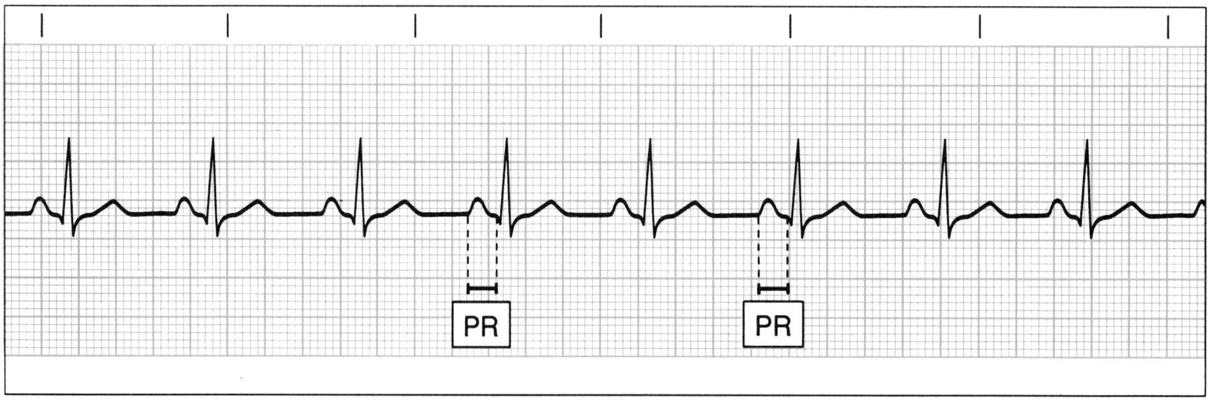

Fig 6-22 PR interval: normal

- Regularly irregular:
    - Where the rate of conduction through the AV nodes varies, e.g. in Second Degree Heart Block type I (Wenckebach phenomenon) in which the rate of AV conduction slows progressively over three or four cycles, until one impulse fails to be conducted through the AV node at all, and so that P wave is not followed by a QRS, after which the cycle is repeated
- Irregularly irregular:
    - Where there is complete blockage of the AV node and both the P waves and QRS complexes occur regularly, but there is no consistent relationship between them, e.g. in Third Degree Heart Block (Complete Heart Block)

Figure 6-23 PR interval: prolonged - 0.28 sec

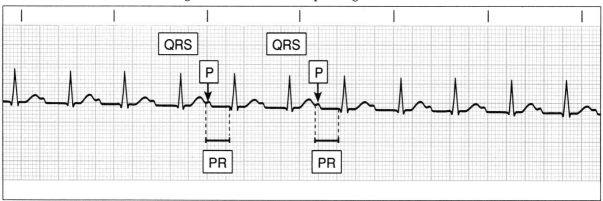

Analyse the QRS complexes (are the QRS complexes normal or abnormal in shape and width?)
- The QRS complex represents ventricular depolarisation (ventricular systole/contraction) and is relatively large, as the muscle mass of the ventricles is relatively large compared to the atria, and the time taken for excitation to spread from the His-Purkinje system through to the ventricular myocardium
- In normal sinus rhythm, the QRS complex should be:
    - Preceded by a P wave
    - < 100 milliseconds: < 2½ small squares

- The QRS will be wide (>2½ small squares/>100 milliseconds) when ventricular depolarisation has occurred via an abnormal and therefore slow pathway as in:
    - Bundle branch block
    - Premature ventricular contractions (PVCs) caused by a ventricular ectopic focus
    - Idioventricular rhythm or ventricular tachycardia
- If the QRS complexes are abnormal and of variable morphology, they arise from multiple ectopic foci

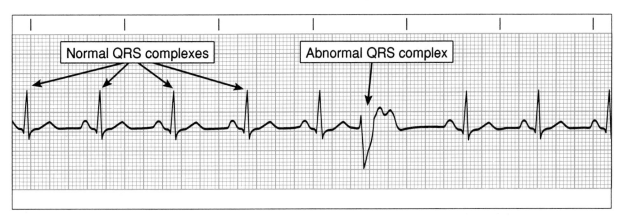

Figure 6-24 QRS complexes: normal and abnormal

Fibrillatory waves
- Waves of random frequency, morphology and amplitude, representing totally disorganised electrical activity arising randomly in the myocardium, e.g. ventricular fibrillation

R waves
- Represent depolarisation in the ventricles.
- Tall R waves in the left ventricular leads may indicate ventricular hypertrophy
- Loss of R wave progression in the chest leads may be an indication of myocardial infarction

Analyse the ST segment
- The ST segment represents the interval during which the myocardium remains at rest in a depolarised state (ventricular diastole/relaxation)
- Should be isoelectric
- The ST segment may be:
    - Convex elevation in acute myocardial injury, e.g. recent infarction
    - Concave elevation in pericarditis
    - Depression, indicating myocardial ischaemia, digoxin toxicity, or left ventricular hypertrophy
- In acute myocardial infarction, the ST segment elevation (or reciprocal depression) occurs in the leads representing the site of the infarction (12-lead ECG):
    - Anterior, it will show in leads V_{1-4}, sometimes in V_5 (and often in I and aVL)
    - Inferior, it will show in leads II, III, aVF
    - Septal, it will show in leads V_{1-4}
    - Lateral, it will show in leads I, aVL, V_{4-6}

Analyse the T waves
- T waves represent ventricular repolarisation
- They should usually be in the same direction as the QRS complex
- If inverted they may be a sign of infarction or ventricular hypertrophy, but are often non specific

Normal sinus rhythm

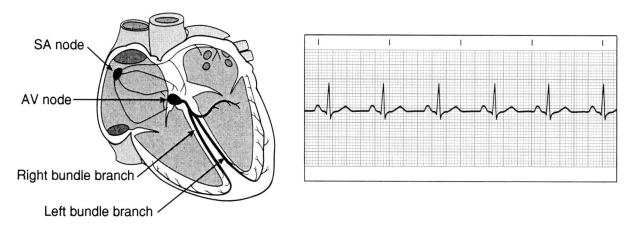

Figure 6-25 Normal sinus rhythm

ECG features

Rhythm: Regular

Rate: 60-100 beats per minute

P waves: Normal, each preceding a QRS complex

Pacemaker site: SA node

PR interval: Normal: 0.12-0.2 sec.

QRS complex: Normal, each preceded by a P wave

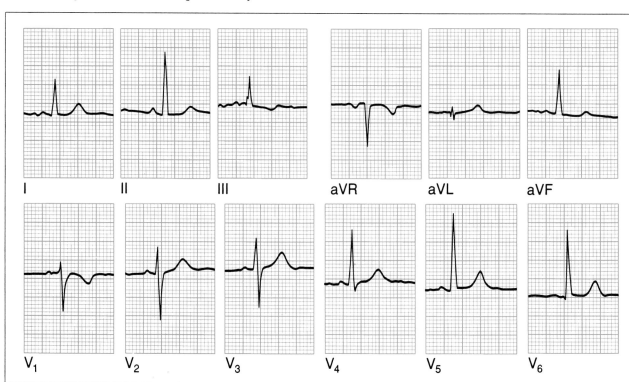

Figure 6-26 Normal sinus rhythm: 12-lead ECG

Obtaining an ECG recording
- In the emergency situation, an ECG rhythm recording may be obtained using either the defibrillator paddles or adhesive chest electrodes

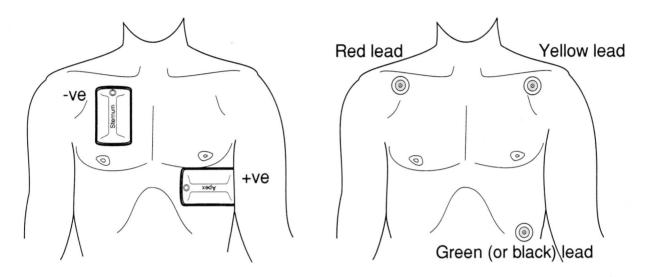

Figure 6-27 Positions of defibrillator paddles and three lead ECG chest leads

Defibrillator paddle placement
- The paddles (with conductive pads or gel) or disposable electrodes should be placed below the right clavicle (-ve) just lateral to the sternal border and over the apex beat of the heart (+ve) covering the V_{4-5} positions of the ECG
- If the positions are inadvertently reversed the tracing will appear upside down, which is of no consequence provided it is recognised
- The ECG tracing obtained will be similar to that from lead II of the standard chest leads

Three lead ECG adhesive chest electrode placement
- Adhesive electrodes should be placed in the appropriate positions and connected to the ECG/ defibrillator leads:

Red: below the right clavicle
Yellow: below the left clavicle } avoiding areas where defibrillator paddles may be placed
Green/black: over left upper abdomen

- A switch will usually allow selection of leads I, II or III
- The best lead to use is that which shows prominent P waves and reasonable QRS complexes (usually lead II):
    - Lead I is good for examining the QRS complexes
    - Lead II is good for examining P waves and the QRS complexes
    - Lead III is good for examining P waves

12-Lead ECG
- This is the standard ECG tracing, and is most valuable as a diagnostic tool when used as an aid to the diagnosis of acute myocardial infarction, as it gives a much more comprehensive view of cardiac electrical activity, which is important when looking for small areas of abnormal myocardium

PRACTICAL POINT: In the emergency situation, especially if there is limited access to the patient, attaching the upper limb leads to the shoulders and the lower limb leads to each side of the lower abdomen/upper thigh, will give very similar results to those obtained from attaching the limb leads to the standard positions, and should give adequate results

Problems with obtaining a satisfactory recording

- Artefact is a common problem, especially in the pre-hospital situation, and may be due to:
    - Patient distress:
        - Reassure and calm the patient if possible
    - Patient movement, shivering or muscle tremor:
        - Make certain that the patient is physically relaxed, warm, and that all their limbs are resting on something
    - Electrical interference from nearby electrical equipment:
        - Switch off unnecessary electrical equipment while the ECG recording is being obtained
    - Poor skin preparation:
        - Remove/wipe off any blood, debris or sweat before applying the electrodes
    - Poor patient contact; the ECG leads may become disconnected or the electrodes fall off:
        - Make certain that the ECG leads are well supported and secured
- If the ECG recording appears grossly abnormal:
    - Check that the limb leads have been connected the right way round
- A wandering baseline (due to respiratory excursions) may be seen in the chest leads, which may cause difficulty in measuring intervals/rates, but is of no other significance

PRACTICAL POINT: The ECG tracing should always be labelled with the patient's name (and the time and date if the ECG machine doesn't do it automatically), as soon as it has been run off

7

Cardiac care: acute myocardial infarction

Acute myocardial infarction (AMI)

Introduction

- The management of acute myocardial infarction (AMI) is something with which all those involved in Immediate Medical Care, both medical and para-medical should be familiar and proficient
- The objective of early treatment is to minimise the mortality and morbidity following an AMI, and many lives could be saved if the interval between the onset of symptoms and the provision of appropriate care, is reduced to the minimum. This requires early symptom recognition and the rapid delivery of treatment

Incidence

- Coronary artery disease is the commonest single cause of premature death in the UK, accounting for nearly 25% of all deaths, and results in an annual total of about 160,000 deaths
- Each year nearly 350,000 people have an acute myocardial infarction, of whom about 50% die as a result. Of these, 80% die within the first 24 hours: 25% in the first 15 minutes, 40% in the first hour
- Two thirds of deaths occur out of hospital; between 3.5-21% of deaths occur in the presence of a General Practitioner and 5% occur during transportation to hospital
- On average a General Practitioner will be called to treat a patient with an AMI only twice a year

Aetiology

- The cause of coronary heart disease is multifactorial and is not yet fully understood, but several factors, including increasing age, smoking, raised serum lipids, diabetes mellitus, obesity and family history are associated with an increased risk of developing the disease, which is characterised by the build up of atheromatous plaques in the coronary arteries. Men are affected 2-4 times more often than women

Pathophysiology

Precipitating factors

- The build up of atheromatous plaques, covered by a thin, fibrous cap in the coronary arteries results in restriction and turbulence of the blood flow
- Enlargement of these plaques occurs due to further atheroma deposition and occasionally intraplaque rupture, which results in cracking, splitting and ulceration of the plaque's fibrous cap, which then forms a surface on which platelets aggregate and fibrin is precipitated
- Increased turbulence and restriction of arterial blood flow occurs and this together with the platelet aggregation triggers coagulation, leading to local progressive intraluminal thrombus (clot) formation
- This intraluminal thrombus may either increase in size resulting in total arterial occlusion, or it may be completely lysed following which the plaque fissure may be resealed
- Thrombus formation may follow an intermittent pattern, which may be reflected by the clinical picture, and it may occlude smaller vessels as it proceeds

- Initially the clot is soft and friable, but becomes firmer as cross links form between the fibrous strands
- Coronary blood flow may be further reduced by swelling of the arterial wall due to intraplaque haemorrhage, by the release of platelet derived vasoconstrictor substances, and the inability of the now inelastic arterial wall to respond to factors which usually result in its relaxation
- Arterial occlusion results in overactivation of the sympathetic nervous system. Consequent coronary spasm may also occur, but this is rarely the sole cause of AMI

Mechanism of infarction

- Occlusion of a main coronary artery by thrombus associated with atherosclerotic changes in the coronary arteries (in >90% of cases), results in infarction and necrosis of the heart muscle supplied by that artery
- Myocardial damage usually starts in the subendocardial layer and spreads progressively outwards
- The rate at which myocardial cell death occurs varies, but may depend on the cardiac work load, previous episodes of ischaemia and the presence of a collateral blood supply. Ischaemic changes begin to develop within 3-5 minutes of arterial occlusion, and myocardial cell necrosis begins within 20 minutes
- Myocardial necrosis is advanced after 2 hours, is irreversible after 4-6 hours and complete in 24 hours

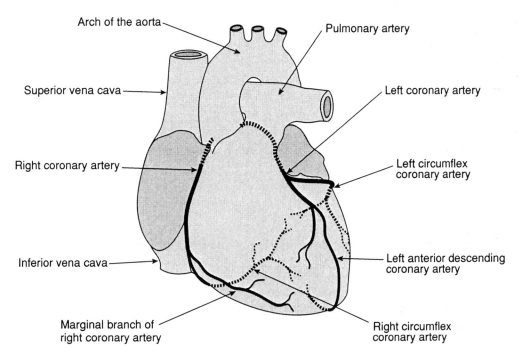

Figure 7-1 Blood supply of the heart

Severity

- The more proximal the site of the arterial occlusion, the greater the amount of potential muscle damage
- The better the collateral blood supply, the less the amount of damage

Location

- Usually, the left ventricle is affected, although in inferior infarction, right ventricular ischaemia and necrosis are relatively common
- The correlation between the site of infarction on the ECG tracing and coronary artery anatomy is poor

Anterior myocardial infarction

- Usually occurs due to occlusion of the left anterior descending coronary artery resulting in infarction of the anterior wall of the left ventricle and the intraventricular septum
- May result in pump failure due to loss of myocardium, ventricular septal defect, aneurysm or rupture and arrhythmias

Inferior myocardial infarction
- May occur due to occlusion of the right or left circumflex coronary arteries resulting in infarction of the inferior surface of the left ventricle
- The right ventricle and the interventricular septum may also be damaged
- Results in bradycardia due to damage to the AV node. Pump failure is less common

Posterior or lateral myocardial infarction
- Usually occurs due to occlusion of the left circumflex or large right coronary artery
- Less common; it results in pump failure and malignant ventricular arrhythmias

Complications of AMI

Death
- 50% of patients, who die from AMI, die in the first 2 hours
- The mortality rate is highest in the elderly, in females, in those who have a history of previous myocardial infarction, in those with extensive infarcts and in those who develop heart failure
- The greater the degree of myocardial damage, the greater the resulting ventricular dysfunction,disability and incidence of complications

Arrhythmias (45%)
- Electrical instability, leading to ventricular fibrillation. May be aggravated by autonomic overactivity
- The major cause of preventable early deaths

Pump failure (45%)
- Decreased strength of muscle contractions, leading to left ventricular failure
- A major cause of late deaths

Other mechanical problems (2%)
- Rupture of:
  - Myocardial wall:
    - Accounts for 10% of all hospital deaths
    - Characterised by the sudden onset of cardiac failure (electro-mechanical dissociation), followed by sudden death due to ventricular fibrillation/asystole
  - Interventricular septum (0.5%), leading to a ventricular septal defect (VSD)
  - Papillary muscles, resulting in acute mitral regurgitation
- Ventricular aneurysm

Thromboembolism (8%):
- Late deep vein thrombosis, pulmonary embolism
- Now rare, due to the routine use of thromolytics and warfarin, in the early management of AMI

Diagnosis

- The diagnosis of acute myocardial infarction is more difficult to make with certainty early after infarction, when the patient will benefit most from early treatment

History
- In the Immediate Care situation, history taking should be as rapid as possible
- Past medical history:
  - Previous myocardial infarction.
  - Angina (20-30%)
  - Risk factors for coronary artery disease

Symptoms/signs
- Many patients who die suddenly have no warning symptoms at all

Malaise
- There may be a history of up to several days general malaise

Angina
- There may be a history of several days increasingly severe angina (crescendo angina)

Cardiogenic shock (pump failure)
- The patient may be:
    - Frightened, ill, pale, breathless and sweating (this decreases with age)
    - Hypotensive (systolic BP <90 mm Hg)
    - Peripherally shutdown with cold extremities
    - Confused (incidence increases with advancing age)

Chest pain/discomfort
- Only occurs in 80-90% of patients, but is more likely to be due to myocardial infarction in the elderly
- May be absent, especially in the elderly

Nature
- Severe, intense, heavy, crushing, "like a heavy weight", tight or frightening

Location
- May be one of or any combination of the following:
    - Precordial *(usual)*
    - Epigastric
    - In either shoulder, arm or in the back
    - In front of the neck or jaw

Radiation
- To neck/jaw, down either arm (usually the left) or through to the back

Duration
- May last many hours

Course
- Continuous, usually without variation, but may be of increasing intensity

Temperature
- May be precipitated by very cold weather (when the blood thickens 'sludging')

Time of day/week
- More likely to occur in the late evening or early morning (the peak is between 6-11 am, possibly precipitated by the blood pressure rising on/before arousing/awakening)

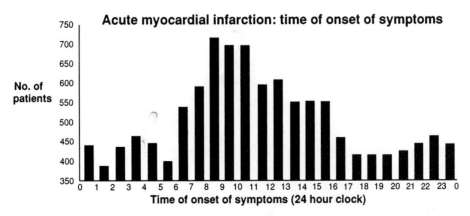

Figure 7-2 Incidence of acute myocardial infarction and time of day

Nausea, vomiting and hiccoughs (more common in inferior infarction): indicate autonomic disturbance

Relationships
- Precipitated by:
    - Physical or emotional stress ⎰ But may often
    - Meals, and micturition or defecation ⎱ occur at rest
- Not usually relieved by rest and nitrates

Pulse
- May be low volume, rapid and irregular

Breath sounds
- Usually normal, but there may be the signs of congestive cardiac failure, e.g. basal crackles

Heart sounds
- Often normal, but there may be a III or IV heart sound

Low grade pyrexia
- This may take a few hours to develop

Investigations: electrophysiology and the ECG

Introduction
- The 12-lead ECG is the most useful investigation for confirming the diagnosis of acute myocardial infarction, locating the site of the infarct and monitoring progress
- The 3-lead ECG may not be sufficiently sensitive to either exclude or confirm the diagnosis of AMI
- The correlation between the ECG tracing and the underlying pathology is poor, especially shortly after infarction:
    - 5-10% of those with a myocardial infarction have no ECG changes
    - 5-10% of those with myocardial infarction have doubtful ECG changes
    - 25% have probable ECG changes, and *only 50% show classical changes*

ECG changes after acute myocardial infarction

Hyperacute changes
- Immediately after infarction, the T waves in the affected area become tall and broad

Acute changes
- ST segment elevation often begins within minutes of the onset of infarction, but may not occur for several hours, and lasts up to 24-48 hours (usually peaking at about 24 hours), before returning to the iso-electric line
- The changes occur over the area of damage and reciprocal changes will be seen in the opposite leads
- Generally the earlier ST elevation occurs and the higher it is; the greater the myocardial damage

Evolving
- Several hours after infarction:
    - Pathological abnormal Q waves begin to form, and persist (may disappear eventually)
- Later:
    - The R wave becomes reduced in size or lost
    - The raised ST segment begins to subside
    - T wave inversion occurs, and may persist for months or years

Resolving
- From day 5 up to 6 weeks:
    - The ST segment returns to the baseline
    - The T wave moves back towards the baseline, or sometimes becomes flattened
- Finally:
    - The T wave becomes upright again, but the Q wave persists indefinitely
    - The loss in height of the R wave persists

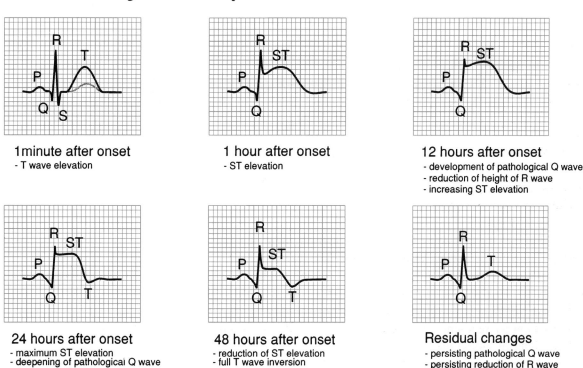

1minute after onset
- T wave elevation

1 hour after onset
- ST elevation

12 hours after onset
- development of pathological Q wave
- reduction of height of R wave
- increasing ST elevation

24 hours after onset
- maximum ST elevation
- deepening of pathological Q wave
- development of T wave inversion

48 hours after onset
- reduction of ST elevation
- full T wave inversion

Residual changes
- persisting pathological Q wave
- persisting reduction of R wave
- return of upright T wave

Figure 7-3 ECG changes after acute myocardial infarction (lead II)

Q waves
- If myocardial infarction results in the death of all the muscle cells from the inner to the outer surface of a ventricle, i.e, it is 'full thickness', this will result in the formation of an electrical window. An electrode placed over that window will record an electrical potential similar to that obtained from an electrode placed within the ventricle. As depolarisation of the ventricles takes place from the inside outwards, an electrode situated within the ventricle will show ventricular depolarisation moving away from it, which will appear on an ECG tracing as a pathological Q wave. Thus full thickness muscle damage shows on the ECG tracing as a pathological Q wave over the area of damage
- If the infarction is not 'full thickness', and so no electrical window is formed, there may be T wave inversion, but no pathological Q waves. This is 'subendocardial' or 'partial thickness' infarction
- Pathological Q waves, indicating myocardial infarction are:
    - Deep: more than 25% of the height of the following R wave
    - Wide: >0.04 seconds in duration (one small square on standard ECG paper recorded at 2.5 cm/sec)
- The leads in which the pathological Q waves appear indicate the part of the ventricle affected
- The development of a pathological Q wave within a few hours of the infarction, indicates irreversible full thickness muscle injury (if present early; this may indicate a previous AMI)
- The absence of a Q wave, indicates that the infarct has not (yet) caused full thickness muscle necrosis.
- Patients who are given thrombolytics early are less likely to have a full thickness infarct and are less likely to have pathological Q waves
- Patients with non Q wave infarctions have lower mortality rates in hospital, but are more likely to have recurrent angina or a second infarction

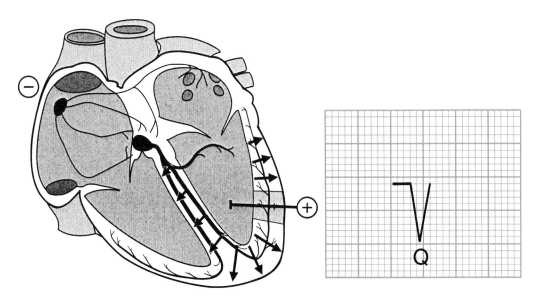

Figure 7-4 Pathological Q wave in full thickness infarction

Arrhythmias
- In addition to the classic ECG signs of infarction, there may also be autonomic dysfunction:
    - Sympathetic overactivity resulting in tachycardia
    - Parasympathetic (vagal) overactivity resulting in bradycardia and frequently in hypotension

Characteristic ECG changes in acute myocardial infarction
- Significant ST segment elevation "acute change" of at least 2 mm in at least two leads:
    - Anterior infarction: I, aVL, V_{2-6}
    - Anterolateral infarction: I, aVL, V_{4-6}
    - Anteroseptal infarction: V_{1-4}
    - Inferior infarction: II, III, aVF
    - Posterolateral infarction:V_1, V_{5-6}.
- ST segment depression (may be reciprocal to ST elevation indicating myocardial ischaemia):
    - Anterior infarction: II, III, aVF
    - Posterior infarction: V_{1-2} (shows reciprocal changes)
    - Inferior infarction: I, aVL, V_{1-2}
- T wave:
    - Elevation: tall broad (hyperacute) in true posterior AMI
    - Inversion (this is a late change, therefore probably indicates an old AMI)
    - Deep symmetrical T waves are found in subendocardial infarction.
- Deep, wide (>0.04 seconds) Q waves
- R wave: progressive loss across the chest (V) leads

Common patterns of acute ST segment change in acute myocardial infarction
- Anterior V_{1-4}, sometimes in V_5 (and often in I, aVL)
- Anteroseptal V_{1-3}
- Anterolateral   I, aVL, V_{5-6}
- Lateral   I, aVL, V_{5-6}
- Inferior   II, III, aVF
- Inferolateral   II, III, aVF, V_{5-6}, sometimes I and aVL
- Inferoseptal   II, III, aVF, V_{1-3}
- Septal V_{1-4}
- Posterior V_{1-2} show reciprocal changes (often associated with inferior infarction)

ECG examples of different types of acute myocardial infarction

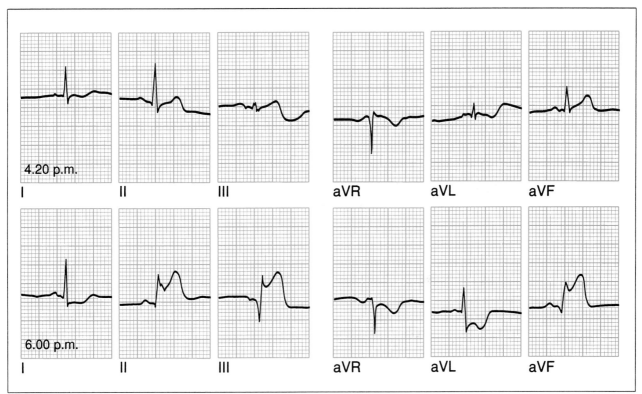

Figure 7-5 Development of inferior myocardial infarction:
4.20: ST elevation in: III, aVF, ST depression in I, aVL
6.00: ST elevation in: II, III, aVF, ST depression in I, aVR, aVL, pathological Q waves in III, aVF

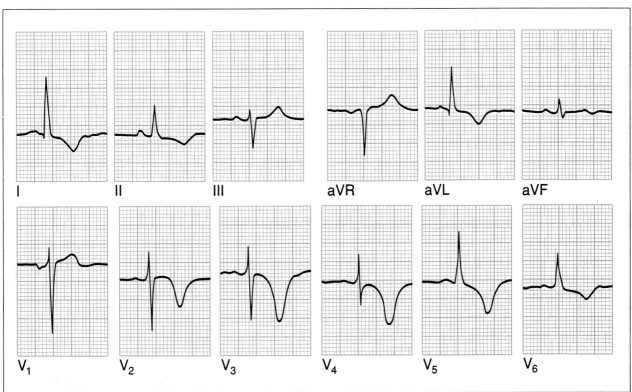

Figure 7-6 Subendocardial infarction: No pathological Q waves
Deep symmetrical T waves

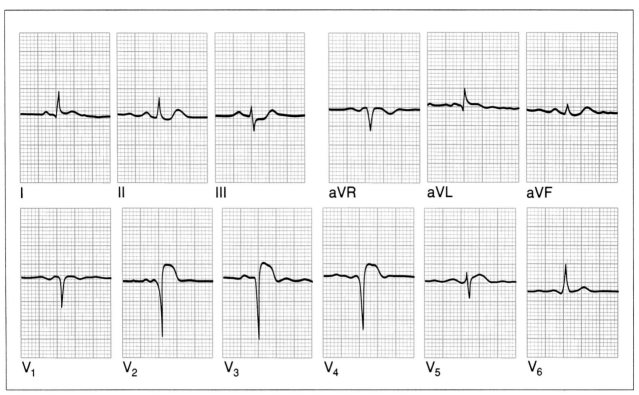

Figure 7-7 Anterior myocardial infarction: ST elevation in: I, aVL, V$_{2-5}$
ST depression in: II, III, aVF

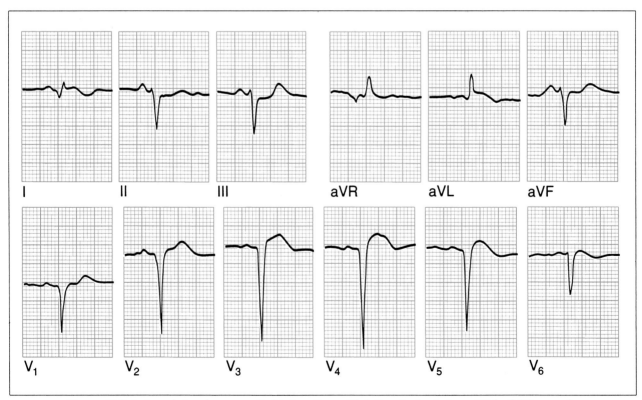

Figure 7-8 Antero-lateral myocardial infarction with left axis deviation: Wide QRS complex
ST elevation: I, aVL, V$_{2-6}$
ST depression: II, III, aVF

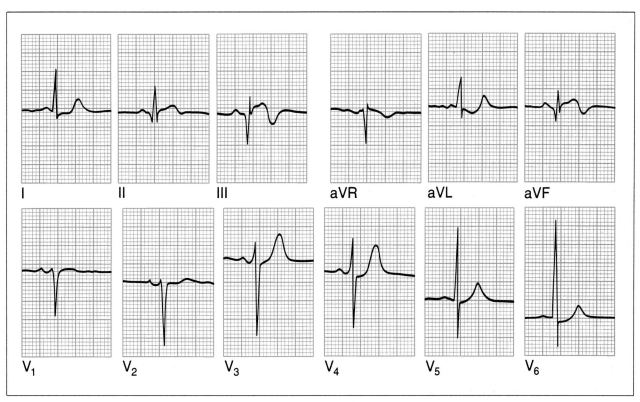

Figure 7-9 Inferior myocardial infarction: ST elevation in: II, III, aVF
ST depression in I, aVL, V₃₋₆
(pathological Q waves in II, III, aVF)

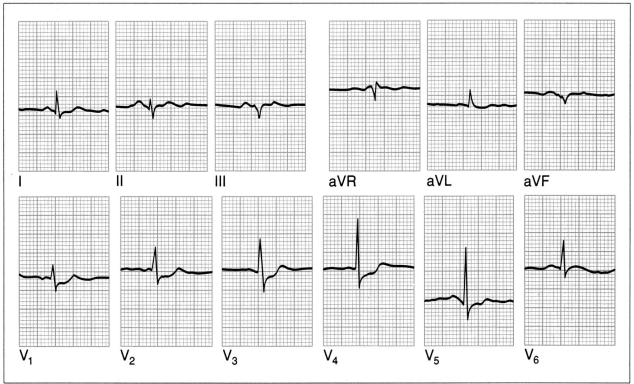

Figure 7-10 Posterior myocardial infarction: ST depression in: V₁₋₅
Dominant R wave in V₁₋₃
(pathological Q waves in inferior leads from associated inf. MI)

Differential diagnosis of chest pain

Chest wall

Herpes zoster
- There may be pain and/or hyperaesthesia up to 7 days before the appearance of the rash

Bornholm disease
- Poorly localised acute pain with pyrexia and tender intercostal muscles

Costal chondritis "Tietze's syndrome"/cough fracture
- Localised tenderness

Trauma/musculoskeletal pain
- History and localised tenderness

Diaphragmatic catch syndrome
- Negative history of trauma
- Pain is transient and "catches the breath"
- There may be tender rib margins

Heart

Myocardial infarction: See above

Stable angina

Aetiology
- Reduced oxygen supply:
    - Partial occlusion of coronary arteries by plaque or congenital narrowing
    - Spasm of coronary arteries
    - Anaemia
- Increased myocardial oxygen demand:
    - Exercise especially after meals
    - Thyrotoxicosis
    - Arrhythmia, e.g. atrial fibrillation, supraventricular tachycardia
    - Stress

Pathophysiology
- Relative impairment of myocardial muscle perfusion resulting in ischaemia

History
- Similar episodes in similar circumstances, e.g. exertion

Symptoms/signs
- Similar to myocardial infarction, with central chest pain, but the pain is:
    - Less severe, though similar in character to AMI
    - Precipitated by and occurs during exertion, and makes the patient stop what they are doing or slow down
    - Relieved completely by:
        - Resting or standing still for a few minutes
        - Glyceryl trinitrate spray or sublingual tablets within 2-3 minutes
- Dyspnoea is common and sometimes the principal feature
- The patient is not usually shocked

ECG diagnosis
- The ECG may be normal or show evidence of:
    - Reversible ischaemic changes:
        - ST segment depression (may be flat or go downwards), T wave inversion or both
    - An old AMI

Management
- Rest and reassurance
- GTN: Spray, sublingual or buccal tablets (best, as slow release and therefore effect is prolonged)
- Oxygen
- If there is no improvement; manage as unstable angina (see below)

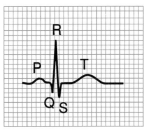

Normal ECG

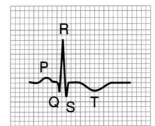

Myocardial ischaemia
- T wave inversion

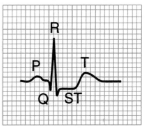

Myocardial ischaemia
- ST depression

Figure 7-11 ECG: ischaemic changes

Unstable angina

Pathophysiology
- Similar to angina, with progression towards infarction
- About 10% of untreated patients progress to acute myocardial infarction (8-15% die within one year)
- Infarction is most likely to occur if there are recurrent episodes of pain with ECG changes lasting more than 24-48 hours in spite of treatment
- 35% are left with persisting angina

Symptoms
- The pain is similar to that of stable angina but it:
    - May be more severe, occurs more frequently, and is less predictable
    - May occur on minimal exertion or even at rest
    - Is more prolonged and may not respond immediately to rest or nitrates
- The recent onset of increasingly painful and frequent episodes of angina
- A change in the pattern of the patient's usual episodes of angina

ECG diagnosis
- Associated with fluctuating ST segment (depression) or T wave changes (inversion)

Management
- Rest and reassurance
- Administer oxygen and buccal or sublingual nitrates
- Give soluble aspirin:
    - Half a 300 mg tablet orally or chewed to reduce the chances of progression to infarction
- Establish intravenous access
- Admit immediately to a Coronary Care Unit
- Consider the administration of analgesia: morphine/diamorphine with an anti-emetic

Pericarditis

Incidence
- May occur at any age

History
- There may be the history and signs of systemic viral infection, and rarely neoplasm or autoimmune disease

Symptoms
- Pyrexia with shallow respiration
- A sharp central chest pain worse on deep inspiration which may be:
    - Reduced by sitting forward
    - Aggravated by deep breathing/coughing and lying flat
- There may be a friction rub, and signs of cardiac tamponade: raised jugular venous pressure (JVP) and pulsus paradoxus

ECG diagnosis
- There may be generalised ST elevation without Q waves

Myocarditis

Incidence
- May be associated with chest pain especially when there is pericarditis

Symptoms
- Usually presents with a pyrexia, malaise and a tachycardia
- Sometimes there may be arrhythmias, cardiac failure and shock

Aorta

Dissecting aortic aneurysm

Incidence
- Non-traumatic dissecting aortic aneurysm is five times more common in men than women and is the third most common cause of cardiovascular death in men over the age of 50; it may simulate or include an AMI

Aetiology
- Pre-existing hypertension and atherosclerosis may be a predisposing factor

Pathophysiology
- Hypertension and associated atherosclerosis results in a tear of the inner wall (intima) of the aorta, usually in the ascending part of the arch of the aorta
- Blood under pressure then enters the tear and dissects a path between the layers of the wall of the aorta. The area affected enlarges and may extend proximally to the aortic valve, resulting in distortion of the valve and distally to the renal arteries. The dissection may involve major arteries branching off the aorta, including the coronary arteries
- Sometimes the dissected channel may re-penetrate the inner wall of the aorta, resulting in re-entry and the formation of a double-barrelled aorta
- Eventually rupture of the aorta may occur resulting in massive haemorrhage into the pericardium, pleura or retroperitoneal space and is usually fatal

Symptoms
- Sudden onset of severe precordial or epigastric searing, tearing pain radiating to the neck, abdomen, legs or back of the chest between the scapulae, which may be similar to the pain of myocardial infarction. The site of the pain may change as the aneurism expands
- May be precipitated by exertion or stress (there may be a history of pre-existing hypertension)

Signs
- *The blood pressure may be raised* and *there may be a machinery murmur on auscultation*
- Evidence of the development of obstruction to blood flow in parts of the body supplied by arteries branching off the aorta:
    - Marked difference in blood pressure and pulses in the upper and sometimes lower limbs on different sides of the body
    - Disturbances in consciousness due to occlusion of the carotid arteries, and sometimes paraplegia due to obstruction of those arteries supplying the spinal cord
    - Myocardial infarction due to occlusion of the coronary arteries
    - Haematuria and gastro-intestinal problems due to occlusion of the renal and mesenteric arteries
    - There may be absent/reduced neck or limb pulses with distended often pulsatile superficial veins
- Patients with an abdominal aortic aneurism may have a pulsatile abdominal mass

Note: The diagnosis of dissecting aortic aneurism is suggested by the sudden onset of severe chest pain, which reaches a crescendo and is followed by the symptoms and signs of developing arterial occlusion as described above

Lungs

Pleurisy

Symptoms
- Frequent coughing, pyrexia and sometimes haemoptysis
- Chest pain which is usually localised and lateral, and may be exacerbated by deep inspiration

Signs
- There is usually a pleural friction rub, and evidence of pneumonia

Pneumothorax (non-traumatic)

Incidence
- Typically seen in:
    - Slim and maybe Marfanoid young males
    - Acute severe asthma, when effective management may be life saving

History
- There may be a history of previous episodes

Symptoms
- Usually the sudden onset of acute pleuritic pain (not always, especially in asthmatics), and dyspnoea

Signs
- There are signs of reduced or absent air entry with hyper-resonance on percussion, and tracheal shift
- If severe, it may mimic a massive pulmonary embolism (see below)

Pulmonary embolism

Incidence
- More common in the, pregnant, elderly and immobile
- May occur after recent pelvic and lower limb surgery, pelvic or long bone trauma, pregnancy, etc.

Pathophysiology
- Occurs when a large clot (thrombus) that has formed in the deep leg or pelvic veins, breaks free and some of it (emboli) is carried via the inferior vena cava and right side of the heart into the pulmonary arterial circulation, part of which becomes occluded, resulting in an increase in pulmonary resistance
- Severe obstruction results in pulmonary hypertension, acute right ventricular failure, tachycardia, and cardiac failure and sometimes in sudden cardiac death

Symptoms/signs
- These will vary according to underlying pathophysiology:
  - *Peripheral embolus:* e.g. a small embolus blocking a peripheral branch of the pulmonary artery:
    - Haemoptysis
    - Pleuritic chest pain
  - *Central embolus:* i.e. a massive embolus blocking a proximal part of the pulmonary artery:
    - Chest pain: may be absent or severe, may mimic an acute myocardial infarction
    - Cyanosis
    - Severe dyspnoea with tachypnoea
    - Tachycardia with evidence of shock, and raised jugular venous pressure
    - Collapse
  - Sometimes there will be evidence of an associated deep vein thrombosis (which should be looked for)

ECG diagnosis
- Often there are minimal or no ECG changes
- May be difficult to distinguish from acute myocardial infarction, but there may be:
  - Atrial tachyarrhythmias (most common)
  - Non-specific ST segment and T wave changes
  - Right axis deviation
  - Right bundle branch block
  - Dominant R in V_1
  - Inverted T wave in $V_{1-3 \text{ or } 4}$
  - Deep S in V_6

Gastrointestinal tract

Reflux oesophagitis/hiatus hernia

Symptoms/signs
- Epigastric/retrosternal burning pain, rarely radiating down the left arm and unrelated to exertion
- Usually related to meals and posture: lying down and bending forward
- May be difficult to distinguish from cardiac pain, especially if unrelated to food and posture
- Usually relieved by food, belching, standing, nitrates or antacids

Oesophageal spasm

Symptoms
- Similar to oesophagitis, but even more difficult to distinguish from AMI
- May be relieved by nitrates

Peptic ulcer, gallstones and pancreatitis
- Usually the history, the site of the pain and physical examination will distinguish these from AMI

Functional

Hyperventilation

Incidence
- Relatively common in young women

Symptoms/signs
- Tight chest, pins and needles in the hands, face and feet
- Anxiety, fear, frequent sighs and dyspnoea
- Tachycardia and tachypnoea

Management of acute myocardial infarction

Object: To resuscitate the patient and reduce myocardial damage and complications following an AMI, prior to rapid evacuation to hospital

Basic Life Support (see chapter on Basic Life Support)
- If the patient is unconscious with no spontaneous respiration, pulse or blood pressure

Position/posture
- The patient should be placed in the position of greatest comfort, usually sitting up, as this may reduce the venous return

Administer high flow rate oxygen via a non-rebreathing mask with reservoir bag
- This is very important for the patient with a suspected AMI

Perform a diagnostic 12-lead ECG
- This is important for the early confirmation of the diagnosis of AMI, especially prior to the administration of a thrombolytic agent (a 3-lead ECG may not give a sufficiently comprehensive view of the myocardium to exclude a diagnosis of acute myocardial infarction)

Establish intravenous access
- Intravenous access may be established with just a cannula or an intravenous infusion may be set up
- This will allow immediate access for administration of intravenous drugs
- If an intravenous infusion is started:
    - Crystalloid, e.g. Hartmann's solution or 5% dextrose, is to be preferred
    - Intravenous fluids should be run in slowly, so as to avoid fluid overload

Monitoring

ECG
- This is very important for the early detection of life threatening arrhythmias

Haemodynamic assessment
- Blood pressure.
- Pulse:
    - Rate, rhythm, and character.
- Breath sounds
- Heart sounds
- The patient's general condition, etc.

Pain relief/sedation

Introduction
- Pain relief following AMI is very important as pain:
    - Causes a rise in the circulating catecholamines and may precipitate "shock"
    - Increases the vagal tone and incidence of arrhythmias (see chapter on Pain management)
- All drugs should be administered intravenously (unless contraindicated) in the management of acute myocardial infarction, as intramuscular drug administration may:
    - Result in less predictable blood levels, especially in shocked patients
    - Cause local muscle damage and as a result complicate the enzymatic assessment of AMI
    - Result in large haematoma formation if thrombolytics are subsequently administered

Analgesics (for details of presentation, dosage, etc., see chapter on Pain management)

Opiates: morphine/diamorphine
- The analgesics of choice for cardiac pain because of their analgesic efficacy and anxiolytic effects

Description
- For principal analgesic action: see chapter on Pain management
- Other beneficial effects for the patient with an AMI include:
    - Dilation of the resistance and capacitance vessels
    - Reduction in the heart rate (sometimes)
    - Reduction in cardiac work and myocardial oxygen demand (beneficial in congestive cardiac failure and AMI)

Disadvantages
- Opiates impair the normal response to changes in posture and may precipitate hypotension
- Care has to be taken if the patient has already taken nitrates or other vasodilators as severe hypotension may occur as a result
- Opiates may cause nausea (which may also be due to increased vagal activity following an AMI)

Dosage
- Diamorphine: 5-10 mg
- Morphine: 10-15 mg

Administration
- This should be by slow intravenous injection, diluted and titrated (1mg/min) to patient response, so as to avoid hypotension or respiratory depression, which is more likely to occur if administration is rapid
- In AMI, opiates should be given together or in combination with an antiemetic to reduce nausea

Pethidine
- More rapid onset of action, shorter acting, less potent, but less likely to cause respiratory depression than morphine
- May be considered in AMI if the pain is not severe

Nalbuphine (*Nubain®*)
- Should be considered if the patient is hypotensive
- May be used by non-medical personnel

Nitrous oxide/oxygen
- Should be considered if opiates are not available, but it only contains 50% oxygen

Antiemetics
- In AMI nausea and vomiting is common and may be due to the autonomic disturbance as a result of AMI itself or as a side effect of opiate analgesics
- Antiemetics used for the relief of nausea and vomiting following an AMI include:
    - Metoclopramide (*Maxolon®*): *probably the antiemetic of choice in AMI*
    - Prochlorperazine (*Buccastem®* buccal tablets)
    - Cyclizine (*Valoid®*), is *not recommended in AMI* as it may cause coronary artery vasoconstriction and an increase in pulmonary artery pressure

Anxiolytics

Diazepam (see chapter on Pain management)
- Diazepam can be beneficial, especially if the patient is very anxious, and may reduce the incidence of arrhythmias following acute myocardial infarction, but is not often used
- Should be used with care when administered intravenously as it may cause respiratory depression

Administration
- Intravenously

Nitrates

Description
- Reduces the myocardial oxygen demand (workload) by causing:
    - Venodilation which reduces the left ventricular filling pressure (preload)
    - A reduction in the afterload
- Increases the coronary blood flow by causing coronary artery vasodilation
- Post infarct, nitrates may help to maintain coronary artery patency during thrombolytic treatment, and improve the prognosis by limiting the infarct size and preserving left ventricular function

Indications
- Cardiac ischaemic pain: angina, AMI and left ventricular failure (LVF)
- Should not be administered if the patient is hypotensive (BP <90 mmHg), or has recently self administered large doses of nitrates

Side effects
- Flushing, headache, dizziness, postural hypotension, tachycardia

Presentation
- Glyceryl trinitrate (GTN):
    - Tablets: 300, 500 and 600 µg
        - Short acting: 20-30 minutes
        - Unstable and once opened, the tablets have a very short life of only 2 months.
    - Buccal tablets (*Suscard*®): 1, 2, 3, 5 mg
        - Rapid onset, longer duration of action
    - Sublingual spray: 400 µg metered dose
        - Rapid onset, short duration of action, long storage life (2 years)
- Isosorbide dinitrate:
    - Tablets/sublingual spray
        - Active sublingually
        - A more stable preparation for those patients who may use it infrequently
        - Long duration of action
- Isosorbide mononitrate:
    - A metabolite of isosorbide dinitrate

Administration
- May be given:
    - Sublingually (spray or tablets):
        - Acts rapidly to cause initial arteriolar vasodilation and subsequent venodilation.
    - By intravenous infusion (not usually administered this way in Immediate Care)
        - Acts predominantly as a venodilator

Aspirin

Description
- Aspirin is an antiplatelet agent which is of additional benefit when it is administered together with a specific thrombolytic
- Used alone aspirin can reduce the long term mortality rate following AMI by up to 25%, saving up to 25 lives per 1000 patients treated, but there is a small additional increase in the incidence of stroke
- Aspirin and thrombolytics administered together can reduce the mortality following AMI by half, if given early after the onset of symptoms to patients with suspected AMI; and could save up to 50 lives per 1000 patients treated

Action
- The precise mechanism of action is unknown, but a reduction in platelet aggregation undoubtedly plays a part in influencing the balance between thrombus formation and growth and spontaneous lysis

Dosage
- One tablet of soluble aspirin (300 mg), chewed to obtain high blood levels rapidly (unless the patient has already taken aspirin in the preceding 24 hours)

Contraindications
- Previous history of gastrointestinal bleed/peptic ulcer disease, and allergy to aspirin or other NSAIDs

Thrombolytics

Introduction
- The use of thrombolytics is now established as a major advance in the management of acute myocardial infarction, and can give a 12-50% reduction in the short term mortality, and up to a 47% reduction in the long term mortality (>1 year)
- Thrombolytics are most effective if given immediately after the onset of symptoms of infarction (and before significant myocardial muscle death occurs), and become less beneficial as time elapses and myocardial damage becomes irreversible)
- Several trials have shown a considerable time saving and increased benefit for pre-hospital thrombolysis, when compared to in-hospital thrombolysis, especially in rural areas
- Thrombolytics are of greatest benefit to those at greatest risk of dying as a result of their infarction:
    - Age: >70 years
    - History of a previous myocardial infarction
    - The hypotensive
    - Females
    - Those with an anterior infarct
    - Those with proven myocardial infarction (ST segment elevation) or new Left Bundle Branch Block
- The greatest benefit occurs if thrombolytics are given together with aspirin (taken for one month)

Action
- Thrombolytics activate the natural endogenous lytic pathways in the circulation. The precursor of this pathway is plasminogen which is converted to an active protease enzyme; plasmin. Plasmin breaks down the fibrin matrix of the thrombus, resulting in dissolution of the clot itself. It has no effect on the underlying atheromatous disease
- Intracoronary clot lysis results in an increase in the patency of the blocked coronary artery, the restoration of blood supply to the infarcted coronary muscle and a reduction in the loss of myocardium
- Reperfusion results in the early release of cardiac enzymes, and may cause cardiac arrhythmias
- After thrombolytic administration there may be early ST segment elevation resolution, the degree of resolution indicating the amount of residual myocardial damage/infarction:
    - Complete ST segment resolution, is associated with a small infarct area and low mortality
    - Lack of early ST segment resolution, indicates failed thrombolysis, and is associated with a large infarct area/late thrombolysis, a relatively high early mortality

Disadvantages
- The overall risk of complications is low
- Severe bleeding (< 1%):
    - 0.5% have a major cerebral bleed, and although there is no overall increased risk of a cerebral vascular accident; this risk is slightly greater:
        - Following administration with alteplase (rtPA) compared with streptokinase
        - In the elderly, those weighing <65 kg, and those with a systolic BP >160 mmHg
    - Most bleeding is minor
- Bradycardia, sudden severe, but transient hypotension ⎤ made worse by
- Life threatening ventricular arrhythmias due to reperfusion of cardiac muscle (rare) ⎟ ambulance ride
- Risk of microemboli due to disintegration of pre-existing clot
- Streptokinase and anistreplase are antigenic, and the antibodies persist indefinitely, so they may only be administered once in a lifetime
- Allergic reactions (rare)
- Expense (apart from streptokinase, which is much cheaper)

Indications
- History strongly suggestive of acute myocardial infarction
- Presentation with:
    - The onset of chest pain of at least 20 minutes to 12 hours duration, unrelieved by nitrates, and:
    - Unequivocal ECG changes diagnostic of AMI:
        - ST elevation of at least 2 mm in two or more leads
- Thrombolysis may be considered:
    - History suggestive of acute myocardial infarction and the patient is severely ill, *and*:
        - There is ECG evidence of:
            - Left Bundle Branch Block (see chapter on Cardiac care: arrhythmias)
        - Short time since onset of symptoms
        - Long travelling time to hospital (more than 45 minutes)

Contraindications
Absolute
- Normal ECG (or ECG not available)
- Cerebrovascular accident in the preceding 3 months leaving residual disability, or transient ischaemic attack within the preceding 6 months
- Known bleeding diathesis, long term anticoagulant therapy, or chronic liver disease with portal hypertension
- Intracranial neoplasm, arteriovenous malformation or aneurysm
- Severe hypertension (BP >200 mmHg systolic and/or >120 mmHg diastolic)
- Known potential site for pre-existing blood clot:
    - Ventricular/aortic aneurism
- Surgery, major trauma, or neurosurgery in the preceding month
- Previous administration of/allergy to streptokinase or anistreplase (but not alteplase or urokinase)

Relative
- Gastrointestinal bleeding, or pancreatitis
- Recent prolonged (traumatic) external chest compressions
- Dental extraction within preceding 14 days
- Non-compressible arterial punctures within the preceding 14 days or required immediately
- Serious organic or psychiatric illness
- Pregnancy

Discussion point: Pre-hospital administration of thrombolytics

Concerns
- The pre-hospital administration of thrombolytics may be dangerous because:
  - Acute myocardial infarction may be difficult to diagnose early with any certainty, when thrombolysis is most effective and beneficial, because of the considerable variation in the onset of definite ECG changes, and the difficulty of differentiating AMI from other conditions, e.g. ruptured aortic aneurism, in which thrombolytic administration could be catastrophic
  - Ventricular fibrillation is common after acute myocardial infarction, and giving a thrombolytic may increase this incidence
- Thrombolytics suitable for pre-hospital administration are very expensive

Evidence
- The Grampian region early anistreplase trial (GREAT) study, although relatively small, but comparing the pre-hospital administration of thrombolytics by General (Medical) Practitioners 'GPs' with the later hospital administration of the same thrombolytic, has shown:
  - GPs are sufficiently capable of making an accurate diagnosis of AMI from the patient's history, examination and 12 lead ECG tracing, and are able to administer thrombolytics effectively, safely, and expeditiously
  - Early GP administration of thrombolytics in rural areas significantly reduces the time from the onset of myocardial infarction to thrombolytic administration, when compared with hospital administration of thrombolytics
  - The early pre-hospital administration of thrombolytics results in a significant reduction in infarct size, left ventricular function (permanent myocardial damage) and mortality following AMI (in patients presenting two hours after the onset of symptoms, each hour's further delay in receiving thrombolysis led to the additional loss of 21 lives per 1000 patients within 30 days, and 69 lives per 1000 patients within 30 months)
  - In some studies the incidence of ventricular fibrillation was lower in those given pre-hospital thrombolysis than those receiving thrombolysis in hospital, and their chances of being successfully defibrillated and leaving hospital alive was also greater
- Meta-analysis of all the randomised trials of pre-hospital versus in-hospital thrombolysis shows a statistically significant benefit with pre-hospital thrombolysis equivalent to 21 lives per 1000 patients within 30 days, for each hour of earlier treatment

Conclusions
- The pre-hospital administration of thrombolytics for the treatment of acute myocardial infarction is safe, and can significantly reduce the mortality and morbidity. The earlier it is performed the greater the benefits
- The pre-hospital administration of a thrombolytic to patients with the ECG signs of acute myocardial infarction, as soon as possible after the onset of the symptoms, should be treated with the same degree of urgency as any other acute life threatening medical emergency, such as cardiac arrest
- As in cardiac arrest the responsibility for initiating treatment should rest with the first qualified person on scene, and GPs should administer thrombolytics if the travelling time to hospital is more than 30 minutes
- All those carrying thrombolytics intended for pre-hospital administration, should be able to record a 12 lead ECG, and carry a defibrillator together with the drugs required for managing the major life threatening peri-arrest and reperfusion arrhythmias
- The injectable forms of thrombolytic treatment suitable for pre-hospital use are more expensive than streptokinase, but this expense is amply justified by the additional lives saved

Streptokinase (SK) (*Streptase®*, *Kabikinase®*)

Description
- Streptokinase is produced from *Streptococcus pyogenes* cultures
- It forms a complex with plasminogen, which converts further plasminogen into (active) plasmin

Presentation
- *Kabikinase*: 1.5 million IU vial of straw coloured powder with human albumin and buffering agents
- *Streptase*: 1.5 million IU vial of purified

Advantages
- The original specific thrombolytic, with which most experience has been gained
- It is less likely to cause cerebral and non-cerebral haemorrhage than either anistreplase or alteplase
- Easy to store (between 2-25°C).

Disadvantages
- Streptokinase is a "foreign" (bacterial) protein and is antigenic. All patients develop antibodies to it within 5-10 days. which persist indefinitely, prohibiting it ever being readministered
- Allergic reactions may occur, but rarely.
- Less effective on old thrombus than fibrin specific activators (see below)

Administration
- Slowly intravenously: 1.5 million units in 50-200 mL normal saline, dextrose 5%, Hartmann's solution, or Haemaccel over 1 hour

Cost
- Cheapest

CONCLUSION
- *Unsuitable for pre-hospital administration* (except possibly using a syringe pump driver), but because it is cheap it is the thrombolytic of choice for hospital use, being administered together with aspirin

Anistreplase (APSAC) (*Eminase®*)

Description
- It is complex molecule containing streptokinase, plasminogen, and an 'anisosoyl' group, which makes the molecule inactive, until *in vivo* hydrolysis occurs and gives it a sustained action after a single bolus. It also has a relatively high affinity for fibrin bound plasminogen

Presentation
- 30 units/5 mL vial, 5 mL water for infusion, syringe and needle

Advantages
- Of proven efficacy and is easy to administer

Disadvantages
- Must be stored between 2-8°C
- Antigenic: antibodies develop within 5-10 days of administration, and allergic reactions may occur rarely (but more frequently than with either streptokinase or alteplase)
- Should not be used after previous administration of streptokinase or anistreplase
- May cause alarming hypotension

Administration
- 30 units/5mL administered intravenously over 4-5 minutes.

Half life
- 90-110 minutes

Cost
- Expensive (in the UK, 7x the cost of streptokinase)

CONCLUSION
- Anistreplase was considered by some to be the *thrombolytic of choice for pre-hospital administration*, but its storage requirements are a major problem. Reteplase is probably better

Alteplase, recombinant human tissue-type plasminogen activator (rtPA) (*Actilyse®*)

Description
- rtPA is a naturally occurring glycoprotein, made in very small quantities by many body tissues. It has a very high affinity for plasminogen in the presence of a fibrin clot, and directly activates the conversion of plasminogen to plasmin
- The commercially available product, rtPA, is manufactured by recombinant gene technology, based on human cell cultures

Presentation
- Pack of 2 x 50 mg vials of dry powder, 2 x 50 mL water for infusion (WFI), 2 transfer devices and 2 hanging bags

Advantages
- Non antigenic, causes less reduction in fibrinogen, and achieves earlier vessel patency
- May reduce the mortality following AMI slightly more than streptokinase

Disadvantages
- More likely to cause cerebrovascular accidents than streptokinase or anistreplase
- It has a very short half-life

Administration
- Given by slow intravenous infusion: 10 mg bolus, 50 mg over 1 hour, then 40 mg over 2 hours

Cost
- The most expensive (in the UK, 11x the cost of streptokinase)

CONCLUSION
- *Difficult to administer in the pre-hospital situation and* is usually reserved for patients who have had streptokinase or anistreplase previously, younger patients with an anterior infarction presenting within four hours of infarction, and possibly those suffering from cardiogenic shock, in whom its ability to achieve early patency is particularly beneficial

Reteplase (rPA) (*Rapilysin®*)

Description
- Reteplase is a genetically engineered deletion mutant of human tPA, modified to result in less high affinity fibrin binding, a longer half-life and a more rapid completion of reperfusion than rtPA

Presentation
- Pack containing 2 each: vial containing 10 U reteplase, as a sterile powder, pre-filled syringe with 10 mL water, reconstitution spike, and intravenous needle

Advantages
- As rtPA, early trials suggest that rPA was associated with higher early patency rates and better ventricular function than alteplase
- Easy to store (between 2-25°C), shelf life 2 years

Disadvantages
- As rtPA

Administration
- Reteplase is administered as a 10+10 U double bolus injection, injected intravenously as a slow intravenous injection over not more than 2 minutes, as soon as possible after the onset of infarction. The second bolus is administered 30 minutes after the first

Cost
- Similar to alteplase

CONCLUSION
- Reteplase is a new thrombolytic, which *may be suitable* for pre-hospital use because of its ease of administration, non antigenicity and lack of special storage requirements, but needs further evaluation

Urokinase (UK) (*Ukidan*®)

Description
- Produced from human adult male urine, it is a enzyme which promotes the activation of plasminogen to form plasmin

Presentation
- Vial containing 1 MIU as a sterile, white, freeze dried powder

Advantages
- Non antigenic, as it is of human origin
- Easy to store (between 2-25°C)

Disadvantages
- Not yet licensed in the UK for myocardial thrombolysis, and only available on a named patient basis
- Has been much less extensively used and evaluated than the other thrombolytics, but it appears to have similar efficacy to rtPA

Administration
- 2 MIU injected intravenously as a bolus

Cost
- Slightly cheaper than anistreplase

CONCLUSION
- *A convenient thrombolytic for pre-hospital administration* because of its ease of administration, and easy storage requirements, but there is concern about the lack of trial evidence of its efficacy and its lack of a licence for use as a coronary artery thrombolytic

---

Discussion point: the best thrombolytic for pre-hospital use

Concerns
- Streptokinase (the cheapest thrombolytic) is not really suitable for pre-hospital use (although it may be used with a syringe pump driver, which is expensive and difficult to set up). All the available alternatives are relatively very expensive
- Anistreplase is easy to administer, but is antigenic, is difficult to store and has a relatively short shelf life. If it is to be readily available, it may need to be stored in several locations, thus increasing the cost
- Urokinase is non antigenic, easy to adminiser and store, but is unlicensed for coronary thrombolysis and is of unproven value in AMI. It is only slightly cheaper than anistreplase, but a lot cheaper than rtPA
- Alteplase is a relatively new, but expensive thrombolytic. It is non antigenic, and easy to store and administer, but has not been evaluated in the pre-hospital situation

Conclusions
- The ideal thrombolytic for pre-hospital use does not yet exist, although reteplase looks promising
- The benefits of early pre-hospital thrombolysis for patients with an AMI easily justify the expense

Complications of acute myocardial infarction

Arrhythmias (see chapter on Cardiac Care: arrhythmias)

Acute left ventricular failure
- This is a common and life threatening medical emergency, and is a major cause of death post AMI

Incidence
- Acute left ventricular failure (LVF) is a common complication of AMI and ischaemic heart disease

Aetiology
- Acute LVF may be caused by:
    - Acute myocardial infarction
    - Ventricular septal defects
    - Heart valve lesions, usually aortic or mitral
    - Cardiac arrhythmias resulting in poor cardiac output, especially in the the presence of pre-existing cardiac disease e.g. atrial fibrillation, acute tachycardias
    - Endocarditis
    - Heart muscle disease of any cause, e.g. cardiomyopathy, ischaemia, etc.

Pathophysiology
- The inability of the left ventricular myocardium to pump blood sufficiently effectively, results in a rise in pulmonary venous pressure and causes pulmonary oedema, resulting in severe breathlessness and orthopnoea

Symptoms/signs
- There is usually an initial dry cough productive of frothy pink sputum
- The patient is pale, distressed, cold, sweaty and tachycardic (due to sympathetic overactivity)
- There is an increase in respiratory rate and depth
- On auscultation of the lungs there are:
    - Basal lung crackles ('creps')
    - A raised jugular venous pressure
    - A third heart sound
    - Wheezing due to airway oedema and bronchospasm (cardiac asthma)

Management
- Sit the patient upright and administer high flow oxygen via a high concentration oxygen mask
- Establish intravenous access and administer:
    - An intravenous loop diuretic, e.g. furosemide *(Lasix®)* (80-120 mg) or bumetanide *(Burinex®)* (2-5 mg)
    - An intravenous opiate, e.g. morphine (5-10 mg), diamorphine (2.5-5 mg), (reduces preload through venodilation and relieves distress) together with an antiemetic, e.g. metoclopramide (10 mg)
    - Sublingual or buccal GTN (reduces left ventricular preload and afterload)
- Monitor the cardiac rhythm
- Identify and treat the cause if possible

Guidelines for the immediate management of AMI

- The overall goal is to reduce mortality and morbidity following AMI
- This may be achieved by reducing the time interval from the onset of symptoms to the provision of resuscitation skills, adequate assessment and diagnosis, administration of adequate analgesia, and where appropriate early administration of a thrombolytic agent
- It may be possible in some circumstances for the patient to commence treatment after the initial call for help and before the arrival of the doctor or ambulance, e.g. administration of aspirin and nitrates

Primary survey

Immediate assessment and management

- *Conscious, breathing, good (carotid) pulse:*
    - Administer high flow oxygen via a high concentration mask
    - Obtain history
    - Monitor heart rhythm
    - Check blood pressure
    - Administer:
        - Sublingual or buccal GTN (unless hypotensive or has already self administered nitrates)
        - Aspirin 300mg (chewed) unless has already self administered in the preceding 24 hours

- *Unconscious, not breathing, no pulse:*
    - Start Basic Life Support immediately followed by Advanced Life Support

Secondary survey

ECG monitor (ideally 12-lead): to confirm diagnosis if possible

Provide rapid treatment of any immediate life threatening arrhythmias or complications

Obtain intravenous access

Administer: Intravenous analgesia (diamorphine up to 10 mg or morphine up to 15 mg) together with an antiemetic (metoclopramide 10 mg): for relief of pain, nausea and vomiting

Thrombolysis: if there are no contraindications

Treat any symptomatic arrhythmia

Admit to hospital immediately

Support and give advice to the patient and their family

Figure 7-12 Guidelines for the management of acute myocardial infarction

Notes

8

Cardiac care: arrhythmias

Arrhythmias

Introduction

- This chapter covers those arrhythmias associated with cardiac arrest, and the more important peri-arrest arrhythmias. There is no attempt to cover all arrhythmias - only those which are most likely to occur acutely in the pre-hospital situation, or those which are similar to these arrhythmias and are included to help in understanding their electrophysiology
- Many arrhythmic cardiac deaths are preventable
- The commonest cause of lethal arrhythmias is acute myocardial infarction, but they may also occur in patients who have no or only minimal myocardial damage:
    - 30% of arrhythmias are not due to an acute myocardial infarction
    - 20% of arrhythmias are not due to coronary artery disease
- The risk of developing a lethal arrhythmia post myocardial infarction is greatest immediately after the onset of symptoms, and falls during the following 24 hours, although up to 95% of patients may develop some kind of arrhythmia. The most common arrhythmia post infarction is premature ventricular contractions
- Arrhythmias, especially ventricular fibrillation, are the usual mode of sudden cardiac death

General principles of management
- *Treat the patient rather than the rhythm*
- Always administer high flow oxygen
- Any arrhythmia causing significant symptoms or haemo-dynamic compromise should be treated immediately, if practicable
- No antiarrhythmic treatment/drugs should be administered without ECG monitoring (3 lead is sufficient)
- If the rhythm changes, go back to the beginning of the guidelines for the new rhythm
- In general:
    - The use of more than one arrhythmic drug is best avoided and may only cause additional problems
    - If first line therapy fails; consider electrical treatment:
        - Cardioversion for tachycardias
        - Pacing (+atropine) for bradycardias
- All antiarrhythmic measures (drug and electrical treatment) may also cause arrhythmias
- No algorithm can cover all eventualities; some situations may arise which may call for different measures than those suggested
- Drug administration must be by the intravenous route; probably via a peripheral vein, in the pre-hospital situation, because it is quicker, easier to obtain, and requires less experience. If the peripheral venous route is used, a flush of 20 mL of 0.9% saline is advised to assist entry of the drug into the central circulation

Note: Some authorities prefer the term dysrrhythmia to describe abnormalities of cardiac rhythm. It appears however that linguistically, arrhythmia is the correct international term

Arrhythmias associated with cardiac arrest

Ventricular fibrillation

Incidence
- This is the most treatable and most common cause of sudden cardiac arrest following acute myocardial infarction
- Responsible for 90% of early cardiac deaths

Aetiology
- Ventricular fibrillation is a common complication of acute myocardial infarction and ischaemia:
    - Occurs in up to 20% of patients (more in some trials, if the patient is administered a thrombolytic)
    - 50% of patients developing ventricular fibrillation do so in first hour
    - The development of ventricular fibrillation is unrelated to the size of the infarct
    - May be precipitated by ischaemia alone (coronary artery spasm)
- May also occur as a complication of:
    - Electric shock, including inappropriate defibrillation
    - Drowning and severe hypothermia
    - Drug overdosage, including tricyclic antidepressants, digoxin and epinephrine
- May be preceded by other arrhythmias, e.g. ventricular tachycardia, bigeminy, or may occur without any previous rhythm disturbance

Pathophysiology
- Ventricular fibrillation is a condition of pulseless chaotic disorganised ventricular rhythm, characterised by an irregular undulating irregular ECG pattern, which varies in size and shape. The chaotic electrical activity results in individual ventricular muscle fibres contracting in a totally uncoordinated fashion
- Ventricular fibrillation may occur as a result of an irritable focus in the ventricular myocardium depolarising spontaneously to produce ventricular depolarisation (a premature ventricular complex) at a critical phase in the preceding cardiac cycle (R on T phenomenon)
- Cardiac output is completely lost, resulting in failure of the blood supply to body. The patient becomes unconscious, and irreversible anoxic brain damage and myocardial muscle damage occur rapidly

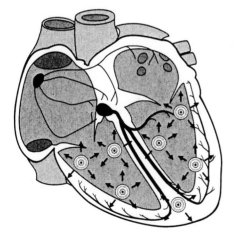 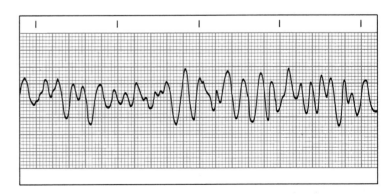

Figure 8-1 Ventricular fibrillation

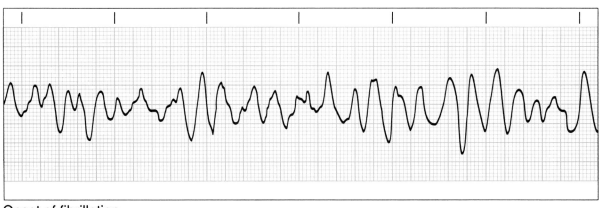

Onset of fibrillation

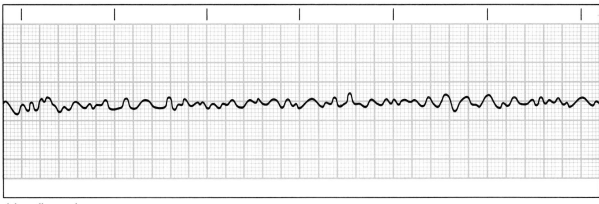

After five minutes

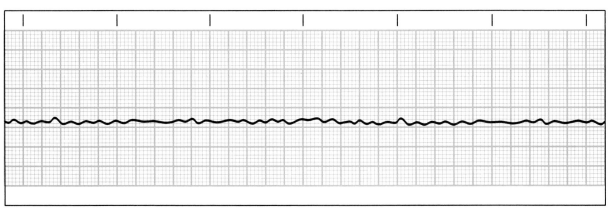

After ten minutes

Figure 8-2 Progression from coarse to fine ventricular fibrillation over time

ECG features

QRS rhythm: There is no true QRS rhythm, the complexes are totally irregular in frequency and amplitude

Rate: Not usually possible to measure, usually >300 uncoordinated waves per minute

P waves: Not visible

Pacemaker site: None

PR interval: None

QRS complex: None:
  - Random fibrillatory waves of differing amplitude, morphology, frequency and duration
  - Initially the waves are relatively coarse, but become finer until finally there is asystole

Management
  - **Administer a precordial thump**, if the cardiac arrest is witnessed and preferably monitored, and immediately afterwards check the ECG monitor, if one is already attached, or the carotid pulse, to see if the rhythm has changed
  - If the arrest was not witnessed, or if the precordial thump was not successful, take the paddles or pads out of the defibrillator. Charge up the defibrillator to deliver a shock of 200 joules as you do so, and place them on the patient's chest in the position shown below
  - **Analyse the ECG tracing**, and if the rhythm is ventricular fibrillation or ventricular tachycardia:
  - **Give a first shock of 200 Joules**. Charge up the defibrillator to 200 joules again, and check the ECG tracing (this should be before Basic Life Support, which does not actually improve the situation and only slows down further deterioration). If there is no improvement in the rhythm:
  - **Give a second shock of 200 Joules**, (transthoracic impedance is reduced with successive shocks, which is why a second shock of the same energy may be successful). Charge up the defibrillator to 360 joules and check the ECG tracing. If there is no improvement in the rhythm:
  - **Give a third shock of 360 Joules**, and analyse the ECG tracing. If there is no improvement in the rhythm:

Note: 1. A pulse check should be performed only, if after a defibrillation, an ECG rhythm compatible with cardiac output is produced. If VF persists, then further shocks in groups of three are given without checking the pulse
  2. After a defibrillating shock there is often a delay of a few seconds before an ECG tracing of diagnostic quality is obtained (with older machines this delay may be even longer)
  3. The defibrillatory shock can result in temporary impairment of myocardial contractility causing a weak or difficult to palpate pulse, even when a rhythm compatible with cardiac output is obtained
  4. If defibrillation is going to be successful, this is usually achieved within the first three shocks. If the patient remains in ventricular fibrillation, the best chance for restoring a perfusing rhythm still lies with defibrillation, although the chances of success are much less. It is now appropriate to treat any reversible causes or aggravating factors for ventricular fibrillation, while still attempting to maintain myocardial and cerebral viability

  - **Perform cycles of 5:1 or 15:2 chest compressions/ventilations** for one minute (to help preserve cardiac and cerebral circulation and to help any drugs to circulate), whilst attempting to:
    - **Intubate the patient.** If this is unsuccessful or the operator is inexperienced in intubation, insert either a Combitube® or a Laryngeal mask® airway
    - **Establish intravenous access**
    - **Attach the chest electrodes for a 3-Lead ECG if you are using paddles** (just outside their usual positions, so that they do not come into contact with the paddles), and switch the ECG monitor to read through the chest electrodes instead of the paddles
    - **Administer epinephrine 1 mg intravenous**ly (or 2-3 times this via a tracheal tube with a *Tracho-Jet*®)
    - **Check the electrode/defibrillating paddle positions and contacts**
    - If there is insufficient time to do all this, try again during the next episode of CPR

  - **After one minute check the ECG tracing**, and if the rhythm is still ventricular fibrillation administer (after first checking that the ECG monitor is reading through the chest leads rather than the paddles if you have just attached them; this is particularly important as movement artefact read through the paddles may look just like ventricular fibrillation!):
  - **Three shocks each of 360 Joules**, checking the ECG monitor after each shock, and if not successful:

- **Repeat the loop, administering epinephrine 1 mg every 3 minutes** or with each cycle of shocks
- Each cycle of shocks should take about 2 minutes (may be difficult with limited numbers of personnel)
- During each episode of CPR, assess the need for administering:
    - Sodium bicarbonate (50 mL of 8.4%)
    - An antiarrhythmic, e.g. lidocaine 100 mg, bretylium or amiodarone
- If further defibrillation is unsuccessful, then consider changing the position of the paddles/pads, e.g. to anteroposterior, trying a different defibrillator and replace the pads

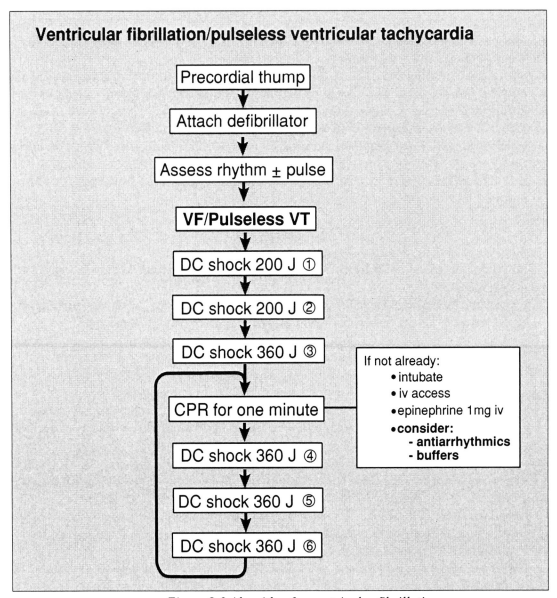

Figure 8-3 Algorithm for ventricular fibrillation

Note: 1. Epinephrine should be administered by the intravenous route, but if this is not possible it may be given by the tracheal route (although research suggests that this is less effective), when the dose should be *doubled or trebled* and diluted in a volume of at least 10 mL of 0.9% saline. Following tracheal administration, give 5 consecutive ventilations to assist absorption from the bronchial tree

2. All doses are based on a 70 kg man

3. Both asystole and electromechanical dissociation can occur transiently after defibrillation for ventricular fibrillation, when the prospects for recovery are much better. The appropriate treatment is continued chest compressions and epinephrine

Precordial thump

- This delivers 8-20 joules of energy, which may be sufficient if delivered immediately after the patient arrests, to convert ventricular fibrillation (the most likely arrhythmia causing cardiac arrest), or ventricular tachycardia into sinus rhythm, and is unlikely to be harmful
- Reported success rates:
    - Ventricular fibrillation: 2%
    - Ventricular tachycardia: 11-40%
- A precordial thump may exceptionally convert ventricular tachycardia into asystole, which is a much less favourable rhythm, and so it is therefore *not considered to be part of bystander BLS*, and is best used for the witnessed (and preferably monitored) cardiac arrest
- A precordial thump may be administered for confirmed ventricular fibrillation when there is no defibrillator immediately at hand
- Precordial thumps reduce the transthoracic impedance, making subsequent defibrillations more effective
- A cough may work as well as a precordial thump, so monitored patients who develop ventricular fibrillation or pulseless ventricular tachycardia, should be encouraged to cough

Method
- Give a moderately hard blow with a clenched fist to the sternum at the junction of its upper two thirds and the lower one third

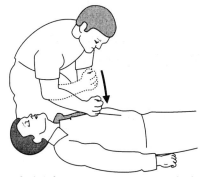

Figure 8-4 Administering a precordial thump

Defibrillation

- This is the only effective treatment for ventricular fibrillation (bystander basic life support helps to prevent immediate death and buys time until defibrillation can be carried out)
- The chance of success is greatest if the defibrillation is given within 90 seconds of the arrest and declines rapidly thereafter, at a rate of 5-10% per minute (see graph overleaf)
- If no ECG monitoring is available, it is best to assume that the patient with a cardiac arrest is in ventricular fibrillation, and manage them accordingly

Safety

- Defibrillation must not place at risk any members of the resuscitation team:
    - Nobody should be in contact with the patient or equipment capable of conducting electricity from the patient at the time the shock is delivered. This includes wet clothing and infusion equipment
    - The defibrillator operator should:
        - Shout "Stand clear" and ensure that everyone has done so before defibrillating
        - Not touch the surface of the defibrillating electrodes
        - Avoid spreading electrode gel across the patient's chest, or on their hands or any equipment
    - The airway carer should ensure that high flow oxygen is not passing near the area of defibrillation
    - Manual defibrillator paddles should only be charged whilst being applied to the casualty's chest or placed in their cradle in the defibrillator. If they are applied to the chest, the operator should advise the other team members whether they are being used to monitor the heart or are about to be charged
    - If manual defibrillator paddles are charged, but there is no need to deliver a shock, they should only be discharged into the air whilst the operator is holding them far apart, with the usual safety checks

Defibrillators
- These are devices which use the energy from batteries or mains electricity to charge a capacitor, and then discharge a high voltage direct current (DC) electric shock through electrodes which are applied to the casualty's chest, over a very short interval of time (4-12 milliseconds)
- The shock passes through the heart, resulting in the instant depolarisation of all receptive myocardial cells. It is hoped that when spontaneous electrical activity resumes, sinus rhythm will return
- The amount of energy stored is adjusted by a control, which shows the energy stored in joules
- Most defibrillators have:
    - An integral ECG monitor display for monitoring the cardiac rhythm
    - A memory for storing details of all important events, which may be downloaded into a computer
    - A printer for printing out the ECG strip and a 'code' summary printout, including the ECG tracing before and after any shocks, together with the date, times and energy selected
- Modern defibrillators are capable of recharging very rapidly following delivery of a shock

Manual defibrillators
- These are defibrillators (often with a computerised memory) which:
    - Depend on the operator to analyse the cardiac rhythm and to deliver the appropriate shock
    - They usually have:
        - Paddles, to which conductive gel is applied, and which have to be held against the anterior chest wall of the patient by the operator. These can be used both for analysing the rhythm and delivering the shock. Some manual defibrillators now use disposable pads similar to those used by semi-automatic external defibrillators (see below). The paddles usually have controls for adjusting the defibrillator, so that charging the defibrillator, defibrillating, recording the ECG tracing, etc. can be performed without taking the paddles off the patient's chest
        - A 3-lead chest electrode attachment for monitoring the heart rhythm more accurately and more easily (hands free) than through the paddles
    - They may also have:
        - A facility for performing a full diagnostic 12-lead ECG
        - A pacing facility
Advantages
- The operator may deliver whatever shock he considers appropriate
- In skilled hands, they are able to deliver a series of shocks as fast as an automated defibrillator
Disadvantages
- Are relatively complicated to use
- Are only suitable for use by skilled trained personnel, who need to be able to:
    - Recognise the ECG rhythm
    - Decide on and select the appropriate energy level and administer the shock

Semi-automatic/advisory external defibrillators (AEDs)
- These are computerised defibrillators, with a display for giving instructions and in most cases showing the ECG tracing, a voice synthesizer for giving verbal instructions, and a memory, which:
    - Analyses the cardiac rhythm and gives appropriate instructions verbally and on the display screen
    - If the rhythm is ventricular fibrillation or ventricular tachycardia, the defibrillator will advise the operator to deliver the appropriate shock, after giving a visual and verbal warning
    - Semi-automatic/advisory defibrillators use disposable adhesive defibrillating electrodes both for analysing the rhythm and delivering the shock
- Some semi-automatic/advisory defibrillators have a facility for a manual override
Advantages
- AEDs are easy to use, and suitable for use by relatively unskilled personnel, as they do not require rhythm recognition on the part of the operator
- Once attached to the patient, semi-automatic/advisory defibrillators, analyse the rhythm automatically, thus freeing one pair of hands for other use in between shocks

Disadvantages
- AEDs may have difficulty recognising fine ventricular fibrillation and refuse to shock
- Some AEDs may be slower to defibrillate than an expertly used manual defibrillator

Biphasic defibrillators
- Standard defibrillators deliver a high energy monophasic damped sinusoidal wave shock
- A recent development is biphasic defibrillators which deliver a lower energy biphasic shock (in some devices, after first measuring the transthoracic impedance)
- The theoretical advantages of this is that the defibrillator needs to deliver a lower energy shock to achieve defibrillation, resulting in less myocardial injury, and the defibrillator requires smaller energy batteries, making it lighter, smaller, more portable and cheaper

Factors affecting the success of defibrillation

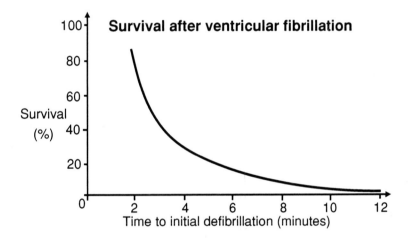

Fig 8-5 Success rate of defibrillation for VF

Time
- The chance of success is greatest if the defibrillation is administered within 90 seconds of the arrest and declines rapidly thereafter
- If defibrillation is delayed:
    - More than 8 minutes, there is a substantial risk of the patient sustaining neurological damage
    - More than 10 minutes, there is very little chance of success
- Time is less critical where the ventricular fibrillation accompanies hypothermia and/or drowning

Transthoracic impedance
- This is the resistance to the flow of electricity caused by the chest wall, lungs and myocardium
- The transthoracic impedance and the voltage delivered by the defibrillator determine the amount of electric current that actually passes through the heart
- The transthoracic impedance depends on:
    - The phase of respiration when the shock is administered
    - The size and placement of the chest electrodes
    - The interface between the electrodes and the skin
    - The number of previous shocks and the speed with which they have been given

The phase of respiration when the shock is administered
- The defibrillation shock should be given at the end of the expiratory phase of respiration, when the amount of air in the lungs is smallest (air is a poor conductor of electricity, and the higher the volume of air in the lungs, the greater will be the resistance to the flow of current)

Paddle/electrode size
- The larger the paddle/electrode size:
    - The lower the resistance to current flow, enabling more current to reach the heart
    - The greater the chance of successful defibrillation
    - The less the amount of myocardial damage caused by the defibrillation shock
- Paddle/electrode sizes should be sufficient to allow good skin contact, but not so large that they touch each other
- Infants and children require smaller paddles/electrodes and lower energy shocks than adults to achieve successful defibrillation
- Once a certain body weight is reached, increasing the size of the paddles/electrodes makes little significant difference, so a standard sized paddle is used for all adults
- Sizes of paddle/electrode:
    - Adults: 13 cm
    - Children: 8-10 cm, but adult paddles should be used if the child's chest is large enough
    - Infants: 4.5 cm

Note: Defibrillator paddles do not make ideal monitoring electrodes, because they have to be kept in position by hand. They are therefore only suitable for the initial rhythm recognition and should be replaced by adhesive chest electrodes after the first cycle of defibrillations

The interface between the electrodes and the skin
- The transthoracic impedance can be minimised by:
    - The use of a conductive gel or gel pads between the paddles and the skin:
        - Gel pads are preferred to gel from a tube, because the gel from a tube may become spread over the chest as a result of chest compressions and cause electrical arcing during defibrillation
    - The application of firm downwards pressure (about 11 kg) to keep the electrodes firmly applied to the chest:
        - This improves the contact between the paddles, gel and skin and reduces the amount of air in the lungs (in spite of the lack of applied pressure, adhesive disposable defibrillating chest electrodes appear to be just as effective as paddles for defibrillation)

The number of previous shocks and the speed with which they have been given
- Transthoracic impedance reduces by about 8% after the first defibrillation, and by about 4% after each subsequent defibrillation
- The reduction in transthoracic impedance will be greatest if the shocks are delivered in rapid succession

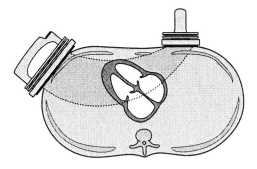
Correct paddle placement
Current passes through the ventricles

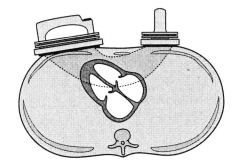
Incorrect paddle placement
Current misses part of the ventricles

Figure 8-6 Positioning the paddles to maximise the passage of current through the ventricles

Position of paddles/electrodes
- The paddles must be placed to allow the maximum flow of electricity through the ventricles
- The polarity of the paddles is probably not important, although paddles may be marked 'Apex' and 'Sternum'
- Do *not* place the paddles near any chest electrodes or within 12.5 cm of a pacemaker
- In adult females place the apex paddle just below or lateral to the left breast, and *not* on the breast, as breast tissue is relatively dense and increases the transthoracic impedance

Antero-apical positioning
- The paddles/pads are placed:
    - Just to the right of the sternum, below the right clavicle
    - Just outside the apex of the heart, covering the V_{4-5} positions of the ECG
- This is the preferred initial paddle position for adults

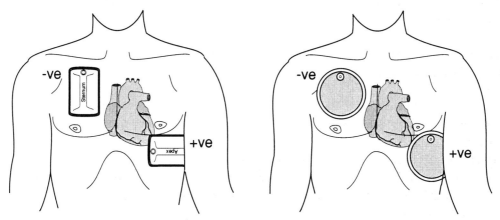

Figure 8-7 Positioning the paddles or disposable adhesive defibrillating electrodes: antero-apical

Antero-posterior positioning
- The paddles are placed:
    - Over the 4th intercostal space, mid clavicular line
    - Just below the left scapula
- Some machines have a special large paddle to fit under the left scapula
- Useful in children because the front of the chest may be too small for two electrodes/paddles
- Can be used in adults, but it may be difficult to turn obese patients sufficiently onto their side to apply the electrodes and to hold standard paddles against a patient who is supported on their side without maintaining contact with the patient during defibrillation

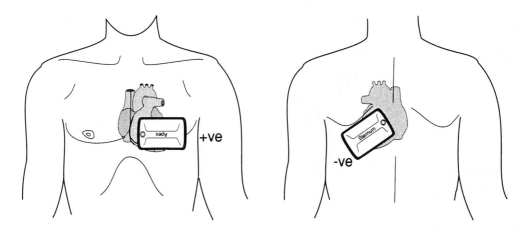

Figure 8-8 Positioning the paddles or defibrillating electrodes: antero-posterior

Method
- Remove any GTN patches, and make sure that the skin is dry
- Switch on the defibrillator, and make certain that the ECG monitor is reading through the paddles/ pads (or if chest leads have already been attached, that the monitor is reading through them)
- Remove the paddles/pads from the defibrillator and apply electrode gel to them or put gel pads on the patient's chest, or attach disposable adhesive defibrillating electrodes
- **Charge** the defibrillator
- Apply the paddles to the skin exerting firm downwards pressure
- **Analyse** the rhythm
- If the ECG tracing shows ventricular fibrillation, or ventricular tachycardia, prepare to **defibrillate** the patient by pressing the appropriate buttons on the paddles
- Before each defibrillation, shout "Stand by to defibrillate: Stand clear" and make certain that nobody is touching the patient or any attached equipment, as they may receive an accidental shock
- If paddles are used the defibrillator should be recharged immediately after each defibrillation, without removing the paddles from the chest, and the next shock given immediately, after checking the ECG tracing, if the post defibrillation rhythm shows that ventricular fibrillation is still present
- Do not interrupt the shock sequence for chest compressions/ventilations (CPR), unless the defibrillator is slow to recharge

CAUTION: Defibrillation should NOT be attempted in a moving vehicle because of the risk of sudden movement, resulting in a paddle or gel coming into contact with the vehicle or another rescuer

Rhythm analysis
- The display and printout from older defibrillators with an ECG monitor is not usually sensitive enough to be used for analysis of ST segment and other fine ECG tracing changes
- A continuous recording should be taken when any anti-arrhythmic drug is administered

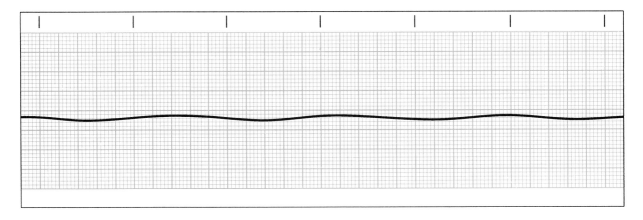

Figure 8-9 Ventricular asystole with baseline shift

Note: After a shock has been delivered, the ECG monitor screen may show an iso-electric line for several seconds. This is usually due to a transient period of 'stunning' of the myocardium, and does not necessarily mean that the cardiac rhythm has converted to asystole, as a coordinated rhythm or a return to VF/VT may subsequently occur. Thus if the ECG monitor screen of a manual defibrillator displays a 'straight' line for more than one sweep immediately post shock, one minute of CPR should be given without administration of epinephrine, and the patient reassessed. If the patient has a non VF/VT rhythm without a pulse, then a dose of epinephrine should be administered, followed by a further two minutes of CPR, after which the patient should be assessed again. Algorithms for AEDs should take this phenomenon into account

Ventricular asystole

Incidence
- Occurs less often than ventricular fibrillation following an acute myocardial infarction accounting for:
    - 10% of arrests outside hospital
    - 25% of arrests in hospital
- Has an extremely poor prognosis except in trifascicular block (where P waves may be seen), extreme bradycardia or where it is a transient rhythm following defibrillation

Aetiology
- Occurs as either a primary arrhythmia or as a secondary arrhythmia following other rhythm disorders in myocardial ischaemia:
    - The end stage of ventricular fibrillation and electromechanical dissociation and other terminal cardiac events and indicates cardiac death
    - The terminal mode of death in most cases of prolonged profound hypoxia following:
        - Respiratory arrest
        - Respiratory obstruction
        - Drowning
        - Severe pulmonary oedema

Pathophysiology
- In asystolic cardiac arrest, there is failure of all the natural (or artificial) pacemakers resulting in the total loss of all electrical and mechanical activity in the ventricles and the failure of myocardial contraction
- In normal circumstances; if either of the supraventricular pacemakers (the SA and AV nodes) or atrioventricular conduction fail (complete heart block), an idioventricular rhythm (produced by an ectopic pacemaker below the AV node), will maintain cardiac (ventricular) output
- This idioventricular rhythm may be suppressed, and asystole result, due to:
    - Myocardial disease
    - Electrolyte disturbance
    - Anoxia
    - Drugs
- Excessive cholinergic activity may suddenly suppress SA or AV node activity, especially when sympathetic tone is reduced, resulting in asystole in:
    - Myocardial ischaemia
    - Myocardial infarction
    - β-blockade

ECG features

QRS rhythm: None: straight line, although in ventricular standstill, some atrial activity may persist briefly until complete asystole ensues (as may artefact, baseline wander and electrical interference)

Rate: None

P waves: None usually, but P waves may be present for a short time after the onset of ventricular asystole

Pacemaker site: None: no ventricular or junctional escape pacemaker and no escape rhythm is present

PR interval: None

QRS complex: None

Management

- **Administer a precordial thump**, if the cardiac arrest is witnessed, and immediately afterwards check the ECG monitor, if one is already attached, or the carotid pulse, to see if the rhythm has changed
- If the arrest was not witnessed, or if the precordial thump was not successful, take the paddles/pads out of the defibrillator, charging up the defibrillator to deliver a shock of 200 joules as you do so, and place the paddles on the patient's chest
- **Analyse the ECG tracing**, and if fine ventricular fibrillation can be excluded and the rhythm is asystole:
- Check that there is clinical cardiac arrest
- Check that the leads, connections, gain and brilliance of the monitor are correct
- **Perform cycles chest compressions/ventilations** for 3 minutes. During this time:
    - **Intubate the patient**. If this is unsuccessful or the operator is inexperienced in intubation, after the first cycle of CPR insert a Combitube® or Laryngeal mask® airway
    - **Establish intravenous access** after the second cycle of CPR
    - **Administer epinephrine** 1/10,000: 1mg in 10 mL intravenously (2-3 times this dose via a tracheal tube)
    - Administer 100% oxygen, especially if hypoxia as a result of e.g. acute severe asthma, is the cause of the asystole
    - **Administer atropine 3 mg** (once *only*, sufficient to produce complete vagal block), and if there is no response:
    - **Consider pacing** if P waves or any other electrical activity is present
- **Perform further resuscitation loops** if there is still no electrical activity, (on the next loop perform any other procedure that has not already been done, i.e. obtain intravenous access, intubate), and if unsuccessful:
- Consider administration of high dose epinephrine (5 mg intravenously), if there is still no response, and if unsuccessful:
- Consider abandoning resuscitation (patients with primary cardiac disease are very unlikely to recover after more than 15 minutes), except in hypothermia, near drowning, or poisoning, when resuscitation should be continued

Note: If numbers of attending personnel are limited (as is usually the case in pre-hospital resuscitation), then 3-4 cycles of 15:2 chest compressions: ventilations is appropriate

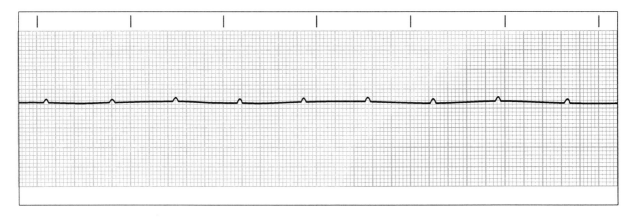

Figure 8-10 Ventricular asystole with P waves

Ventricular standstill

- May occur in complete heart block (Stokes-Adams attacks) or as an agonal rhythm
- In ventricular standstill:
    - There is no ventricular activity, but atrial activity may be recorded
    - There are P waves, but no QRS complexes

Stokes-Adams attacks

Aetiology
- These may occur in patients with some pre-existing degree of heart block or arise de novo

Pathophysiology
- In this condition the underlying rhythm may be sinus rhythm or there may be some degree of heart block, which is interrupted suddenly by ventricular standstill (asystole), before reverting after a short interval to the original rhythm
- This results in a transient loss of cardiac output producing dizziness, followed after about 5 seconds by loss of consciousness, then epileptiform movements and apparent death after about 30 seconds. If the heart does not revert to a rhythm with an adequate cardiac output, death will follow (unless the patient is resuscitated)

ECG features
- The original rhythm (usually sinus rhythm or some degree of heart block), is followed by ventricular asystole (with or without P waves), followed by a return to the original rhythm

Symptoms/signs
- Sudden onset of unconsciousness and pallor (syncope) during the episode of ventricular arrest/asystole, followed by flushing and the rapid return of consciousness

Management
- CPR or pacing (or defibrillation for ventricular fibrillation) if the period of asystole is prolonged (to minimise hypoxic cerebral damage)

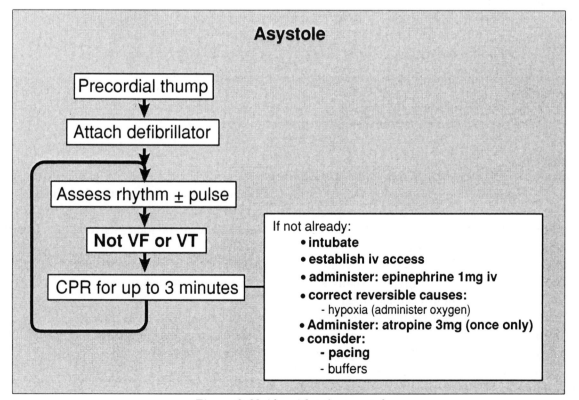

Figure 8-11 Algorithm for asystole

Note: Epinephrine and atropine should be given by the intravenous route, but if this is not possible they may be given by the tracheal route, when the dose should be *doubled or trebled*

Electromechanical dissociation (EMD)

Incidence
- Outside hospital:
    - Uncommon: accounts for less than 3% of cardiac deaths
    - Commonest cause is trauma
- Common in hospital: 30-70% of cardiac deaths
- Treatment is only rarely successful

Aetiology
Primary EMD
- Due to failure of excitation-contraction coupling as a result of:
    - Myocardial infarction (especially inferior wall)
    - Drugs, e.g. β-blockers, calcium antagonists and poisoning (overdosage of tricyclics)
    - Electrolyte abnormalities (hypocalcaemia, hyperkalaemia)
    - Hypothermia

Secondary EMD
- Due to mechanical impairment of ventricular filling or cardiac output as a result of:
    - Hypovolaemia due to trauma, concealed haemorrhage, etc.
    - Tension pneumothorax
    - Pericardial tamponade after ventricular rupture or trauma
    - Cardiac rupture
    - Pulmonary embolism
    - Prosthetic heart valve occlusion
    - Atrial thrombus or myxoma

Pathophysiology
- Loss of effective cardiac output in spite of normal or near normal electrical activity

ECG diagnosis
- The ECG may show normal sinus rhythm or any other rhythm, e.g. atrial fibrillation, which is usually consistent with an effective cardiac output

Management
- **Administer a precordial thump**, if the cardiac arrest is witnessed, and immediately afterwards check the ECG monitor, if one is already attached, or the carotid pulse, to see if the rhythm has changed
- If the arrest was not witnessed, or if the precordial thump was not successful, take the paddles/pads out of the defibrillator, charging up the defibrillator to deliver a shock of 200 joules as you do so, and place the paddles on the patient's chest
- **Analyse the ECG tracing**, and if fine ventricular fibrillation can be excluded and the rhythm appears to be sinus rhythm or another rhythm usually associated with a normal cardiac output:
- Check that there is clinical cardiac arrest
- **Perform cycles of chest compressions/ventilations** for 3 minutes. During this time:
    - **Intubate the patient.** If this is unsuccessful or the operator is inexperienced in intubation, insertion of a Combitube® or Laryngeal mask® airway is an alternative
    - **Establish intravenous access**

- Identification and treatment of the underlying cause if possible:
    - Hypovolaemia: intravenous infusion
    - Hyperkalaemia and electrolyte imbalance:
        - Consider calcium chloride (10 mL of 10%), but be aware that it it may cause hypercalcaemia and calcium overload, resulting in cardiac or cerebral cell death, for:
            - Known or suspected hyperkalaemia
            - Known or suspected hypocalcaemia
            - Calcium antagonist use or overdose
            - Wide QRS complex EMD
    - Hypothermia: start rewarming
    - Tamponade: pericardiocentesis
    - Tension pneumothorax: needle thoracocentesis
    - Thromboembolic/mechanical obstruction: ? administration of thrombolytics

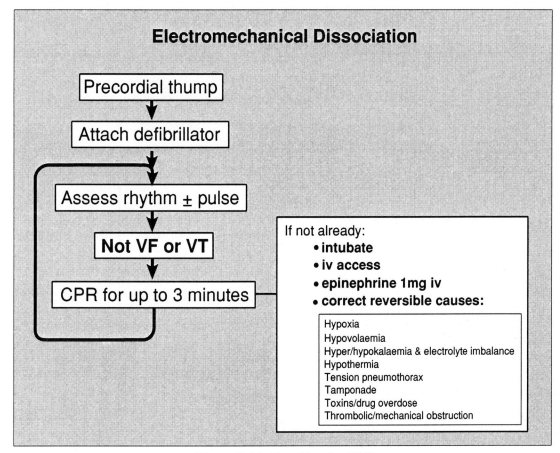

Figure 8-12 Algorithm for EMD

*Note:*1. If attending personnel are limited (as is usually the case in pre-hospital resuscitation), and there is only one basic life support provider, then 3-4 cycles of 15:2 chest compressions: ventilations is appropriate
2. All drugs should be administered by the intravenous route, but if this is not possible epinephrine may be given by the tracheal route, when the dose should be *doubled or trebled*
3. All doses are based on a 70 kg man
4. Electromechanical dissociation can occur transiently after defibrillation for ventricular fibrillation, when the prospects for recovery are much better. The appropriate treatment is continued chest compressions and epinephrine

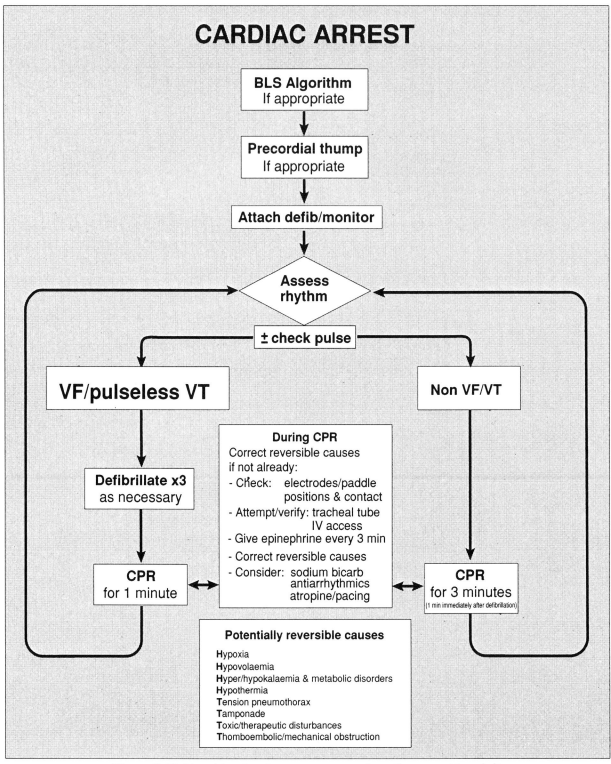

Figure 8-13 Algorithm for the management of cardiac arrest in adults
(copyright of the European Resuscitation Council, reproduced with permission)

Note:1. Each successive step is based on the assumption that the one before has been unsuccessful
  2. *Epinephrine* (adrenaline) and atropine should be given by the intravenous route, but if this is not possible they may be given by the tracheal route, when the dose should be *doubled or trebled.*
  3. All doses are based on a 70 kg man
  4. Both asystole and electromechanical dissociation can occur transiently after defibrillation for ventricular fibrillation, when the prospects for recovery are much better. The appropriate treatment is continued chest compressions and epinephrine
  5. Following successful defibrillation consider a lidocaine infusion of 3 mg/minute

Peri-arrest arrhythmias

- These are the arrhythmias, some of them potentially lethal, that may precede cardiac arrest or complicate the period after resuscitation

Bradyarrhythmias

Definition: Any arrhythmia where the heart (ventricular) rate is less than 60 beats per minute

Incidence
- These arrhythmias are common after inferior myocardial infarction

Aetiology
- If they occur after:
  - Inferior myocardial infarction:
    - The prognosis is good, as the treatment is usually simple and successful and the rhythm will usually revert to sinus rhythm, although temporary pacing may be necessary
    - The arrhythmia is often transient and occurs as a result of reversible ischaemia or vagal overactivity
  - Anterior myocardial infarction:
    - Bradycardia is a sign of extensive infarction involving the interventricular septum, and has a poor prognosis unless it is due to vagal overactivity alone
    - Death is the usual outcome due to the development of cardiogenic shock as a result of the extensive muscle damage
- May occur as a result of:
  - Previous treatment with β-blockers
  - AV nodal and conduction system disease

Electrophysiology

Aetiology
- Occurs most commonly after an inferior myocardial infarction (in 20% of all patients)

Incidence
- May be caused by:
  - Vaso-vagal slowing, or impairment of sino-atrial function, i.e. sinus bradycardia
  - First degree AV block (may not cause a bradycardia)
  - Second degree AV block (may not cause a bradycardia)
  - Third degree/complete AV block

Symptoms/signs
- The patient's condition depends on the underlying aetiology and the rate, and may vary from their being:
  - Relatively well with few or no symptoms
  - Very unwell with:
    - Chest pain due to cardiac ischaemia or even infarction
    - Dyspnoea
    - Confusion
    - Hypotension

Sinus bradycardia

Incidence
- Often found in normal fit young men, especially athletes
- Commonly occurs after inferior myocardial infarction

Aetiology
- May be caused by normal doses of:
    - β-blockers
    - Digoxin
    - Opiates
- May occur in:
    - Myxoedema
    - Hypothermia
    - Raised intracranial pressure

Pathophysiology
- Arises as a result of a slow rate of discharge from the sinoatrial node
- As the ventricular rate falls, the heart will attempt to compensate by increasing the stroke volume
- If the heart rate drops below 50 bpm, there is a risk of hypotension, especially in the elderly with ischaemic heart disease (IHD)
- Following AMI, sinus bradycardia indicates an increase in vagal (para-sympathetic) tone
- After an anterior infarction it does not have the same poor prognosis as the development of heart block

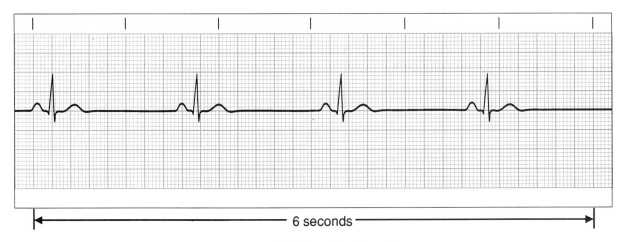

|← ———————————————— 6 seconds ————————————————→|

Figure 8-14 Sinus bradycardia

ECG features

Rhythm: Regular or very slightly irregular with a prolonged R-R interval between R waves

Rate: <60 beats per minute

P waves: Normal: each followed by a QRS complex

Pacemaker site: SA node

PR interval: Normal (0.12-0.2 sec.)

QRS complex: Normal: each preceded by a P wave

Sinus arrest

Incidence
- Relatively common

Aetiology
- Commonest cause is sino-atrial disease
- Often occurs as a result of ischaemic heart disease or rarely following AMI

Pathophysiology
- Caused by a defect in the SA node

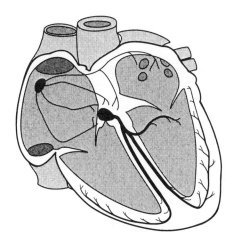
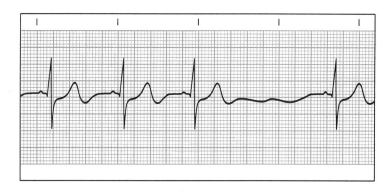

Figure 8-15 Sinus arrest

ECG features

Rhythm: Irregular (regular underlying rhythm with dropped beats)

Rate: Normal or slow

P waves: Normal, when they are present, preceding a QRS complex (abnormal, if an atrial escape beat occurs)
However, if the SA node is blocked or does not discharge, the entire sequence of P-QRS-T is missed, unless an ectopic escape focus takes over and an escape beat occurs

Pacemaker site: SA node

PR interval: Usually normal (0.12-0.20 sec)

QRS complex: Normal, each preceded by a QRS complex ⎫ absent during SA block
⎬
⎭

Heart block

Incidence
- Occurs in 5% of patients following AMI

Aetiology
- Usually results from ischaemic heart disease and inferior acute myocardial infarction

Pathophysiology
- Caused by conduction defects in the AV node and Bundle of His, which may be partial (first and second degree heart block) or complete (third degree or complete heart block)

First degree AV block

Incidence
- Common after acute myocardial infarction, when it may herald more advanced degrees of heart block

Aetiology
- Damage to the AV node due to organic heart disease
- Hypoxia
- Increased vagal (parasympathetic) tone
- Toxicity from cardiac drugs: β-blockers, digoxin, quinidine, procainamide

Pathophysiology
- There is a problem at the AV junction resulting in the slowing of conduction through the AV node

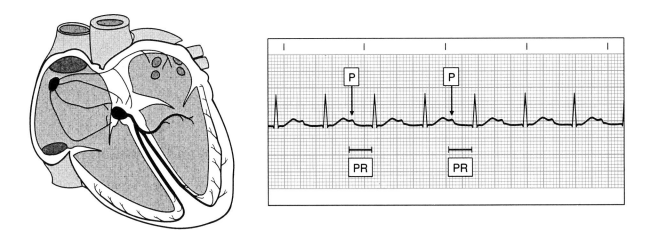

Figure 8-16 First degree AV block

ECG features

Rhythm: Regular

Rate: Normal or slow

P waves: Normal, preceding each QRS complex

Pacemaker site: SA node

PR interval: Prolonged PR interval: >200 milliseconds (5 small squares)

QRS complex: Usually normal each preceded by a P wave

Second degree AV block: Mobitz type I, Wenckebach phenomenon

Incidence
- A relatively common rhythm following acute myocardial infarction

Aetiology
- Ischaemic heart disease

Pathophysiology
- The conduction defect usually occurs at the AV junction, usually in or near the AV node itself
- There is a progressive increase in the delay of the transmission of impulses through the AV node, until one impulse fails to be transmitted (usually every third or fourth impulse)
- This rhythm is usually transient and reversible and does not always progress to a higher degree of block

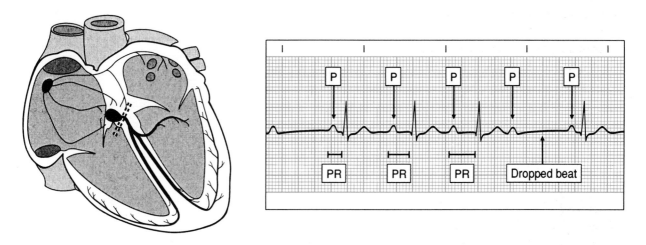

Figure 8-17 Second degree AV block: Mobitz type I: Wenckebach phenomenon

ECG features

Rhythm: Atrial (P wave) regular
        Ventricular (QRS) rhythm is regularly irregular

Rate: Atrial rate : Normal.
        Ventricular rate: Regularly irregular with dropped beats

P waves: Normal and regular

Pacemaker site: SA node (when sinus rhythm present)

PR interval: Progressively increases until a QRS complex is dropped as AV conduction fails completely; the process is then repeated

QRS complex: Usually normal: each QRS complex is preceded by a P wave, unless an escape beat occurs. The R-R interval usually decreases as the PR interval increases, but this is not easy to detect

Second degree AV block, Mobitz type II

Aetiology
- May follow a large anterior AMI, and is caused by damage to the conducting system below the AV node, in the bundle of His
- May be associated with bundle branch block
- Often *not* associated with ischaemic heart disease
- May be aggravated by use of β-blockers

Pathophysiology
- An intermittent failure of AV conduction results in the occasional failure of ventricular contraction
- It may progress rapidly and without warning to complete heart block

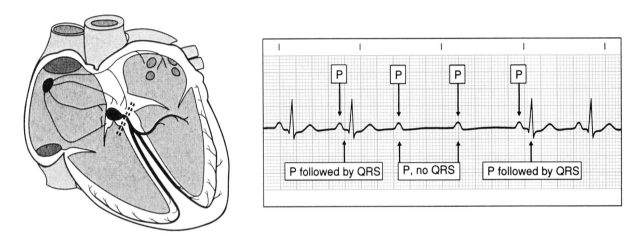

Figure 8-18 Second degree AV block: Mobitz type II

ECG features

Rhythm: Atrial (P wave) rhythm regular
Ventricular (QRS) rhythm is regular with missed complexes

Rate: Atrial rate normal.

P waves: Normal, but not every P wave is followed by a QRS complex
There are more P waves than QRS complexes
The ratio of P waves to QRS complexes may be 2:1, 3:1, etc., or may follow no regular pattern

Pacemaker site: SA node

PR interval: Normal or prolonged, but constant.

QRS complex: Usually normal, but may be widened: each is preceded by a P wave, unless escape beats occur

Third degree AV block: complete heart block

Aetiology
- May occur in the elderly due to non-ischaemic causes
- May occur following acute myocardial infarction

Pathophysiology
- Atrial contractions may occur normally, but there is a complete failure of AV conduction. In the absence of normal stimulation, the ventricles are excited by a subsidiary depolarising focus in the AV junction or ventricular muscle, resulting in a slow escape rhythm, so that there is no relationship between atrial and ventricular contractions
- If the ventricular rate is below 35-50 beats per minute, cardiac output may be significantly compromised
- Additionally, occasionally there may be poor ventricular filling, due to the non co-ordination between atria and ventricles

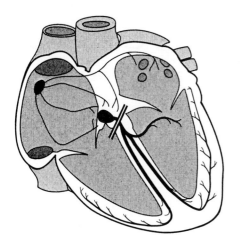
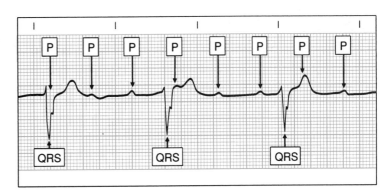

Figure 8-19 Third degree AV block

ECG features

Rhythm: Regular

Rate: Atrial (P waves) rate: regular in sinus rhythm (the atrial rhythm may also be atrial fibrillation with f waves or atrial flutter with F waves)
Ventricular (QRS) rate: regular: 30-40 beats per minute

P waves: Normal, but they do not have a constant relationship to the QRS complexes, i.e. there is AV dissociation (except in atrial flutter, when there may be a constant relationship with 2:1, 3:1 or 4:1 block)

Pacemaker site: SA node, but impulses are blocked at the AV junction, and so do not reach the ventricles
An ectopic focus in the AV junction or the ventricle then takes over
The lower the focus in the ventricles, the slower the rhythm, and the more abnormal the ventricular complexes appear

PR interval: There is no true PR interval

QRS complex: Usually wide and bizarre, although if the escape focus is in the AV node or junction they may appear normal

Management
- Administer oxygen
- If the patient is well: observe
- If the patient is unwell, i.e. pale, sweaty, shocked and is haemodynamically compromised (pulse rate <55 bpm, systolic blood pressure <100 mmHg), consider:
  - Atropine (more likely to be successful if the QRS complex is narrow): 0.5-0.6 mg given intravenously in incremental doses up to 2.0 mg over 5 minutes
  - Bolus of isoprenaline (50 µg), followed by an isoprenaline infusion (2-4 µg/min)
  - External pacing (if available)
  - Early evacuation to hospital

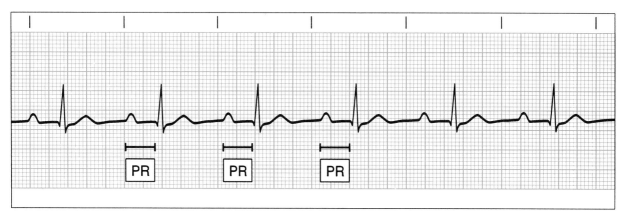

Figure 8-20 First degree AV block

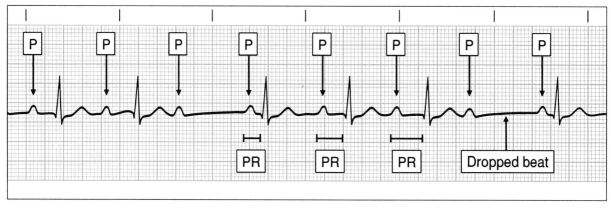

Figure 8-21 Second degree AV block: Mobitz I: Wenckebach

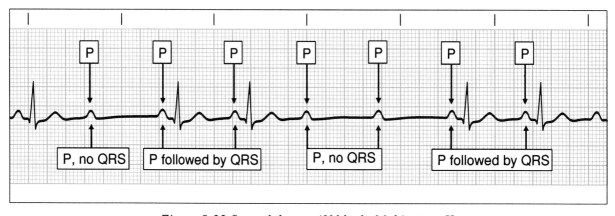

Figure 8-22 Second degree AV block: Mobitz type II

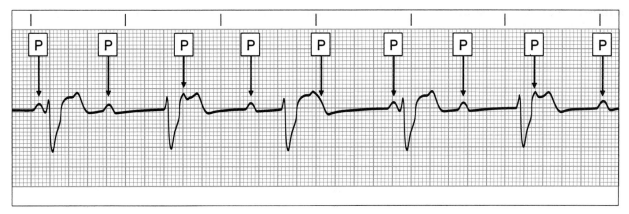

Figure 8-23 Third degree AV block: Complete heart block

Management of brady arrhythmias

- It should be borne in mind that bradycardia and conduction problems may precede cardiac arrest, and that their early recognition and correct management may prevent the subsequent cardiac arrest. This is especially important following acute myocardial infarction, when lesser degrees of conduction disturbance may develop into complete heart block

Principles of management

- The management of any patient depends on their clinical state, rather than on the arrhythmia alone
  - Oxygen
  - Relief of pain
  - Treatment of significant arrhythmias

Administer oxygen

Establish intravenous access

Provide adequate analgesia

- Nitrates:
  - Sublingual or buccal preparations
- Morphine/diamorphine (administered together with an anti-emetic):
  - Administered slowly and titrated to patient response to avoid respiratory depression

If there is a risk of asystole as indicated by:

- History of asystole
- Mobitz II AV block
- Any pause of 3 or more seconds
- Complete heart block, wide QRS complex

Administer atropine:

- *Atropine sulphate:* 0.5-3.0 mg administered intravenously in incremental doses of 0.5 mg, up to a maximum of 3 mg, over 5 minutes, is indicated if the patient is symptomatic

Administer external pacing, and if the patient is still symptomatic:

Administer isoprenaline

- *Isoprenaline:* 200 μg as an initial bolus, followed by an infusion of 2 mg in 500 mL of 5% dextrose or Dextro-saline, the infusion rate being titrated against heart rate

If there is no risk of asystole; assess whether there are any adverse clinical signs as indicated by:
- Evidence of low cardiac output:
    - Pallor
    - Sweating
    - Syncope
- Hypotension with a systolic blood pressure of 90 mmHg or less
- Heart failure
- Heart rate of 40 bpm or less
- Presence of a ventricular arrhythmia requiring suppression

If there are any adverse signs:
- **Administer atropine**. and if the patient is still symptomatic:
- **Administer external pacing**. and if this does not work:
- **Administer isoprenaline**

If there is no risk of asystole and no adverse clinical signs:
- Observe/monitor

External/non invasive cardiac pacing
- An artificial pacemaker is a device which administers an electric current to the myocardium to stimulate depolarisation and thereby to cause cardiac contraction
- Although external pacing is not yet widely available in the pre-hospital situation, many new defibrillators incorporate an external pacing facility, using adhesive chest electrodes
- External pacing is:
    - A temporary emergency procedure, until transvenous pacing can be instituted
    - Extremely effective, but can only be used for a short time, due to patient discomfort (it may cause contraction of the chest wall and pectoral muscles under the pacing electrodes)
    - Easy to carry out and can be performed by both trained paramedics and Immediate Care doctors
- Pacing can usually be achieved very rapidly, and without having to move the patient
- If external pacing is indicated, but the necessary equipment is not available, it is advisable to forewarn the hospital to which the patient is being sent, that pacing will be required, and attempt fist pacing

Fist pacing (external cardiac percussion)
- This may generate QRS complexes together with an effective cardiac output, especially when myocardial contractility is not impaired

Method: Make a fist and deliver a blow over the heart (not the sternum) at a rate of about 100 thumps/minute, with a force just a little less than that required for a pre-cordial thump. Start CPR if unsuccessful

Indications
- Bradycardias:
    - Failure of the sinoatrial (SA) node to generate an impulse:
        - Sinus arrest
    - Failure or partial failure of conduction in the atrioventricular node or His-Purkinje system:
        - Second degree heart block type II
        - Third degree heart block
    - Asystolic cardiac arrest, when there is any electrical activity suggestive of sporadic atrial or ventricular (QRS complexes) function
- *Note:* Hemiblock
    Bundle branch block $\left.\right\}$ do not require pacing
    First degree heart block
    Second degree heart block type I

Pacemakers
- All pacemakers used for external ventricular pacing consist of a pulse generator and two pacing electrodes

Pulse generator
- This has a power source (rechargeable batteries in the case of pacemakers incorporated in defibrillators) and electrical circuitry, for delivering the pacing stimulus
- There are controls for adjusting:
    - Rate (of discharge)
    - Sensitivity
    - Output

Pacing stimulus
- When the pacemaker discharges, the voltage rises almost instantaneously to the desired (preset) output voltage of the generator (usually about 5 volts), then decays relatively slowly over about 5 milliseconds, before falling rapidly
- This shows up on the ECG tracing as a single small spike

Capture
- 'Capture' is said to occur when the pacing stimulus causes sufficient myocardial depolarisation to result in depolarisation (systole) of the whole myocardium
- On the ECG monitor this will show as the spike of the pacing stimulus being followed by a broad QRS complex, as the initial ventricular depolarisation acts as an ectopic ventricular focus

Threshold
- The ventricular threshold is the minimum output from the pacemaker generator that results in capture

Rate
- The pacing generator produces stimuli at regular intervals, which can be set by a separate control

Pacing modes
- Asynchronous (or fixed rate) pacing:
    - An asynchronous pacemaker delivers stimuli at the selected rate, regardless of the patient's intrinsic cardiac activity
    - If the stimulus is given during the heart's vulnerable period (during repolarisation, represented by the T wave on the ECG), there is a danger of it causing ventricular tachycardia or fibrillation
    - In the pre-hospital setting, the asynchronous mode may have the advantage that it avoids the possibility of movement artefact interfering with the sensing of beats required in demand pacing
- Demand pacing:
    - This delivers a pacing stimulus only when needed (usually when the heart rate drops below the preset level, e.g. 60 bpm.)
    - The device senses when there is an intrinsic QRS complex, and inhibits the pulse generator from discharging until the preset coupling interval is again exceeded

Overdrive (burst) pacing
- This is used for the management of atrial or ventricular tachycardias
- Uses a burst of atrial or right ventricular pacing at a greater rate than the ventricular rate. The pacing impulses penetrate and break the re-entry circuit responsible for the tachycardia, permitting the re-establishment of sinus rhythm

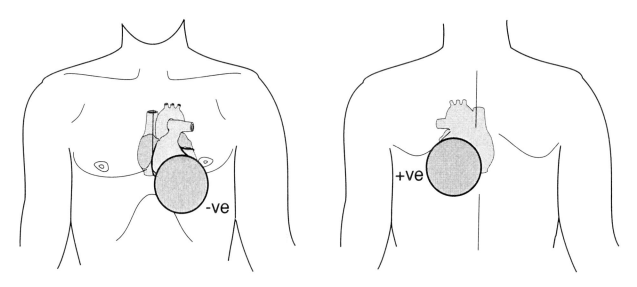

Figure 8-24 Position of the electrodes for external cardiac pacing

Electrode positions
- Anterior-posterior:
  - The negative electrode pad is applied to the anterior chest wall over the V_3 position of the 12-lead ECG, and the positive electrode pad to the left side of the back of the chest beneath the scapula
- Anterior-axillary (less desirable as there is a greater risk of pectoral muscle stimulation):
  - The positive electrode pad is placed just below the right clavicle in the mid clavicular line, and the negative electrode in the 4th intercostal space in the mid axillary line

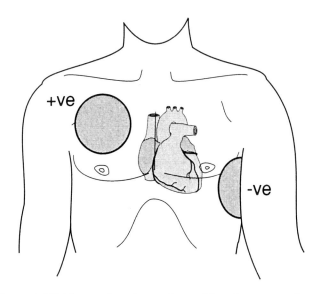

Figure 8-25 Alternative electrode position for external pacing

Method
- Apply the two adhesive electrode pads
- If the patient is conscious, warn them that they are likely to feel some discomfort
- Turn the pacing device on in 'demand' mode (if available), at a rate of about 80 beats per minute
- Adjust the output control until there is 'capture' and then increase it to 10-20 mA
- Continue to monitor the patient's haemodynamic state

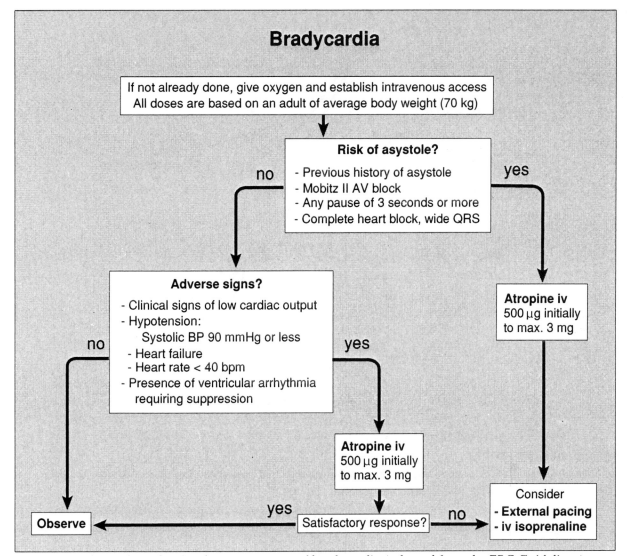

Figure 8-26 Algorithm for the management of bradycardia (adapted from the ERC Guidelines)

Bundle Branch Blocks
- Bundle branch and fascicular blocks have been included here because of their relationship to complete heart block and acute myocardial infarction, although they are not usually considered to be peri-arrest arrhythmias

Incidence
- Abnormalities of conduction may develop in any part of the conducting system

Aetiology
- Right bundle branch block often indicates right ventricular problems, but may be found as an incidental finding in otherwise fit individuals
- Left bundle branch block nearly always indicates serious conducting system or diffuse ventricular disease, including:
    - Hypertension
    - Myocardial ischaemia
    - Acute myocardial infarction
    - Cardiac failure
    - Cardiomyopathy

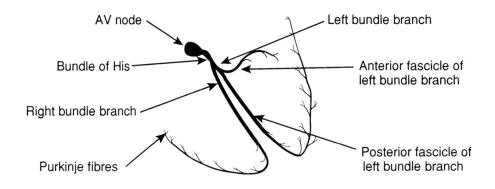

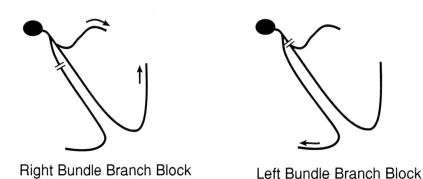

Right Bundle Branch Block   Left Bundle Branch Block

Figure 8-27 Right and left bundle branch blocks

Pathophysiology
- Bundle branch block occurs when there is a failure of transmission of conduction down one of the bundle branches in the interventricular septum
- Complete block of a bundle branch deprives the corresponding ventricle of its normal conduction pathway, so it is depolarised from the other ventricle via an abnormal (and slow) pathway. This results in delayed depolarisation of the affected ventricle
- Block of both bundle branches results in complete heart block

Symptoms/signs
- These depend on the underlying aetiology

ECG features
QRS rhythm: Regular

Rate: Normal.

P waves: Normal preceding each QRS complex

Pacemaker site: SA node

PR interval: Normal (0.12-0.2 sec.)

QRS complex: Abnormal morphology, and broad (> 100 milliseconds/>2.5 small squares)

Chest (V) leads: V_1 looks at the right ventricle
V_6 looks at the left ventricle

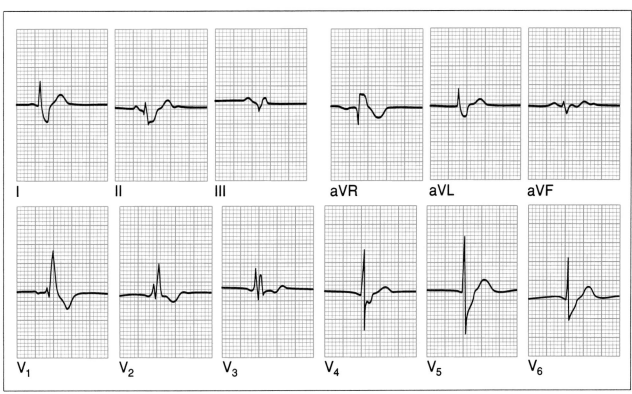

Figure 8-28 Right bundle branch block

Right bundle branch block

- Septal and left ventricular depolarisation occur normally, resulting in an R wave in V_1 and a small Q wave in V_6
- Left ventricular depolarisation then occurs normally, resulting in an S wave in V_1 and an R in V_6
- Right ventricular depolarisation occurs in response to a wave of depolarisation spreading across from the left ventricle, resulting in a second R wave (R^1) in V_1, and a wide, deep S wave in V_6
- Best seen in V_1, where the QRS complex forms an RSR^1 pattern

Management
- Usually none necessary

Left bundle branch block

- As normal septal depolarisation cannot take place, septal depolarisation takes place from right to left, resulting in a small Q wave in V_1 and an R wave in V_6
- The right ventricle then depolarises normally and in spite of its relatively small muscle bulk, this shows up as a small R wave in V_1 and a small S in V_6 (which often looks like a small notch)
- At the same time a wave of depolarisation passes from the right ventricle to the left causing its depolarisation, resulting in an S wave in V_1 and a second R wave (R^1) in V_6
- This is best seen in V_6, where the QRS complex looks like an 'M'

Note: 1. Bundle branch block with a supraventricular tachycardia may be confused with ventricular tachycardia, as both have wide QRS complexes and a rapid ventricular rate
2. Left bundle branch block may appear similar to:
   - Premature ventricular contractions
   - Pacemaker rhythm (but there is no pacing spike)

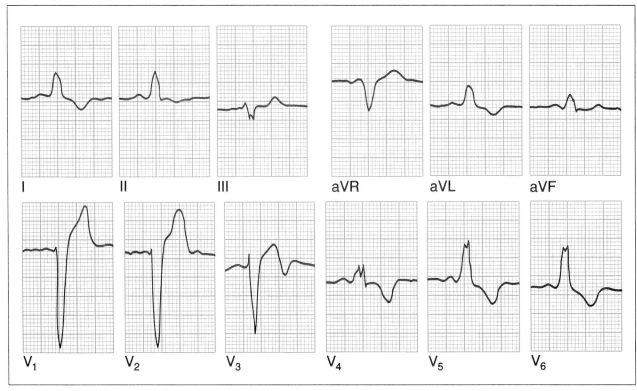

Figure 8-29 Left bundle branch block

Management
- In the context of Immediate Care, the patient with the sudden onset of chest pain, who is found to have left bundle branch block should be presumed to have had an acute myocardial infarction, and managed accordingly (including the administration of a thrombolytic)

Bundle branch blocks and cardiac axis deviation
- The cardiac axis depends on the mean direction of the vector representing depolarisation of the ventricles
- If one of the branches or fascicles fails to conduct, it will result in depolarisation taking place in a different direction from normal, which may show up on the ECG tracing as a change in the cardiac axis

Left anterior fascicular block
- If the anterior fascicle of the left bundle branch fails to conduct; the left ventricle will be depolarised via the posterior fascicle alone
- This results in the cardiac axis rotating to the left, and is called 'left axis deviation'

Left posterior fascicular block
- If the posterior fascicle of the left bundle fails to conduct (rare), the left ventricle will be depolarised via the anterior fascicle alone
- This results in the cardiac axis rotating to the right, and is called 'right axis deviation'

Right bundle branch block
- If the right bundle branch fails to conduct, the cardiac axis is usually normal, as the left ventricle with its large muscle mass depolarises normally

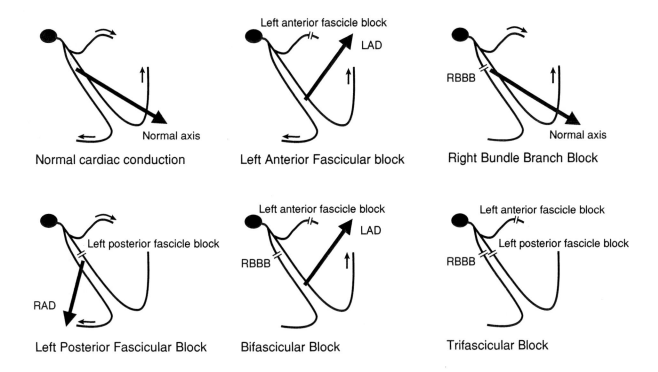

Figure 8-30 Fascicular blocks and the cardiac axis

Bifascicular block
- This occurs when both the right bundle branch and the left anterior or posterior fascicle fail to conduct
- The ECG tracing will show right bundle branch block and left axis deviation

Aetiology
- May occur in patients:
    - Following an infarct
    - Asymptomatically

Pathophysiology
- Associated with large infarcts which have a high mortality
- Following AMI, this may progress suddenly to more severe degrees of heart block, including complete heart block
- May often be an incidental finding

Management
- Following AMI, the patient requires careful cardiac monitoring in case the block suddenly progresses to a more severe degree of heart block, especially complete heart block

Trifascicular block
- This occurs when the right bundle branch and one of the left fascicles fail to conduct, while the other left fascicle still conducts, but with partial block
- Has the features of bifascicular block with first degree AV block in addition (prolonged PR interval)
- Is a warning block and may progress to complete heart block

Management
- Careful monitoring of the patient's haemodynamic state

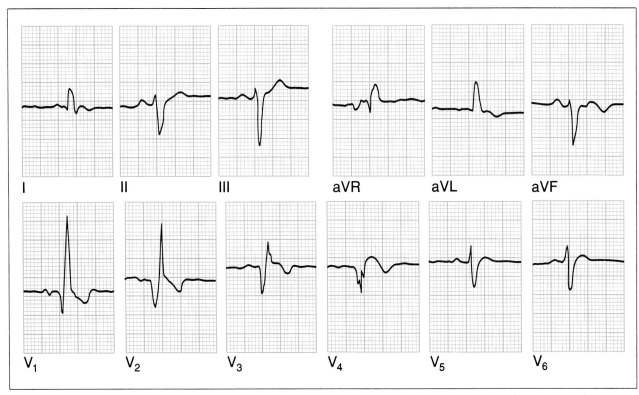

Figure 8-31 Bifascicular block (right bundle branch block with left axis deviation) and anterior infarction

Tachyarrhythmias:
Narrow complex tachycardias/supraventricular tachyarrhythmias

Definition: A supraventricular tachycardia is any tachyarrhythmia originating above the bifurcation of the bundle of His

- Typically supraventricular tachycardia will produce narrow QRS complexes (100 milliseconds or less)

Sinus tachycardia

Incidence
- Relatively common after/during AMI, occurring in up to 15% of patients
- A sinus tachycardia is normal in infants and young children

Aetiology
- May be caused by:
    - Pain, exercise and emotion
    - Pyrexia and heat
    - Anaemia and hypoxia
    - Hyperthyroidism
    - Left ventricular failure
    - Acute myocardial infarction and pulmonary embolism
    - Hypovolaemic shock
    - Drugs: epinephrine, atropine, isoprenaline and salbutamol

Pathophysiology
- In sinus tachycardia there is an increased rate of discharge/depolarisation from the SA node
- A very fast heart rate results in:
    - An increase in cardiac work, which results in further ischaemia and infarction
    - Inadequate ventricular filling and reduced cardiac output, resulting in a fall in blood pressure
    - Cardiac failure
- Following AMI, the heart rate is often related to the severity of the infarct

Symptoms/signs
- Usually none

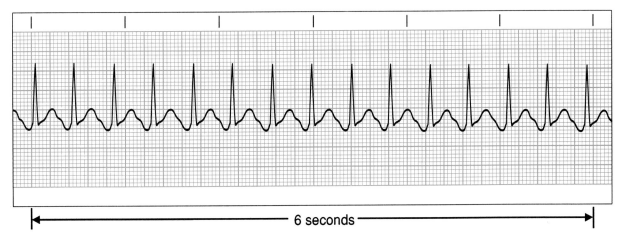

6 seconds

Figure 8-32 Sinus tachycardia

ECG features

QRS rhythm: Regular

Rate: 100-160 beats per minute

P waves: Normal preceding each QRS complex
    The P waves may be lost in the previous T wave if the heart rate is very fast

Pacemaker site: SA node

PR interval: Normal (0.12-0.2 sec.)

QRS complex: Normal: each preceded by a P wave

Management
- Follow the usual protocol:
    - Airway
    - Breathing with administration of oxygen
    - Circulation
- Treatment of the underlying cause:
    - Left venticular failure
        - Diuretics:
            - Furosemide
            - Bumetanide
        - Opiates
            - Morphine
    - Pain:
        - Analgesia

Premature atrial contractions (PACs)

Incidence
- Commonly found in normal individuals, especially with increasing age, although tends to occur more often in organic heart disease and after acute myocardial infarction

Aetiology
- May be precipitated by tobacco and coffee and excess use of some drugs, e.g. salbutamol, digoxin

Pathophysiology
- Premature atrial complexes are caused by an ectopic atrial focus, which fires before the SA node and causes the atria to contract prematurely

Symptoms/signs
- Rarely cause any symptoms other than an awareness of an irregular heartbeat or pulse (which may be distressing for the patient)

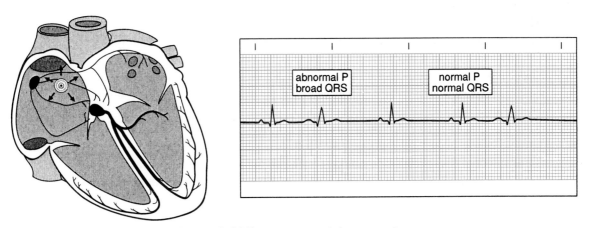

Figure 8-33 Premature atrial contractions

ECG features
- There are abnormal premature P waves, which may be hidden in the preceding T wave
- The abnormal P wave is usually followed by a normal QRS complex, although it may sometimes be broad, if there is bundle branch block

QRS rhythm: Irregular (regular basic rhythm, with occasional superimposed extra complexes)

Rate: Depends on the number of premature supraventricular beats and the underlying rate

P waves: The premature P waves often have a different size and shape from normal P waves

Pacemaker site: The pacemaker for the premature supraventricular beat is an ectopic focus in some part of the atria or the AV junction (junctional ectopic focus) other than the SA node

PR interval: Varies depending on the rate of conduction between the ectopic pacemaker and the ventricles

QRS complex: Usually normal, but aberrant conduction may occur
            May be absent, if there is a failure of AV conduction

Management
- Active treatment is not usually indicated

Atrial fibrillation

Incidence
- Atrial fibrillation is:
    - The commonest (and often asymptomatic) arrhythmia, especially over the age of 55, occurring in:
        - 0.5% of patients aged 50-59 years
        - 5% of patients over 75 years old
        - 8.8% of patients aged 80-89 years
    - A major cause of cardiac and cerebrovascular death
- Atrial fibrillation may be paroxysmal or established

Aetiology
- Cardiac causes include:
    - Ischaemic heart disease, resulting in angina, cardiac ischaemia and heart failure
    - Acute myocardial infarction, after which atrial fibrillation:
        - Occurs in 10-15% of cases
        - Indicates ischaemia of the SA node or atria
    - Hypertension;
        - Atrial fibrillation contributes to the complications of stroke, especially if left ventricular hypertrophy is present
    - Rheumatic (now a relatively rare cause in developed countries) and non-rheumatic heart disease, especially mitral valve disease, which increase the risk of stroke about 18 times
    - Sick sinus and pre-excitation syndromes
- Non cardiac causes include:
    - Thyrotoxicosis occurring in about 10-15% of patients
    - Acute infections, especially pneumonia, being present in about 7% of cases
    - Alcohol abuse, which can precipitate atrial fibrillation in those with otherwise normal hearts
    - Carcinoma of the lung
    - Pericardial disease
- 'Lone' atrial fibrillation:
    - This is said to occur when there is no obvious cause for the atrial fibrillation
    - It accounts for 3-11% of all patients with atrial fibrillation
    - Patients under the age of 60 probably have a low risk of thromboembolic problems, but older patients (over 65) have a significant risk of stroke

Pathophysiology
- There is random irregular atrial activity possibly arising from a focal re-entry circuit, which leads to uncoordinated atrial activity
- Atrial fibrillation may be paroxysmal, lasting minutes or hours, or may be continuous (established)
- Due to the lack of co-ordination between atrial and ventricular contractions, there may be incomplete ventricular filling, which may result in up to a 25% reduction in cardiac output and a lowered blood pressure
- If the ventricular response is rapid, cardiac output is further reduced, and cardiac workload increased

Symptoms/signs
- These may vary from insignificant to life threatening
- The commonest emergency presenting features in Western countries include:
    - Heart failure precipitated by the sudden onset of atrial fibrillation with a rapid ventricular response, especially if left ventricular function is already impaired by coexisting heart disease, e.g. ischaemic heart disease or valve disease
    - Stroke due to emboli (atrial fibrillation increases the risk of stroke five times that of the normal population or by 5% a year, increasing with age)
- Other less serious symptoms may include:
    - Palpitations
    - General fatigue with a greatly reduced exercise tolerance
- The patient will have:
    - An irregularly irregular pulse
    - The symptoms and signs of heart failure and other complications may be present

ECG features
- Irregular QRS complexes with f waves

QRS rhythm: Irregularly irregular

Rate: Atrial rate is 350-600 per minute, but this is not measurable on the rhythm strip
The ventricular rate is 100-160 (or more) beats per minute if untreated, but may be slower if the patient is taking digoxin or other drugs active at the AV node, e.g. β-blockers, verapamil

P waves: Absent. Instead there are fibrillatory (f) waves, which may be coarse or so fine that atrial activity is not apparent

Pacemaker site: Multiple ectopic pacemaker sites throughout the atria

PR interval: Does not exist

QRS complex: Usually normal (but may be broad), but not preceded by P waves

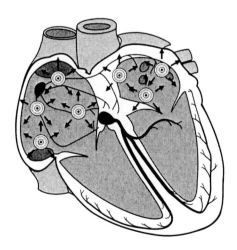
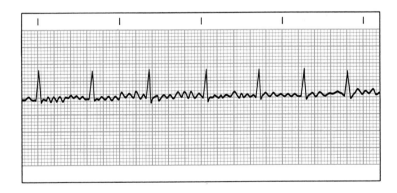

Figure 8-34 Atrial fibrillation

Management

- Administer:
    - Oxygen
    - Establish intravenous access
- Assess whether or not there are any adverse signs:
    - Hypotension with a systolic BP 90 mmHg or less
    - Chest pain
    - Heart failure
    - Impaired consciousness
    - Heart rate of 200 bpm or more
- If there are *no* adverse signs, consider:
    - Administration of amiodarone 300 mg intravenously over one hour, repeated as necessary
- If the *are* adverse signs:
    - Sedate
    - Consider synchronised DC cardioversion; 100 joules, 200 joules, 360 joules, and if no better:
    - Administer amiodarone 300 mg intravenously over 5-15 minutes, followed by 300 mg over one hour
    - *Administer further cardioversion*

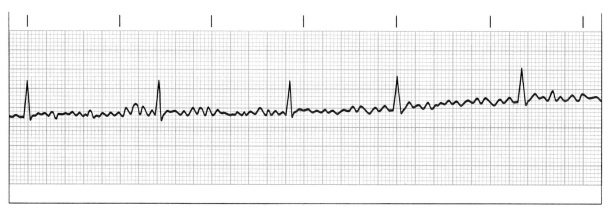

Atrial fibrillation with a slow ventricular response

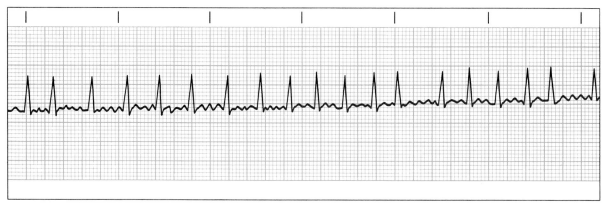

Atrial fibrillation with a rapid ventricular response

Figure 8-35 Atrial fibrillation with differing ventricular response

Atrial flutter

Incidence
- Relatively common, increasing with age

Aetiology
- Usually caused by significant underlying ischaemic heart disease, or by metabolic abnormalities
- May occur in paroxysms varying in length from hours to days
- May progress to atrial fibrillation

Pathophysiology
- Atrial flutter is caused by a re-entry tachycardia, leading to an actual atrial rate of about 300 depolarisations per minute
- The AV node is usually unable to conduct impulses at rates of more than about 200 per minute, so at rates higher than this, AV block occurs resulting in 2:1 (commonest), 3:1 or 4:1 block, but variable block may also occur
- If the ventricular response is rapid, the cardiac workload is increased and the cardiac output may be reduced

Symptoms/signs
- Palpitations
- Dizziness and syncope, if the ventricular rate is very rapid
- Left ventricular failure (in the early stages of an acute myocardial infarction)

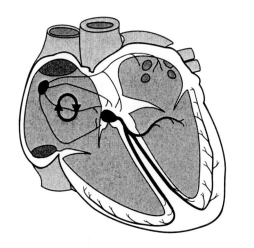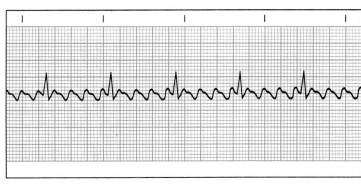

Figure 8-36 Atrial flutter with 4:1 block

ECG features
- A narrow complex tachycardia, with a rate of 150 bpm should be considered to be atrial flutter until proven otherwise (consider carotid sinus massage to slow AV conduction, reduce the ventricular response and reveal the F waves of atrial flutter, as an aid to diagnosis)

QRS rhythm: Atrial rhythm is regular (or almost so)
> The ventricular rhythm is usually fairly regular, with 2:1, 3:1 or 4:1 block, but it will be irregular when the AV block is variable

Rate: The atrial rate is often 240-360 per minute
> The ventricular rate is 140-160 per minute with 2:1 block, but may be slower with higher degrees of block, for example when the patient is taking digoxin or β-blockers

P waves: Absent; instead there are flutter (F) waves, often in a jagged or "saw tooth" pattern, especially in inferior leads

Pacemaker site: A re-entry circuit in the atria

PR interval: Not measurable

QRS complex: Usually normal, following every second, third or fourth F wave

Management
- As atrial fibrillation
- Atrial flutter is often very responsive to low voltage DC cardioversion

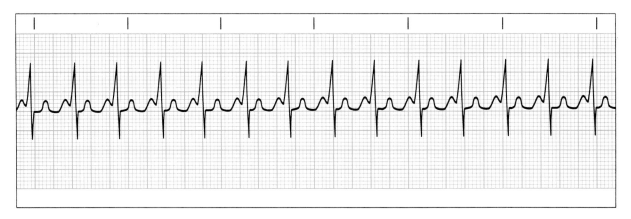

Figure 8-37 Atrial flutter with 2:1 block

- Administer:
    - Oxygen
    - Establish intravenous access
- Assess whether of not there are any adverse signs:
    - Hypotension with a systolic BP 90 mmHg or less
    - Chest pain
    - Heart failure
    - Impaired consciousness
    - Heart rate of 200 bpm or more
- If there are *no* adverse signs, consider:
    - Administration of amiodarone 300 mg intravenously over one hour, repeated as necessary
- If the *are* adverse signs:
    - Sedate
    - Consider synchronised DC cardioversion; 100 joules, 200 joules, 360 joules, and if no better:
    - Administer amiodarone 300 mg intravenously over 5-15 minutes, followed by 300 mg over one hour
    - *Administer further cardioversion*

Supraventricular tachycardia

Incidence
- A fairly common arrhythmia, but uncommon following AMI

Aetiology
- Supraventricular tachycardia may be:
    - Non-paroxysmal:
        - Rare but may occur due to digoxin toxicity
    - Paroxysmal, beginning and ending suddenly, lasting from seconds to hours and (rarely) days:
        - May be precipitated in susceptible individuals by stress, coffee (caffeine), alcohol, heavy smoking, and hyperventilation
        - May occur in the young who have a history of similar attacks, and macroscopically structurally normal hearts, although in many cases a bypass track may exist between the atria and ventricles, e.g. in Wolff Parkinson White syndrome
        - May be caused by structural abnormalities or damage to the AV node

Pathophysiology
- Usually due to a re-entry circuit involving the AV junction
- Persistent paroxysmal atrial tachycardia may result in left ventricular failure

Symptoms/signs
- Sudden onset of palpitations and dizziness, occasionally resulting in syncope/collapse, but may be self limiting
- Angina and cardiac failure in patients with ischaemic heart disease
- Adverse signs include:
    - Hypotension: systolic BP <90 mmHg with heart failure and syncope
    - Chest pain
    - A heart rate >200 bpm.

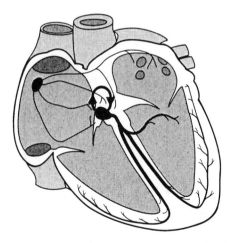
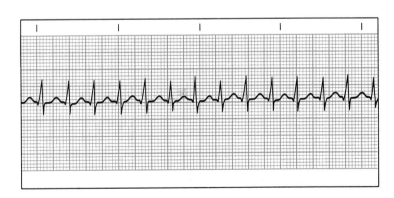

Figure 8-38 Paroxysmal supraventricular tachycardia

ECG features (rapid regular narrow QRS complexes)

QRS rhythm: Usually regular

Rate: 140-220 beats per minute

P waves: Absent or abnormal in morphology and position (usually present in some leads)

Pacemaker site: An ectopic focus in the atria or AV junction above the bifurcation of the Bundle of His. If there is a bypass tract between the atria and ventricles, a cycle of excitation occurs between the atrial and ventricular myocardium and perpetuates the tachycardia (Wolff Parkinson White and several other types)

PR interval: May be none.

If a P wave precedes/follows a QRS complex, the PR interval is usually short. Where atrial depolarisation occurs from retrograde activation of the ventricles the P wave will usually follow the QRS complex and will be evident in the T wave

QRS complex: Usually normal (depending on the heart rate)

Management
- Establish intravenous access
- Assess whether or not the patient has adverse signs:
    - Hypotension with a systolic BP 90 mmHg or less
    - Chest pain
    - Heart failure
    - Impaired consciousness
    - Heart rate of 200 bpm or more
- If the patient has *no* adverse signs, administer:
    - Vagal stimulation (caution if there is possible digoxin toxicity, acute ischaemia or a carotid bruit):
        - Valsava manoeuvre (forcibly breathing out against a closed glottis)
        - Carotid sinus massage
        - Face in cold water or bag of frozen peas held to the face
        - Pressure applied to the eyeballs
        - Cough/deep breath
    - Adenosine:
        - Initial intravenous bolus of 3 mg administered as rapidly as possible
        - If this does not terminate the rhythm within 1-2 minutes, this may be followed by 6 mg administered as rapidly as possible
        - If this does not terminate the rhythm within 1-2 minutes, a bolus of 12 mg may be administered as rapidly as possible
        - If this does not terminate the rhythm within 1-2 minutes, a further bolus of 12 mg may be administered as rapidly as possible
    - Amiodarone 300 mg over 5-15 minutes, then 600 mg over one hour
    - Consider overdrive pacing (see below)
- If the patient *has* adverse signs, administer:
    - Oxygen
    - Consider sedation with a small dose of diazepam/midazolam if the circumstances permit
    - Administer synchronised DC cardioversion:
        - 75-100 Joules
        - 200 Joules
        - 360 Joules
- If conversion is successful, but the paroxysmal supraventricular tachycardia (PSVT) reoccurs, repeated cardioversion is not indicated:
    - Sedate the patient and monitor their haemodynamic state during transportation to hospital

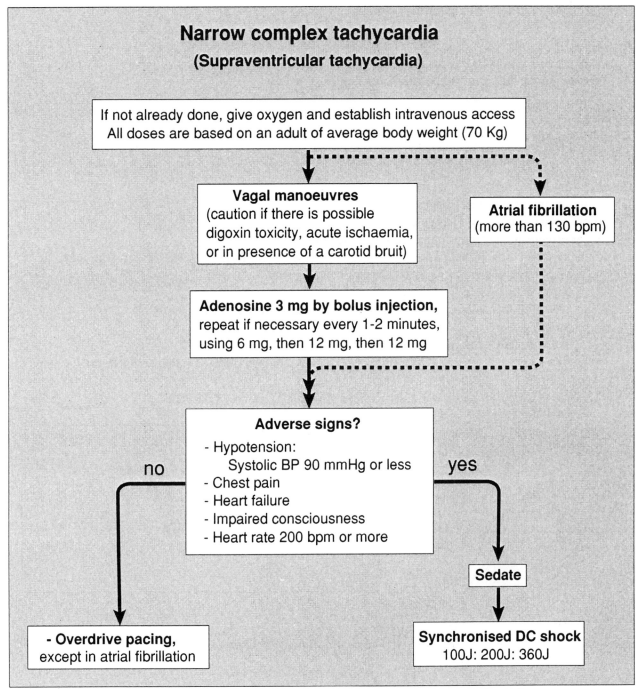

*Figure 8-39 Algorithm for the management of narrow complex tachycardias
(adapted from the ERC guidelines)*

Premature ventricular contractions (PVCs)

Incidence
- May occur in normal individuals
- Very common after acute myocardial infarction

Aetiology
- Damage to the myocardium following AMI
- Digoxin, hyperkalaemia

Pathophysiology
- Indicates increased ventricular excitability
- If only occasional: of little importance
- If very frequent: they may compromise cardiac output
- Some types are of particular importance, because if they occur following AMI, the rhythm may deteriorate to ventricular tachycardia or ventricular fibrillation:
    - In salvos
    - R on T phenomenon: important as this may initiate ventricular fibrillation
    - Multifocal
    - Frequent PVCs (more than 6 per minute)
    - PVCs with every second beat: bigeminy (this rhythm may often be stable and benign)

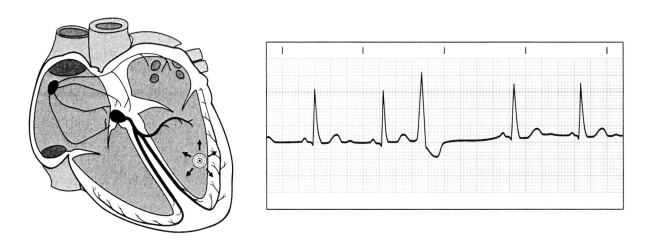

Figure 8-40 Premature ventricular contractions

ECG features

QRS rhythm: Irregular if the PVCs occur randomly, but may be regularly irregular with bigeminy, trigeminy, etc.
The PVC complex is separated from the preceding normal complex by a shorter than normal R-R interval
Most PVCs are followed by a compensatory pause

Rate: The ventricular rate is unaffected

P waves: Usually absent before the PVC, but may follow a QRS if retrograde atrial activation occurs

Pacemaker site: The origin of the PVC is an ectopic focus in one of the ventricles

PR interval: None for the PVC, because it is not usually preceded by a P wave

QRS complex: Distorted, bizarre and wide (0.12 seconds: three small squares or more)
The T wave is usually in the opposite direction to the main QRS deflection

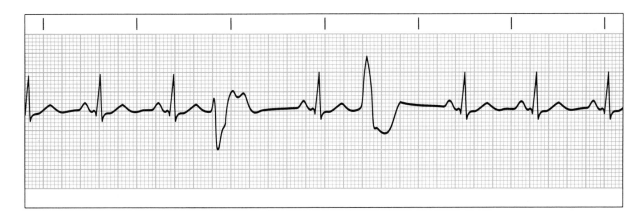

Figure 8-41 Multifocal PVCs: different sizes/shapes: indicate ectopic ventricular foci from different sources

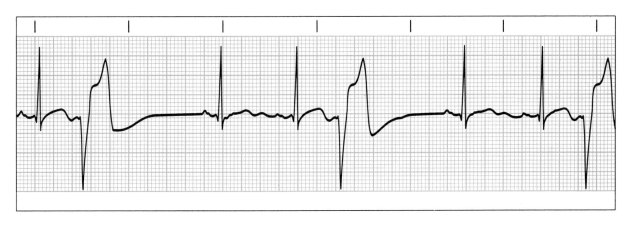

Figure 8-42 Frequent PVCs: Ventricular trigeminy: a PVC follows two successive sinus beats

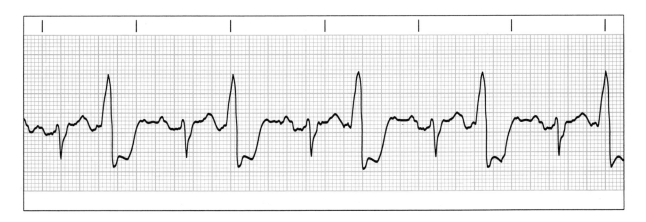

Figure 8-43 Ventricular bigeminy: when PVCs occur every second beat

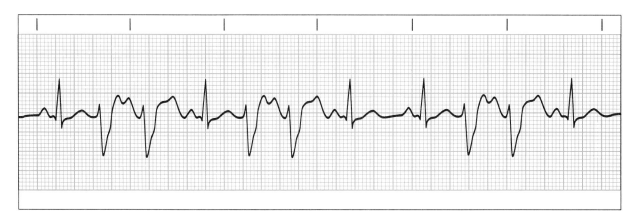

Figure 8-44 Two PVCs in a row (couplets) or more (salvos): may progress to ventricular tachycardia

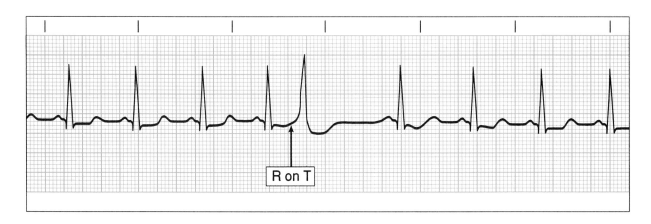

Figure 8-45 R on T pattern (a PVC falling on a T wave): may precipitate ventricular fibrillation

Management
- Observation only as, with the exception of immediately post AMI, these are unlikely to progress to VT
- Bigeminy may respond to an increase in the heart rate, e.g. with atropine or pacing
- Immediately post AMI, when there is a risk that these rhythms may progress to ventricular tachycardia or ventricular fibrillation, administer:
    - A lidocaine infusion beginning at a rate of 2 mg per minute for the first 2 hours, reducing to a maintenance dose of 1 mg per minute thereafter

Note: Although some of these arrhythmias may deteriorate to ventricular fibrillation, ventricular fibrillation may appear without any prior arrhythmia

Broad complex tachycardias

Ventricular tachycardia

Incidence
- A common and life threatening arrhythmia after acute myocardial infarction

Aetiology
- An ectopic focus or a focal re-entry circuit in a ventricle

Pathophysiology
- May progress to ventricular fibrillation
- Slow VT (100-130 beats per minute):
    - May cause little haemodynamic compromise, unless there is impaired left ventricular function e.g. in AMI
- Rapid VT (160->250 beats per minute):
    - May result in collapse

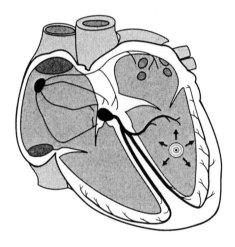 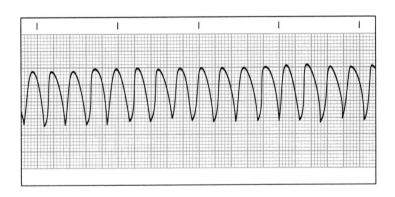

Figure 8-46 Ventricular tachycardia

ECG features
- In the context of ischaemic heart disease, a patient with a broad complex tachycardia should be presumed to have a VT

Rhythm: Regular or slightly irregular

Rate: 100-200 beats per minute or faster

P waves: Often not seen as they are obscured by the QRS complexes
When they are seen, they usually have no consistent relationship to the QRS complexes, i.e. there is AV dissociation (can be associated if retrograde activation of the atria occurs)

Pacemaker site: An ectopic focus in a ventricle

PR interval: None

QRS complex: Distorted, wide (0.12 seconds or more)

ECG criteria used to differentiate VT from SVT with aberrant conduction
- Features which tend to indicate ventricular tachycardia, rather than supraventricular tachycardia:
  - *Diagnostic*:
    - AV dissociation (independent atrial activity)
    - Fusion beats (bizarre complexes formed by the fusion of sinus and ventricular beats) or capture beats (sinus beats seen during broad complex tachycardia)
    - RSR' in V_1 with the primary R wave being taller than the secondary R' wave
    - Deep S wave in V_6
    - Concordant pattern in the precordial leads, i.e. QRS vector is in the same direction in all the chest leads (V_1-V_6)
    - Abnormal QRS axis, especially left axis (compare with a previous normal ECG, if available)
  - *Suggestive*:
    - History of:
      - Ventricular tachycardia
      - Ischaemic heart disease
    - >45 years old
    - Severe haemodynamic compromise

Note: If in doubt, assume that any alert patient with a broad complex tachycardia has an SVT and manage with adenosine

Management
- Assess whether the patient has a palpable pulse
- If there is no pulse:
  - Treat as ventricular fibrillation
- If there is a pulse:
  - Administer oxygen
  - Establish intravenous access
  - Administer analgesia (if the patient has just had an AMI)
- Assess whether the patient has any adverse clinical signs:
  - Systolic BP is 90 mmHg or less
  - Chest pain
  - Heart failure
  - Heart rate of 150 bpm or more
- If there are adverse clinical signs, treat the arrhythmia as an emergency:
  - Sedate if circumstances permit and the patient is conscious
  - Perform synchronised direct current cardioversion at 100 Joules, 200 Joules, 360 Joules
  - If this is unsuccessful or the arrhythmia reoccurs administer:
    - Lidocaine hydrochloride 50-100 mg intravenously over 2 minutes, repeated every 5 minutes, to a total dose of 200 mg
  - If successful:
    - A lidocaine infusion should be started beginning at a rate of 2 mg per minute for the first 2 hours, reducing to a maintenance dose of 1 mg per minute
  - If unsuccessful:
    - Further synchronised DC cardioversion
  - If still unsuccessful consider:
    - Bretylium
    - Overdrive pacing

- If there are no adverse signs:
    - Administer lidocaine hydrochloride:
        - 50-100 mg intravenously over 2 minutes, repeated every 5 minutes, to a total dose of 200 mg
    - If successful:
        - A lidocaine infusion should be started beginning at a rate of 2 mg per minute for the first 2 hours, reducing to a maintenance dose of 1 mg per minute
    - If this fails or the patient becomes unstable, consider:
        - Synchronised direct current cardioversion at 100 Joules, 200 Joules, 360 Joules
    - If unsuccessful, consider:
        - Amiodarone: 300 mg administered intravenously over 5-15 minutes, then 300 mg over 1 hour

Synchronised external direct current (DC) cardioversion

- This uses a direct current (DC) electrical discharge to depolarise the myocardium, allowing the SA node to reassert itself and establish sinus rhythm (as in defibrillation)

Synchronisation
- The shock is synchronised (unlike defibrillation, in which there are no QRS complexes with which to synchronise), so that it is delivered at the same time as the the R wave (of the QRS complex), thus avoiding the T wave, and the possibility of triggering ventricular fibrillation, in the management of:
    - Broad complex tachycardias, e.g. ventricular tachycardia
    - Atrial fibrillation
    - Atrial flutter

Indications (in the pre-hospital situation)
- DC cardioversion is used in the management of persistent tachyarrhythmias causing significant and persistent haemodynamic compromise:
    - Hypotension (systolic BP <90 mmHg)
    - Chest pain or dyspnoea
    - Heart failure (signs of pulmonary oedema)
    - Heart rate 150 bpm or more
    - Failure of drug therapy

Note: In the hospital setting DC cardioversion is used electively for managing some stable arrhythmias, e.g. atrial fibrillation

Sedation
- Administer a small dose of a sedative, e.g. midazolam, if the patient is conscious

Power levels
- The power level selected depends on the arrhythmia:
    - Broad complex tachycardias: 100J, 200J, 360J
    - Atrial fibrillation: 200 J (much lower if the patient is taking digoxin)
    - Atrial flutter: 10/50 J

Method (using a manual defibrillator)
- Make certain that the skin is dry
- Switch on the defibrillator, select the synchronisation mode ('Sync'), and make certain that the ECG monitor is reading through the paddles (or if chest leads have already been attached, that the monitor is reading through them)
- Remove the paddles from the defibrillator and apply electrode gel to them or put gel pads on the patient's chest, or attach disposable adhesive defibrillating electrodes

- **Charge** the defibrillator
- Apply the paddles to the skin exerting firm downwards pressure, and **analyse** the rhythm
- If the ECG tracing confirms the arrhythmia, prepare to **cardiovert** the patient by pressing the appropriate buttons on the paddles
- Before each cardioversion, shout "Stand by to cardiovert: Stand clear" and make certain that nobody is touching the patient or any attached equipment

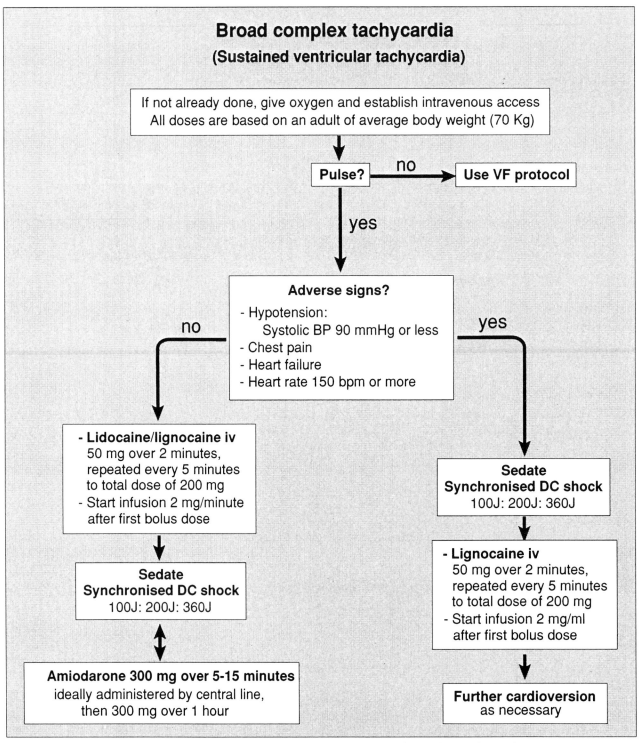

Figure 8-47 Algorithm for the management of broad complex tachycardias

Organisation of the team for advanced life support

- This is a method of team management of cardiac arrest and/or life threatening arrhythmias first developed in the USA. It is also used for practising/testing performance
- The minimum number of people necessary to carry out effective Advanced Cardiac Life Support is three; four is better
- The whole situation is fluid and constantly changing as the initial response is replaced by more effective and efficient methods of patient management, which themselves change according to the patient's need and the treatment carried out

Team leader

- Manages the resuscitation team
- Takes an overview of the resuscitation effort/monitors all pertinent information
- Assesses the patient's condition
- Monitors the team's performance
- Monitors the ECG screen and provides the rhythm recognition
- Is in control of defibrillation
- Manages the post arrest care

Team member 1: airway carer

- Maintains the airway:
  - Head tilt/chin lift
  - Jaw thrust
  - Oropharyngeal airway
  - Laryngeal mask airway
  - Tracheal intubation
- Provides oxygenation and ventilation:
  - Mouth to mouth/nose
  - Mouth to mask
  - Bag and mask
  - Ventilator

Team member 2: circulation carer

- Monitors a central pulse.
- Provides circulatory support:
  - External chest compressions

Team member 3 *(team leader if only three rescuers are in attendance)*

- Establishes and maintains an intravenous infusion.
- May administer any cardiac drugs.
- Acts as a runner.
- Gets additional equipment as requested.
- Assists the other members of the team.
- Provides help with transport.
- Keeps record of:
  - Time elapsed
  - Shocks/drugs given

Drugs used in cardiac emergencies

Introduction

- This is a brief list of most of the drugs used in the early treatment of cardiac emergencies, together with a description of their basic pharmacology
- Analgesics and sedating agents are described in the chapter on Pain management, and nitrates, β-blockers, diuretics, anti-platelet agents and thrombolytics in the chapter on Cardiac care: acute myocardial infarction
- Not all the drugs listed are used in Immediate Care, but those that are not, are included so as to provide a reasonable overview of the subject
- The two first line drugs: epinephrine and atropine, should be carried by all those involved in Immediate Cardiac Care

Note: Caution should be exercised in the use of negatively inotropic drugs in patients with cardiac disease as they may have impaired left ventricular function and the use of these drugs may precipitate sudden heart failure (as they may in normal hearts, if tachycardia conversion does not occur)

Adrenergic receptor agonists

Action
- Stimulate adrenoreceptors resulting in:
    - α_1 *and* α_2 *receptors:*
        - Arterial and arteriolar constriction: an increase in the systemic vascular resistance, resulting in an increase in coronary and cerebral perfusion during CPR (mostly an α_2 effect in cardiac arrest)
        - Venoconstriction: a reduction in venous pooling and an increase in the venous return
        - (Pupillary dilation)
    - β_1 *receptors:*
        - An increase in myocardial contractility and systolic pressure, i.e. a positive inotropic effect
        - An increase in aortic diastolic pressure and blood flow, coronary perfusion pressure and coronary and cerebral blood flow
        - An increase in pacemaker rates: increase in heart rate
        - An increase in spontaneous electrical activity (converts fine ventricular fibrillation to coarse ventricular fibrillation)
        - An increase in myocardial oxygen demand
    - β_2 *receptors:*
        - Smooth muscle vasodilation:
            - Bronchodilation
            - Tremor
        - Increased glycogenolysis and a subsequent increase in oxygen requirement and hypokalaemia

Epinephrine (adrenaline) (*Min-I-Jet® Adrenaline*)

Description
- Epinephrine is a natural catecholamine

Action
- α, β_1, β_2 adrenoceptor agonist action
- In cardiac arrest, epinephrine has been shown to have positive haemodynamic effects, increasing the systolic blood pressure and myocardial and cerebral perfusion
- Some animal studies suggest that the administration of epinephrine may increase the chances of a successful defibrillation

Indications
- All forms of cardiac arrest because of its ability to improve the cerebral and coronary blood supply:
    - VF and failed DC shock
    - Electromechanical dissociation
    - Asystole, when it may have the added advantage of coarsening fine VF
- Anaphylaxis (see chapter on Circulation care: shock)

Presentation:
- Prefilled syringe (*IMS, Aurum*): 3, 10 mL of 1:10,000, 1 mL of 1:1,000 (for anaphylaxis)

Dosage for cardiac arrest (for anaphylaxis see chapter on Circulation care: shock)
- Adults: Intravenous injection: 0.5-1mg (5-10 mL of epinephrine 1:10,000)
          Via tracheal tube: 2-3 mg (20-30 mL of epinephrine 1:10,000)
- Children: 10 µg/kg
- Administration may be repeated every loop (at 2-3 minute intervals) during cardiac arrest according to the patient's response, until resuscitation is successful or abandoned.
- An increased dose of 5 mg may be given as a fourth dose in EMD or asystole

Note: It has been reported that absorption of drugs administered by the tracheal route may be as little as one tenth of that if the drug is administered via a central vein (even if the dose is doubled)

Half life
- 1-2 minutes

Side Effects
- Hypertension and cardiac arrhythmias

CONCLUSION: Epinephrine is the catecholamine of choice in the management of cardiac arrest, although there is no conclusive evidence that its administration increases the overall rate of survival

Dopamine (*Intropin®*)

Description
- The naturally occurring precursor of epinephrine and norepinephrine

Action
- Essentially sympathomimetic and inotropic: agonist effect on dopamine, α and β_1 receptors. The predominant action depends on the dosage (see below)

Indications
- Drug of choice for inotropic support in low output states, i.e. hypotension not due to simple hypovolaemia:
    - Cardiogenic shock
    - Infective shock

Contraindications
- Tachyarrhythmia, marked increase in blood pressure

Presentation
- Dopamine hydrochloride:
    - In 5% Dextrose: 250 mL containers of 200, 400, and 800 mg (800, 1,600 and 3,200 µg/mL)
    - IMS: 40 mg/mL: 5, 10, 20 mL

Dosage
- 1-4 µg/kg/min:
    - Dopamine receptor effects:
        - Renal and gut vasodilation and increased urinary output
- 4-10 µg/kg/min:
    - Above + β_1 effects:
        - Increase myocardial contractility resulting in an increase in cardiac output and heart rate
- >10 µg/kg/min:
    - Above + α effects:
        - Vasoconstriction and may exacerbate cardiac failure and precipitate arrhythmias
- Paediatric: 2-10 µg/kg/min

Administration
- This should be by intravenous infusion and the dose adjusted according to the patient's response
- Must be given via a central line, and therefore not usually used in Immediate Care

Half life
- A few minutes

Side effects
- Nausea and vomiting
- Hypertension, tachycardia

Dobutamine (*Dobutrex®*)

Description
- A synthetic analogue of dopamine

Action
- Dobutamine is a positive inotrope, mainly affecting β_1 receptors
- Increases myocardial contractility, raising cardiac output, stroke volume and at higher doses pulse rate
- Overall it improves the myocardial oxygen supply and demand balance, if tachycardia is avoided

Indications
- As dopamine

Presentation
- Dobutamine hydrochloride: 12.5 mg/mL: 20 mL vials

Dosage
- 2.5 µg/kg, titrated to patient response

Administration
- As dopamine, but may be given via a peripheral line

Advantages
- Tends to lower the cardiac filling pressure, and usually reduces the peripheral resistance

Note: Often a combination of these two drugs (dopamine 5 µg and dobutamine 5-20 µg/kg) are given to maintain urine output and blood pressure in hospital

Isoprenaline (*Saventrine®, Min-I-Jet® Isoprenaline*)

Description
- A synthetic catecholamine

Action
- Potent β_1 and β_2 effects with no α effects
- More chronotropic than inotropic, it reduces the systemic vascular resistance, resulting in a drop in the systemic and diastolic blood pressures
- Improves myocardial contractility and produces a marked rise in heart rate and cardiac output
- Diverts blood supply from cerebral and coronary vessels to gut, muscle and skin

Indications
- Second line antiarrhythmic when atropine (and external cardiac pacing, if available) has not been effective, in the management of:
    - AV heart block
    - Symptomatic sinus bradycardia

Presentation
- 10 mL prefilled syringe (IMS): 20 µg/mL
- 2 mL ampoule: 1 mg/mL

Dosage
- Intravenous injection: 0.2 mg
- Intravenous infusion: 2-10 µg/minute

Half Life
- 2 minutes

Side effects
- May convert bradycardia to a tachycardia
- Increases myocardial excitability resulting in arrhythmias, hypotension
- Sweating, headache

Atropine sulphate (*Min-I-Jet® Atropine sulphate*)

Description
- A naturally occurring alkaloid

Action
- Competitive muscarinic antagonist, which causes vagal inhibition at the SA and AV nodes
    - SA node: increase in automaticity, resulting in a rise in heart rate (and rate related cardiac output). Blood pressure may rise as a result
    - AV node: increases cardiac conduction by blocking inhibitory effects and increasing automaticity
    - Atrial and ventricular muscle: opposes vagal depression

Indications
- Symptomatic bradycardia: sinus and nodal (especially following acute, usually inferior, myocardial infarction)
- Asystole (after failure of epinephrine)
- Symptomatic AV block
- Bradycardia related ventricular ectopics
- Hypotension: if the cardiac rate is slow
- Overdosage:
    - Neostigmine, physostigmine
    - Organophosphates

Presentation
- 10, 20, 30 mL prefilled syringe (IMS): 100 µg/mL, 10 ml prefilled syringe (Aurum) 300 µg/mL
- 1 mL ampoule of 600 µg/mL

Dosage
- Bradycardia:
    - Incremental doses of 0.5-0.6 mg over 5 minutes up to a maximum of 2 mg repeated as required
- Asystole:
    - 3 mg intravenously, 6-9 mg via tracheal tube

Half life
- A few hours

Side effects
- Excessive tachycardia
- Pupillary dilation (making interpretation of pupil sizes difficult), blurred vision, acute glaucoma
- Dry mouth, urinary retention, flushed, dry skin
- Confusion and restlessness (especially in the elderly, with higher doses)

Calcium chloride (*Min-I-Jet® Calcium chloride*)

Action
- Increases myocardial contractility
- (Cerebral and coronary artery vasoconstriction)
- May slow the heart rate and precipitate arrhythmias

Indications
- Cardiac arrest in patients with acute hypocalcaemia, hyperkalaemia or following an overdosage of calcium antagonists

Presentation
- Prefilled syringe (IMS): 10%: 1 g/10 mL

Dosage
- 10 mL as a bolus intravenously

CAUTION
- Calcium chloride should *never* be mixed with sodium bicarbonate
- A high serum calcium will aggravate digoxin toxicity

Sodium bicarbonate (*Min-I-Jet® Sodium bicarbonate*)

Indications
- Used to try to correct metabolic and respiratory acidosis in the prolonged resuscitation situation (after 20 minutes)

Presentation
- Prefilled syringe (IMS): 8.4% in 50 mL: 1 mEq/mL

Dosage
- 50 mL 8.4% intravenously (*never* by tracheal tube)

CONCLUSION: Although theoretically useful for correcting the metabolic and respiratory acidosis following cardiac arrest, the administration of sodium bicarbonate may in fact be positively harmful: it is much more important to ensure that oxygenation and ventilation are adequate

Anti-arrhythmic drugs

Introduction
- All anti-arrhythmic drugs may also cause arrhythmias; and in general the more powerful a drug is, the more likely it is to be pro-arrhythmogenic
- In the emergency situation anti-arrhythmic drugs may be used in two ways:
    - To convert the arrhythmia to sinus rhythm
    - To prevent a recurrence or deterioration of an arrhythmia (usually a tachycardia)
- In patients with early post infarction arrhythmias, although administration of an anti-arrhythmic may appear to help with the initial management of an arrhythmia, there is no evidence that any of them (except β-blockers and amiodarone) increase survival rates (and in many cases may be associated with decreased survival). Because of this there is a trend away from their use towards (safer and ?more effective) electrical treatment

Classification
- Anti-arrhythmic drugs may be classified:
    - Clinically, according to where and for what type of arrhythmia they are used:

Supraventricular arrhythmias	Verapamil
Supraventricular and ventricular arrhythmias	Disopyramide
Ventricular arrhythmias	Lidocaine

   - According to their effect on the myocardial action potential; the Vaughan-Williams classification:

Class I: membrane stabilising or 'local anaesthetic' agents:
- All oppose the fast inward sodium channel and reduce the rise in the action potential

Ia :	-	Also prolong the action potential	Disopyramide, procainamide
Ib:	-	Do not extend the refractory period	Lidocaine, Mexiletine
Ic:	-	Also reduce conduction velocity	Flecainide

Class II: antisympathetic drugs:
- Competitive β-blockade   All β-blockers

Class III:
- Prolong the refractory period, but have   Amiodarone
  no effect on the initial action potential   Bretylium
                                        Sotalol

Class IV: Calcium channel blockers:
- Block the calcium channel   Verapamil, diltiazem

Class I: Membrane stabilising drugs

Introduction
- These drugs are negatively inotropic and should be avoided in patients with impaired left ventricular function and a systolic blood pressure less than 95 mmHg.
- Usually divided into three classes according to their effect on the duration of the action potential

Class Ia

Disopyramide (*Rythmodan*®)

Action
- Suppresses the excitability of atrial and ventricular myocardium
- Slows conduction in the His-Purkinje system and in myocardial cells
- May also have an anticholinergic effect (causing an increase in AV conduction rate)

Indications
- Ventricular arrhythmias (VT) especially after myocardial infarction, not responsive to lidocaine
- Paroxysmal atrial fibrillation

Presentation
- 50 mg/5 mL ampoules

Dosage
- Initially 2 mg/kg by slow intravenous injection over 5-20 minutes; maximum 150 mg regardless of body weight, repeated after one hour if necessary, if there is no response
- A maintenance infusion may then be set up at a rate of 20-30 mg/hour, ceasing as soon as sinus rhythm returns

Side effects
- May impair cardiac contractility, and aggravate heart failure (this effect will be increased by the concurrent administration of any other anti-arrhythmic drugs including β-blockers)
- Anticholinergic side effects include:
    - Dry mouth, urinary retention, and an increase in intraocular pressure (in glaucoma)

CONCLUSION: Class Ia *drug of choice* for the management of paroxysmal atrial tachycardia including atrial fibrillation, but not the the drug of choice overall

Procainamide (*Pronestyl*®)

Description
- A powerful anti-arrhythmic drug with a strongly negative inotropic effect

Action
- Reduces the automaticity of ectopic pacemakers
- Slows interventricular conduction
- Has a stronger anti-fibrillatory effect than lidocaine

Indications
- Ventricular and supraventricular arrhythmias

Presentation
- 100 mg/mL ampoules

Dosage
- 20-50 mg/min, administered as 50-100 mg boluses every 5 minutes (500 mg maximum in the first hour), until the arrhythmia is suppressed or blood pressure begins to drop

Half life
- Short, and therefore the drug needs to be topped up frequently

Side effects
- Myocardial depression, heart failure and arrhythmias
- Nausea, diarrhoea

Contraindications
- Heart block, heart failure, hypotension

CONCLUSION: Rarely used in the UK, because of its short duration of action and pro-arrhythmic effect

Class Ib

Mexilitene (*Mexitil®*)

Indications
- Ventricular tachyarrhythmias, resistant to lidocaine (in hospital only)

Contraindications
- Heart block

Side effects
- Nausea, vomiting, dizziness and tremor

Presentation
- 10 mL ampoules 25 mg/mL

Dosage
- Intravenous bolus of 250 mg or 5-10 mL, followed by 250 mg/hour for the first hour and 125 mg/hour for the second hour

CONCLUSION: Not often used because of its side effects, but does have a role in the management of ventricular arrhythmias in hospital

Lidocaine/lignocaine hydrochloride (*Xylocard®*, *Min-I-Jet® Lignocaine*)

Description
- Stabilises cell membranes by reducing the excitability of myocardial cells and the rate of depolarisation. This decreases ventricular automaticity, suppresses ventricular ectopic activity, and raises the threshold for VF (this may reduce the incidence of primary VF following AMI, but does not alter the overall mortality)
- Acts selectively in diseased and ischaemic myocardium interrupting and preventing re-entry circuits
- Good local anaesthetic, but may cause serious myocardial depression

Indications
- Conversion or prevention of recurrent ventricular tachycardia
- Frequent symptomatic PVCs as a result of acute myocardial ischaemia/infarction

Contraindications (relative)
- Should not be given in the presence of AV block
- Sinoatrial disorders

Advantages
- Fewer proarrhythmic effects

Presentation
- 10 mL IMS prefilled syringe: 1% lidocaine hydrochloride: 10 mg/mL
- 5 mL IMS prefilled syringe: 2% lidocaine hydrochloride: 20 mg/mL
- 5 mL prefilled syringe: 2% lidocaine hydrochloride: 20 mg/mL

Dosage
- Rapidly metabolised and initial dose may only last 10 minutes, half life is then 2 hours
- Give an initial bolus of 100 mg (10 mL of 10 mg/mL) over 2-3 minutes followed by a repeat bolus of 50-100 mg after 5-15 minutes, and an infusion of 2-4 mg/min for 24 hours (maximum 3 mg/kg)
- Paediatric: 1mg/kg

Side effects (more marked in the elderly and those with hepatic impairment)
- Parasthesiae, dysphasia, drowsiness, dizziness, hypotension, confusion, muscle twitching and fits
- Reduction in heart rate, myocardial depression, greater resistance to defibrillation

CONCLUSION: Drug of choice in the management of ventricular tachycardia

Class Ic

Flecainide (*Tambocor®*)

Description
- This is one of the more effective new drugs available for the management of ventricular and supraventricular arrhythmias

Action
- Suppresses atrial and ventricular myocardial excitability
- Slows conduction throughout the heart, increasing the length of the PR interval, and widening the QRS complex; it does not lengthen the QT interval or T wave, unlike many other anti-arrhythmics

Indications
- Ventricular and supraventricular tachycardias
- Ventricular extra systoles
- Arrhythmias associated with the Wolff Parkinson White syndrome
- Ventricular fibrillation refractory to lidocaine and electricity

Contraindications (relative)
- Heart failure
- PVCs following AMI
- SA disorders
- AV block

Presentation
- 15 mL ampoules of 10 mg/mL

Dosage
- 2 mg/kg intravenously over 10-30 minutes (max. 150 mg) with ECG monitoring, then as required by intravenous infusion

Half life
- Long

Side effects
- Has proarrhythmic effects, especially if administered with other drugs which prolong the QT interval.
- Flecainide is negatively inotropic and may aggravate cardiac failure (associated with an increased mortality when used orally to suppress ventricular activity in impaired left ventricular function)
- Visual disturbance and dizziness

CONCLUSION: Its is *reserved for treating life-threatening or refractory ventricular arrhythmias*, because although it is a powerful anti-arrhythmic, it is also highly pro-arrhythmic

Class II: β-adrenergic receptor blockers

β-blockers (see under chapter on Cardiac care: acute myocardial infarction)

Class III: Repolarisation inhibitors

Description: Widen the direct action potential duration, and therefore the QT interval

Amiodarone (*Cordarone®*)

Action
- As well as Class III effects, amiodarone has some Class I activity (inhibits the fast sodium channel)
- Has a mild negative inotropic effect
- Amiodarone is a coronary artery dilator (making amiodarone especially useful in the management of patients with impaired left ventricular function)

Indications
- Arrhythmias associated with the Wolff Parkinson White Syndrome
- In the management of serious arrhythmias when other drugs have been ineffective or are contraindicated for:
    - Supraventricular (narrow complex) and ventricular (broad complex) tachycardia
- Atrial fibrillation and flutter, recurrent ventricular fibrillation (very effective for preventing paroxysmal atrial fibrillation, and ventricular tachycardia/fibrillation)

Contraindications
- Sinus bradycardia, AV block, (thyroid problems)
- If administered concurrently with other drugs which prolong the QT interval, amiodarone may paradoxically become arrhythmogenic

Side effects
- Skin photosensitivity resulting in erythema, pulmonary fibrosis, thyroid dysfunction (both over and under activity), peripheral neuropathy, hepatotoxicity (with long term use only)
- Nausea (even at low doses)
- Concurrent administration of β-blockers or verapamil may result in an increased degree of nodal block
- Asymptomatic reduction in pulmonary gas transfer (significant lung toxicity is rare),
- Potentiation of the action of digoxin and warfarin

Presentation
- 150 mg/3 mL ampoules

Dosage
- Up to 5 mg/kg in 100 mL 5% dextrose (not saline) intravenously over 1-4 hours (onset of full description may take several hours)
- For Wolff Parkinson White Syndrome: may be given orally

Half life
- Long (>90 days).

CONCLUSION: Amiodarone is the only anti-arrhythmic which has been shown to increase survival rates, when used in the management of post infarction arrhythmias

Bretylium tosylate (*Bretylate®, Min-I-Jet® Bretylium tosylate*)

Description
- Bretylium is a unique adrenergic neuron blocking agent, with direct and indirect modes of action

Action
- Direct action:
    - Has a direct beneficial effect on VF by raising the fibrillation threshold (in a similar way to lidocaine). It prolongs the refractory period to a greater extent in normal myocardium, than in damaged or ischaemic myocardium and may therefore prevent re-entry circuits in ischaemic tissue
- Indirect action:
    - Initial action is to stimulate adrenergic neurons resulting in the release of norepinephrine, which may result in transient hypertension and tachycardia
    - This is followed about 20 minutes later by full adrenergic blockade, which peaks after 45-60 minutes

Indications
- Recurrent or refractory VF
- VT after lidocaine and DC version/defibrillation have failed

Presentation
- 50 mg/mL: 10 mL ampoule, IMS prefilled syringe

Dosage
- 400-500 mg (5-10 mg/kg) diluted in 5% dextrose administered by slow intravenous injection over 8-10 minutes; this may take 20-30 minutes to be effective
- If successful; this may be repeated after 20 minutes and again 1-2 hours later or followed by an infusion of 1-2 mg/kg/hr

Half life
- 7-9 hours

Side effects
- Severe postural hypotension (usually transient), nausea, vomiting

Disadvantage
- If used, may commit the rescuer to 30 minutes further resuscitation

Class IV: calcium channel blockers/calcium antagonists

Description:
- Inhibit the slow calcium channel in the AV node
- Reduce myocardial oxygen consumption

Verapamil (*Cordilox®*)

Action
- Inhibits the action potential in the SA and AV nodes, resulting in an increase in AV block and an increase in the refractory period of the AV node
- Causes arteriolar vasodilation and reduces cardiac contractility (has a negative inotropic effect)

Indications
- Atrial fibrillation and flutter
- Paroxysmal supraventricular tachycardia (drug of choice if adenosine is not available)
- Relief of cardiac ischaemic pain: angina (orally)
- Hypertension

Contraindications
- Bradycardia, sick sinus syndrome, pre-existing AV nodal disease, heart block, heart failure, atrial flutter or fibrillation complicating the Wolff Parkinson White syndrome
- Patients taking:
    - High doses of β-blockers (may precipitate severe refractory hypotension)
    - Quinidine or disopyramide

Note: Verapamil may safely be administered to patients already on digoxin, when it will enhance digoxin's AV node suppression

Presentation
- 5 mg/2 mL ampoules

Dosage
- SVT:
    - 5-10 mg intravenously rapidly over 30 seconds initially (which will produce its peak therapeutic effect within 3-5 minutes), followed 15-20 minutes later by 5-10 mg intravenously if required

Side effects
- Headache, flushing
- Hypotension, bradycardia, heart block, asystole
- May precipitate heart failure and exacerbate conduction disorders especially in children

Note: The negative inotropic effects of these antiarrhythmic drugs tend to be cumulative, so care should be exercised if they are used together
Their tendency to cause as well as treat arrhythmias may be aggravated by hypokalaemia

Adenosine (*Adenocor®*)

Description
- A naturally occurring purine nucleotide found throughout the body; formed by the breakdown of adenosine triphosphate (ATP) and S-adenosylhomocysteine

Action
- When given intravenously, it acts at the adenosine A_1 (myocardial) and A_2 (coronary artery) receptors.
- At the A_1 receptors this interaction results in an outward shift of intracellular potassium and hyperpolarisation of the cardiac cell membranes, resulting in depression of the AV node and the blocking of conduction
- Effective at terminating episodes of paroxysmal supraventricular tachycardia including those involving the AV node in re-entry pathways
- Half-life is very short, so that a blocked arrhythmia may re-emerge

Indications
- Paroxysmal supraventricular tachycardias including those associated with AV node re-entry circuits, e.g. Wolff Parkinson White syndrome
- As an aid to the diagnosis of broad complex tachycardias where the rhythm is uncertain (VT v SVT with aberrant conduction):
    - If it stops the tachycardia, it is likely to be junctional in origin and involve the AV node
    - If there is transient AV block with specific ECG changes (P waves, f waves or F waves), the arrhythmia is likely to be due to atrial tachycardia, flutter, or fibrillation
    - If there is no effect, the arrhythmia is likely to be ventricular tachycardia

Contraindications
- Asthma (adenosine is a bronchoconstrictor)
- Second or third degree AV block
- Sick sinus syndrome (unless a pacemaker is fitted)

Side effects (occur in about 20-25% of patients and last less than one minute)
- Most common:
    - Transient facial flushing, dyspnoea, bronchospasm, a choking sensation, nausea, light headedness, chest pain and a peculiar unpleasant feeling
- Less common:
    - Sweating, palpitations, hyperventilation, headache, blurred vision, burning sensation
    - Severe bradycardia requiring pacing
    - Transient ECG rhythm disturbances
- Antagonised by methylxanthenes, e.g. aminophylline, theophylline and caffeine

Presentation
- 3mg/mL: 2 mL ampoules

Dosage
- Initial intravenous bolus of 3 mg administered as rapidly as possible into a large vein, e.g. antecubital fossa vein, with cardiac monitoring, followed by a saline flush
- If this does not terminate the rhythm within 1 minute, this may be followed by a further bolus of 12 mg after 1-2 minutes, administered as rapidly as possible
- Additional doses are not recommended
- Further increments should not be given if high level AV block develops

Half-life
- Very short: 2-15 seconds

Advantages
- It is safe to administer to patients with a broad complex tachycardia (unlike verapamil)
- It exhibits no negative inotropic effects
- It is safe to administer to patients on β-blockers (unlike verapamil)
- It is safe in children (unlike verapamil): dosage: 0.0375 mg/kg

CONCLUSION: *Drug of choice for the management of supraventricular tachycardias*
Useful as an aid in the diagnosis of tachycardias of unknown type
Should only be administered to monitored patients with full resuscitation facilities available
Not licensed (yet) for pre-hospital use

Loop diuretics

Introduction
- Loop diuretics are used for the treatment of acute left ventricular failure resulting in pulmonary oedema

Action
- Loop diuretics inhibit resorption of water and potassium from the ascending loop of Henle in the renal tubule and are powerful diuretics. They also reduce the cardiac pre-load sooner than would be expected if their only effect is as a diuretic
- Intravenous administration produces relief of breathlessness and a dose related diuresis which is maximal within about 30 minutes

Indications
- Acute left ventricular failure

Side effects
- If administered too rapidly intravenously there is a risk of hypotension
- Urinary retention in elderly males with prostatism

Furosemide (frusemide) (*Lasix®*)

Presentation
- 10 mg/mL in 2, 5 and 25 mL ampoules
Dosage
- By slow intravenous injection (no more than 4 mg per minute) of 80-120 mg (less in the elderly)

Bumetanide (*Burinex®*)

Presentation
- 500 µg/mL in 2 and 4 mL ampoules
Dosage
- By slow intravenous injection of 1-2 mg, repeated as required after about 20 minutes, up to a maximum of about 5 mg (less in the elderly)

9

Medical emergencies

Medical emergencies

Introduction
- The pre-hospital assessment and management of medical emergencies should be performed in the same way as any other pre-hospital emergency. The subjective interview and medical history are of particular importance
- Many pre-hospital medical emergencies will occur in the patient's home, which is a much less hostile environment than outside, and may permit more active intervention (management of their problem) before the patient is conveyed to hospital
- Some medical emergencies are immediately life threatening, and must be managed before the patient is conveyed to hospital
- Patients suffering from trauma may also be suffering from an acute medical problem:
    - What was the cause of the accident?
    - Are the injured also suffering from hypothermia?

Assess the scene, scene safety

Triage if there is more than one casualty

Primary Survey
- Airway
- Breathing and ventilation
- Circulation
- Disability
- Exposure and control of the environment

Secondary Survey
- **Subjective interview**
    - This is most important and useful in medical emergencies
    - If possible try to obtain information from relatives/partners/bystanders as well as the patient
    - Try to ascertain:
        - What has happened?
        - What is the patient complaining of?
        - The patient's significant past medical history
- **Medical history (AMPLE)**
    - Allergies;
        - Has the patient any known allergies?
    - Medicines:
        - What medicines is the patient currently taking?

- Past medical history:
    - Obtain a brief history of any major illness (especially those involving hospital admission) or operations that the patient has had, in chronological order
- Last meal:
    - When did the patient last eat or drink?
- Events leading up to the illness.
    - What has happened to the patient, and what symptoms did they have just before they were taken ill?
    - Has the patient had an illness or symptoms similar to this before?
- **Objective examination and management**
    - Appearance
    - Head (including neurological status)
    - Neck
    - Chest
    - Abdomen
    - Pelvis
    - Extremities
    - Spine
    - Back.
- **Pain** assessment and management

Unexplained deterioration
- If there is any sudden, severe or unexplained deterioration in the patient's condition:
    - Go back to the primary survey

Monitoring/reassessment of the patient
- This should be continuous and repeated, so as to detect any changes in the patient's condition and will allow modification of their management accordingly
- Is their condition:
    - Improving?
    - Deteriorating?: if so why? what can be done to improve it?
    - The same

Monitor
- Airway patency.
- Breathing:
    - Appearance/colour
    - Respiratory rate
    - Chest expansion
    - SpO_2
    - Peak expiratory flow rate
- Circulation:
    - Pulse rate
    - Blood pressure
    - Capillary refill
    - Peripheral pulses
- Disability/neurological status:
    - Glasgow coma scale
- Pain severity

Acute severe asthma

Definition: Acute potentially reversible expiratory airways obstruction, unresponsive to the patient's usual medication, resulting in a reduction in the peak flow to 40% or less of its predicted value

Introduction
- Acute severe asthma is one of the most common medical emergencies, and is increasing in incidence
- It is a life threatening condition, causing approximately 2000 deaths per year in the UK, which necessitates immediate recognition and requires rapid, aggressive and effective management
- Most deaths occur in older people, but are more preventable in the young (80-90%) in whom the severity of the attack is often not recognised either by the patient, their parents/partner, or by their own doctor
- The onset of an attack may be either rapid or insidious, but by the time an Immediate Care doctor or extended trained ambulanceman is involved, the patient is usually extremely ill

Incidence
- Usually occurs in known asthmatics
- One of the commonest medical emergencies encountered outside hospital
- Death may occur quickly and with little warning
- Occurs most often at night or in the early hours of the morning
- May be precipitated by a viral or rarely a bacterial upper or lower respiratory tract infection
- May be exacerbated by stress
- In atopic individuals, it may be caused by a sudden rise in the pollen count/airborne moulds, e.g after thunderstorms

Aetiology
- Over reliance on bronchodilators
- Under use of inhaled/oral steroids
- Failure to make objective measurements of severity of an attack
- Inadequate medical supervision
- Those particularly at risk include:
    - Patients with psychosocial problems including social and economic deprivation
    - Patients hospitalised for asthma within the previous year, especially during the last few days/weeks
    - Patients with a previous history of acute severe asthma
    - Patients who require the administration of oral steroids and/or nebulised drugs intermittently or regularly
    - Patients with a history of worsening symptoms (especially at night)
    - Patients with progressively worsening of their peak flow readings
    - Patients who have an increasing variation (especially diurnal) in their peak flow readings
    - Patients who are experiencing an increase in their exposure to seasonal aero allergens (pollens, mould, etc.), to an environment known to make their asthma worse or a decrease in air quality, (especially a combination of these)
    - Adolescents and young adults
    - Immigrants, temporary residents and those on holiday

Pathophysiology
- Asthma is an acute inflammatory reaction of the airways resulting in:
    - Bronchospasm
    - Mucus secretion resulting in:
        - Plugging of bronchioles and alveoli (mucus gland hyperplasia)
    - Desquamation of the epithelium with thickening of the basement membrane
    - Narrowing of the airway, which causes a reduction in airflow and oxygenation
    - Tachypnoea and sometimes hyperventilation, aggravated by fear and respiratory centre stimulation

- Dehydration: combination of inadequate fluid intake and increased fluid loss (increased ventilation)
- Hypoxia caused by an impairment of gaseous exchange, leading to a reduction in PaO_2 and SpO_2
- $PaCO_2$ may fall initially due to the tachypnoea, but as the airways become narrower, it may return to normal and then rise as respiration fails
- Complications may include:

Spontaneous pneumothorax
- This is an uncommon (only found in 0.5% of those admitted to hospital with acute severe asthma), but potentially fatal complication of asthma characterised by sudden circulatory collapse, and sometimes by pain
- May be bilateral, and is very difficult to detect clinically

Mediastinal or subcutaneous emphysema
- Relatively common in acute severe asthma, especially in the ventilated patient, when it often indicates the presence of a pneumothorax
- Is usually of relatively little consequence by itself

History
- Previous history of asthma or atopy

Signs/symptoms

Unstable/uncontrolled asthma
- Normal speech
- Tracheal tug with intercostal recession and use of the accessory muscles
- Pulse <110 beats per minute
- Hyperinflation with a respiratory rate <25 breaths/minute
- Peak expiratory flow rate (PEFR) >50% of best or predicted

Acute severe asthma
- Increasing wheeze and breathlessness
- Difficulty with speaking (unable to complete a sentence in one breath), get up from a chair/bed, or feed
- A persistently increased respiratory rate: >25 breaths per minute (>50 breaths per minute for children)
- Tachycardia: >110 bpm (>140 bpm for children)
- Reduced peak expiratory flow rate: <50% of the predicted value or if not known <120 l/m in adults
- Reduced SpO_2

Life threatening asthma
- "Silent Chest" or severe wheezing
- Cyanosis
- Bradycardia
- Exhaustion, restlessness, agitation, confusion and unconsciousness
- Reduced peak expiratory flow rate: <33% of predicted
- Very reduced SpO_2

Note: **In young children:**
- Asthma can be very difficult to diagnose
- The differential diagnosis includes:
    - Croup
    - Inhaled foreign body
    - Acute viral pneumonitis
    - Cystic fibrosis

Management
- Needs to be rapid and aggressive, if lives are going to be saved
- Can be especially difficult in children under the age of 18 months as they may respond poorly to treatment
- Monitor the patient's response to treatment, observing changes in appearance and vital signs:
    - Obtain serial peak flow meter readings (and SpO_2 percentages) initially and after treatment

Breathing/ventilation: hypoxia

Oxygen
- Oxygen *is mandatory*
- Use a high concentration oxygen mask with a high flow rate, as most patients who die, do so as a result of hypoxia
- Retention of carbon dioxide is not aggravated by oxygen therapy in patients with acute severe asthma

Bronchospasm/mucus plugging

β_2 adrenergic stimulants (salbutamol, terbutaline)
- These are best administered via a nebuliser (preferably oxygen driven)
- Great care should be exerted as a transient fall in PaO_2 may occur, resulting in a respiratory arrest in the severely hypoxaemic patient. This is thought to be due to a direct vascular effect, and is caused by a reversal of the compensatory pulmonary vasoconstriction in poorly ventilated areas of the lung which leads to an increase in the ventilation/perfusion mismatch. The fall in PaO_2 is usually transient and ends once the bronchi dilate and ventilation becomes more homogeneous, but in the severely hypoxaemic patient the additional reduction in PaO_2 may lead to a respiratory arrest. *Oxygen, should therefore always be administered before giving β-agonists*, if the nebuliser is not oxygen driven
- If a nebuliser is not available:
    - Consider using an inhaler fitted with a large spacer (a plastic cup or even a soft drinks bottle may suffice for children) filled with the inhalant from 20 puffs from the inhaler
- If there is minimal response to the nebulised preparation (possibly due to mucous plugging), then administration by slow intravenous and/or subcutaneous injection, may be tried
- In severe refractory cases an intravenous infusion may be considered and the infusion rate titrated against the patient's response (the value of parenteral administration has not yet been proven and may only increase the incidence of side effects)

Salbutamol (*Ventolin*®)

Presentation
- Nebules: 2.5 mg, 5.0 mg
- Injection: 50 µg/mL in 5 mL ampoules, 500 µg/mL in 1 mL ampoules

Dosage
- By nebuliser: 2.5-5 mg (recommended maximum: 15 mg)
- By subcutaneous or intramuscular injection: 500 µg, repeated every four hours as required

Terbutaline (*Bricanyl*®)

Presentation
- Respules: 5 mg in 2 mL
- Respirator solution: 100 mg in 10 mL

Dosage
- By nebuliser: 5-10 mg (recommended maximum 10 mg)
- By subcutaneous, intramuscular or slow intravenous injection: 250-500 µg, eight hourly

Note: Intravenous preparations of both salbutamol and terbutaline are available, but are associated with a high incidence of side effects and are not usually used in pre-hospital care

Anticholinergics

Ipratropium bromide (*Atrovent®*)
- May be particularly useful in young children under 1 year, who may not have fully developed β-receptors, and in whom β-agonists may be relatively ineffective
- Can also be useful in the treatment of residual bronchoconstriction after using an inhaled β-agonist, without causing the side effects of β-agonists, and in COPD

Presentation
- Nebuliser solution 0.025% (0.25 mg/mL)

Dosage
- Adults: 0.4-2.0 mL solution (0.1-0.5 mg)
- Children (3-14 years): 0.4-2.0 mL solution (0.1-0.5 mg)

Administration
- Usually administered by nebuliser
- May either be administered together with a β-agonist in the same nebuliser, or given separately afterwards
- May take longer to be effective than β-agonists (30-60 minutes), but has a longer duration of action

Note: Patients who have severe asthma benefit more from combination therapy than those who do not

Steroids

Hydrocortisone (sodium succinate/phosphate)

Presentation: See under anaphylactic shock

Dosage
- Adults: 200 mg   Children: 100 mg

Administration
- By intravenous injection

Side effects
- Paraesthesiae, which may be painful and unpleasant, and is often experienced in the genital area, but is occasionally generalised, and is usually short lived

Prednisolone
- Considered by many to be a better alternative to hydrocortisone (unless the patient is unable to take oral medication), and may be given alone or in combination with hydrocortisone 200 mg intravenously

Presentation
- Tablets 5 mg

Dosage
- Adults: 30-60 mg orally
- Children: 2 mg/kg initially (maximum 40 mg)

Note: All steroids are slow to take effect and have a short duration of action. They should therefore be administered as soon as possible

Epinephrine (adrenaline)
- This may have a role in the management of acute severe asthma, where there is a major atopic element (buys time in case the patient needs ventilating)
- For further details see the chapter on Circulation care: shock

Methylxanthenes
- The use of these are well established, but they have a narrow therapeutic range, and serious toxic side effects, such as arrhythmias and convulsions may occur before other less serious symptoms of toxicity: nausea, vomiting and tachycardia (intravenous salbutamol is proved to be more effective than aminophylline)

Aminophylline (*Min-I-Jet® Aminophylline*)

Presentation
- Ampoules of 250 mg/10 mL
- Prefilled syringe (IMS)

Dosage
- Adults: 250-500 mg (5 mg/kg)
- Children: 5 mg/kg initially

Administration
- Should be administered by slow intravenous injection over 20 minutes

Note: Aminophylline should *never* be administered to the patient already receiving a methylxanthene (aminophylline, theophylline) as fatal overdosage may occur

Assisted ventilation
- Intermittent positive pressure ventilation may be needed in a small number (0.5-1%) of patients, but can be difficult to achieve due to the high inflation pressures which may be necessary, and the need to suppress the patient's spontaneous ventilatory effort, which may necessitate heavy sedation
- In the past the mortality rate has been 9-38%, but this has been reduced recently by using "Controlled hypoventilation", a technique which uses high inspired oxygen concentrations and low flow rates and inflation pressures

Pneumothorax
- Insertion of a chest drain (see chapter on Chest injuries)

Dehydration
- This is caused by a combination of inadequate fluid intake and increased fluid loss due to increased ventilation

Intravenous fluids: crystalloid

Hartmann's/Ringer-Lactate solution: Sodium lactate intravenous compound (see chapter on Shock)

- An intravenous infusion may be started in all patients with prolonged acute severe asthma as significant dehydration may occur

Monitoring
- Serial peak expiratory flow rates
- Oxygen saturation:
  - Try to maintain SpO_2 >92%
  - A sudden fall in SpO_2 may indicate a pneumothorax

Guidelines for the emergency management of asthma

Unstable/uncontrolled asthma
- Nebulised β_2 stimulant:
    - Salbutamol 5 mg or terbutaline 10 mg (half doses in very young children), using an oxygen driven nebuliser if available (if no nebuliser is available, use an aerosol inhaler with a spacer)
- Observe and if there is *minimal response after 15-30 minutes*, i.e PEFR >50-70% predicted or best:
- Administer oral prednisolone 30-60 mg and step up usual treatment

Acute severe asthma
- Oxygen (in as high a flow rate as possible), using a high concentration oxygen mask
- Salbutamol 5 mg or terbutaline 10 mg (half doses in very young children), using an oxygen driven nebuliser if available (if no nebuliser is available, use an aerosol inhaler with a spacer)
- Steroids:
    - Oral prednisolone 30-60 mg or intravenous hydrocortisone 200 mg (both if the patient is very ill)
    - For children administer prednisolone 1-2 mg/kg body weight (maximum 40 mg) initially
- Observe and if there is *minimal response after 15-20 minutes*:
    - Repeat nebulised β_2 stimulant and add nebulised ipratropium 500 μg
    or Administer subcutaneous terbutaline (or salbutamol)
    or Give intravenous aminophylline 250 mg (5mg/kg for children) slowly over 20 minutes (if the patient is not already taking a methylxanthene)

Life threatening asthma
- Oral prednisolone 30-60 mg or intravenous hydrocortisone 200 mg (children:100 mg) *immediately*
- Nebulised β_2 stimulant:
    - Salbutamol 5 mg or terbutaline 10 mg (half doses in very young children), using an oxygen driven nebuliser together with nebulised ipratropium bromide 0.5 mg (0.25 mg for children or 0.125 mg for very young children) added to the nebulised β_2 stimulant
    or Administer subcutaneous terbutaline (or salbutamol)
    or Give intravenous aminophylline 250 mg (5mg/kg for children) slowly over 20 minutes (if the patient is not already taking a methylxanthene)
    - Consider the administration of
- If there is *little or no improvement*, consider intubation and ventilation

Note: Consider use of intravenous epinephrine if there is a major atopic element of the patient's asthma

Hospital admission

- Admit to hospital *without delay* if:
    - Any immediately life threatening features are present
    - Any potentially life threatening features persist in spite of treatment
    - The PEFR 15-30 minutes after treatment is still 40% below the predicted/best
- Consider hospital admission if:
    - Attack is in the afternoon or evening
    - Recent onset of nocturnal or worsening symptoms
    - There have been previous severe attacks, especially if they have been of rapid onset
    - The patient or their relatives are unlikely to respond appropriately to any deterioration in the patient's condition
    - There is concern over the patient's social circumstances

Figure 9-1 Guidelines for the emergency management of asthma

Acute epiglottitis

Introduction
- This is an acute life threatening condition, and rapid effective treatment can save lives

Incidence
- Occurs much less often than croup, and is becoming increasingly rare, due to the recent successful *Haemophilus influenzae* vaccination programme
- Usually occurs in children between 18 months and 7 years old (peak incidence 2-3 years)
- Much less common in adults
- Boys are more often affected than girls

Aetiology
- Usual causative pathogen:
    - Children: *Haemophilus influenzae* type b
    - Adults: *Haemophilus influenzae, Streptococcus pyogenes*

Pathophysiology
- Infection results in acute inflammation of the supraglottic structures of the larynx, resulting in the rapid development of severe pharyngeal oedema and consequent airway obstruction
- There is a generalised septicaemia

Symptoms/signs
- *History:*
    - Sore throat with the rapid (usually less than 6 hours) development of respiratory distress and severe dysphagia
- *General appearance*
    - Very unwell, anxious, toxic with a temperature often >40 ºC
- *Tripod position:*
    - Chin forward, extended neck, with mouth open, protruding tongue and often drooling saliva (as swallowing is so painful)
    - The child resists attempts to make him lie down
- *Airway:*
    - Stridor:
        - Soft low pitched, with the rapid onset of inspiratory wheeze *only.*
    - There is *no* cough, and the voice is muffled (in croup the voice is abnormal or absent)
    - Severe dysphagia with saliva tending to pool in the pharynx
- *Breathing:*
    - Intercostal, subcostal, costal and sternal recession, with reduced air entry
    - Tachypnoea, tachycardia, cyanosis, use of the accessory muscles:
        - Ala nasae
        - Sternomastoids
    - Respiratory arrest may occur suddenly and without warning
- *Circulation:*
    - Poor peripheral perfusion, proceeding to shock

Note: It is best to examine the child naked lying on its parent's lap, so as to avoid distressing it

CAUTION: If acute epiglottitis is suspected do *not* attempt to examine the child's throat by depressing the tongue with a spatula or other instrument, as this may push the epiglottis down onto the larynx and provoke total airway obstruction

Management
- Strong reassurance to keep the child as calm as possible
- Administer high flow oxygen via a high concentration oxygen mask
- Give nebulised:
    - Epinephrine: 3-5 mL of 1:1000, repeated after 30 minutes (stop if the pulse rate >120 bpm)
    - Budesonide (*Pulmicort®*) 2mg as a single dose (*or* as two 1 mg doses separated by 30 minutes)
- If acute respiratory distress develops; perform a cricothyrotomy
- Do *not* delay transportation to hospital:
    - *Always accompany the child to hospital* (they may develop severe respiratory distress proceeding to respiratory arrest *very* rapidly)
- If transportation time to hospital is long administer antibiotics:
    - Amoxycillin/co-amoxiclav
    - Erythromycin/clarithromycin

Note: Tracheal intubation should *only* be attempted by the very experienced if the child is moribund, as it can exacerbate an already critical situation, and is probably *not appropriate* in Immediate Care
  If intubation *is* attempted:
    - The tracheal tube should be non cuffed, and two sizes smaller than that normally used in children of that age, to prevent later pressure necrosis of the subglottic region
    - It is advisable to pass an introducer, e.g. a gum elastic bougie, first

Differentiating features of croup and epiglottitis

Feature	Croup	Epiglottitis
Incidence	Very common	Rare and becoming more so
Aetiology	Mostly *para-influenzae* viruses	*Haemophilus influenzae* type b
Onset	Over several days (spasmodic: sudden)	Over a few hours
Preceding coryza	Yes	No
Appearance	Unwell	Toxic and very ill
Position	Irritable, active	Tripod position
Stridor	Harsh, rasping	Soft
Cough	Severe barking	Slight or absent
Drooling	No	Yes
Temperature	<38.5°C	>38.5°C
Voice	Hoarse, croaky	Reluctant to speak, muffled
Able to drink	Yes	No
Wheeze	Inspiratory wheeze often present	Absent

Figure 9-2 Differentiating features of croup and epiglottitis

Bacterial laryngotracheobronchitis (bacterial or membranous LTB/croup)

- This is a rare, but life threatening illness

Incidence
- Uncommon
- Occurs mostly in children >5 years old

Aetiology
- Often caused by *Staphylococcus aureus* secondary to a viral infection
- May also be caused by Streptococci or *Haemophilus influenzae* (becoming rarer)

Pathophysiology
- Inflammation and ulceration of the glottis
- Necrosis of the tracheal mucosa
- Production of copious purulent secretions and a thick, crusting exudate (pseudomembrane)

Symptoms/signs
- Similar to acute viral LTB, but the systemic disturbance is much greater
- Barking cough with copious sputum production
- Signs of increasing airways obstruction:
    - Severe stridor or stridor at rest
    - Evidence of respiratory distress:
        - A steadily increasing respiratory rate
        - Intercostal recession
        - Exhaustion
        - Cyanosis
    - Increasing pulse rate
- Evidence of septicaemia, e.g. appears toxic, pyrexia >39.5 °C, tachycardia

Management
- Initially similar to acute viral LTB
- Reassurance
- Administer high flow oxygen via a high concentration oxygen mask
- Consider:
    - Nebulised:
        - Epinephrine: 3-5 mL of 1:1000, repeated after 30 minutes (stop if the pulse rate >120 bpm)
        - Budesonide (*Pulmicort*®): see below
    - Oral dexamethasone (0.15 mg/kg)
- Cricothyrotomy, if total airway obstruction appears imminent or the child becomes unconscious
- Antibiotics:
    - Flucloxacillin
    - Co-amoxiclav
- Rehydration with frequent small volumes of clear fluid
- Admit to hospital immediately

Budesonide (*Pulmicort*® respules)

Presentation
- 2 mL ampoules of 0.25 mg/mL or 0.5 mg/mL budesonide in a suspension for nebulisation

Dosage (croup)
- 2 mg as a single dose (*or* two 1 mg doses separated by 30 minutes)

Viral laryngotracheobronchitis (viral LTB/croup)

Incidence
- Viral croup is one of the more common childhood respiratory illnesses, occurring more often in boys
- Usually (6%) occurs in children aged 2 months to 9 years (usually 6 months to 6 years, peak 18 months)
- The peak incidence is between October and March in temperate climates

Aetiology
- Viral croup:
    - Most commonly:
        - *Para-influenzae* types I and II (commonest)
        - *Influenza A+B*
    - Less commonly:
        - *Respiratory syncytial* virus (may also cause bronchiolitis)
        - *Echo* virus
        - *Coxsackie A* virus
        - Rhinovirus
- Recurrent or spasmodic croup:
    - Some children develop croup suddenly and repeatedly at night without evidence of infection
    - Thought to be allergic as it is more common in atopic children, and will often resolve within hours

Pathophysiology
- Acute inflammation of the larynx, trachea and bronchi with subglottic oedema resulting in airway narrowing, and respiratory embarrassment in young children because of the small calibre of their airway

Symptoms/signs
- History of prodromal (usually 48-72 hrs) viral upper respiratory tract illness
- The child is not usually toxic and the temperature is usually <39.5 °C
- The child is usually restless, but not acutely ill
- Harsh inspiratory or biphasic stridor, of gradual onset
- Sore throat, with a *barking "seal like" cough* and an abnormal hoarse voice
- The chest is clear, and there is no intercostal recession

Management (the great majority of children may be managed quite safely at home)
- Reassurance
- Nebulised water/steam
- Rehydration with frequent small volumes of clear fluid
- If the child develops signs of increasing airways obstruction; admit to hospital immediately:
    - Severe stridor or stridor at rest
    - Evidence of respiratory distress:
        - A steadily increasing respiratory rate
        - Intercostal recession
        - Exhaustion
        - Cyanosis
    - Increasing pulse rate
- Administer high flow oxygen via a high concentration oxygen mask
- In persistent or severe croup consider:
    - Nebulised:
        - Budesonide (*Pulmicort®*): 2 mg as a single dose (*or* two 1 mg doses separated by 30 minutes)
        - Epinephrine: 3-5 mL of 1:1000, repeated after 30 minutes (stop if the pulse rate >120 bpm)
    - Oral dexamethasone (0.15 mg/kg)
    - Cricothyrotomy, if total airway obstruction appears imminent or the child becomes unconscious

Angio-oedema

Incidence
- This a relatively uncommon problem, which can present as an acute medical emergency

Aetiology
- Occurs in individuals who are allergic to a variety of stimulants including:
  - Food and medication
  - Toxins, e.g. β-haemolytic streptococcal infection
- Occurs in hereditary angio-oedema (HANE), due to a deficiency of complement C-1 enterase inhibitor

Pathophysiology
- Localised allergic type I reaction affecting parts of the face and upper airway, with severe oedema and swelling, which may result in upper airway obstruction

Symptoms/signs
- There is usually a personal or family history of allergy/atopy and sometimes of previous attacks
- There may be swelling of the face, lips, tongue and sometimes the tissues surrounding the airway

Management
- If any airway obstruction is present or looks as if it might develop:
  - Treat as anaphylactic shock, administer:
    - Epinephrine *(treatment of choice)*:
      - 0.5-1.0 mL of 1:1000 administered subcutaneously or intravenously slowly over 5 minutes if they have collapsed
    - Antihistamines:
      - Chlorpheniramine *(Piriton®)*: 2-5 mg administered intravenously
    - Steroids:
      - Prednisolone 30-60 mg orally
      - Hydrocortisone: 100-200 mg administered intravenously
  - Consider tracheal intubation/cricothyrotomy
- Patients with hereditary angio-oedema, may carry a solution of the missing complement for immediate injection during an attack and those with known angio-oedema may carry epinephrine for self-injection

Differential diagnosis for a child with acute cough, dyspnoea and stridor

Common
- Croup (viral laryngotracheobronchitis)
- Asthma: expiratory stridor/wheeze

Less common
- Recurrent or spasmodic croup

Rare
- Bacterial laryngotracheobronchitis: LTB
- Acute epiglottitis
- Inhalation of foreign body: sudden onset coughing/choking, followed by cough and stridor

Very rarely
- Angio-oedema/anaphylaxis
- Retropharyngeal abscess
- Dihptheria
- Steam inhalation burn

Figure 9-3 Differential diagnosis for a child with acute cough, dyspnoea and stridor

Diabetic emergencies
- Diabetic comas are a very serious complication of diabetes, with a high mortality if not managed correctly

Hypoglycaemic coma
- Mortality rate for severe hypoglycaemic coma is 2-4%
- Rapid effective management is necessary to prevent permanent cerebral damage

Incidence
- This is a relatively common occurrence in type I diabetic patients, especially those whose diabetic control is difficult, including the newly diagnosed, the young, the alone, the long term and the elderly:
  - Severe hypoglycaemia affects about 20-30% of patients annually with an incidence of 1.1-1.6 episodes per patient per year
- Only rarely occurs in type II diabetics (tends to be at night due to long acting sulphonylureas)

Aetiology
- A fall in blood glucose levels below the normal physiological range caused by:
  - Accidental or deliberate administration of excess insulin
  - Excessive exercise resulting in rapid glucose metabolism, without extra carbohydrate intake
  - Starving, i.e. missing carbohydrate intake, whilst still using insulin/hypoglycaemics
  - Ingestion of too high a dose of oral hypoglycaemics, especially sulphonylureas (longer acting ones may cause prolonged/severe attacks, resulting in permanent neurological damage)
  - Natural over production of insulin, e.g. the rare insulin secreting tumour of islets of Langerhans
- Hypoglycaemia may be precipitated by prior alcohol consumption
- Hypoglycaemia may be caused by renal or hepatic disease
- Drug interactions:
  - The hypoglycaemic effects of sulphonylureas may be potentiated by: salicylates, warfarin, MAO inhibitors, fibrates, alcohol, NSAIDs, antibiotics, phenothiazines, miconazole, H_2 antagonists and sulphinpyrazone

Pathophysiology
- Blood glucose levels below the patient's normal range may result in:
  - Compensatory sympathetic overactivity (may be masked in those taking β-blockers)
  - Continued hypoglycaemia resulting in altered cerebral function, and eventually permanent damage

Symptoms/signs
- These may develop very quickly with little or no warning, especially in Type I diabetic patients who may lose those warning signs of hypoglycaemia which are due to sympathetic overactivity
- Diabetics particularly at risk because they may also lose their warning signs include:
  - Well controlled diabetic patients, who have been managed with insulin for a long time (>15 years)
  - The elderly
  - Those diabetic patients who have developed an autonomic neuropathy
  - Those who have developed tolerance due to to repeated hypoglycaemic attacks
  - Those taking β-blockers, clonidine, reserpine and guanethidine

Initially
- Shaky, trembling, perioral paraesthesiae, sweaty with
- Headache, emptiness, hunger and palpitations

Later
- Double vision, poor concentration, slurred speech with confusion, drowsiness, irritability, aggression
- Appearance of intoxication, and sometimes hypothermia

Finally
- May become unconscious, unrousable and lapse into fits, coma, and death

Investigation
- Blood sugar level testing with test strips and blood glucose testing meter to confirm low blood sugar

Management
- If the patient is *conscious*, administer:
    - Glucose: 10-20 gm orally in a solution, e.g. *Lucozade® or*
    - Carbohydrate in a readily absorbable form, e.g. glucose tablets

Glucose gel (*Hypostop®*) a convenient glucose preparation carried by many diabetics:
- This is a glucose gel, which can be squeezed from the container onto the gums or the space inside the cheek and massaged in. Honey or non-diabetic jam are alternatives

- If the patient is *unconscious,* provide care of the airway, administer oxygen and:

Glucose (*treatment of first choice, because of its rapid effect*)
Presentation
- 50% glucose; 25, 50 mL ampoules or IMS system

Dosage
- Adults: 50 mL   Children: 0.5-1.0 mg

Administration
- By careful intravenous injection (may cause thrombophlebitis or localised tissue necrosis if extravasation occurs)
- If intravenous access is difficult because of fitting, restlessness, aggressive behaviour or peripheral venous shutdown, administer:

Glucagon
Action
- Increases plasma glucose levels by mobilising glucose (stored as glycogen in the liver)
- Repeated administration will result in exhaustion of these (glycogen) stores in about 45 minutes

Presentation
- 1,2 mg vial with diluent

Dosage
- 0.5-1 mg (acts more slowly than dextrose)
- May be repeated after 10 minutes

Administration
- 1 mg/mL administered intramuscularly, intravenously or subcutaneously (particularly useful if the patient's veins are difficult to inject or the patient is restless)
- If the patient fails to respond after 15-20 minutes, administer glucose

Side effects
- May cause nausea (may make it difficult to persuade the patient to eat), vomiting and headache

- Blood sugar levels should be monitored during and after treatment
- Feed the patient after apparent recovery (especially after glucagon administration)
- If the patient has been unconscious for some time, the response to treatment may be slow (probably due to cerebral oedema or brain damage)
- *Always* admit to hospital if hypoglycaemia is due to oral hypoglycaemics, alcohol, over-administration of a long-acting insulin, after deliberate overdosage, if rapid recovery does not occur, or if unsupervised

Note: In hypoglycaemia due to sulphonylureas:
- Coma may be prolonged and is likely to reoccur after treatment, so a glucose infusion is advisable.
- Glucagon treatment may be contraindicated as it can stimulate insulin secretion in those non-insulin dependent diabetics with some residual B-cell function

Hyperglycaemia
- Mortality rate is 5-10%: due to cerebral oedema and irreversible brain damage (risk increases with age)
- Diabetic ketoacidosis (DKA) is the commonest cause of death in diabetics aged less than 40 years

Incidence
- Diabetic ketoacidosis (DKA):
  - Occurs in Type I diabetic patients, more commonly in women than men
  - Occurs about once per 100 diabetic patients per year (recurrence rate is 10%)
- Hyperosmolar non-ketotic coma (HONK):
  - Occurs in Type II diabetic patients
  - Less common than DKA
  - Has a higher mortality rate due to greater age of patients and presence of severe concurrent disease

Aetiology
- May be the presenting feature of diabetes mellitus (insidious onset)
- Reduction in, failure to increase or accidental omission of insulin dose (often associated with problems with personality, or compliance, or to have social or psychiatric problems)
- May be precipitated by stress or concurrent illness (commonest cause):
  - Upper and lower (65% of cases) respiratory tract infection
  - Skin abscess
  - Urinary tract infection
  - Mental stress
  - Menstruation
  - (Cerebrovascular accident)
  - Trauma

Pathophysiology
- Hyperglycaemia may be ketoacidotic (DKA) or hyperosmolar non ketoacidotic (HONK)

Ketoacidotic hyperglycaemia (DKA):
- Occurs in Type I diabetic patients in whom there is an absolute deficiency of insulin
- Insulin is necessary for glucose to be transported from the blood into cells.
- The absence of insulin therefore results in:
  - An increase in blood glucose (as absorption of glucose from the gut is not affected)
  - The absence of cellular glucose results in:
    - A failure of the sodium and potassium pumps resulting in a raised serum potassium
    - Potassium is preferentially excreted by the kidneys to preserve sodium, resulting in potassium loss and a low cellular potassium, which may precipitate cardiac arrhythmias and death
    - The metabolism of fats and protein, which is much less efficient than glucose metabolism results in the production of ketone bodies which cause a metabolic acidosis and compensatory hyperventilation, causing further fluid loss
- As a result:
  - Blood glucose and serum potassium levels increase and the pH falls
  - There is an overall deficiency of insulin, sodium, potassium, chloride and water
  - The patient becomes dehydrated, although the serum osmolarity is often normal

Hyperosmolar non ketoacidotic hyperglycaemia (HONK):
- Occurs in Type II diabetic patients, in whom there is a relative deficiency of insulin (insulin resistance), but there is enough intracellular activity to avoid ketoacidosis
- This may result (compared to DKA) in a more marked hyperglycaemia and extracellular increase in osmolarity and cellular dehydration. There may be a minor degree of ketoacidosis (small amounts of ketones may be produced in starvation)

Symptoms/signs
- The gradual onset of polydypsia, polyuria, malaise, thirst, and weight loss
- Often associated with infection, nausea and vomiting (and a failure to increase the dosage of hypoglycaemic agents in known diabetics)
- Ketoacidosis: smell of acetone on breath (DKA only, unless the patient has starved)
- Warm, dry skin and mucous membranes
- Hyperventilation, or deep sighing "Kussmaul" respiration (DKA)
- Dehydration and salt depletion: rapid, weak and irregular pulse, and hypotension
- Constipation, abdominal pain/cramps (often severe enough to mimic an acute abdomen) and diplopia

Diagnosis
Urine: Glycosuria, ketonuria (not usually in HONK)
Blood sugar: Levels raised on testing with blood glucose testing meter and test strips:
- Patients with HONK may have blood glucose levels up to 60 mmol/litre and above
- Patients with DKA usually have blood glucose levels of at least 30 mmol/litre

Management
Airway
- Intubation and gastric emptying may be indicated to protect the airway in the unconscious patient, as vomiting is a common complication and cause of death

Breathing
- Ventilation
- Hypoxia:
  - All unconscious patients may suffer from hypoxia, and should therefore be given oxygen

Circulation
- Dehydration:
  - If transfer to hospital is delayed or likely to take several hours, an intravenous infusion of normal saline should be administered, rather than a buffered solution, e.g. Hartmann's solution, which may precipitate catastrophic falls in serum potassium
  - Infuse 1 litre of fluid over the first hour, followed by a further 1 litre administered over 2 hours and a further 2 litres each administered over 4 hours (over-infusion may precipitate cerebral oedema)
  - This should be reduced in the young, the elderly, or if there is renal or cardiac impairment

Hyperglycaemia
- Although insulin is needed, administration is not appropriate in the Immediate Care situation

Infection
- Consider administration of broad spectrum antibiotics if a precipitating infection is suspected and evacuation to hospital is delayed

Evacuation
- The patient should be transferred to hospital without delay

Epilepsy

Incidence
- This is a relatively common cause of collapse, and is one of the situations with which all those involved in Immediate Care should be familiar
- The overall mortality for people with epilepsy is 2-3 times that of the general population and is even higher in the younger age groups
- Common causes of death in epileptics include:
    - Accidents, e.g. drowning, head injury, and road traffic accidents
    - Status epilepticus
    - Neoplasia
    - Cerebrovascular disease
    - Chest infections
    - Sudden unexpected death

Aetiology
- The likely cause of fitting varies according to age:
    - *All ages*
        - Infection:
            - Meningitis
            - Encephalitis
        - Trauma
        - Congenital cerebral lesions
    - *Neonatal*
        - Birth trauma
        - Metabolic:
            - Hypoglycaemia
            - Hypocalcaemia
        - Congenital cerebral lesions
    - *6 months to 5 years*
        - Febrile convulsions
    - *Young adult*
        - Alcoholism
        - Drug abuse
        - Cerebral tumour
    - *Elderly*
        - Cerebrovascular disease
        - Cerebral tumour
        - Subdural haematoma

Generalised seizures

Aetiology
- Usually, but not always occurs in known epileptics.
- May be precipitated by:
    - Illness
    - Stress
    - Poor management of medication: deliberate or accidental
    - Reduced efficacy of medication; due to altered hepatic metabolism, e.g. as a result of:
        - Other drugs
        - Alcohol
        - Hepatic disease

Pathophysiology
- A spontaneous cortical discharge which may be generalised or localised
- The focal point may be scar tissue, tumour, etc.

Symptoms/signs
- Previous history of epilepsy
- May be preceded by aura/visual disturbance
- Sudden collapse with generalised or localised (focal Jacksonian) tonic and/or clonic fitting
- May bite tongue, and/or be incontinent of urine and/or stools
- After fitting may be drowsy and disorientated, complaining of a headache and will usually go to sleep

Differential diagnosis
- Hypoglycaemia: Check the blood sugar level testing with test strips and blood glucose testing meter
- Poisoning
- Tetany with carpopedal spasm
- Head injury:
    - Always examine the head carefully, as head injury may be either the cause of fitting or occur as a result of fitting
- Hysteria
- Cerebral space occupying lesion:
    - Tumour
    - Cerebral abscess
- Collapse:
    - Think of all possibilities

Management
- Most fits are self limiting and do not require medical treatment

Safety
- Move the patient away from hard objects and other hazards, e.g. fires
- Loosen the patient's clothing

Airway
- Make sure that the airway is not obstructed by false teeth, etc.
- There is very little danger of the tongue causing airway obstruction, and attempts to prevent this or tongue biting, often only damage the patient's teeth

Prolonged convulsions
- Administer diazepam *(Valium®, Diazemuls®, Stesolid®)*, midazolam *(Hypnovel®)* or clobazam *(Rivotril®)* by:
    - Slow intravenous injection
    - Rectally *(Stesolid®)*: this is the route of choice in children
- Titrate the dose against ptosis, and beware of apnoea, which may be delayed

Clobazam *(Rivotril®)*
- May be used as an alternative to diazepam, and is apparently equally effective, but there has been little experience in its use in Immediate Care

Presentation
- 1 mg in solvent/1 mL diluent ampoules

Administration
- By slow intravenous injection

Dosage
- Children: 0.5 mg
- Adults: 1 mg

- If fitting continues; sedate heavily and be prepared to intubate and ventilate
- After fitting has ceased, put the patient into a safe position:
    - The recovery position
    - In small children, across their mother's knees

Generalised convulsive status epilepticus (GCSE)

Definition: Prolonged fitting lasting more than 10 minutes, or consisting of two or more distinct concurrent episodes of fitting without regaining consciousness

Introduction
- This is a life threatening condition; the longer fitting continues, the more difficult it is to control, and the higher the morbidity and mortality
- The mortality in patients admitted to an intensive care unit with GCSE is 5-10%

Aetiology
Known epileptic (occurs in those with any type of epilepsy, but more often with frontal lobe abnormalities)
- Poor anti-convulsant compliance
- Recent change in medication
- Alcohol withdrawal/pseudostatus
- Intercurrent illness or fever

New presentation (60%)
- Acute cerebrovascular accident (commonest cause in the elderly)
- Acute head injury (commonest cause in adolescents and young adults)
- Meningo encephalitis and fever (commonest cause in young children)
- Cerebral neoplasm
- Metabolic disorders:
    - Renal failure, hypoglycaemia, hypercalcaemia
- Drug overdose:
    - Tricyclics, phenothiazines, theophylline
- Inflammatory arteritides:
    - Systemic lupus erythematosus

Pathophysiology
- Tonic/clonic status.
- Permanent neuronal damage may occur if fitting is very prolonged
- Complications depend on the underlying aetiology and include; death, permanent neurological deficit and the subsequent development of chronic epilepsy

Symptoms/signs
- These may vary from repeated clonic seizures to subtle convulsive movements and coma

Management
Airway care
- Airway maintenance and the administration of oxygen

Breathing
- Intubate and ventilate if there is evidence of respiratory impairment (reduced SpO_2), after appropriate sedation, but do not attempt this while the jaw is still clenched

Fitting
- Control fitting with diazepam (*Stesolid*® or *Diazemuls*®), which may be repeated if necessary

Note: Check the blood sugar if the patient is unknown, and administer 50% glucose if appropriate

Febrile convulsions/fits

Definition: A convulsion or fit occurring in a child aged from 6 months to 5 years, precipitated by fever arising outside the nervous system in a child who is otherwise neurologically normal

Incidence
- In the United kingdom, over 3% of all children will have at least one febrile convulsion without evidence of intracranial infection or defined cause (other than infection outside the central nervous system), and of these, just over one third will have one further convulsion
- Febrile convulsions are the most common cause of fitting in children. The parents usually think that the child is dying
- Age: usually 6 months to 5 years. The patient can be older, but there is nearly always a previous history

Aetiology
- Cause of pyrexia:
    - Usually a virus infection
- Family history:
    - There is sometimes a family history of febrile convulsions

Pathophysiology
- This is not fully understood as the fits are not clearly associated with either the level or the duration of the pyrexia, but may be associated with a rapid rise in temperature. The immature brain responds with a generalised cortical discharge
- With increasing age, this tendency is outgrown, although some children take longer than others.
- Very few (2.4% of those previously normal) go on to develop epilepsy

Symptoms/signs
- Prior to a fit the child may appear jittery
- Tonic-clonic type of fitting, usually lasting <20 minutes, with complete recovery within 1 hour
- The tonic phase may be characterised by a frightened cry followed by abrupt loss of consciousness with muscular rigidity. During this phase, which may last up to 30 seconds, breathing may cease and the child be incontinent of urine and faeces
- The clonic phase which follows consists of repetitive jerking movements of the limbs or face

Management
- *Aim:* to prevent a prolonged fit (lasting more than 15 minutes), which may result in permanent brain damage, epilepsy, and developmental delay

Airway
- Make sure that the child has a clear airway, by lying them on their side or prone with their head on one side, so as to avoid aspiration following vomiting

Cooling
- Remove clothing, put in cool room with window open, but do not allow to shiver.
- Consider:
    - Tepid sponging
    - Putting in a cool, but not cold, bath (but not if they are still fitting)
- If appropriate administer copious clear oral fluids
- Administer oral or rectal (if still fitting) paracetamol elixir in the maximum recommended dose for the child's age

Convulsions
- Rectal diazepam (*Stesolid®*) 1 mg + 1 mg for each year of age

Admit to hospital if:
- First febrile convulsion/fit in a child
- Child under 6 months old
- Prolonged fitting (>15 minutes)
- Focal fit
- Repeated fits in same episode of an illness
- Incomplete recovery (residual impaired consciousness) one hour after the onset of fitting
- Any evidence suggestive of meningitis
- Suspicion of non accidental injury

Breath holding

- Benign apnoeic attacks in toddlers

Incidence
- Usually begins at 9-18 months, ceases by 5 years

Aetiology
- Usually after a painful or frustrating experience

Pathophysiology
- The infant cries vigorously, and suddenly holds his breath
- He may then become cyanosed, and in severe cases lose consciousness
- The limbs may become rigid (rarely), with a few clonic movements, lasting a few seconds
- The infant then begins breathing and regains consciousness

Management
- Exclude other conditions
- Reassure the mother

Differential diagnosis of fitting in a child

Febrile convulsions/fits

Meningitis/encephalitis

Hypoglycaemia
- Test blood with Dextrostix/BM stix.

Breath holding

Septicaemia

Figure 9-4 Differential diagnosis of fitting in a child

Meningitis

Bacterial meningitis

- Bacterial meningitis is a significant cause of morbidity and mortality in children and young adults, and is an example of a potentially life threatening illness, where early diagnosis and rapid effective management can make a major difference to outcome
- Bacterial meningitis still tends to be under-diagnosed and under-treated in the community

Incidence
- In the UK, bacterial meningitis is more prevalent in the winter between October and March
- All age groups may be affected, but the highest incidence occurs in children aged between one and five and in late adolescence. Children under one year old are the most susceptible and have the highest mortality rate (30% in neonates). Many survivors are left with mental or physical handicap
- Bacterial meningitis is more common among poor families, who live in over-crowded conditions
- The incidence of meningitis caused by *Haemophilus influenzae* type b in the UK has declined dramatically since the introduction of an effective immunisation campaign
- The incidence of meningococcal infection has increased over the last 5 years with nearly 2,500 notified cases each year in the UK, including over 900 with meningitis, 450 with septicaemia, and 250 deaths)

Aetiology
- Bacterial meningitis is commonly caused by:
    - *Neisseria meningitidis*: meningococcus (accounting for 70% of bacterial meningitis in the UK):
        - The many different strains of this gram-negative diplococcus are divided into serogroups:
            - Type B, accounting for up to 70% of meningococcal infections in the UK
            - Type C, accounting for 25-30% of meningococcal infections in the UK, and is increasing
            - Types A or C in tropical Africa and South America, Saudi Arabia and India
        - Person to person transmission occurs by droplet spread as a result of prolonged close contact
        - Only a very small percentage of people carrying the organism actually become ill, the illness usually develops in these susceptible individuals within seven days of acquiring the organism
        - Meningococcal infection may result in:
            - Meningitis alone: 15% ; mortality 5%
            - Septicaemia alone: 25%; mortality 30-60% (when recognition/management is delayed)
            - Mixed meningitis and septicaemia: 60%
    - *Streptococcus pneumoniae* (accounting for 25% of bacterial meningitis infections in the UK)
    - *Haemophilus influenzae* (type b used to be the most common infecting organism in the UK in pre-school children, until the current immunisation campaign, but is now rare)
- Rarely caused by:
    - *Eschericia coli*
    - Streptococci Group B, *Listeria monocytogenes* (neonates, pregnant, elderly, immunocompromised)
    - *Mycobacterium tuberculosis* or Leptospira

Pathophysiology
- Bacterial cell wall material induces the release of cytokines (low molecular weight proteins which act locally as chemical messengers), by host cells
- These cytokines initiate meningeal inflammation and brain swelling
- Complications of bacterial meningitis:
    - Cochlear damage (10% of survivors), which occurs very early in the illness
    - Sensineural deafness
    - Epilepsy (7% of survivors), which is often complex and difficult to manage
    - Behavioural and learning difficulties
    - Neurological deficits and hydrocephalus

- Mortality rates:
    - Meningococcal meningitis: 10% overall
    - *Haemophilus influenzae* meningitis: 5%
    - Pneumococcal meningitis: 20-35%

Symptoms/signs
- Bacterial meningitis alone is often difficult to diagnose with any certainty in the pre-hospital situation.
- Symptoms and signs may appear very suddenly, with rapid deterioration in the patient's condition
- Only a small number of patients exhibit the typical features of bacterial meningitis, which tend to vary depending on the causative organism.
- In the early stages of the illness, there are *no* features which can distinguish reliably between bacterial and viral meningitis
- Signs of focal cerebral disease are more common in pneumococcal and influenzal meningitis and carries a relatively poor prognosis

Infants:
- Non specific:
    - Floppiness, drowsiness, irritability, distress on being handled
    - Off feeds, vomiting and/or diarrhoea
    - Pyrexia, non responsive to paracetamol
- More specific:
    - Neck stiffness/rigidity with positive Kernig's sign and Brudzinski's signs (often absent in the very young)
    - Tense or bulging fontanelles
    - In meningococcal septicaemia only, a purpuric/petechial rash that does not blanch under pressure (a positive 'Tumbler test'); which may be localised initially, but later can become generalised
    - Febrile convulsions (most frequently occurs in *H. influenzae* meningitis)
- Late:
    - High pitched or moaning cry
    - Deafness
    - Coma
    - Neck retraction
    - Shock
    - Widespread purpuric/haemorrhagic rash with a positive 'Tumbler test' (meningococcal septicaemia)

Older children/adults:
- Non specific:
    - Pyrexia with headache, vomiting
    - Back or joint aches/pains
- More specific:
    - Neck stiffness/rigidity with evidence of meningeal irritation (may be absent in the very old or severely obtunded):
    - Positive Kernig's and Brudzinski's signs (in children this is the inability of a child sitting with their knees drawn up, to touch their knees with their nose).
    - Photophobia
    - Confusion
    - Purpuric/petechial rash that does not blanch under pressure (meningococcal septicaemia only)
- Late:
    - Coma and shock
    - Widespread haemorrhagic rash with a positive 'Tumbler test' (meningococcal septicaemia only)

Note: **Tumbler test:**
- If a tumbler is pressed firmly against a septicaemic rash; the rash will not fade, but will remain visible through the glass

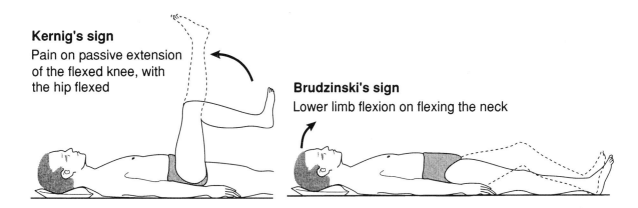

Kernig's sign
Pain on passive extension
of the flexed knee, with
the hip flexed

Brudzinski's sign
Lower limb flexion on flexing the neck

Figure 9-5 Signs of meningeal irritation/inflammation

Discussion point: management of meningitis

Concerns
- In the management of meningitis:
    - Pre-hospital antibiotic administration may interfere with or prevent identification of the
      causative organism, making later treatment more difficult
    - The early administration of steroids (dexamethasone) may block cytokine release and can be
      more beneficial than antibiotics in the management of meningitis alone
    - There is a theoretical risk, that in meningococcal infection, antibiotic administration will result
      in massive endotoxin release and the development of overwhelming and fatal toxic shock

Evidence
- The early administration of dexamethasone (before the administration of intravenous penicillin) has
  been shown to reduce meningeal and cerebral inflammation and brain swelling, and the incidence of
  neurological and audiological sequelae in bacterial meningitis as a whole, and specifically for
  Haemophilus influenzae meningitis
- The early administration of dexamethasone has shown *no* benefit in meningococcal septicaemia, and
  in fact may make matters worse
- The principal cause of death in meningococcal disease is meningococcal septicaemia (septic shock);
  patients with meningococcal meningitis without septicaemia have a much better prognosis
- Early high dose penicillin has been shown to reduce the mortality rate in meningococcal disease
  by up to 50%

Conclusion
- The distinction must be made between patients with meningitis alone, those with meningitis and
  signs of septicaemia, and those with septicaemia and no meningitis:
    - If treatment is delayed for any reason, the patient should *always* be accompanied to hospital
    - If a rash develops, penicillin (or an alternative) should be administered intravenously
      immediately
    - For patients with definite meningitis, but no evidence of a rash, consideration may be given to
      administering dexamethasone after the immediate administration of intravenous penicillin, if
      evacuation to hospital is likely to take a long time, e.g. in remote areas

Management
- Administer high flow oxygen using a high concentration oxygen mask
- If the patient is unconscious; intubate and ventilate them
- Obtain intravenous/intraosseous access and if unconscious, have a raised respiratory rate or are shocked:
  - Start an intravenous infusion of colloid
- Administer *intravenous* antibiotics *immediately*:
  Benzyl penicillin (penicillin G) immediately by slow intravenous injection

  Presentation
  - 600 mg powder for reconstitution
  Dosage
  - Infants under 1 year: 300 mg
  - Children 1-9 years old: 600 mg
  - Adults/children 10 years old and over: 1200 mg

- If there is a history of *penicillin anaphylaxis* (rare in children), administer intravenous:
  Chloramphenicol

  Presentation
  - 300 mg, 1.2 g (*Chloromycetin®*), 1 g (*Kemicetine®*) vials of powder for reconstitution
  Dosage

- 25 mg/kg :	- Infants	<3 months	(approximately 5 kg)	125 mg
		3 months-1year	(approximately 10 kg)	250 mg
	- Children	1-5 years	(up to 15 kg)	500 mg
		5-10 years	(up to 30 kg)	750 mg
		10-15 years	(up to 55 kg)	1000 mg

- Alternatively, especially if there is a history of *penicillin allergy*, administer intravenous
  Cefotaxime (*Claforan®*)

  Presentation
  - 500 mg, 1, 2 g vials of powder for reconstitution
  Dosage
  - Neonates: 100-125 mg initially, up to 500 mg in severe cases
  - Children: 750 mg initially, up to 1 g in severe infections
  - Adults: 1 g initially in moderate infection, increasing up to 2 g in severe infections

Note: About 10% of patients who are allergic to penicillins are also allergic to cephalosporins

- If there is definite meningitis and no rash, and transportation to hospital is going to take a long time, consider the prior administration of:
  Dexamethasone (as the phosphate ester)

  Presentation
  - 1 mL ampoule, 2 mL vial of dexamethasone phosphate 4.8 mg/mL (*Dexamethasone®*)
  - 2 mL vial of dexamethasone phosphate 4 mg/mL (*Decadron®*)
  - 5 mL vial of dexamethasone 20 mg/mL (*Decadron Shock-Pak®*)
  Dosage
  - Children: 0.4 mg/kg
  - Adults: 10 mg initially

- Admit *immediately* (always accompany the sick child to hospital, as very rapid deterioration may occur)

Meningococcal septicaemia

Incidence
- Occurs less commonly than meningococcal meningitis, but is associated with a much greater mortality, with death sometimes occurring within a few hours of the first symptom

Aetiology
- As meningococcal meningitis

Pathophysiology
- The pathophysiology is very complex and is not fully understood
- Meningococci and their products including endotoxin, trigger an intense host inflammatory response
- Macrophage, neutrophil and platelet activation occur, together with the activation of the coagulation cascade resulting in:
    - Severe capillary leak with loss of albumin and other proteins from the intravascular compartment, causing hypovolaemia, a reduction in the venous return and pulmonary oedema
    - Dysregulation of vascular tone with an initial intense vasoconstriction, followed later by vasodilation, a wide pulse pressure, hypotension and progressive acidosis
    - Intravascular thrombosis
    - Myocardial depression
- All this results in cardiorespiratory failure, with multiorgan failure, disseminated intravascular coagulation and a complex metabolic disorder with acidosis and electrolyte imbalance

Symptoms/signs
- *Early*
    - Nausea and vomiting with abdominal pain and a headache
    - Myalgia with shivering and rigors
    - Pyrexia with toxic appearance
    - Tachycardia
- *Later*
    - Circulatory failure and shock with:
        - Cold peripheries
        - Delayed capillary refill and an increasing tachycardia
        - Tachypnoea
        - Altered mental status with confusion and drowsiness
        - Hypotension (a pre-terminal sign in children)
    - Rapidly progressive purpuric rash (may appear early, and sometimes is the first sign of infection)
- A particularly poor prognosis is indicated by:
    - Petechiae evolving into echymoses in less than 12 hours
    - Evidence of shock (delayed capillary refill and low systolic blood pressure)
    - *Absence of meningitis*
    - High core temperature (>40°C)
    - Stupor or coma

Management
- Meningococcal septicaemia may be very rapidly fatal and is one of the *most acute medical emergencies*
- Administer high flow oxygen using a high concentration oxygen mask
- Intubate and ventilate if there is any respiratory distress or the patient becomes unconscious
- Establish an intravenous infusion with colloid (via the intraosseous route in young children and babies)
- Administer high dose intravenous/intraosseous antibiotics: penicillin, chloramphenicol, cefotaxime
- Monitor carefully for any evidence of developing shock, and infuse aggressively if indicated
- *Always* accompany to hospital

Prophylaxis of meningococcal infection

- Prophylaxis is indicated for everyone who has had intimate (kissing) contact with someone with meningococcal infection in the preceding 10 days (household contacts of those with meningococcal disease are 1,000 times more likely to develop the disease than the general population; this is greatest immediately after the initial case, and persists for up to a year), and should be administered within 24 hrs of the first diagnosis
- If resuscitation of the patient has been necessary, this may include medical, ambulance and nursing staff
- Prophylaxis may reduce the risk of secondary cases, but there is still a 1% chance of infection in the household of a patient with meningococcal disease

Ciprofloxacin (*Ciproxin®*)
- Preferred prophylaxis
Presentation:
- 250 mg tablets
Dosage:
- Adults: 500 mg as a single dose

Rifampicin (*Rifadin®/Rimactane®*)
- May also be given to close contacts of patients with *Haemophilus influenzae* type b infection (Hib)
Presentation:
- 150, 300 mg tabs, 100 mg/mL syrup
Dosage (ideally one hour before meals):
- Infants (3 months-1 year): 5 mg/kg every 12 hours for 2 days
- Children: 10 mg/kg every 12 hours for 2 days (20 mg/kg once daily for Hib prophylaxis)
- Adults: 600 mg every 12 hours for 2 days (600 mg once a day for 4 days for Hib prophylaxis)

Ceftriaxone (*Rocephin®*)
- Antibiotic of choice for the pregnant patient, and for children who refuse oral medication
Presentation:
- 250 mg vial of powder for reconstitution
Dosage:
- Adults: 250 mg as a single dose
- Children under 12 years: 125 mg
Administration:
- Intramuscularly (may be painful due to the large volume)

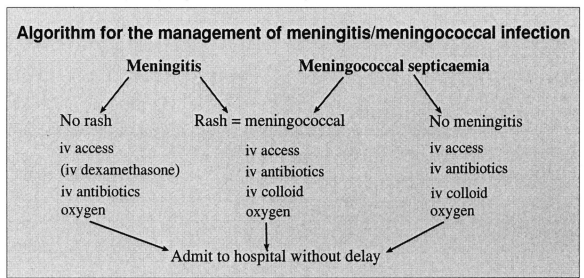

Figure 9-6 Algorithm for the management on meningococcal infection

Viral meningitis

Incidence
- More common than bacterial meningitis
- Maximum incidence is in children < 5 years (except mumps meningitis)
- "Meningism" is common in many acute viral infections, e.g. influenza

Aetiology
- May be caused by the following viruses:
    - Enteroviruses:
        - Echo
        - Coxsackie
    - Mumps (rare in the UK since the introduction of MMR - Mumps, Measles and Rubella vaccination)
    - Poliomyelitis (very rare)
    - Herpes simplex (very rare)

Symptoms/signs
- Usually slower onset than bacterial meningitis (prodromal period is 3-4 days)
- The patient is not so ill
- There is no rash
- Consciousness is not usually impaired

Management
- Admit to hospital for confirmation of diagnosis
- Symptomatic relief of symptoms

Rectal bleeding

Incidence
- Nearly always only found in the elderly

Aetiology
- Bleeding from colonic diverticulae is usually the cause
- Haemorrhage may also (rarely) be from carcinoma or polyps of the rectum/sigmoid colon

Symptoms/signs
- There may be profuse fresh blood loss

Management
- Treatment of hypovolaemic shock:
    - High flow oxygen via a high concentration mask
    - Intravenous fluid replacement with colloid/crystalloid via wide bore cannulae (14 gauge)
    - Monitor the patient's haemodynamic state continuously

Haematemesis

Incidence
- Usually occurs in the over sixties, and increases with increasing age
- Mortality is >10%, and increases rapidly with increasing age
- Is an important cause of emergency admission to hospital

Aetiology
- Commonly occurs as a result of:
    - Peptic ulceration
    - Erosive gastritis
    - Mallory Weiss tears
- Less commonly:
    - Gastric or oesophageal carcinoma
    - Oesophageal varices
    - Oesophageal ulceration, oesophagitis
    - Cardiovascular malformation
    - Bleeding dyscrasias
    - Systemic disease: renal failure, connective tissue disease
    - Rupture of the aorta or other artery into the gastrointestinal tract

Symptoms/signs
- *History*
    - Alcohol abuse
    - Melaena stools
- *Forceful vomiting:*
    - With history of alcohol abuse in males: Mallory Weiss tears
    - Other causes of protracted vomiting:
        - Migraine
        - Alcoholic gastritis
        - Medication, e.g. NSAIDs
        - Intestinal obstruction
- *Hypovolaemic shock:*
    - Pale, sweaty
    - Rapid, weak, irregular pulse, hypotension
- *Liver disease:*
    - Liver palms, spider naevi, jaundice
    - Blood vessel malformation in skin and mucosa
- *Anaemia:*
    - Skin pallor with pale sclera
- *Malignancy:*
    - Emaciated, cachectic

Management
- Administer high flow oxygen via a high concentration mask
- If the patient has lost a significant amount of blood set up two intravenous lines with large bore cannulae
    - If the patient is shocked, administer:
        - Colloid followed by crystalloid
    - If the patient is not shocked, administer:
        - Crystalloid slowly
- If the patient has only lost a little blood, set up one intravenous infusion of crystalloid and infuse slowly
- Observe the patient for any further blood loss and monitor their haemodynamic state continuously

Massive haemoptysis

Definition: The expectoration of 200-1000 mL of blood in 24 hours

- Massive haemoptysis has a high mortality rate (30-50% in hospital)

Incidence
- Relatively rare

Aetiology
- Usually occurs due to erosion of bronchial blood vessels secondary to:
    - Cavitating lung disease: tuberculosis, aspergilloma
    - Bronchiectasis (including cystic fibrosis)
    - Lung abscess
    - Neoplasia of lung, mediastinum and associated structures.
- May rarely occur secondary to severe thoracic trauma

Pathophysiology
- The usual cause of death is asphyxia as a result of aspiration, rather than hypovolaemic shock
- The greater the rate of haemorrhage, and the poorer the quality of the underlying lung, the higher the mortality:
    - In patients with poor pulmonary reserve as a result of underlying lung disease, a relatively small haemorrhage may have disproportionately severe consequences

Symptoms/signs
- The amount of obvious haemorrhage is an unreliable guide as to the severity of the problem, as a relatively small haemorrhage may cause asphyxiation
- Careful monitoring of the patient's respiratory state:
    - Respiratory rate
    - Oxygen saturation: SpO_2

Management
- *Aim:* To prevent asphyxiation and treat hypovolaemia
    - Administer high flow oxygen via a high concentration mask
    - Position:
        - If the side of the bleeding can be lateralised:
            - The patient should lie head down on the side of the haemorrhage to prevent aspiration of blood into the unaffected lung
    - Do not suppress any cough:
        - Patients should be encouraged to clear their airway with gentle coughing
    - If the patient is unconscious or in danger of asphyxiation:
        - Consider intubation
        - Ventilation
        - Suction
    - Intravenous infusion, if the patient is significantly hypotensive (slight hypotension may aid resolution)

Hyperventilation

Definition: Physiologically inappropriate over-breathing

Incidence
- Relatively common especially in the young, female and asthmatic

Aetiology
- Hysteria:
    - Mostly occurs in younger women
    - Asthmatics may feel/fear that they have an asthma attack starting, and begin to fight to breathe
- May be precipitated by:
    - Pain.
    - Metabolic acidosis (rare):
        - Diabetic ketoacidosis
        - Aspirin overdose
        - Hypoxaemia
        - Uraemia, hepatic cirrhosis/coma and Gram negative septicaemia
    - Organic central nervous system disturbance

Pathophysiology
- Anxiety and subjective dyspnoea results in hyperventilation, which in turn results in an increase in anxiety and so a vicious cycle develops
- Hyperventilation results in an increased minute volume and an acute respiratory alkalosis, with a fall in the arterial PCO_2, and elevation of PO_2 and blood pH.
- The plasma HCO_3^- is reduced by renal excretion causing hypocarbia, and tetany occurs due to a fall in the serum ionised plasma calcium levels

Symptoms/signs
- The patient will be anxious, fearful, possibly with a history of emotional problems and/or asthma
- The patient may be complaining of:
    - A strange feeling/paraesthesiae/coldness in the hands, face (especially around the mouth), and feet (this may be bilateral or unilateral)
    - Dyspnoea, palpitations, atypical chest/abdominal pains/tightness, faintness/lightheadedness or dizziness
    - Poor memory/concentration, and/or a feeling of unreality
- Tachypnoea with rapid deep sighing breathing
- Tachycardia
- Carpopedal spasm, tetany
- SpO_2 of 100% (always), and a low end-tidal CO_2 level

Management
- Massive reassurance
- Treatment of the cause (if appropriate)
- Rebreathing using a paper/plastic bag: this results in a rise in the inspired CO_2 and corrects the respiratory alkalosis
- Nitrous oxide/oxygen via an *Entonox*® or *Nitronox*® apparatus

Note: 1. Monitoring of the SpO_2 is useful, especially if the rebreathing method of treatment is used and the patient is asthmatic. The patient should rebreathe until the SpO_2 begins to fall below 100%
2. If the patient is asthmatic and has difficulty using their inhaler, several puffs of salbutamol, etc. may be squirted into the paper or plastic bag, before they start to use it for rebreathing

Sudden focal neurological deficit
- This may be transient or permanent, and may be subdivided accordingly:

Transient ischaemic attack (TIA)

Definition: This is the sudden or gradual onset of a focal neurological deficit lasting *for less than 24 hours* caused by a cerebrovascular disorder

Cerebrovascular accident (Stroke)

Definition: This is the sudden or gradual onset of a focal neurological deficit lasting *for more than 24 hours, or leading to death*, caused by a cerebrovascular disorder

Incidence
- Sudden focal neurological deficit is common in the elderly, hypertensive and diabetic
- Stroke is the third most common cause of death in the UK; and is the most common cause of disability
- Subarachnoid haemorrhage is rare; affecting 10-15 in 100,000 people including the young and fit. It is associated with a mortality of 40-60% from the initial haemorrhage, and a high morbidity

Aetiology
- Sudden onset of localised brain damage caused by:
    - Cerebral infarction (90%) caused by:
        - Cerebral thrombosis from:
            - Arterial atherosclerosis
            - Temporal arteritis (rare)
        - Arterial embolism from:
            - Atrial fibrillation
            - Mitral stenosis
            - Post myocardial infarction (mural thrombus)
    - Cerebral haemorrhage (10%) caused by:
        - Intracerebral haemorrhage secondary to:
            - Hypertension (commonest)
            - Intracranial tumour
            - Bleeding disorders, including anticoagulation
        - Subarachnoid haemorrhage due to ruptured berry aneurism or arteriovenous malformation

Pathophysiology
- Cerebral infarction:
    - This occurs as a result of complete or partial blockage of part of the arterial blood supply to a part of the brain; the mechanism is similar to that of acute myocardial infarction
    - Large aterial emboli usually cause sudden and complete blockage of relatively large vessels, whereas small emboli (microemboli) may only cause a small and sometimes temporary blockage
    - Complete blockage results in brain cell ischaemia and death (infarction) within a few minutes
    - Cerebral thrombosis usually results initially in partial blockage, but this may then spread backwards and the size of the neurological deficit increase
    - The brain usually has a good collateral blood supply and after the intial blockage adjacent blood vessels may open up and the eventual amount of brain damage may be fairly small
- Cerebral haemorrhage:
    - The side wall of an artery bursts and aterial blood rushes out causing a local increase in pressure resulting in local brain cell injury and death
- Brain cell injury and death results in local brain swelling, causing an increase in intracranial pressure (ICP), and a rise in blood pressure and a slowing of the pulse rate

Symptoms/signs
- These may vary depending on the aetiology and underlying pathophysiology, but it is usually not possible to distinguish between them clinically (except possibly subarachnoid haemorrhage)

Cerebral thrombosis
- This is often preceded by a transient ischaemic attack
- The neurological deficit usually develops slowly

Cerebral embolism
- Sudden onset of a complete neurological deficit

Intracerebral haemorrhage
- Sudden onset of:
    - Headache, vomiting, stupor or coma
    - A progressive neurological deficit
    - Raised blood pressure and reduced pulse rate

Subarachnoid haemorrhage
- Sudden onset of a very severe (usually occipital) headache, often after exertion or straining, sometimes preceded by a mild 'sentinel' headache, often followed by collapse with loss of consciousness
- Some patients may die instantly, whilst others may remain comatose (rare and carries a very poor prognosis), and others may regain (or never lose) consciousness, but develop:
    - Meningism with photophobia, neck stiffness with a positive Kernig's sign and nausea/vomiting
    - Focal neurological deficit (rare and carries a poor prognosis)
    - Raised blood pressure and reduced pulse rate
- Complications include cardiac arrhythmias (35%) and pulmonary oedema (22%).
- ECG changes include abnormal ST segments or T waves (25%) with profound myocardial dysfunction in 3%, possibly as a result of a 'sympathetic storm' occurring as a response to the rapid increase in ICP

Note: The sudden loss of consciousness may result in collapse and a secondary head injury

Management
- Administer high flow oxygen via a high concentration mask
- Check their gag reflex
- If the patient is unconscious:
    - Airway care with an oropharyngeal airway (tracheal tube if the gag reflex is absent or reduced)
    - Ventilate the patient if they are not breathing (preferably via a tracheal tube)
    - Put them into the recovery position if they are breathing satisfactorily
- If the patient is conscious:
    - Reassure them (they may be confused and frightened, and apart from any humanitarian considerations; an increase in blood pressure is undesirable!)
    - Establish intravenous access and monitor the cardiac rhythm
- Measure the blood glucose level, as hypoglycaemia may mimic stroke, and if it is low administer 50 mL 50% dextrose intravenously
- Keep the patient cool (those with a low body temperature; may suffer less brain injury)
- Administer aspirin, 300 mg orally, if the history/examination suggests cerebral thrombosis/embolism (particularly the latter), but *not* if it suggests haemorrhage (will make the bleeding worse). Medium dose aspirin has been shown to produce a small but significant reduction in early death from stroke
- If the history suggests that the patient has had a subarachnoid haemorrhage, they should be admitted to hospital without any delay, as treated early there is a good possibility of a full neurological recovery
- Recent evidence suggests that all stokes due to cerebral infarction should be admitted immediately and treated urgently with a thrombolytic (e.g. rtPA), unless it is contraindicated

Differential diagnosis of collapse (classified according to aetiology)

Airway/breathing
- Upper airway obstruction:
    - Foreign body
    - Laryngeal oedema
    - Epiglottitis
- Lower airway:
    - Asthma
    - Anaphylactic shock
    - Pneumothorax

Circulatory
- Cardiac:
    - Acute myocardial infarction
    - Arrhythmias:
        - Ventricular fibrillation
        - Ventricular tachycardia
        - Complete heart block
    - Electrocution
- Vascular:
    - Neurogenic shock (syncope):
        - Vasovagal
        - Micturition
        - Cough
        - Carotid sinus hypersensitivity
    - Pulmonary embolism
    - Hypovolaemic shock
    - Bacteriological shock (peritonitis, pelvic infection)

Disability (CNS)
- Epilepsy
- Infections: meningitis, encephalitis
- Stroke:
    - Cerebrovascular accidents
    - Transient ischaemic attacks
    - Sub-arachnoid haemorrhage
- Cerebral tumours and abscesses
- Head injury
- Poisoning and drug overdosage: accidental/deliberate, including alcohol
- Hysteria

Endocrine/metabolic
- Diabetes:
    - Hypoglycaemia
    - Hyperglycaemia
- Thyroid disease
- Renal failure
- Liver failure
- Adrenal failure
- Hypercalcaemia
- Hypothermia and hyperthermia

Figure 9-7 Differential diagnosis of collapse

10

Poisoning and overdosage

Poisoning and overdosage

Introduction

- Although this topic may not be an obvious part of Immediate Care, it is part of emergency medicine and the management of poisoning and overdosage is a subject with which the Immediate Care doctor should be familiar

Definitions:
- **Non-Drug Poisoning:** Exposure to substances that are intrinsically harmful in a dose sufficient to cause clinical signs and symptoms

- **Overdosage:** Exposure to substances that are only harmful when taken in excess

Incidence
- Very common in children under the age of 5 years (50%):
    - Usually accidental, although non-accidental poisoning may occur
    - Deaths are very rare (under 10 per year)
- Self poisoning/non accidental overdosage:
    - Accounts for about 5% of all emergency medical admissions
    - Most common in the 15-19 year old age group
    - Analgesics, especially paracetamol are involved in over 50% of cases
    - Hypnotics and tranquillisers (usually benzodiazepines) are the next most commonly involved
    - 50% have taken alcohol in addition to their primary poison
    - Carbon monoxide is an important cause of death (motor vehicle exhaust fumes: 1000 deaths per year)

Aetiology
- Accidental non-drug poisoning is often caused by ordinary household chemicals:
    - Detergents, bleaches, etc.
- Non-drug poisoning may be accidental:
    - Children, the elderly
- Non-drug poisoning may be deliberate:
    - Suicide, parasuicide: drugs, carbon monoxide
- In self-poisoning more than one substance may be involved, especially alcohol and drugs

Pathophysiology

- The substances involved may produce both systemic and local effects depending on the route of absorption

Through the dermis

- Absorbed: chemicals
- Bite: insect, snake
- Injected: plants, intravenous drug abuse

Effects

- *Local:*
  - Erythema, blistering, etc.
- *Systemic:*
  - Bee stings: anaphylactic shock
  - Organophosphates

Inhaled

- Noxious gases, etc.

Effects

- *Local:*
  - Upper and lower respiratory tract: rhinitis, laryngeal and bronchial oedema
  - Lungs: pulmonary oedema
- *Systemic:*
  - Specific to the poison

Ingested

Effects:

- *Local:*
  - Burning of lips, mouth, oesophagus, vomiting, and abdominal pain
- *Systemic:*
  - Specific to the poison

Systemic effects

- **Blood**
  - Reduce available oxygen in the circulation:
    - Carbon monoxide
    - Cyanide
- **Brain**
  - Produce generalised cerebral depression
    - Narcotics
    - Tricyclic antidepressants
    - Alcohol
  - Produce specific effects
    - Respiratory depressants
- **Heart**
  - Arrhythmogenic:
    - Tricyclic antidepressants
    - β-blockers
    - Calcium antagonists

- **Chest wall**
    - Respiratory muscle paralysis:
        - Snake bite
        - Organophosphates
        - Botulinus toxin
- **Lungs**
    - Bronchospasm
        - β-blockers in those who are asthmatic
- **Liver**
    - Hepatic damage:
        - Paracetamol
        - Amanita mushrooms
- **Kidneys**
    - Renal damage:
        - Paracetamol
- **Tissues**
    - Cyanides
- **Multisystem**
    - Anaphylactic shock:
        - Insect bites

Guidelines for the management of poisoning/overdosage

Assess the scene

Rapidly assess what has happened

Look for and protect yourself from any obvious danger

Move the casualty away from direct contact with the poison/source of danger to a place of safety
- Remove any contaminated clothing and wash/hose down the skin with water

Primary survey

Assess the patient's vital signs, including pupil size and perform basic/advanced life support:
- Airway:
    - Airway care is important in poisoning as the casualty may be unconscious
- Breathing:
    - Tracheal intubation will be required if the patient is deeply unconscious, requires ventilation due to respiratory depression or respiratory muscle paralysis, or there is a risk of aspiration
    - High flow oxygen should be administered by a high concentration mask in poisoning with carbon monoxide and irritant gases, or if the patient has impaired ventilation or is hypotensive, but *not* in paraquat poisoning
- Circulation:
    - Hypotension sufficient to cause irreversible brain injury may occur in severe poisoning with central nervous system stimulants:
        - Transport the patient in the head down position
        - Administer high flow, high concentration oxygen
        - Establish an intravenous infusion with colloid
    - Fluid depletion without hypotension may occur in prolonged coma and after aspirin poisoning, due to vomiting, sweating and hyperventilation

- Some drugs, e.g. tricyclic antidepressants may cause cardiac conduction problems and arrhythmias. These may respond to correction of any underlying hypoxia or acidosis by ensuring adequate ventilation: but otherwise they are probably best left untreated until the patient reaches hospital
- Hypothermia:
    - This may be a problem in patients who have been unconscious for any length of time, especially following overdosage with barbiturates or phenothiazines:
        - Wrap the patient in warm blankets and insulate, but do not use hot water bottles as these may cause burns
- Fitting:
    - Single short-lived fits do not require treatment
    - Prolonged or multiple fits should be treated with diazepam or midazolam (see chapter on Medical emergencies: management of epilepsy)

Secondary survey

Identify the cause of the poisoning, and the quantity (may not be possible in children or if the casualty is unconscious) from:
- Medicines:
    - Shape, colour of pills/capsules
    - Labels of container/bottle
- Chemicals;
    - Container labels
    - HAZCHEM code
- Dead snake/insect
- Uneaten food, leaves, fruit, berries, etc.

Management
- Consider treatment for removing or eliminating ingested poisons, prior to evacuation to hospital (depends on the travelling time to hospital and the speed of onset of the poison)

Induction of emesis or gastric emptying
- Generally seldom practicable until the patient has reached hospital, and not now generally recommended, as there is good evidence that gastric emptying does not affect the amount of substance absorbed, but there is still disagreement about its value even amongst the experts!
- The dangers of gastric emptying (pulmonary aspiration of gastric contents) have to be weighed up against the toxicity of the suspected poison, which will depend on:
    - The quantity of poison ingested
    - The inherent toxicity of the poison
    - The time since ingestion
- This is of *doubtful value* more than 1-2 hours after ingestion except for:
    - Salicylates (4-6 hrs)
    - Tricyclics (8 hrs)
- It is *dangerous* in drowsy/comatose patients unless there is:
    - A good cough reflex
    - Airway protection with a cuffed tracheal tube
- *Not advised* for:
    - Petroleum products (more dangerous in the lungs than the stomach: aspiration pneumonitis).
    - Corrosive compounds
    - Pregnant patients
- If the patient is unconscious, their airway should always be protected by a cuffed tracheal tube to prevent pulmonary aspiration of the gastric contents

Emesis
- Used to be used in children, but is now considered to be of limited value, as there is little evidence that it prevents clinically significant absorption, and its adverse effects may complicate diagnosis
- Should *not* be used if the child is unconscious or semi-conscious, or after ingestion of corrosive or volatile substances, e.g. petroleum distillates, essential oils

Method
- Administer **Paediatric Ipecacuanha Emetic Mixture BP** (*not* tincture)

Dosage
- Children: 6-18 months: 10 mL
          18 months-14 years: 15 mL
- Adults: 30 mL
- The dose should be followed by a glass of water or orange juice and may be repeated once after 20 minutes as necessary

Prevention of absorption

Adsorbants: activated charcoal (charcoal that has been treated with chemical activators or in a stream of gas to increase its surface area, and thus its ability to absorb small molecules on its surface)
- Activated charcoal given orally can bind and reduce the absorption of many poisons
- Most effective if given as soon as possible after ingestion of the poison, but may be effective if given within 4 hours; longer in the case of modified-release preparations or of substances with anticholinergic properties.
- Relatively safe and is particularly useful for preventing absorption of poisons which are toxic in relatively small amounts, e.g. tricyclic antidepressants.
- Ineffective and should not be administered for poisoning by:
  - Lithium
  - Cyanide
  - Corrosive agents (strong acids/alkalis)
  - Iron salts
  - Organic solvents
  - Petroleum distillates
- Activated charcoal absorbs ipecacuanha, rendering it ineffective
- Activated charcoal should be considered if indicated, but should not be given if the patient requires an oral antidote, e.g. in iron ingestion

Activated charcoal powder (*Carbomix*®)

Presentation
- Packs 25, 50g powder to which 400 mL of tap water or other liquid is added

Dosage
- Children: 25 g.
- Adults: up to 50 g.

Side effects
- Nausea, vomiting and constipation

Activated charcoal granules (*Medicoal®*)
- Also contains povidone and sodium bicarbonate

Presentation
- 5g sachets of granules in packs of 5 and 30

Dosage
- Initially 1-2 sachets every 15-20 minutes, until dose is 5-10 times the amount of drug ingested (if known) or if not known up to a maximum of:
  - Children: 25 g
  - Adults: up to 50 g

Side effects
- Nausea, vomiting and constipation

Active elimination
- Repeated doses of oral activated charcoal may enhance the elimination of some drugs after they have been absorbed and is useful following overdosage with:
  - Aspirin
  - Barbiturates
  - Carbamazepine
  - Cyclosporin
  - Dapsone
  - Digoxin
  - Phenobarbitone
  - Phenytoin
  - Quinine
  - Theophyllines
- The usual dose is 50 g initially, then 50 g every 4 hours. If the dose has to be repeated, it is advisable to administer a laxative as well

Skin contamination
- Consider washing the poison off contaminated skin with copious volumes of water

Specific treatment
- Use specific antidotes if applicable/available
- Information should be obtained from the local Poisons Information Centre (see list at the end of this chapter)

Inform receiving hospital of
- The cause, effects, and treatment of poisoning
- The time of:
  - Ingestion/exposure
  - Onset of symptoms
  - Treatment carried out
- The quantity of poison/drug ingested

If possible send to hospital
- The chemical/pill container/syringe
- The chemical code number
- Dead snake/insect
- Uneaten fruit/mushrooms, etc.
- Any suicide note
- A sample of vomit

Specific problems

Ant, bee and wasp (hymenoptera) stings
- The toxin injected by the insect is not usually itself dangerous or life threatening; but may be dangerous if an acute allergic reaction, especially anaphylactic shock, occurs, or if a bite in the mouth or on the tongue causes upper airway obstruction and respiratory distress

Incidence
- Life threatening problems are rare, but there are more deaths from anaphylaxis in the UK and USA as a result of a bee or wasp sting than from all other venomous bites and stings put together
- Bee keepers may be at risk of sensitisation to bee venom
- Greatest risk of fatality occurs in those aged over 40 years (with more males than females in some countries)
- Most deaths occur after a single sting (systemic toxic effects are seen after multiple stings, but are rarely fatal)
- Wasp stings cause twice as many deaths as bee stings
- Stings to the head and neck have a greater mortality, due to airway obstruction
- The risk of non fatal systemic reactions is greater in bee than wasp stings

Aetiology
- Stings from Hymenoptera:
    - Formicids:
        - Venomous ants including fire ants and harvester ants
    - Apids:
        - Honey bees (*Apis mellifera*):
            - Not aggressive, but may sting to protect their colony
        - Bumble bees (*Bombus* species):
            - least aggressive and sensitisation to their venom is uncommon
    - Vespids:
        - Wasps (vespula):
            - highly aggressive and will sting without provocation, especially in early autumn, when food is scarce
            - Sensitisation is common as wasps scavenge around food waste in populated areas
        - Hornets
        - Paper wasps:
            - These live in small colonies in temperate climates
            - Major cause of sensitisation in southern Europe

Symptoms/signs
- Local:
    - Pain and tenderness.
    - A circle of erythema and swelling sometimes with a haemorrhagic centre (especially if it has been sucked!)
- Systemic:
    - Development of an anaphylactic reaction:
        - Facial oedema
        - Abdominal pain
        - Dyspnoea
        - Hypotension and collapse

Mueller classification of allergic reactions to hymenoptera

Large local reactions
- Swelling at site of sting greater than 10 cm in diameter lasting over 24 hours

Systemic reactions

Grade I
- Urticaria, itching, malaise and anxiety

Grade II
- Angio-oedema

or - A combination of any grade I symptoms *plus* two or more of:
- Chest tightness, nausea, vomiting, diarrhoea, abdominal pain, dizziness

Grade III
- Dyspnoea, wheeze or stridor

or - A combination of grade II symptoms, *plus* two or more of:
- Dysphagia, dysarthria, hoarseness, weakness, confusion, feeling of impending disaster

Grade IV
- Any of the above, *plus* two or more of:
- Hypotension, collapse, syncope, incontinence (urine or stool), cyanosis

Note: Grades I and II are mild to moderate reactions, grades III and IV are severe
Other reactions may occur, including:
- Serum sickness, nephritis, neuritis, fits, thrombocytopaenia, haemolysis, Disseminated intravascular coagulation and myocardial ischaemia

Figure 10-1 Mueller classification of allergic reactions to hymenoptera

Management
- Large local reactions:
    - Bee sting:
        - Remove by scraping the sting off with a knife
        - Do *not* try to remove sting with fingers or tweezers as this may result in further injection of venom
    - Cleanse area, apply cooling lotion or topical antihistamine
    - Oral antihistamine, eg. chlorpheniramine *(Piriton®)*, cetirizine *(Zirtec®)*, terfenadine *(Triludan®)*
    - If the mouth is affected: sucking ice may be helpful
    - Subsequent large local reaction:
        - Antihistamines and a short course of prednisolone
- Systemic reactions:
    - Anaphylactic shock:
        - Basic/advanced life support, epinephrine, etc. (see Circulation care: anaphylactic shock)
    - Respiratory obstruction:
        - Consider cricothyrotomy

Note: Venom immunotherapy is indicated for those who have had a Grade III or IV reaction, to prevent anaphylaxis on subsequent exposure

Spider bites

Incidence
- Species of venomous spiders occur throughout the world in both temperate and tropical regions
- Although there are no venomous spiders indigenous to the UK, exotic escapees may cause bites

Aetiology
- Two main species of spider are responsible for most toxic spider bites:
  - *Lactrodectus* (commonest):
    - Black widow spider (South America)
    - Redback spider (Australia)
  - *Loxosceles*:
    - Brown recluse spider

Symptoms/signs
- *Lactrodectus*:
  - Local:
    - Severe 'agonizing' pain (which may also be generalised), muscle cramps and spasm
  - Systemic:
    - Abdominal pain, nausea, vomiting, headache, sweating, and occasionally severe hypertension
- *Loxosceles*:
  - Local:
    - Severe pain
    - A characteristic haemorrhagic pustule 'bull's-eye' lesion, with slowly evolving tissue necrosis

Management
- Analgesia with opiates or injection of local anaesthetic
- Muscle relaxants: diazepam
- Bradycardia: atropine
- *Lactrodectus*:
  - Antivenom
- *Loxosceles*:
  - Oral macrolide (erythromycin, clarithromycin) plus dapsone

Scorpion stings
- Several thousand people worldwide are killed by scorpion stings each year, especially in the Americas, North Africa, the Middle East and South Asia

Incidence
- Relatively common in the countries where scorpions are indigenous

Symptoms/signs
- Severe pain at the site of the sting
- Hyperexcitability with sweating, lacrimation and excessive salivation
- Hypertension, cardiac arrhythmias and tachypnoea
- Muscle spasms

Management
- Analgesia with injection of local anaesthetic
- Antivenom may be available locally for some species
- The most dangerous species is *Mesobuthus tamulus*, for which no antivenom is available. The recommended treatment is with a selective α adrenergic blocker, prazosin (*Hypovase*®)

Snake bite

Incidence
- Rare in the UK; the only indigenous venomous snake is the adder (*Vipera berus*):
    - Usually only occurs in warm weather, as the adder hibernates in winter
    - Systemic envenomation occurs in less than half of all patients with snake bite
    - Rarely fatal, except in the very debilitated patient who receives a large amount of venom
- May be an important cause of death in some countries, especially in tropical and subtropical areas:
    - In Sri Lanka and Burma, the annual mortality from snake bites may be as high as 5-15/100,000 population
- May result in severe limb damage, resulting in disability, especially in the tropics

Aetiology
- Bites may occur as a result of:
    - Trying to pick up the snake
    - A sudden encounter with a snake, as a result of which it feels threatened and responds by striking, (usually the lower limb)

Pathophysiology
- Venom is usually deposited subcutaneously by the hollow fangs of the snake
- The components of venom usually reach the circulation via the lymphatics, although some components may enter the capillaries directly
- Most venoms are a complex mixture of different toxins:
    - Proteases:
        - Act as cytotoxins, causing a severe local reaction with swelling and tissue damage
    - Neurotoxins:
        - Interfere with neuromuscular transmission (some also damage muscle)
    - Haemorrhagins:
        - Break down endothelial barriers and cause bleeding
    - Substances which act on different sites in the coagulation pathway, causing anti- and pro-coagulation effects, leading to a state similar to disseminated intravascular coagulation, and also act directly on platelets

Symptoms/signs
- As the clinical effects of envenomation vary from one species to another, accurate identification of the species, ideally from examination of the dead snake, is essential:
    - Kraits and cobras (elapid snakes):
        - Most commonly cause neurotoxicity
    - Viper, pit vipers, rattlesnakes (viperine snakes):
        - Usually cause tissue damage and coagulopathies
- The patient should be carefully examined before treatment is administered as up to one third of all bites caused by venomous snakes do not result in envenomation
- Bite:
    - Two puncture marks about a centimetre apart, usually situated on the extremity of a limb
- Local reaction (usually develops within minutes):
    - Swelling (which may spread rapidly to involve the whole limb)
    - Erythema
    - Ecchymosis
    - Local pain
    - Painful enlargement of the regional lymph nodes
    - Local tissue breakdown

- Systemic (most signs develop within a few hours, but neurotoxicity may sometimes take over 12 hours to develop):
    - Nausea, vomiting, colicky abdominal pain and diarrhoea
    - Tachycardia, bradycardia and early transient hypotension with syncope
    - Angio-oedema
    - Dizziness, restlessness, agitation, confusion, fits and coma.
    - Later there may be:
        - Persistent or recurrent hypotension
        - ECG abnormalities
        - Coagulopathy with bleeding from venepuncture sites and wounds
        - Haemorrhagic diathesis with bleeding from the gums and other sites
        - Adult respiratory distress syndrome
        - Renal failure
        - Progressive paralysis:
            - Ptosis occurs initially progressing to bulbar muscle involvement and later to paralysis of the diaphragm
        - Death (most at risk are the elderly and the very young)

Management
- Get a good description of the snake, and try to identify it if possible:
    - Zagreb antivenom is available in specialist centres for adder envenomation and is indicated in severe local and systemic reactions
- Local:
    - Remove all rings, etc. from the affected limb so as to avoid impairment of the peripheral circulation, if swelling occurs
    - Clean and cover the bite with a dressing and firmly (but not occlusively) bandage the affected limb:
        - This increases the systemic vascular resistance, and reduces the lymphatic return, thus reducing local and lymphatic spread and the possibility of the venom causing systemic side effects (do *not* use this method for bites from snakes which cause local tissue necrosis)
    - Immobilise the limb in a sling or splint, and keep it below heart level, but not dependent (to reduce the venous return)
    - Do *not*:
        - Allow the patient to walk on the affected limb as muscle activity will increase the blood supply and aids the systemic absorption of venom, (ideally do not allow the patient to move at all)
        - Allow the patient to drink alcohol as this may exacerbate any CNS depression
        - Apply a tourniquet
        - Lance, squeeze or suck the bite
        - Remove the bandage once it has been applied
- Systemic:
    - Administer oxygen
    - Intubate and ventilate the patient if there is evidence of bulbar involvement (indicated by the inability of the victim to swallow secretions)
    - Establish intravenous access
    - Monitor the heart rhythm with an ECG
    - Consider using antihistamines for an acute local reaction
    - Treat any early anaphylactic reactions with epinephrine

Marine animals

Incidence
- Venomous jellyfish occur throughout the world, but are particularly common in the tropical waters of the Indo-Pacific region
- Several species of hazardous marine animals may be found in the coastal waters of the UK

Aetiology
- *Jellyfish*
    - Portuguese man-of-war, sea nettle, compass
    - A mechanical stimulus causes nematocysts on the tentacles to discharge, injecting venom into the victim
- *Poisonous fish* (poisonous spines)
    - Lesser weaver fish
    - Sting ray
- *Sea urchin*
    - Injury is caused by many tiny spines breaking off after penetrating the skin and underlying tissues including the deep palmar and plantar spaces and joint cavities

Symptoms/signs
- *Jellyfish*
    - Local:
        - Burning pain and oedema
    - Systemic (very rare):
        - Myocardial toxicity
- *Poisonous fish*
    - Local:
        - Extreme pain
        - Oedema
    - Systemic:
        - Respiratory depression
        - Hypotension
        - Diarrhoea
- *Sea urchin*
    - Local:
        - Excruciating pain
        - Oedema
    - Systemic:
        - Cardiorespiratory failure

Management
- *Jellyfish stings*
    - Rinse the affected part in sea water
    - Remove any adherent tentacles
    - Prevent any further nematocyst discharge with vinegar (acetic acid)
    - Provide cardiorespiratory support
- *Poisonous fish and sea urchin stings*
    - Relieve pain by immersing the affected part in hot water to denaturise the poison or administer a local anaesthetic block
    - Consider administration of an oral antibiotic, e.g. co-trimoxazole, and tetanus prophylaxis
    - Provide cardiorespiratory support

Medicines

Non steroidal anti-inflammatory drugs (NSAIDs)

Salicylates (aspirin)
- More likely to cause adverse effects and more dangerous in overdosage than ibuprofen

Incidence
- Accidental poisoning is commonly encountered in young children
- Used to be a very popular method of overdosage in adults, and although deliberate salicylate poisoning is declining it still accounts for about 5,000 admissions and 50 deaths per year in the UK

Pathophysiology
- Produces an initial respiratory alkalosis caused by hyperventilation, followed by a metabolic acidosis
- Pulmonary oedema and renal failure

Symptoms/signs
- These may not occur for up to 24 hours post ingestion due to gastric mass formation delaying absorption
- Flushed appearance (vasodilation), pyrexia, sweating, hyperventilation and dehydration
- Nausea, vomiting, haematemesis
- Tinnitus, deafness, vertigo, headache
- Restlessness, confusion, coma, and fits or cardiac arrest (very severe poisoning only)

Management
- Administer activated charcoal (gastric emptying may achieve worthwhile recovery of salicylate up to 4 hours post ingestion)
- Rehydrate with an intravenous infusion of crystalloid
- Fits: treat with diazepam or midazolam

Mefenamic acid (*Ponstan®*)

Incidence
- A relatively uncommon cause of overdosage

Symptoms/signs
- Fits, usually brief, (rarely status epilepticus may develop) occurring 30 minutes to 12 hrs post ingestion

Management
- Fitting: intravenous diazepam/midazolam
- Consider gastric emptying

Ibuprofen

Incidence
- Serious overdosage is uncommon (there are documented cases of full recovery after major overdoses)

Symptoms/signs
- Nausea, vomiting, tinnitus
- Large overdoses may result in renal failure, a metabolic acidosis, hypotension, and pulmonary oedema

Management
- Consider gastric emptying or induction of emesis, if more than 10 tablets have been ingested

Paracetamol

Incidence
- Often used in deliberate overdosage (commonest cause of parasuicide in young people, accounting for over 45% (30-40,000) of all hospital admissions and 35% of all deaths (100- 150 deaths/year) due to poisoning in those under 20 years old in the UK), and in accidental overdosage in children

Pathophysiology
- As few as 20-30 tabs may cause delayed hepatic (hepatocellular) necrosis, and less commonly renal tubular necrosis

Symptoms/signs
- Often the patient does not appear ill
- Nausea, vomiting (usually settles within 24 hours, but persistent vomiting is usually associated with right subcostal pain/tenderness, and indicates hepatocellular necrosis)
- Liver damage is usually maximal 3-4 days after ingestion and may lead to jaundice, encephalopathy haemorrhage, hypoglycaemia, cerebral haemorrhage and death

Management
- All cases should go to hospital, even if they appear well, so that appropriate treatment may be started
- Basic and Advanced Life Support in extreme cases as indicated
- Perform gastric lavage/emptying followed by activated charcoal within 4 hours of ingestion
- Hepatic protection may be provided within 24 hours of ingestion by:

N-Acetylcysteine (*Parvolex®*) in 5% dextrose as an intravenous infusion
Dosage: 150 mg/kg in 200 mL over 15 minutes then 50 mg/kg in 500 mL over 4 hours, followed by 100 mg/kg over 16 hours

Methionine: administered orally (do *not* administer activated charcoal as well)
Dosage: 2.5 g initially followed by a further 2.5 g every 4 hours, up to a total of 4 times (10 g)

Note: Paracetamol levels should be obtained if available

Co-proxamol: Dextropropoxyphene and paracetamol

Incidence
- Commonly used in overdosage

Pathophysiology
- Initial effects are those of opiate overdosage (see below), followed by the effects of paracetamol toxicity
- Respiratory arrest is very common
- Sudden cardiovascular collapse may also occur within the first few hours post ingestion

Management
- Basic and Advanced Life Support in extreme cases as indicated
- Consider induction of emesis/gastric emptying
- As opiate and paracetamol overdosage
- Administer intravenous naloxone (see under opiates)

Narcotic analgesics: opiates: morphine, heroin, methadone, codeine, and dextropropoxyphene

Incidence
- Overdosage is relatively rare in the UK, except amongst drug addicts, due to the difficulty in obtaining these drugs, legally and in any quantity, except for dextropropoxyphene, which is widely prescribed in combination with paracetamol (co-proxamol)

Pathophysiology
- Cause respiratory and central nervous system depression (exacerbated by alcohol)
- Death may result very rapidly

Symptoms/signs
- Vomiting
- Bradypnoea leading to apnoea, pulmonary oedema
- Hypotension
- Constricted pupils, drowsiness, unconsciousness and coma
- Needle marks, thrombosed veins in drug addicts

Management
- Basic Life Support
- Oxygen

- **Naloxone** (400 µg/mL: 1/2 mL ampoules):
  Dosage: 0.8-2.0 mg given as an intravenous bolus. This may need to be repeated, as naloxone has a short half life

Note: Reversal of symptoms should begin within about 1 minute, but beware of "recovery" followed by further collapse (for more information: see chapter on Pain management)

- Circulatory support with an intravenous infusion
- Consider use of activated charcoal if the opioid has been ingested

Note: There is some debate as to whether the patient should be given intramuscular naloxone or be given no naloxone, but ventilated and allowed to wake up on their own

Antimalarials (chloroquine, hydroxychloroquine, quinine)

Incidence
- Rarely taken in deliberate overdosage

Symptoms/signs
- Rapid onset of arrhythmias

Management
- Symptomatic
- Contact a poisons centre for specific advice

Tricyclic antidepressants

Incidence
- Often used in deliberate overdosage, and are an important cause of poisoning deaths, accounting for about 14% of successful suicides

Pathophysiology
- Tricyclics:
    - Have a marked anticholinergic effect
    - Inhibit reuptake of catecholamines in peripheral nerves
    - Have a membrane stabilising effect
    - Overdosage may result in a metabolic acidosis and hypokalaemia

Symptoms/signs
- Peripheral:
    - Warm dry skin and hyperpyrexia due to vasodilation and impairment of sweating
    - Blurring of vision with dilated pupils
    - Dry mouth
    - Urinary retention
- Central nervous system:
    - Drowsiness/unconsciousness and coma associated with increased muscle tone, myoclonus, hyperreflexia and extensor plantar responses.
    - Convulsions
    - Respiratory failure, metabolic acidosis
    - Hypothermia
- Cardiac:
    - Hypotension
    - Sinus tachycardia (occurs in >50% of patients)
    - Cardiac conduction defects with a prolonged PR or QT interval, and QRS widening (occurs in <6% of patients)
    - Cardiac arrest

Management
- Care of the unconscious patient
- If the patient is conscious:
    - Administer activated charcoal orally immediately
- If the patient is unconscious:
    - Intubate them to protect the airway
    - Perform gastric lavage, up to 6 hours post ingestion
- Monitor the patient's ECG tracing and haemodynamic state:
    - If there is hypotension or ECG changes, e.g. a prolonged PR or QT interval, QRS widening or arrhythmia:
        - Administer high flow oxygen via a high concentration oxygen mask
        - Ventilate via a tracheal tube
        - Consider administration of sodium bicarbonate 8.4% (0.5-1 mmol/kg) intravenously
    - If there is a serious arrhythmia, it is best to administer sodium bicarbonate 8.4% (0.5-1 mmol/kg) intravenously for its cardioprotective effect, and transfer rapidly to hospital
- If the patient is fitting or delirious:
    - Administer intravenous diazepam/midazolam

β-blockers

Incidence
- Deliberate overdosage with β-blockers is relatively rare

Pathophysiology
- β-blockers are β-adrenergic receptor blockers and their effects may be cardioselective or non-cardioselective
- The individual response to β-blockers varies from one individual to another; patients with pre-existing cardiovascular disease are more at risk, whilst those already on β-blockers may have some resistance

Symptoms/signs
- Therapeutic overdosage, especially in patients with pre-existing conduction disorders or impaired myocardial function may cause:
    - Lightheadedness, dizziness and syncope due to bradycardia and hypotension
    - Heart failure may be precipitated or exacerbated
- Bradycardia
- CNS effects include:
    - Respiratory depression
    - Dilated pupils
    - Hallucinations, drowsiness, and convulsions
- Massive overdosage of β-blockers may cause various different effects:
    - Propranolol may cause coma and convulsions
    - Sotalol may sometimes cause ventricular tachyarrhythmias (including torsades de pointes)

Management
- *General:*
    - If the patient is unconscious:
        - Provide airway support, i.e. oxygen, ventilation, etc.
    - Administer activated charcoal
    - Convulsions should not be treated if they are short-lived and infrequent
    - Severe bradycardia and hypotension:
        - Administer atropine 3 mg for adults or 40 μg/kg for children intravenously (which may be repeated if necessary) with continuous cardiac monitoring
- *Cardiotoxicity:*
    - Glucagon 5-10 mg administered intravenously in glucose 5% is the treatment of choice for serious cardiotoxicity, and is thought to work by activating adenylcyclase
    - In severe poisoning the response to glucagon may be transient, so an infusion of 4mg/hr should be set up and the dose gradually reduced as the patient responds to treatment
- *β-adrenoceptor agonists (isoprenaline):*
    - Although these may seem to be the logical antidotes to poisoning with β-blockers, their usefulness is reduced by the length of time involved in giving a sufficient amount safely, as the dose must be carefully titrated against the clinical response
    - An isoprenaline infusion should be set up and the rate of administration slowly increased until there is an adequate increase in pulse rate and blood pressure

Hypnotics and anxiolytics

Barbiturates

Incidence
- Used to be commonly used in overdosage, but now uncommon in the UK as their prescribing has almost ceased, except for epileptics

Pathophysiology
- Depressants of nervous tissue especially the central nervous system, resulting in depression of the level of consciousness
- May also cause severe respiratory depression

Symptoms/signs
- Drowsiness, confusion, unconsciousness, coma
- Pupil size may vary
- Respiratory depression, bradypnoea, with shallow respirations, or Cheyne Stokes respiration
- Vomiting and aspiration, resulting in pneumonia
- Signs of shock, hypotension, etc.
- Erythema, skin blisters (barbiturate blisters)
- Hypothermia
- Metabolic acidosis

Management
- If unconscious:
    - Airway support, i.e. oxygen, ventilation, etc.
- If conscious:
    - Activated charcoal orally immediately
- Cardiac monitoring

Benzodiazepines: temazepam, nitrazepam, lorazepam, diazepam, chlordiazepoxide

Incidence
- Still a relatively popular drug of overdosage (involved in 20-40% of cases in the UK)
- Taken more often by women than men
- Often taken combined with alcohol

Pathophysiology
- Benzodiazepines are general CNS depressants but causes less severe respiratory depression
- Rarely fatal by themselves
- May potentiate effects of other CNS depressants if taken at the same time, especially alcohol

Symptoms/signs
- Ataxia, dysarthria (slurred speech)and nystagmus
- Drowsiness, unconsciousness and coma (uncommon unless combined with other sedatives, alcohol or in the elderly)
- Hyporeflexia, hypotension
- Respiratory depression

Management
- Care of the unconscious patient including administration of oxygen.
- Administer activated charcoal if the patient remains unconscious
- Consider administration of flumazenil as an aid to diagnosis in mixed overdosage if there is respiratory depression:
    - Flumazenil should be administered with care and titrated against the patient's response (for details of administration see chapter on Pain management)
    - Flumazenil should *not* be administered if:
        - The patient has also taken tricyclics (indicated by history and ECG changes, i.e. prolonged PR or QT interval, and QRS widening, and a tachycardia >100 bpm), at it may cause convulsions
        - The patient is an epileptic (may precipitate fits)

Iron compounds: Ferrous sulphate, ferrous gluconate, etc.

Incidence
- Common in accidental poisoning of children
- Has an appreciable mortality

Pathophysiology
- Hepatocellular necrosis

Symptoms/signs
- Nausea, vomiting, abdominal pain, diarrhoea, haematemesis and rectal bleeding
- Leukocytosis and hyperglycaemia
- Hypotension and shock with apparent recovery between 8-24 hours, but later there may be profound hypotension, coma, and hepatocellular necrosis resulting in renal failure

Management
- Gastric emptying:
    - Gastric lavage

Desferrioxamine (chelating agent)

> *Dosage:* By mouth: 5-10 g in 50-100 mL of water
> By intravenous infusion: Up to 15 mg/kg/hour (maximum: 80 mg/kg)

Note: Intravenous desferrioxamine may cause hypotension and an anaphylactic reaction

Lithium salts

Incidence
- Acute poisoning is uncommon

Aetiology
- Poisoning may be deliberate or accidental
- Most cases of lithium poisoning occur as a result of long-term therapy or deterioration in renal function, infection, dehydration, diuretics, poor compliance or poor monitoring, as the therapeutic and toxic levels are very close

Symptoms/signs
- Severe effects are rare following acute overdosage, in spite of there being very high blood levels, which are a poor indication of toxicity
- The development of symptoms may be delayed more than 12 hours after ingestion
- Early symptoms are often non-specific, but may include:
    - Non specific apathy, restlessness, polyuria, thirst, vomiting, diarrhoea
    - Ataxia, muscle weakness, blurred vision, dysarthria (slurred speech), muscle twitching/tremor, hyperreflexia
- Severe poisoning:
    - Cardiac arrhythmias, convulsions, coma, hypotension, renal failure and electrolyte imbalance

Management
- Induction of emesis/gastric emptying if under 2-4 hours post ingestion
- Dehydration: intravenous infusion of buffered solution of crystalloid, e.g. Hartmann's solution
- Convulsions: intravenous diazepam/midazolam

Phenothiazines

Incidence
- Fairly commonly used in self poisoning

Pathophysiology
- Centrally acting dopamine antagonists

Symptoms/signs
- Hypotension
- Hypothermia
- Sinus tachycardia, cardiac arrhythmias
- Dystonic reactions (these can also occur with therapeutic doses)
- Convulsions (severe cases only)

Management
- Arrhythmia control
- Hypotension:
    - Intravenous fluids
- Convulsions:
    - Intravenous diazepam/midazolam
- Dystonic reactions:
    - Orphenadrine
    - Procyclidine

Methylxanthenes (aminophylline, theophylline)

Incidence
- Therapeutic overdosage is now becoming rarer as these drugs are used less often, and the problems of a narrow therapeutic range, and early toxicity are appreciated, but may be a problem in the emergency management of acute severe asthma, when methylxanthenes may be administered intravenously, without checking first whether the patient is already taking one of these drugs

Pathophysiology
- Overdosage with methylxanthenes causes:
    - Gastrointestinal irritation
    - CNS stimulation with an increase in arousal
    - Catecholamine release, resulting in hyperglycaemia and glycosuria and the rapid onset of profound hypokalaemia
    - Hyperventilation resulting in an initial respiratory alkalosis; which is followed by the development of a metabolic acidosis
    - Tachycardia

Symptoms/signs
- Most oral preparations are sustained-release, which may delay recognition and complicate the management of overdosage.
- Gastrointestinal irritation causing nausea, severe and intractable vomiting with haematemesis and occasionally diarrhoea
- Agitation, restlessness and hyperactivity with pressure of speech
- Dilated pupils with tremor and hyperventilation
- Myoclonus, erratic jerky limb movements, increased muscle tone, hyperreflexia and eventually fits and unconsciousness
- Sinus tachycardia progressing to supraventricular and ventricular arrhythmias including ventricular fibrillation
- The blood pressure may rise a little before falling

Management
- If the patient is unconscious:
    - Airway support, i.e. oxygen, ventilation, etc.
- Consider gastric lavage, if the patient presents within 2 hours of the overdose
- Elimination of the methylxanthene may be enhanced by the repeated administration of activated charcoal (always protect the airway with a tracheal tube if the patient is unconscious)
- Monitor the patient's ECG:
    - Consider the administration of propranolol for the management arrhythmias (unless the patient is asthmatic)
- Treat convulsions and agitation with intravenous diazepam/midazolam

Antihistamines

Incidence
- Acute poisoning with antihistamines is relatively uncommon, but occurs more often in children than adults

Aetiology
- Accidental poisoning

Symptoms/signs
- Most of the older antihistamines have sedating and anticholinergic effects:
  - CNS depression:
    - Drowsiness (very common)
    - Nausea, vomiting
    - Lethargy, ataxia, slurred speech, dry mouth, dilated pupils, irritability, flushing, tachycardia
- Some antihistamines may cause paradoxical CNS stimulation with:
  - Hyperactivity
  - Excitement
  - Tremors
  - Disorientation
  - Hallucinations
  - Pyrexia
  - Tonic/clonic convulsions
- Terfenadine and astemizole lack the anticholinergic effects of the older antihistamines, but may cause:
  - Cardiac arrhythmias and ECG changes:
    - Prolongation of the QT interval
    - Ventricular arrhythmias including torsades de pointes

Management
- Care of the unconscious patient
- If the patient is conscious:
  - Administer activated charcoal orally immediately, followed by administration of activated charcoal
- If the patient is unconscious:
  - Intubate them to protect the airway
  - Perform gastric lavage, up to 6 hours post ingestion
- Monitor the patient's ECG tracing and haemodynamic state:
  - If there is hypotension or ECG changes, e.g. a prolonged PR or QT interval, QRS widening or arrhythmia:
    - Administer high flow oxygen via a high concentration oxygen mask
    - Ventilate via a tracheal tube
    - Consider administration of sodium bicarbonate 8.4% (0.5-1 mmol/kg) intravenously.
  - If there is a serious arrhythmia, it is best to observe and transfer rapidly to hospital
- If the patient is fitting or delirious:
  - Administer intravenous diazepam/midazolam

Other poisons

Cyanide
- May cause cardiac arrest and death very rapidly and poisoning is therefore an acute medical emergency

Incidence
- Cyanide poisoning usually occurs as a result of inhalation of cyanide gas given off by burning plastics, foam, and fabrics in accidental house fires
- Poisoning in industry is rare and usually occurs as a result of skin contamination and/or inhalation

Aetiology
- May occur by ingestion, absorption or inhalation

Pathophysiology
- Cyanide ions bind very strongly to the ferric component of cytochrome oxidase, preventing cellular oxygen utilisation, and resulting in severe cellular hypoxia

Symptoms/signs
- Cyanides act relatively quickly, and symptoms of poisoning will appear almost immediately after poisoning, whichever the route. If symptoms do not appear within 30 minutes, poisoning is unlikely
- Skin contact:
    - Irritation, erythema and local pain
    - Burns can also occur
- Ingestion:
    - Burning sensation in the throat, with nausea and vomiting
- Inhalation:
    - Odour of almonds on the patient's breath
    - Chest pain
- Systemic (most of the systemic symptoms of cyanide poisoning are due to severe hypoxia)
    - Absence of pallor and cyanosis
    - Chest tightness and respiratory distress with dyspnoea, and a tachypnoea leading to bradypnoea
    - A rapid and/or irregular, weak pulse
    - Red discolouration of the venous blood (on fundoscopy; arteries and veins look the same colour)
    - Dizziness, anxiety, mental confusion, verbal incoherence, coma, convulsions and death

Management
- Protect yourself from contamination
- Remove the patient away from any toxic atmosphere to fresh air as soon as possible
- Take off any contaminated clothing, and thoroughly wash down any exposed skin
- If ingestion of cyanide has occurred; induce emesis and perform gastric lavage
- If the casualty is breathing:
    - Break two amyl nitrite capsules beneath the casualty's nose, so that they inhale the vapour
- If the patient is unconscious or is losing consciousness:
    - Administer 1.5% dicobalt edetate (*Kelocyanor*®) 300 mg/20 mL intravenously over 1-5 minutes, followed immediately by 50 mL 50% dextrose (if no response, may be repeated up to three times)
- Maintain the airway
- Administer high flow, high concentration oxygen
- If the casualty is not breathing: ventilate with a bag and mask
- Provide circulatory support: intravenous infusion of colloid
- Monitor the cardiac rhythm
- If possible obtain 'before' and 'after' treatment blood samples to send for laboratory analysis

Note: Dicobalt edetate can cause flushing, vomiting, tachycardia, hypotension with collapse and convulsions if the patient *does not* have cyanide poisoning, and should therefore *only* be used when there has been *definite* cyanide poisoning

Noxious gases

Carbon monoxide: Colourless, odourless and tasteless gas (Domestic gas in mainland Britain is CO free)

Incidence
- Commonest inhaled agent involved in causing death: up to 1000 deaths every year, up to 200 occurring during the winter months and at home
- Often used in successful suicide: motor vehicle exhaust, etc. (over 800 deaths per year)

Aetiology
- Produced by incomplete combustion of fossil fuels, e.g. gas, petrol
- Accidental poisoning:
    - Inhalation of smoke, car exhaust or fumes caused by blocked flues from fires and boilers or the incomplete combustion of gases in confined spaces

Pathophysiology
- Carbon monoxide has a very high affinity for haemoglobin, with which it combines to form carboxyhaemoglobin, displacing oxygen and causing tissue hypoxia
- Levels of carbon monoxide do not need to be high to cause poisoning

Symptoms/signs (may be difficult to recognise initially)
- Lethargy, muscular weakness, a throbbing headache, nausea and vomiting
- Dizziness, confusion and disorientation, followed by convulsions and coma
- A bounding pulse, dilated pupils, cyanosis and pallor (the cherry red colour of the lips, so often described is in fact rarely seen during life)
- Pulmonary oedema, with respiratory depression
- (Investigation: Take blood and put into EDTA or lithium heparin bottle for carboxyhaemoglobin estimation. Do *not* get it spun down, or take blood for blood gas analysis, as many blood gas analysers will also give carboxyhaemoglobin levels)
- ECG: ischaemic changes
- About 12% of those recovering from CO poisoning develop a neuropsychiatric syndrome 2-8 weeks after apparently recovering, which presents with the acute onset of dementia and parkinsonism

Note: 1. Chronic low dose CO poisoning may cause gastrointestinal symptoms with general malaise, and is often missed in patients. The possibility of chronic CO poisoning should always be borne in mind, especially in cold weather
2. Pulse oximetry will give a false high reading in carbon monoxide poisoning, as the photo-detector is unable to distinguish oxy- from carboxy-haemoglobin

Management
- High flow oxygen with a tight fitting high concentration mask and a circuit which minimises rebreathing
- Respiratory support

Freons

Incidence
- Rarely encountered except in solvent abuse which is an increasing problem in some parts of the UK and is usually found in children and young adolescents

Aetiology
- Used as refrigerants and propellants in aerosols
- The mortality rate is high with significant exposure, usually in solvent abusers

Pathophysiology
- Usually only cardiotoxic when inhaled

Symptoms/signs
- Dyspnoea
- Headache, nausea, drowsiness, and unconsciousness
- Hyperactivity
- Cardiac arrest

Management
- Basic Life Support
- Oxygen
- Cardiac monitoring
- Intravenous infusion
- Consider using lidocaine for tachycardias

Toluene

Incidence
- This is the major substance involved in child solvent abuse (glue sniffing), resulting in the deaths of up to two children per week in the UK. May also be ingested

Aetiology
- Used as a solvent in: glue, paint, cleaning fluids, nail varnish remover
- Poisoning usually occurs as a result of accidental overexposure

Pathophysiology
- Hallucinogenic, can cause intoxication
- Nervous system depressant: may cause respiratory and cardiac arrest

Symptoms/signs
- Dry throat with cough, and chest tightness
- Dyspnoea and pulmonary oedema
- Drowsiness, confusion and unconsciousness, fits, coma and death

Management
- Oxygen/fresh air
- Airway care, with monitoring of the vital signs
- Reassurance
  (Recovery is usually fairly rapid and may be full within 20 minutes)

Sulphur dioxide, chlorine, phosgene

Incidence
- Relatively rare, but poisoning may be fatal
- Chlorine poisoning is the most common

Aetiology
- Inhalation is the usual mode of poisoning.
- Usually only found in accidental industrial poisoning
- Chlorine poisoning may occur:
    - In the home when lavatory cleaner and bleach are mixed
    - In public swimming baths

Pathophysiology
- Acidic gases causing:
    - Lung tissue damage resulting in pulmonary oedema, etc.

Symptoms/signs
- Coughing, choking (except phosgene)
- Breathlessness and cyanosis (this may develop suddenly up to 36 hr following exposure)

Management
- Observation for more than 36 hrs.
- If symptomatic:
    - Oxygen
    - Steroids

Note: For poisoning with other dangerous chemicals please refer to:
- "Substances Hazardous to Health: Emergency First Aid Guide" *and/or*
- Contact the nearest Poisons Information Centre (see end of this chapter)

Pesticides

Paraquat

Incidence
- Used to be responsible for a considerable, but now rapidly decreasing number of deaths

Aetiology
- Used to be a commonly used chemical in farming and market gardening
- Only toxic when ingested, but highly irritant to the eyes and skin

Pathophysiology
- Local cytotoxic effect
- Causes pulmonary fibrosis due to proliferative alveolitis and bronchiolitis
- Renal failure

Symptoms/signs
- Eyes:
    - Corneal and conjunctival ulceration
- Skin:
    - Irritation, blistering, and ulceration
- Inhalation of spray mist or dust:
    - Epistaxis, sore throat
- Ingestion:
    - Nausea, vomiting, diarrhoea
    - Ulceration of the lips, tongue and fauces within 36-48 hrs.
- Large overdose:
    - Multiple organ failure (hepatic and renal failure with myocarditis and pulmonary oedema within 6-48 hr
- Milder overdose:
    - Dyspnoea and hypoxia after initial recovery

Management
- Eyes:
    - Copious washing, antibiotic eyedrops
- Ingestion:
    - Activated charcoal, Fuller's earth or bentonite to adsorb the poison and reduce absorption
    - Careful gastric lavage/emptying (not emesis), and then further Fuller's earth/magnesium sulphate
    - Intravenous fluid replacement and analgesia

Note: Do *not* administer oxygen as this increases the pulmonary toxicity

Organophosphates
- Poisoning may be fatal

Incidence
- Found in many insecticides as powders or dissolved in organic solvents and in chemical warfare "nerve" agents

Aetiology
- May be absorbed accidentally through intact skin, accidentally or deliberately ingested or accidentally inhaled (rarely)

Pathophysiology:
- Causes parasympathetic stimulation; by inhibition of cholinesterase activity, leading to a build up of acetylcholine at muscarinic and nicotinic receptors
- May be absorbed through the skin, with symptoms similar to inhalation or ingestion
- May cause pulmonary oedema and general muscular paralysis

Symptoms/signs
- Skin contact:
    - Mild local erythema and irritation, followed by systemic effects
- Muscarinic effects:
    - Nausea, excessive sweating, and profuse salivation *(early)*
    - Epigastric and retrosternal discomfort, with abdominal cramps, vomiting and diarrhoea
    - Rhinorrhoea, bronchoconstriction with profuse bronchial secretion, dyspnoea, respiratory distress, pulmonary oedema and hypoxia, leading to respiratory arrest
    - Bradycardia, arrhythmias and finally asystole
    - Urinary and faecal incontinence
- Nicotinic effects:
    - Muscle twitching, followed by weakness, convulsions and flaccid paralysis, including ocular and respiratory muscle paralysis (in approximately 6 hours)
- Central nervous system effects:
    - Anxiety, restlessness, dizziness, confusion and headache *(early)*
    - Pupil constriction *(early)*
    - Convulsions

Management
- Oxygen (100%) with frequent suction to remove bronchial secretions
- Consider ventilation
- Remove clothing and decontaminate the skin with water and possibly use soap
- Consider induction of emesis after ingestion
- Start an intravenous infusion
- If the patient is symptomatic, administer:
    - Atropine 2 mg intravenously immediately
        - Repeat the intravenous dose every 5-10 minutes, until there are signs of atropinisation, i.e. dilated pupils, dry mouth, pulse rate >80 bpm
    - Pralidoxime 1g every 4 hours (only available at specialist centres), administer slowly intravenously
    - Diazepam: 2-15 mg intravenously, if fitting

Note: Never administer morphine or aminophylline as these exacerbate the effects of organophosphates

Acids

Aetiology
- Found in rust removers, car batteries, toilet cleaners, descalers, etc.

Pathophysiology
- Skin:
    - Produces localised burns.
- Ingestion (tend to burn the stomach):
    - Burning/pain around the mouth and oesophagus, with dysphagia
    - Abdominal pain, nausea and vomiting
- Inhalation:
    - Dyspnoea

Symptoms/signs
- As for burns

Management
- Ingestion:
    - Do *not* induce vomiting or perform gastric lavage
    - Give copious water immediately
- Burns:
    - See chapter on Burns

Alkalis

Aetiology
- Found in bleach (which is irritant and only corrosive in large quantities), washing soda, drain cleaner, ammonia and oven cleaner

Pathophysiology
- Skin:
    - Produces localised burns
- Ingestion
    - Tends to cause oesophageal burns, which may occur in the absence of oral burns
    - Burning/pain around the mouth
    - Retrosternal pain with heartburn with dysphagia
    - Abdominal pain, nausea and vomiting
- Inhalation:
    - Dyspnoea

Symptoms/signs
- Burning/pain around mouth and oesophagus
- Pain/difficulty in swallowing

Management
- Do *not* induce vomiting or perform gastric lavage
- Administer milk or water orally

Note: Never administer neutralising chemicals, as the neutralising reaction is highly exothermic and the heat produced may cause further significant injury

Petrol and petrol distillates

Incidence
- Accidental petrol ingestion is a rare problem in the UK
- Inhalation of petrol distillates is relatively common

Aetiology
- Petrol ingestion is usually caused by siphoning petrol
- Petrol distillates are a common constituent of many household products, e.g. lighter fuel, furniture polish, white spirit and turpentine

Pathophysiology
- Only toxic when ingested or inhaled in high concentrations
- Highly irritant to the respiratory mucosa, and may cause pulmonary oedema
- May result in vomiting and an aspiration pneumonia
- Absorption may result in cerebral and cardiac toxicity

Symptoms/signs
- Respiratory distress with cough, choking, cyanosis and pulmonary oedema
- Severe abdominal pain
- Cerebral irritability, convulsions and coma
- Hypoglycaemia may occur
- Cardiac arrhythmias may occur

Management
- Do *not* induce vomiting, as this may result in aspiration pneumonia
- Oxygen
- Airway care with intubation to protect the lungs from pulmonary aspiration
- Suction of any secretions (which may be copious)
- Circulatory support:
    - Intravenous infusion
- Cardiac monitoring
- All patients should go to hospital, even if they appear well initially

Poisonous plants and fungi

Incidence
- This is a relatively common cause of accidental poisoning
- Fungi: accidental ingestion is a relatively uncommon cause of poisoning in the UK
- Abuse of hallucinogenic fungi "magic mushrooms", e.g. *Amanita Psylocybus*, is fairly common
- It is relatively difficult to distinguish a Liberty Cap mushroom, which is non poisonous, but is used by some people for its hallucinogenic effects, from the amanita mushrooms

Aetiology
- Young children are most at risk from ingesting poisonous plants accidentally
- Adults may accidentally ingest poisonous fungi in the mistaken belief that they are edible
- Young adults may ingest hallucinogenic fungi deliberately, or poisonous mushrooms accidentally being under the mistaken impression that they are Liberty Cap mushrooms

Symptoms/signs
- Can be almost anything depending on the plant/fungus
- Symptoms of poisoning with Amanita mushrooms may be very delayed (main effect is hepatic failure)

Management
- Resuscitate as necessary.
- Reassure and obtain history:
    - Botanical or common name of plant/fungus if known
    - If possible sample of plant/fungus, or if not possible obtain a good description
    - Type and severity of exposure: skin contact, ingestion, etc.
    - If ingested, how much and which parts of the plant/fungus were eaten
    - Time of exposure/ ingestion, onset of symptoms and any treatment carried out
    - Age of patient
    - Symptoms
- Decide whether or not plant/fungus is toxic
- Contact your local poisons centre
- Induce emesis if advised.
- Activated charcoal (5-10 g) will bind most plant toxins, and reduces the severity of poisoning

Crowd control agents
- These substances are used by some Police forces for the control of major crowd problems/riots

Incidence
- The most commonly used agents are:
    - o-chlorobenzylidene malonitrile (CS)
    - l-chloroacetophenone (CN, constituent of Mace)
    - dibenzoxapine (CR)
    - oleoresin capsicum (OC, pepper spray)
- All these chemicals are crystalline in their natural state, but are packaged as liquid aerosols for convenient and relatively safe projection and dispersal

Note: The abbreviations are code names, and are not derived from the chemical names or formulae

Pathophysiology
- These chemicals cause severe irritation, which in most cases is short-lived and self limiting, of the:
    - Eyes
    - Skin
    - Mouth and upper respiratory tract
    - Lower respiratory tract (rare as these gases are highly water soluble and usually dissolve in secretions, before they reach the alveoli)
- There is some variation between the various chemicals in their effects:

o-chlorobenzylidene malonitrile (CS)
- Produces ten times more lacrimation than CN, but is less toxic

l-chloroacetophenone (CN, Mace)
- This is the most toxic of these agents; with reports of some deaths from respiratory problems/asphyxia

Dibenzoxapine (CR)
- This is the most potent lacrimator, but has the least systemic effects

Symptoms/signs
- Onset:
    - Virtually immediate
- Duration of action:
    - Usually 15-30 minutes after removal from exposure
    - Ocular and mucous membrane effects may occasionally last up to 24 hours
- Eyes:
    - Profuse secretion of tears (lacrimation), with blepharospasm, conjunctival erythema and periorbital oedema
    - Pain and blinking
- Skin:
    - Erythema and a burning sensation, which usually settles within 24 hours
    - Prolonged exposure may result in chemical burns, especially if the skin is wet
    - CR exposure may result in the skin becoming painful on contact with water up to 48 hours later
    - CN sensitises the skin and may cause an allergic contact dermatitis with pruritus, weeping and a papulovesicular rash, within 72 hours of exposure
    - CS may also cause an allergic contact dermatitis

- Mouth:
    - Burning sensation or stinging
    - Salivation
    - Nausea, vomiting (occasionally)
- Upper respiratory tract:
    - Sore throat, cough and laryngospasm
    - Sore nose with discomfort or a burning sensation, sneezing and rhinorrhoea
- Lower respiratory tract (patients with pre-existing respiratory disease, e.g. asthma, COPD, may be more severely affected):
    - Tight chest with bronchospasm
    - Pulmonary oedema may occur 12-24 after excessive exposure

Management
- In the majority of cases, the effects of these agents resolve spontaneously within 15-30 minutes after removal from exposure, and medical treatment is not usually indicated
- All medical staff involved should avoid any exposure and wear protective clothing including latex gloves

Removal of the cause
- All casualties should be removed from exposure to the gas, preferably in the fresh air
- Any contaminated clothing should be removed dry *if possible*, and placed in bags, which are immediately sealed

Eyes
- Tear secretions are usually sufficient to remove the chemical from the eye
- Symptomatic relief may be provided by blowing dry air onto the eyes with a fan
- Irrigation with N-Saline is indicated if the ocular effects are persistent

Skin
- Chemical burns should be managed in the same way as thermal burns
- Contact dermatitis may be treated with topical steroids

Respiratory tract
- Nebulised oxygen may provide some symptomatic relief before admission to hospital

Clothing
- This may be decontaminated by washing it several times in a conventional washing machine using normal washing powder or liquid, before it is worn again

Dangerous chemicals/medicines and their specific antidotes

Drug	Antidote	Action
β-blockers	Isoprenaline Glucagon	Pharmacological antagonist Stimulates myocardial adenylcyclase
Cyanide	Dicobalt edetate	Chelating agent
Methanol/Glycol	Ethanol	Competes with alcohol dehydrogenase
Organophosphates	Atropine	Acetylcholine antagonist
Opioids	Naloxone	Pharmacological antagonist
Paracetamol	N-Acetylcysteine Methionine	Glutathione precursors
Phenothiazines	Orphenadrine Procyclidine	Antiparkinsonism agents
Iron compounds	Desferrioxamine	Chelating agent
Sympathomimetics	β-blockers	Pharmacological antagonist

Figure 10-2 Dangerous substances and their specific antidotes

Poisons information centres in the UK

Centre	24 hour telephone number
Belfast	01232 240 503
Birmingham	0121 507 5588/9
Cardiff	01222 709 901
Dublin	0110 837 994/6
Edinburgh	0131 536 2300
Leeds	0113 243 0715 *or* 292 3547
London	0171 635 9191 *or* 955 5095
Newcastle	0191 232 5131

Figure 10-3 Poisons information centres in the United Kingdom

Notes

11

Heat related injury, drowning and dysbarism

Heat related injury

Introduction

- Heat related injury and illness is being encountered more and more due to the increased leisure time that many people enjoy, spending it on outdoor pursuits, when with inadequate experience and wearing inappropriate clothing, they may be unexpectedly exposed to the extremes of temperature and climate

Sunburn

Incidence
- Common in the summer months, and in those on snow and ice, especially at high altitudes
- More likely to occur in those who are unaccustomed to exposure to the sun

Aetiology
- Caused by excessive exposure to ultraviolet light
- Gradual exposure can lessen the effect due to tanning
- People with a fair complexion are the most at risk

Pathophysiology
- Similar to burns
- If large areas are involved, sunburn may result in heat hyperpyrexia

Symptoms/signs
- **Initially**
    - Erythema and itching
- **Later**
    - Pain, oedema and bullae
    - Malaise, headache and nausea

Management

Shock
- Rehydration: usually oral fluids are sufficient

Pain
- Sedation and antihistamines, e.g. chlorpheniramine

Dermal injury
- Calamine lotion

Note: Snow blindness caused by excessive ultraviolet radiation may affect those climbing on snow or ice at high altitudes. The management includes padding and analgesia

Heat illness

Heat cramps

Incidence
- Uncommon in the UK except in very hot weather and with prolonged vigorous exercise, e.g. marathon running, troops in training

Aetiology
- Occurs with vigorous exercise in hot climates

Pathophysiology
- Profuse sweating results in salt and water depletion
- This results in muscle cramps

Symptoms/signs
- The sudden onset of pain and cramps in the extremities
- There may be nausea and hypotension
- Hyperventilation

Management
- Move the patient to a cool environment
- Give copious oral fluids with added glucose, provided that nausea is not present
- If there is nausea or hypotension, establish an intravenous infusion with normal saline or dextrose 5%
- Treatment of hyperventilation (see under Medical Emergencies)

Heat exhaustion

Incidence
- Quite common after physical exertion, even in moderate temperatures

Aetiology
- Progression from heat cramps, i.e. it is a more severe condition
- This condition is more likely in the dehydrated, the unfit, the elderly and the hypertensive

Pathophysiology
- Salt and water loss, with additional peripheral pooling

Symptoms/signs
- Headache, fatigue, dizziness, confusion, nausea and abdominal cramping
- Syncope, collapse
- Profuse sweating, pale, with clammy skin
- A rapid, weak pulse, with hypotension and tachypnoea
- Normal or slightly elevated (<39°C) body temperature

Management
- Move the patient to a cool environment
- Cooling:
    - Fan
    - Tepid sponging
    - Immersion in lukewarm water
- Administer copious fluids (water) unless nausea is present
- Establish an intravenous infusion:
    - Crystalloid: Hartmann's solution or normal saline

Heat hyperpyrexia/heat stroke
- This is an *acute medical emergency* with a mortality rate of 25-50%

Incidence
- Rarely encountered in temperate climates, except for those taking part in physical activities requiring extreme exertion, even in relatively cool conditions
- Most commonly occurs in the young

Aetiology
- The same as heat exhaustion

Pathophysiology
- Begins as heat exhaustion.
- As the body's attempts to lose heat fail, the core temperature rises rapidly, and irreversible tissue damage occurs principally affecting the brain, kidneys and liver
- Circulatory collapse

Symptoms/signs
- Headache, dizziness, dry mouth
- Hot, flushed, and sometimes dry skin
- Hyperpyrexia (typically >40°C):
    - It is very important to take an accurate temperature, preferably with a tympanic membrane or rectal probe
- Strong, bounding pulse initially, followed by collapse
- Convulsions, coma and death

Management
- Rapid cooling:

Method 1
- Put the patient in a cool environment, e.g. a tepid bath (do *not* use ice)
- If the periphery is cooled too rapidly, however, peripheral cutaneous vasoconstriction may occur and this may prevent further core cooling

Method 2 (method of choice)
- Evaporative cooling in which the skin is kept moist while it is fanned strongly. This may be achieved with the patient lying on their side or supported in the hands and knees position, whilst the skin is wet with a spray of atomised water under pressure at 15 °C and fanned with warm air
- This maintains a high water pressure gradient from skin to air, facilitating rapid heat loss, without causing peripheral vasoconstriction

- Fluids:
    - Oral fluids (water or special glucose and electrolyte solution), if possible (may cause vomiting)
    - Intravenous infusion:
        - Rapid infusion of large volumes of crystalloid, plus colloid if there is any haemorrhage, with careful and continuous haemodynamic monitoring to avoid overinfusion or fluid shift
- Cardiac monitoring
- Treatment of fits

Hypothermia
- Exists when the body core temperature is <35°C

Incidence
- Wet hypothermia: immersion is a major cause in the UK
    - The North Sea is warmest in August and coldest in March, Even in Summer the temperature of the sea rarely goes above 15°C at which temperature many casualties will not survive for more than 2-3 hours. In winter the sea temperature often goes below 5°C, at which temperature most casualties will not survive for more than 2-3 minutes
- Dry hypothermia:
    - Incidence and mortality are doubled with each 5°C fall in ambient outside temperature
    - Males are more likely to die than females

Aetiology
- Occurs when the rate of heat produced by metabolism is less than the rate of heat loss from the body
- Can affect any age or fitness group
- Water immersion
- Dry hypothermia usually occurs in the elderly:
    - Following a fall, they may be unable to get up
    - May be due to poor heating and impaired cold perception
    - May occur due to diabetes mellitus
- May be due to cold exposure:
    - Accidents in bad weather/hostile environments
    - Alcoholic intoxication
    - Sporting events: mountaineering, climbing, marathons in cold wet weather

Pathophysiology
- The elderly (less efficient metabolism, myocardium and circulation) and the young (greater relative surface area and small subcutaneous fat and energy stores) are particularly susceptible
- A fall in the body temperature results:
    - *Initially:*
        - In increased heat production: shivering
        - In reduced heat loss: peripheral vasoconstriction
    - *Later* (at body temperatures below 35°C):
        - Shivering stops
        - A reduction in ventilation and later ventilatory arrest
        - Slowing of body metabolism: reduction in oxygen requirement/carbon dioxide production
        - Cardiovascular:
            - Hypotension
            - The myocardium becomes electrically unstable: cardiac arrhythmias (usually VF)
            - Sludging of the blood
            - Cardiac arrest
        - A metabolic acidosis

Symptoms/signs

Moderate hypothermia (body temperature between 35 and 32ºC)
- Behavioural/personality changes, slurred speech, incoordination, confusion, drowsiness, apathy/lethargy.
- Shivering, pallor, cold skin
- Stumbling and slowing of physical activity
- Low rectal/oral temperature (use a low reading thermometer)

Pathophysiology of hypothermia

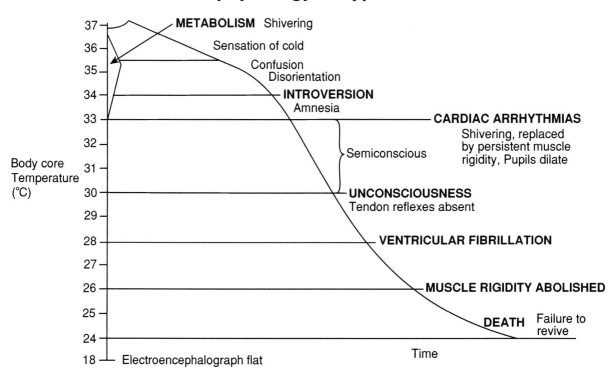

Figure 11-1 Pathophysiology of hypothermia

Severe hypothermia (body temperature below 32 ºC)
- The patient may be unconscious or stuporose, with non reacting pupils
- The skin may be ice cold
- They may be bradypnoeic
- They may have no detectable pulse or blood pressure, with inaudible heart sounds

Management
- Protect yourself: do not expose yourself to the risk of becoming a cold casualty:
    - Do not become exhausted
    - Do not donate your protective clothing to others, including the casualty you are trying to help

All cold casualties
- Lay the casualty flat, treat any significant injuries and resuscitate if indicated
- Prevent further heat loss by enclosing the casualty (including the head, but allowing for ventilation) in:
    - Heavy gauge plastic bags (if available)
    - Sleeping bag
    - Space blankets (need a heat source inside to be effective, not so robust and may not be effective in a hostile environment, i.e. difficult to make airtight)
- Insulate the casualty from the ground and provide overall wind and waterproof protection, as necessary

- Provide further protection from the elements by finding/creating a shelter if possible
- Remove the casualty, lying flat, to a warmer environment, so as to reduce any further heat loss
- Gently rewarm the casualty, without removing their insulation (so as to avoid rapid surface rewarming):
  - Consider "airway insulation" with a heat and moisture exchanger. If this is not available, a scarf over the mouth and nose will help
  - Oxygen may be beneficial, but should not be used if the cylinder is very cold
- Consider body surface rewarming with hot water bottles or hot packs (beware of direct contact as this may cause burns), and be careful as rapid rewarming of the surface may result in severe hypotension
- Carefully monitor the patient's respiration and pulse

Cold, conscious or confused casualties
- Once under shelter:
  - If their clothing is wet, replace it with dry clothing
  - If their clothing is dry, keep them wrapped up and allow them to rewarm slowly
- Give the casualty a warm sweet drink (but no alcohol), but only if they are able to swallow easily (may have little effect on body temperature, but can be comforting)
- Obtain any significant medical history, e.g. diabetes mellitus, epilepsy
- If immediate evacuation to a hospital is not possible:
  - Immerse the casualty up to the neck in warm water (maintained at approximately 40°C, which is comfortable both for your elbow and the casualty)
  - Remove any heavy outer clothing before immersion and any remaining clothing later after the casualty has been put into the bath
  - Cessation of shivering should occur shortly after immersion, but this is *not* an indication for removal from the hot water
  - When the casualty is comfortably warm, remove them from the bath, encourage them to lie down flat, dry them and then cover them with blankets (if they complain of feeling hot or dizzy, make them get out of the bath)
  - Keep the casualty lying flat until they feel warm, and have a near normal body temperature

Unconscious or semiconscious casualties
- Remove the casualty from the cold to a warm environment, wrapped up in blankets or a sleeping bag.
- Gently remove wet clothing (be very careful, as rough handling may precipitate ventricular fibrillation)
- Carefully place the casualty in the recovery position, until they regain consciousness, and then keep them lying down until they are warm

Cardiopulmonary resuscitation of cold casualties
- In spite of appearing to be dead, patients with severe hypothermia can survive, and every effort should be made to continue the attempt to resuscitate them, until they have been rewarmed to normal body temperature. The patient should not be confirmed deceased until the body temperature has been brought up to near normal or attempts to raise core temperature have failed
- Full neurological recovery is possible even after prolonged arrest, as hypothermia reduces cerebral oxygen requirements

Basic Life Support
- Maintain a clear airway and administer oxygen
- If breathing is absent, is less than 5 breaths per minute, becomes obstructed or stops, perform expired air ventilation at a rate of 8-12 ventilations per minute
- *Only* start chest compressions if:
  - There is no carotid pulse detectable after palpating for at least one minute (the pulse is often slow and weak in severe hypothermia)
  - Cardiac arrest is observed, i.e. a pulse was present, but has subsequently disappeared
  - There is a reasonable possibility that the cardiac arrest occurred within the previous 2 hours

- There is a reasonable expectation that effective CPR can be provided continuously (or with only brief interruptions to allow for movement of the casualty), until they can be removed to a location where full ALS can be provided
- If at any time a pulse is detectable, chest compressions should be stopped
- Hypothermia may cause stiffness of the chest wall, which can result in increased resistance to chest compression

Advanced Life Support
- Monitor the cardiac rhythm:
    - If the patient is in asystole or ventricular fibrillation, start Basic/Advanced Life Support
- Defibrillation may not be effective at temperatures below 30°C.
- Drugs should be administered in a reduced dosage during rewarming, so as to reduce the amount of peripheral pooling
- Use bretylium (5 mg/kg) instead of lidocaine, which is not effective at low temperatures
- Arrhythmias other than VF tend to revert to normal sinus rhythm spontaneously as the core temperature rises, and do not require treatment
- Continue ALS until the patient is fully rewarmed, or until effective respiration and circulation return.
- Administer an intravenous infusion of warmed fluid at 40°C, preferably via a central vein:
    - Use a buffered solution of crystalloid, with sodium bicarbonate if cardiac arrest is prolonged
- Insert a nasogastric tube
- Monitor the patient's rectal temperature, using a low reading thermometer or thermocouple
- Convey to hospital in the head down position
- Remember that no victim of hypothermia is dead until their core is warm and dead

Frostbite

Incidence
- Rarely encountered in the UK, except in extreme weather conditions

Aetiology
- Exposure of the extremities to subzero temperatures (with or without windchill) may occur in cold climates, or may be due to exposure to very cold liquids/gases

Pathophysiology
- The heat injury is very similar to burns as the mechanism of injury is similar
- Usually affects the fingers, toes and exposed extremities (may also very rarely affect the male genitalia)

Symptoms/signs
- Pricking pain, loss of sensation, followed by severe pain as the affected part warms up
- Skin discolouration: waxy white, mottled blue
- Blistering
- Hardness
- Impaired movement

Management
- Removal of the patient from the cold
- Management of hypothermia
- Gentle removal of clothing, avoiding damage to the skin, or bursting of blisters, etc.
- Rewarm in warm water at about 40°C (checked with a thermometer) until completely rewarmed
- Analgesia, as required, from aspirin up to and including morphine
- Do *not* allow the patient to smoke as nicotine may cause peripheral vasoconstriction

Near drowning

Introduction

- The problems associated with swimming is a relatively specialised part of Immediate Care and only something that those who live on or near the coast, or near large inland waterways, will experience with any regularity. However, all of us go on holiday, often near the sea, and so should have some idea as to the problems involved

Drowning

- Children often survive after near drowning in the British Isles, especially if they have been hypothermic (30% of children with fixed dilated pupils may survive fully neurologically intact)

Incidence
- Usually occurs in summer, particularly in children and teenage males
- Drowning is the third most common cause of accidental death in the UK, responsible for about 1000 deaths and over 5,000 near drownings per annum in the UK (most occurring inland)
- 50% occur within 5m of land, 75% occur in an unsupervised area

Aetiology
- In young adults alcohol plays a major part

Pathophysiology
- Deaths are due to:
  - Cold Shock
  - Drowning
  - Hypothermia
- Unlike other situations respiratory arrest occurs before cardiac arrest

Cold challenge
- The colder the temperature; the longer the heart can remain stopped without major problems. The main limiting factor is the development of ventricular fibrillation

Lung injury
- Water inhalation: 10% have no water in the lungs, and there is rarely more than 1.5 litres in the lungs

Brain injury
- Hypoxia, resulting in cerebral oedema
- The lower the temperature, the less the injury
- Cerebral oedema may increase as the patient warms up

Electrolyte changes
- Relatively unimportant
- Hypokalaemia: salt and fresh water
- Hypernatraemia: salt water
- Hyponatraemia: infants in fresh water

Cold water drowning (temp <10 °C or below)
- Initial response (**cold shock**):
    - The patient gives an inspiratory gasp followed by hyperventilation
    - This can precipitate death by inhalation of water and wet drowning
    - May also precipitate sudden hypertension and severe cardiac arrhythmias and arrest
- Short term (up to 15-20 minutes):
    - Inability to cope with cold shock:
        - Hyperventilation continues and swimming/breathing becomes uncoordinated, leading to water inhalation and wet drowning
- Long term:
    - Hypothermia:
        - Wet drowning
        - Ventricular fibrillation
- Post rescue circulatory collapse:
    - During immersion, the hydrostatic pressure of the water supports an otherwise compromised circulation (hydrostatic squeeze)
    - When the body is removed from the water, and the patient is subjected to gravity, this support is suddenly removed. This may result in catastrophic circulatory collapse (similar to suddenly deflating a PASG)
    - This effect may be exacerbated by rapid rewarming

Management
- All those casualties suffering from hypothermia should be handled very carefully to avoid precipitating cardiac arrythmias

Respiratory problems

No apparent water inhalation
- If some water is aspirated:
    - Adult respiratory distress syndrome (ARDS) may develop 0-72 hours later
        - *Signs:*
            - Cough, rising respiratory rate, crackles on chest auscultation.
        - *Management:*
            - Observation for 24 hours:
                - If they develop signs of ARDS: early aggressive ARDS management (O_2, PEEP)

Note: 12-20% of patients with no apparent water inhalation die for no known reason --"dry drowning":
- This may possibly be due to a primitive diving reflex:
    - Results in laryngeal spasm and bradycardia.
In children, spontaneous respiratory effort is associated with a full recovery

Some water inhalation, but adequate ventilation

Incidence:
- Commonest group

Signs:
- Respiratory distress, cyanosis and painful wheezy breathing

Management:
- Oxygen
- Admit for observation

Water inhalation and inadequate ventilation

Management:
- Clear the airway: if it is blocked by water consider:
    - Inversion
- Mouth to mouth/mask, expired air resuscitation
- Oxygen (100%) using an oxygen reservoir (because of the severe hypoxia resulting from drowning)
- Ventilation: high pressures may be needed due to increased pulmonary compliance
- Frequent suctioning (or turn the patient onto their side to allow drainage of fluid from the mouth).
- If the patient is unconscious consider:
    - Intubation
    - Insertion of a nasogastric tube

Note: Most water is usually in the stomach; getting it out by any method other than by a nasogastric tube risks causing pulmonary aspiration of the gastric contents

No ventilation or cardiac output

Management
- Basic Life Support (this should be started in the water if possible)
- Advanced airway and cardiac management

Cardiovascular problems

Cardiac arrest
- This may often be delayed
- Ventricular fibrillation is the usual mode of death

Symptoms/signs
- Pulse: feel for the carotid pulse for at least 10 seconds
- The skin colour is often misleading

Management
- Basic life support:
    - If the heart restarts, the survival rate increases from 8% to 70%
    - This should be started only if it can be continued for at least 1 hour or until the body temperature is greater than 32 °C (34 °C core temperature), and you are reasonably near a hospital
- ECG and temperature monitoring should be carried out continuously
- Advanced Cardiac Life Support:
    - Defibrillation should be performed for ventricular fibrillation, but not until the patient's temperature >32 °C (the myocardium is not responsive to defibrillation at very low temperatures).
- If the patient has poor peripheral perfusion, with signs suggestive of hypovolaemia, then administer an intravenous infusion of colloid (with sodium bicarbonate 8.4%, if resuscitation is prolonged)

Circulatory collapse

Management
- The body should be held horizontally with the legs elevated before removal from the water, to minimise the effects of the hydrostatic squeeze and kept in this position, until they have recovered (at least 30 minutes)
- If there are signs of circulatory collapse, put up an intravenous infusion and monitor the BP and pulse
- Rewarming should be carefully controlled

Cold injury

Management
- If the patient is conscious:
    - Rapid rewarming, e.g. in a bath, is indicated, if immersion has been brief
    - Gradual rewarming, for prolonged immersion (the temperature may fall initially for 5-10 minutes)
  - If the patient is unconscious:
    - Rewarm slowly in clothing with insulation (plastic bag, etc.). This reduces the risk of increasing any cerebral oedema, or circulatory collapse
- Monitor the patient's temperature continuously with an aural or rectal thermometer or thermocouple

Note: Too rapid warming may result in rewarming collapse:
    - Remove the casualty from the heat, lower the head and elevate the legs

Brain injury

Management
- Basic and Advanced Life Support (to improve/maintain cerebral oxygenation)

Associated problems
- Head/Neck injuries:
    - Immobilise the neck in a rigid cervical collar, if there is *any* possibility of a cervical spine injury
- Myocardial infarction
- Cerebrovascular accidents
- Epilepsy
- Hypoglycaemia
- Alcoholic intoxication/drug abuse
- Diving dysbarism
- Secondary drowning: acute pulmonary oedema

Guidelines for the management of near drowning

Basic Life Support (this should be started in the water if possible)
- Airway management: with stabilisation of the cervical spine if injury is suspected (cervical collar)
- Breathing: expired air ventilation
- Circulation: external chest compressions

Remove from the water: without allowing the casualty to pull you in!

Advanced airway management

Hypothermia: Dry and start rewarming

Monitor temperature continuously

Advanced Cardiac Life Support: as the temperature rises and it is likely to be effective

Treat any associated problems

Resuscitation should be continued for at least 45 minutes and/or until the body temperature is near normal

---

Figure 11-2 Guidelines for the management of near drowning

Dysbarism

Introduction

- This is a condition caused by rapid changes in the environmental pressures to which the patient is subjected
- Many patients suffering from dysbarism may also be suffering from other associated problems, e.g. near drowning, hypothermia, injury accidents
- Dysbarism is a relatively rare problem and is only something that military doctors and those who have an interest in diving, climbing or flying will come across in normal circumstances

High altitude: low pressure dysbarism

Incidence
- Virtually unknown in the UK, as there are no mountains over 1500 m high, but may occur due to sudden depressurisation in aircraft
- Occurs equally in the old, young, male, female, fit and unfit
- Those who have experienced problems once are more likely to suffer again

Aetiology
- A significant reduction in atmospheric pressure may occur during flying/climbing at altitudes greater than 3500 m (aircraft cabin pressures go up to 2750 m)

Pathophysiology
- At high altitudes, there is less oxygen due to the reduced atmospheric pressure, and hypoxia develops
- Too rapid an ascent does not allow physiological compensation to occur
- Acute mountain sickness, due to mild cerebral oedema, may occur at heights >2500 m, affecting 70% of people at heights between 3500-4000 m.
- At heights above 4000 m, about 2% of people develop high altitude pulmonary oedema (HAPE) resulting in cardio-respiratory failure and cardiac arrest
- At heights above 4500 m, about 1% of people will develop high altitude cerebral oedema (HACE), usually resulting in death
- Above 5000 m, 50% of people will suffer from flame shaped retinal haemorrhages, leading to blindness

Symptoms/signs

Acute mountain sickness (AMS)
- Dyspnoea, tachycardia, lethargy and insomnia
- Headache, nausea, anorexia, vomiting and diarrhoea

High altitude pulmonary oedema (HAPE)
- Rapid onset of severe breathlessness, nocturnal dyspnoea, chest pain and cough with haemoptysis

High altitude cerebral oedema (HACE)
- Worsening headache, drowsiness, ataxia, nystagmus and papilloedema
- Irrationality, hallucinations, unconsciousness, coma and death

Note: Recent research suggests that a rise in body temperature after rapid ascent to high altitude is a sign of acute mountain sickness, and is associated with the severity of hypoxaemia

Management
- Removal to a low altitude
- Oxygen
- Mountain sickness:
    - Antiemetics: prochlorperazine buccal preparation (*Buccastem®*), metoclopramide
    - Oral electrolyle replacement: *Dioralyte®*, *Rehidrat®*, *Electrolade®*
- High altitude pulmonary oedema:
    - Diuretics, e.g. furosemide
    - Intubation and ventilation (possibly with PEEP)
    - Nifedipine 20 mg S/R 6 hourly
- High altitude cerebral oedema:
    - Dexamethasone: 8 mg initially followed by 4 mg 6 hourly, or betamethasone

Note: Portable pressure chambers may have some value in the management of acute mountain sickness

Diving diseases: low altitude: high pressure dysbarism

- Diving is a very popular sport with over 100,000 participants in the UK
- Some 200-250 cases of serious dysbarism occur annually in the civilian population
- Although most patients present to coastal centres, a significant number present to their GP or local Accident and Emergency department as the onset of symptoms may be delayed and not recognised as being diving related
- Diving to deeper than 50 metres is usually done only by professional divers, who have their own specialist occupational health and medical backup offshore. Any problems that they may encounter are beyond the scope of this book.

Compression barotrauma (compression dysbarism)

Aetiology
- Only found in divers or fliers

Pathophysiology
- As a diver descends in the water the pressure around him increases by 1 atmosphere for every 10 metres (33 ft) descended
- As the pressure increases, gas becomes compressed
- Human tissues are incompressible, but hollow spaces, e.g sinuses, the lungs, etc. are not
- Unless extra gas enters these spaces, either:
    - The space will either collapse (lungs, chest or abdomen) *and/or*
    - Extra fluid or tissue will be drawn into the space (sinuses)

Ear compression barotrauma

Incidence
- This is a relatively common problem, especially in inexperienced divers

Pathophysiology
- If the pressure on one side of the tympanic membrane is very much greater than that on the other side, injury to the membrane will result
- This may be:
    - Haemorrhage
    - Rupture, sometimes with obliteration of the middle ear space by a serosanguinous exudate

Symptoms/signs
- Pain in the ear: usually very severe

Management
- Prevention:
    - Clearing the ears (Valsalva manoeuvre): this allows pressure equalisation on both sides of the tympanic membrane
- Analgesia:
    - Oral analgesics are usually adequate
    - Do *not* use nitrous oxide when there is any indication of decompression sickness

Round window rupture

Incidence
- Rare

Symptoms (similar to those from inner ear decompression illness)
- Tinnitus
- Deafness
- Disorientation
- Giddiness

Management
- Urgent assessment by an ear, nose and throat specialist

Sinus compression barotrauma

Pathophysiology
- If the openings to the sinuses become blocked due to catarrhal swelling, polypi or a deviated nasal septum, pressure equalisation between the sinuses and the upper respiratory tract cannot take place
- On descent, the volume of air in the sinus decreases and because the bone of the sinus is rigid, a negative pressure develops inside the sinus, which then becomes filled with transudate
- During ascent, the air in the sinus re-expands, and aggravates the injury to the previously traumatised mucosa (lining) of the sinus
- If large vessels are involved there may be severe haemorrhage
- May (rarely) result in facial nerve neuropraxia

Symptoms/signs
- There may be severe pain
- Haemorrhage from nose
- Facial weakness (may be difficult to distinguish from weakness caused by gas embolism, or cranial nerve involvement in decompression illness)

Management
- Pain relief (do *not* use nitrous oxide/oxygen mixture, if there is *any* indication of decompression illness)
- Treatment of shock, if the haemorrhage is severe

Pulmonary compression barotrauma

Incidence
- Only occurs in breath holding divers and is very rare

Pathophysiology
- As the diver descends, the volume of gas (air) in the lungs decreases and it becomes more dense, due to the increase in pressure:
  - At 30 metres (99 ft) depth the pressure increases to 4 atmospheres (atmospheric pressure + 3 atmospheres)
- In the breath holding diver, the lung volume gets smaller until it approaches the residual volume, resulting in a change in the chest configuration from one of inspiration to one of expiration. Further descent and resulting pressure increase will result in haemorrhage into the alveoli (*chest squeeze*).
- In order to overcome these problems, the diver needs to be supplied with air, which is at the same pressure as the surrounding water. This is done either by:
  - Supplying air at the appropriate pressure via an air line *or*
  - A self-contained underwater breathing apparatus (SCUBA), which supplies air at the appropriate pressure via a demand valve.

Symptoms/signs
- Dyspnoea, with respiratory distress and cyanosis.
- Ventilatory insufficiency, and pulmonary oedema.

Management
- Careful evacuation to the surface.
- Oxygen.
- Artificial ventilation, using PEEP, if there is low arterial oxygen tension.

Decompression illness

Aetiology
- Occurs on return to atmospheric pressure following significant exposure to increased pressure (depth and time) as a consequence of inert gas bubble formation or air embolism due to pulmonary barotrauma (see below):
  - Too rapid an ascent from depth without due regard to the Diving Tables. These dictate the speed of ascent and the number of stops necessary, depending on the depth dived and the time spent at that depth:
    - Poor diving discipline
    - Following equipment failure
    - Accident and panic
    - Submarine escape
    - May occur from *any* dive in which air is breathed from a SCUBA
  - May even (rarely) occur if standard decompression procedures (Diving Tables/Computers) are followed rigorously
  - Sudden decompression in an aircraft

Pathophysiology
- As pressure is reduced, gases expand
- If the reduction in pressure is too rapid, it may cause problems for the human body in two ways:

Inert gas disease: the "bends"
- Gases which are usually dissolved in the blood and tissues, form bubbles
    - These bubbles may be intravascular and/or extravascular, and they cause problems in two ways:
        - Have a mechanical effect: blocking arterioles, etc.
        - There is a reaction at the bubble/tissue interface resulting in:
            - Protein denaturation
            - Lipid emboli
            - Red cell sludging
            - Platelet aggregation
            - Activation of clotting mechanisms
            - Histamine release

Pulmonary decompression barotrauma: air embolism
- As the diver ascends, the air in the lungs expands. He should breathe out, but if he does not, or if a mucus plug obstructs an alveolus, pressure builds up in the alveoli and alveolar rupture may occur.
    - The rupture may extend:
        - Through the visceral pleura to cause a pneumothorax
        - Anteriorly to cause a pneumopericardium, mediastinal emphysema and subcutaneous emphysema
        - Into the pulmonary veins to cause a pulmonary air embolism, resulting in an arterial air embolism usually in the brain or limbs, but it may affect any part of the body

Note: In practice the disease has a wide spectrum of symptomatology, and it is frequently not possible to distinguish between inert gas disease and pulmonary decompression barotrauma, which are together referred to as decompression illness

Symptoms/signs
- These may vary very considerably depending on the individual patient's physiology, the rate of ascent, and the duration and depth of the dive

Mild decompression illness
- Symptoms usually begin within the first hour of surfacing, but may be delayed for up to and occasionally more than 24 hours
- Unexplained fatigue, malaise and anorexia
- Transient pruritus especially of the shoulders and trunk
- Musculoskeletal pain around synovial joints (*Limb or joint bends*):
    - This usually begins as an ache, and initially is often attributed to physical exertion, lifting heavy equipment, etc.
    - '*Niggles*', flitting pains between joints may occur (tend to be associated with deep or saturation dives), before becoming poorly localised in the limb around the joints and more severe.
        - Most common sites:
            - Shoulder
            - Knee
    - It is rare for there to be associated tenderness; if this is present, consider another cause
- Skin rashes:
    - Trunk/abdomen:
        - Patches of cutaneous venous stasis and cyanosis
    - Limbs:
        - Cutaneous and subcutaneous oedema, occasionally with swelling and tenderness of the regional lymph nodes
    - Any part of the body:
        - Local oedema due to bubble formation in lymphatics (rare).

More severe decompression illness
- Usually appears within a few minutes of surfacing, but may be delayed for several hours

Neurological effects (the most common)
- Usually affects the brain or spinal cord, and very rarely the peripheral nerves
- Any neurological deficit or combination of lesions may occur (often from more than one site)
    - Cerebral decompression illness:
        - Unconsciousness
        - Visual disturbance, particularly of peripheral vision
        - Migraine-like headaches
        - Behavioural alteration: cognitive dysfunction, personality and mood changes
        - Symptoms/signs of a cerebrovascular accident: ataxia
    - Spinal decompression illness:
        - Paralysis or paresis of limbs (commonly)
        - Paraesthesiae
        - Girdle pains of the trunk
        - Bladder, sphincter or sexual dysfunction
    - Inner ear decompression illness:
        - Vertigo with nausea and vomiting (*Staggers*)
        - Tinnitus (this may be difficult to distinguish from barotrauma to the inner ear)

Pulmonary effects (*Chokes*)
- May develop slowly, and are rarely associated with neurological damage:
    - Chest pain due to:
        - Pneumothorax
    - Retrosternal pain on inspiration due to mediastinal emphysema
    - Dyspnoea
    - Signs of hypoxia in severe cases

Circulatory effects (occurs due to the rise in capillary permeability)
- Hypovolaemia
- Haemoconcentration
- Hypotension
- Peripheral circulatory failure

Dermatological effects
- Subcutaneous emphysema (additional symptoms include change of voice quality)

Management
- Recompression (treatment of choice):
    - This should be done as soon as possible; the patient will be recompressed and treated with hyperbaric oxygen
    - Any delay may lead to deterioration in the patient's condition
- Prior to and during transport:
    - Oxygen:
        - 100% which may displace the less soluble nitrogen from the air bubbles
    - Intubation:
        - If the patient requires intubation, the cuff should be filled with water rather than air (volume change during recompression)
    - Ventilation:
        - Should be done with great care, and if symptomatic, chest drains inserted immediately if there is any evidence of a pneumothorax

- Intravenous infusion:
    - In every severe case
    - If there is evidence of hypovolaemia
    - Crystalloid is generally preferred to colloid, although some think that Dextran 40 may have specific advantages due to its low molecular size, in spite of the risk of it causing renal tubular necrosis
- Steroids:
    - Dexamethasone: 16 mg administered intravenously immediately followed by 10-12 mg 6 hourly may be considered for patients with cerebral problems.
- Analgesia:
    - Not often used
    - Paracetamol is preferred (aspirin make aggravate capillary bleeding within the nervous system)
    - Nitrous oxide/oxygen mixture (Entonox/Nitronox) is *absolutely contraindicated*
- Sedation/fits
    - Intravenous midazolam or diazepam
- Catheterisation
    - It is prudent to assess whether or not the patient can empty his bladder. If not, he should be catheterised, and the catheter balloon filled with water and *not* air

Note: *Any symptoms presenting within 36 hours of a dive should be considered to be due to dysbarism until proven otherwise*

Transportation of the patient with high pressure dysbarism
- If air transport is used, e.g. helicopter:
    - The pilot should fly below 300 metres, if possible, as any significant reduction in pressure will aggravate the patient's condition
- With road transport:
    - In mountainous areas the lower altitude route is to be preferred
- In order to assist the doctor receiving the patient for recompression, the following information should be supplied:
    - Depth and duration of last two dives
    - Any problems with ascent or descent
    - Whether the patient became unduly cold or worked particularly hard during their dive
    - Was the patient's diving discipline good or did he omit any decompression procedures (stops)
    - Whether the patient's symptoms worsened, if they have flown following the dive.
    - Whether there has been any change in the patient's symptoms following the administration of 100% oxygen

Note: All the diving equipment used and the patient's diving partner "buddy" should always accompany the patient to the treatment (recompression) facility

Other diving problems
- Diving dysbarism in particular may be associated with other problems, which may considerably complicate management:
    - Near drowning
    - Hypothermia
    - Breathing bad air: carbon monoxide is the commonest

Advice on medical diving problems in the UK

- The Royal Navy provides a **24 hour emergency advice service**, which will give information on:
    - The location of the nearest medical diving problem treatment facility (recompression chamber)
    - The emergency management of diving related illness

- The **emergency telephone number** is: **0831 151523** (cellular telephone)
    - If there is difficulty in obtaining a reply, use:
    Portsmouth (01705) - 768026 (direct line) during the working day (0800 - 1600)
    - 818888 out of hours

- Please state that you have a medical diving problem

Figure 11-3 Advice on medical diving problems in the United Kingdom

12

Kinetics and Mechanisms of injury

Kinetics and mechanisms of injury

Introduction

- In the pre-hospital situation, it is seldom appropriate or indeed possible to take a complete and accurate history and perform a full head to toe examination of the casualty
- Casualties may not be capable of giving an accurate history, because of their injuries and the emotional shock of what has happened to them, and may not be aware of significant and sometimes life threatening injuries
- It is therefore essential that the Immediate Care practitioner is able to make deductions about the casualty's probable injuries from observing the accident scene and working out the mechanism of injury. To do so he must have an understanding of the physics involved and the way in which impacts occur, how energy is transferred and the types and patterns of injury that can result

Mechanics of injury

- To understand the mechanics of injury, a knowledge of the relevant physical principles and laws is essential
- Energy cannot be created or destroyed, but can be changed in form. The form of energy may be mechanical, thermal, electrical or chemical:
    - When a body stops moving as a result of impacting with another body, some of its energy may be transferred to that other body (causing it to move), and some of it may be changed in form to thermal and chemical energy (resulting in deformity/damage to both bodies)

Newton's First Law of motion
- A body will remain at rest, and a body in motion will remain in motion, unless it is acted upon by some other outside force

Newton's Second Law of motion
- The rate of change of momentum is proportional to the force producing that change, and takes place in the same direction as the applied force

Newton's Third Law of motion
- To every active force, there is always an equal and opposite reactive force

Kinetic energy
- **Kinetic energy = ½ mass x (velocity)^2**
    - Mass is the body weight and velocity is the speed of that body:
        - Velocity (speed) increases the production of kinetic energy more than mass, thus the speed of impact is more important than the mass (weight) of the impacting objects

Force
- **Force = mass x acceleration or deceleration**
- **Impact energy**: energy used up in deforming the objects involved in an impact
- The effect of the release of energy following an impact will depend on:
    - The nature of the materials and the way in which energy is dissipated/dispersed through them:
        - A fall into snow, which is soft will cause less damage than a fall onto concrete. The body will penetrate the snow and deceleration will be relatively slow as it takes place over a greater distance. If a body falls onto concrete, which is hard and non penetrable; deceleration will be very rapid as it occurs immediately
    - The area over which the impact takes place and the energy that is released:
        - If the area of impact is small, the amount of energy released per unit area will be greater than if the area is large: impact with a sharp instrument will cause more local damage than with a blunt one
    - Whether the release of energy (deceleration) is gradual or sudden:
        - If all the energy is transferred suddenly; it will cause more damage than if it is transferred gradually, e.g. before an impact, the driver of a vehicle will be moving at the same speed as the vehicle. If the vehicle stops suddenly due to an impact, car and driver will decelerate to a standstill almost simultaneously, with most of the considerable decelerative force being transmitted to the driver. If the stopping distance is increased, the deceleration will be less, resulting in proportionately less decelerative force, vehicle damage and injury

Cavitation
- In blunt trauma:
    - Injury is caused by compression of the tissues under the area of impact
- In penetrating trauma:
    - Injury is caused by compression and separation of the tissues along the track of the penetrating object
- Both types of trauma will result in cavity formation, as the tissues are forced out of their usual position
- Cavitation occurs as the tissues which have impacted with the penetrating object, move away from the point of impact and the track of that object as it penetrates further into the body
- The cavities thus created may form and reform several times until all the kinetic energy transferred from the penetrating object has been dissipated
- The amount of cavitation produced and hence the extent of the injury (tissue damage) caused is directly proportional to the amount of impact energy transferred and will depend on:
    - The density of the tissues with which the penetrating object impacts and through which it passes
    - The size of the frontal area of the penetrating object
    - The elasticity of the various body tissues involved
- In blunt trauma there is only a temporary cavity formation
- In penetrating trauma (especially gunshot injury) there is both permanent and temporary cavity formation:
    - When a fast moving object (high kinetic energy) with a small frontal area impacts with a tissue, it releases its kinetic energy over a small area
    - If this exceeds the tensile strength of the tissue, the object will penetrate that tissue, resulting in permanent cavity formation
    - At the same time a temporary cavity will be formed both in front of the object and to the side of its track through the tissue

Blunt trauma

- In blunt trauma, injury occurs as a result of the release or transfer of energy produced by:
    - Compression of tissues
    - A sudden change in velocity: acceleration or deceleration
    - Shearing forces

Compression injuries

- Occur when tissue damage is caused by crushing or squeezing
- May affect both the body surface and its internal organs
- Compression is the most common mechanism of injury

Head

- Compression of the head may result in:
    - Skull fractures, which in turn may cause:
        - Vascular injury; including extradural and subdural haemorrhage
        - Cerebral contusion

Thorax

- Compression of the thorax may result in:
    - Fractured ribs, including flail chest
    - Pulmonary contusion and pneumothorax
    - Cardiac contusion as a result of compression of the heart between the sternum and the dorsal spine

Abdomen

- Compression of the abdomen may result in:
    - Crushing of organs between the anterior abdominal wall and the posterior thoracic cage and lumbar spine, rupturing them resulting in damage to the spleen, liver, pancreas and sometimes the kidneys
    - A sudden rise in intra-abdominal pressure, usually from a frontal impact, resulting in rupture of the diaphragm (the weakest wall of the abdomen), which in turn may result in:
        - Loss of use of the diaphragm as a respiratory muscle
        - Herniation of intra-abdominal organs, e.g. large bowel into the thoracic cavity, causing respiratory impairment
        - Aortic valve rupture (rarely) as a result of retrograde arterial flow
    - Fractures of the pelvic ring, which may (in 10% of cases) be associated with injury of the bladder and urethra, and the pelvic blood vessels

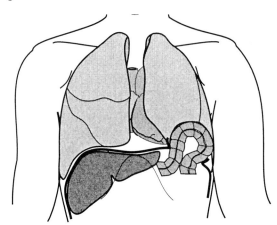

Figure 12-1 Blunt injury: abdominal compression resulting in rupture of the diaphragm and herniation of the bowel into the thoracic cavity

Limbs

- Compression of limbs may result in bony fracture

Change of speed (acceleration, deceleration, shear) injuries
- This occurs when there is a sudden change in speed (acceleration or deceleration), of a body composed of two separate but connected parts. One of the parts stops moving relative to the other which results in stretching and then tearing of the tissue or material connecting the two parts, or one part impacting with the other. Occurs where a fixed part joins a mobile part, e.g. duodenojejuneal junction, descending aortic arch, ileocaecal junction
- Usually only occurs when the acceleration or deceleration is very considerable, and is relatively uncommon as a mechanism of injury
- Injuries caused in this way are not usually visible and are easy to miss initially, if not looked for

Head
- A sudden change in speed may result in:
    - Brain contusion caused by the brain continuing to move at its previous speed until it impacts with the skull
    - Vascular shearing injury with stretching and tearing of blood vessels resulting in:
        - Temporal or frontal lobe bruising/haematoma formation
        - Subdural haematomas
    - Shearing injury to the spinal cord or brainstem

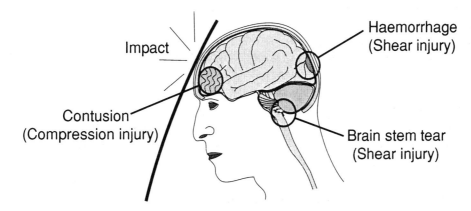

Figure 12-2 Blunt injury to the head resulting in compression and shear injury

Cervical spine
- Sudden changes in speed of the casualty's body may result in significant injury to the cervical spine and its associated soft tissue structures, including the spinal cord, similar to shearing injury
- The body may be considered to be similar to two balls one (the thorax and abdomen) much larger than the other (the head) connected by a short piece of string (the neck):
    - If the body suddenly decelerates, the head will continue to move forwards flexing the neck as it does so, until the head impacts with something or until the neck can flex no further. This may result in a hyperflexion injury of the cervical spine including anterior wedge fractures, fracture dislocations and ligamentous disruption
    - If the body suddenly accelerates the head will tend to be left behind, resulting in neck extension until it can extend no further, and the head is then pulled forwards by the body. This may result in a flexion injury of the cervical spine ("whiplash injury") including, fracture dislocations and anterior ligament disruption
    - Sudden sideways acceleration or deceleration will similarly cause lateral flexion to the side opposite to the direction of the movement. This often occurs in association with a rotational injury The cervical spine has relatively good anterior/posterior stability, but is less able to resist lateral and rotational movements, especially the two combined, and severe injuries to the cervical spine and its ligaments may result, including injury to the spinal cord sufficient to result in neurological deficit

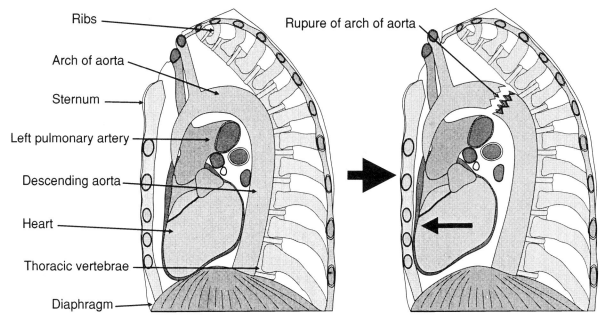

Figure 12-3 Shear injury: rupture of the arch of the aorta due to severe frontal impact

Thorax
- Sudden deceleration as a result of a severe frontal impact or a fall from a considerable height, or acceleration occurring as a result of a severe side (lateral) impact, may result in a shearing injury with:
    - Rupture (partial or complete) of the arch of the aorta, occurring most commonly at the site of the ligamentum arteriosum because:
        - Distal to this point the aorta is tethered firmly to the thoracic spine
        - Proximal to this point the aorta is attached to the heart and is mobile

Abdomen
- Sudden deceleration, or less commonly sudden acceleration may result in:
    - Shearing injury to those abdominal organs which are not firmly attached close to the abdominal wall, as they continue to move forward within the abdominal cavity, although the body itself has stopped moving:
        - This usually occurs at the site of the attachment of the organ to its mesentery and results in stretching and then tearing of the mesentery and its blood vessels
        - Organs which may be affected in this way include: the kidneys, spleen, small and large bowel
    - The liver impacting with the ligamentum teres, as it continues to move forwards and downwards , resulting in severe hepatic laceration

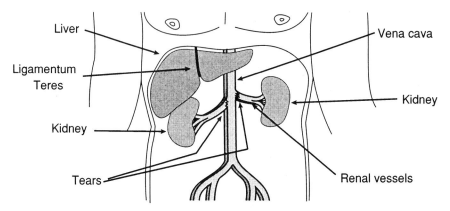

Figure 12-4 Shear injury: tearing of the renal blood vessels

Road traffic accidents: impacts and injuries

- In road traffic accidents and other accidents in which there is sudden deceleration, three impacts may occur:
    - The vehicle and the object with which it collides
    - The casualty with the interior of the vehicle or the pedestrian with the road
    - The casualty's internal organs with the abdominal wall or thoracic cage (compression injury)
- There may also be shearing injury as the tissues/materials tethering mobile organs stretch and then tear
- In order to assess the injuries that a casualty is likely to be suffering from, a knowledge of the mechanism of all three impacts is necessary

Vehicle damage
- Modern cars are designed with
    - Impact or crumple zones at the front and rear of the vehicle, which collapse progressively, absorbing much of the kinetic energy of an impact (impact energy).
    - A passenger compartment which is designed to be rigid and minimise any intrusion into it, 'the passenger safety cell'
- The result of this is that:
    - Less impact energy is transmitted to the passenger compartment, which helps to preserve its integrity
    - There is a reduction in intrusion into the passenger compartment and consequently a reduction in blunt injury to vehicle occupants caused by intrusion alone
    - There is a reduction in the impact energy transmitted to the vehicle occupants, when they impact with the interior of the vehicle
- An increasing number of cars also have side impact bars in the doors to prevent side intrusion

Injuries in road traffic accidents
- Vehicle occupants or riders will be subjected to the same direction and type of force as the vehicle in or on which they are travelling.
- The amount of energy transferred to the vehicle occupant will depend on:
    - How much impact energy has been absorbed by the vehicle, when it was deformed by the impact
    - Whether the deformation of the vehicle occurred over a relatively long or short interval of time
- Large vehicles tend to be safer than smaller ones, because there is usually:
    - More of the vehicle to help absorb the impact energy
    - More interior space, so that the occupants have more room to move in without impacting with the vehicle interior
    - More safety features
- If a large vehicle impacts with a smaller one, the mass of the larger vehicle will affect the movement of the smaller vehicle to a greater extent than the mass of the smaller vehicle will affect the movement of the larger vehicle
- Injuries sustained by vehicle occupants will depend on:
    - The amount and direction of the impact force transferred to them
    - The nature of that part of the body absorbing the force
- The injuries sustained may be subdivided into those caused by:
    - Compression
    - Shearing
    - Penetration (very rare)

Types of impact

Frontal impact (70%)
- Occurs when the front or front corner of the vehicle collides with another vehicle or object which may or may not be mobile itself, causing the first vehicle to cease movement, suddenly or gradually
- Frontal impact will result in rapid deceleration of the vehicle and everything in it, including its driver and any passengers

Vehicle damage
- Part or all of the front of the vehicle will be involved in the initial impact and will absorb most of the impact energy, resulting in frontal deformity with:
    - Exterior damage:
        - Shortening of the front of the vehicle. This will vary depending on the amount of the impact energy (the vehicle's kinetic energy and the kinetic energy of the object/vehicle with which it impacts, and the area of impact, e.g. an impact with another car will cause less intrusion/ shortening than an impact with a motor cycle with the same kinetic energy, but a much smaller profile/area of impact)
        - The front of the vehicle and its engine compartment are usually designed to absorb most of the impact energy and to collapse progressively, without involving the passenger compartment, which only becomes deformed in very severe impacts
        - Rearward displacement of:
            - The front wing body panels (which may impact with the front of the front doors making opening them difficult or impossible)
            - The front wheels
            - The front doors
        - Buckling of the vehicle's floor pan or roof may be caused by very severe impacts

Effects of severe frontal impact

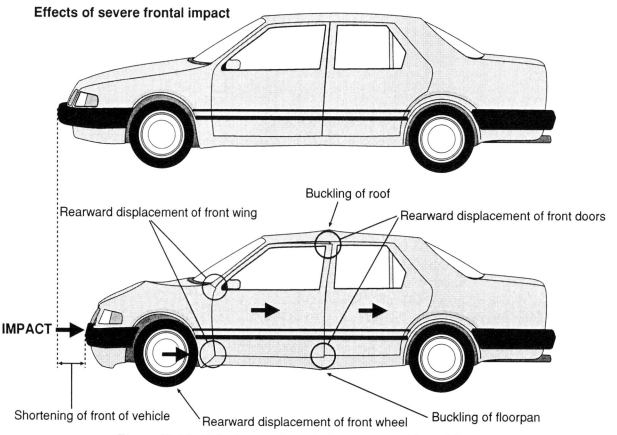

Figure 12-5 Vehicle damage (exterior) as a result of frontal impact

- Interior damage:
  - Intrusion of a wheel arch (occurs most often when the impact is offset or oblique rather than full frontal (when the engine helps prevent wheel arch intrusion)
  - Rearward displacement of the front fascia and steering wheel (rare)
  - Upward displacement and buckling of the floor pan
  - Downwards displacement and buckling of the roof
  - Forward movement of insecure seating (rare)
- Impact with the front seat occupants may also occur, and cause:
  - Steering wheel deformity: pushing it forwards and upwards
  - Rear view mirror damage: bent or broken off
  - Windscreen damage
  - Front shelf damage
- Impact with the rear seat occupants may result in:
  - Damage to front seats
  - Windscreen damage if they are not restrained by seat belts

Vehicle occupant movement

Unrestrained occupants
- After the impact, unrestrained car occupants will continue to move forward relative to the vehicle, until they impact with the vehicle interior. It is only then that they will experience deceleration, and the remaining impact force will be transmitted to them
- The first significant force will transmitted through the feet in the foot well. If the impact is anticipated and the knees braced, forward movement may be resisted
- At low speeds:
  - Knee bracing (and arm bracing by drivers) may be successful in preventing forward body movement and further body impact with the vehicle interior may not occur
- At higher speeds:
  - Forward movement is not prevented
  - Initially the whole body pivots about the feet, until the knees impact with the front parcel shelf or front fascia
  - This is followed by the upper abdomen, thorax and neck impacting with the steering wheel (in the case of the driver) and the head impacting with the windscreen, including the rear view mirror, or car roof
  - Each successive impact occurs with increasing velocity (and therefore force), as the body flexes progressively about the last point of impact
  - This may result in ejection of the front seat passenger (but not usually the driver whose ejection may be prevented by the steering wheel)

Injury prevention devices

Anti-submarining seats
- The occupant of a seat may slide forwards (under the seat belt, if worn), on impact, if the seat squabs are too soft, and suffer very severe lower limb injuries as a result. Modern car seats are designed to prevent this

Collapsible steering column
- These are designed to telescope on impact to prevent the steering wheel intruding further into the passenger compartment in frontal collisions, causing injury to the driver's head and chest, by telescoping on impact

Restraining devices
- Seat belts:
    - Inertia reel seat belts lock a few milliseconds after a frontal impact restraining the casualty (some cars are now fitted with seat belt pre-tensioners, which actively tighten the belt during the first milliseconds of a crash, thus pulling the the occupant back into the seat)
    - Stretch during severe deceleration increasing the time interval before the body ceases forward movement, and reducing the force of deceleration
    - Reduce forward movement of the pelvis, and to a lesser extent the thorax and abdomen, and help to prevent injuries caused by impaction with the steering wheel
    - Prevent forward (but not sideways or backwards) ejection
    - Spread the compressive forces over a greater area, reducing the force applied per unit area, and hence reduce the severity of injury caused by compression
    - May cause some injuries (which are much less severe than if no seat belt was worn), which may show up as a line of bruising (pattern bruising) or a weal where the seat belt strap passes over parts of the bony skeleton, e.g. clavicle, iliac crest
    - Restrained occupants tend to flex their cervical spine more than unrestrained car occupants and may hit the windscreen with their heads
    - Incorrectly worn seat belts may cause some injuries:
        - Shoulder strap too high:
            - Neck injury
        - Lap strap loose or too high (above the pelvis):
            - Compression of the soft intra-abdominal organs between the seat belt and the posterior abdominal wall;
                - Injury to the spleen, liver and pancreas
            - Sudden rise in intra-abdominal pressure:
                - Diaphragmatic rupture with herniation of intra-abdominal organs into the thoracic cavity
            - Anterior compression (wedge) fracture of the lumbar spine (T12, L1, 2) due to hyperflexion (similar to when the lap belt is worn alone)
- Airbags:
    - These are being fitted to an increasing number of new cars, following their successful use in the USA
    - Only deploy in medium and high speed frontal and oblique frontal impacts (above 18 mph, in European cars, where seat belts are worn by more than 95% of front seat occupants; at 10-12 mph in the USA, where seat belts are not commonly worn)
    - Are fitted in the steering wheel boss (or front fascia in front of the front seat passenger), and are triggered by a sensor, resulting in a very rapid chemical reaction (controlled explosion) which produces a large volume of gas, and inflates the bag within a few seconds of a frontal/oblique frontal impact. There are vents in the side or top seams which allow the bag to deflate almost immediately after inflation, releasing the driver or passenger
    - They spread the decelerative forces over a large area, reduce forward movement, and prevent impact with the front of the interior of the vehicle
    - Airbags are not effective in preventing secondary injury in multiple impacts, due to their rapid deflation after the primary impact
    - May sometimes cause friction burns, usually of the forearms and neck, due to their rapid inflation or heat burns, usually of the forearms, due to release of very hot gases

Driver movement on frontal impact

Unrestrained   **Seatbelt**   **Airbag**

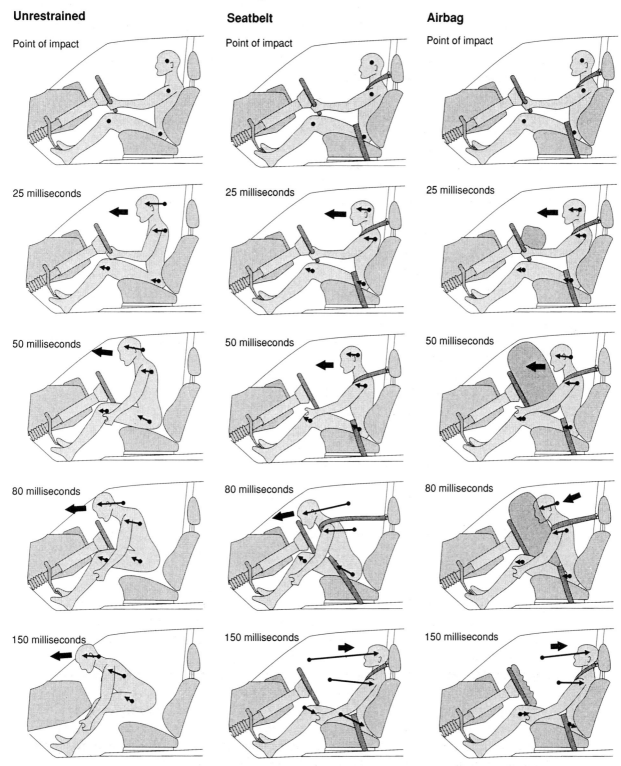

Figure 12-6 Frontal impact: movement of driver: unrestrained, restrained with seat belt and restrained with seat belt and airbag (at 150 milliseconds the unrestrained front seat passenger may be ejected, whereas the unrestrained driver will tend to impact with the steering wheel preventing ejection)

Vehicle occupant injuries

Front seat occupants:
- The front seat passenger often suffers more severe injuries than the driver, as they are usually less prepared for the impact than the driver, who may anticipate the impact and can also use the steering wheel to reduce forward movement (high speed impacts may result in bilateral forearm/wrist fractures)
- Compression injuries as front seat occupants impact successively with:
    - The front parcel shelf or dashboard, resulting in the transmission of impact energy through the knee and along the femoral shaft to the pelvis, causing:
        - Knee injuries:
            - Fractures of the patella and disruption of the patellar ligament
            - Dislocation of the knee (risk of popliteal artery injury)
        - Fractures of the shaft of femur
        - Backwards displacement (posterior dislocation) of the hip and acetabular fracture

Frontal impact: lower limb injuries

Fractured patella   **Dislocation of the knee**   **Fracture of the shaft of femur**

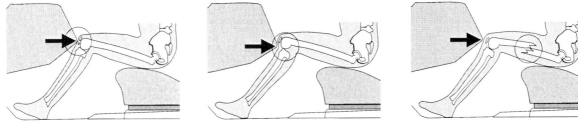

Posterior dislocation of the hip   **Fracture of the tibial plateau**

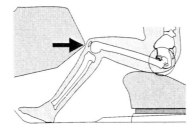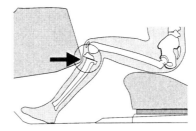

Figure 12-7 Frontal impact: injuries to the knee, and femur

- The steering wheel, with the upper abdomen, resulting in compression of the anterior abdominal wall against the spine and posterior abdominal wall, causing:
    - Compression and rupture of hollow abdominal organs: stomach, and large and small bowel
    - Compression injuries of solid viscera: the liver, spleen, kidneys and rarely the pancreas
- The steering wheel with the thorax resulting in compression of the anterior thorax against the spine and posterior thorax, causing:
    - Anterior chest wall injuries: fractured ribs, including anterior flail chest, and sternum
    - Contusion of the heart and lungs (lung tissue is elastic and compressible and so is not so easily damaged)
    - If the casualty anticipates the accident and holds their breath, closing the glottis in the process. When the impact occurs and the thorax is suddenly and forcibly compressed, the lungs burst (like a paper bag full of air), resulting in a pneumothorax

- The windscreen glass/frame or side pillars with the head, resulting in :
    - Injuries of the forehead, including scalp lacerations, skull fracture, cerebral contusion and intracranial haemorrhage (relatively rare since the introduction of seat belts, which have dramatically reduced the severity of this type of injury)
- The rear view mirror:
    - Person in the front right hand seat:
        - Laceration of the left side of the forehead.
        - Injury of the left eye
    - Person in the front left hand seat:
        - Laceration of the right side of the forehead
        - Injury to the right eye
- Unrestrained occupants may be ejected through the windscreen, sustaining injuries similar to ejected motor cyclists (see below), but in addition may suffer from severe facial injuries if they impact with a hard (road) surface, due to their not wearing a helmet
- Shearing injuries of:
    - The liver and kidneys may also occur with tearing of the vessels and tissues tethering them to the posterior abdominal wall, due to the sudden cessation of forward movement as the abdomen impacts with the steering wheel, resulting in;
        - Stretching and then tearing of the renal veins and arteries near where they join the inferior vena cava and thoracic aorta
        - Tearing of the liver caused by impact with the ligamentum teres
    - The thoracic aorta, where it becomes tethered to the posterior thoracic wall, due to the sudden cessation of forward movement of the thorax when it impacts with the steering wheel, resulting in:
        - Transection of the aorta or more commonly a partial tear of the wall of the aorta resulting in a traumatic aortic aneurism
    - The cervical spine due to cervical hyperflexion and hyperextension, resulting in:
        - Severe soft tissue injury to the soft tissues of the neck
        - Fractures of the cervical spine and damage to its ligaments
    - The blood supply to that part of the brain furthest from the impact
- Front seat car occupants may be hit by unrestrained rear seat passengers resulting in:
    - Head and neck injuries
    - Back injuries (from the rear seat passengers hitting the back of the front seats with their knees)

High speed frontal impact
- May result in:
    - Buckling of the roof and floor of the passenger compartment, resulting in compression and spinal injuries
    - Deceleration (shear) injury: tearing of thoracic aorta (especially in the young), which may not be obvious initially
    - Fractures of the wrist/forearms as the driver braces the arms to try to prevent forward movement

Offset frontal and oblique frontal impact
- May result in front wheel arch intrusion:
    - Fractured ankles/lower legs (more common and more severe in car drivers, as their feet and ankles can become tangled around the control pedals, especially the right ankle, which is used for braking)

Seat belt injuries
- Chest strap:
    - For those in the right front seat:
        - The line of injury may extend down across the chest from the right shoulder to the left costal margin and loin, and may result in:
            - Subluxation of the acromio-clavicular joint
            - Fracture of the right clavicle
            - Fracture of the sternum
            - Fracture of the left lower ribs
            - Injury to the spleen and left kidney
    - For those in left front seat; this will be reversed with injury to the liver instead of the spleen
    - Injury to the neck may be caused by a seat belt which is anchored too high up
- Lap strap:
    - Direct injury to the lower abdominal viscera and bladder
    - Sudden rise in intrathoracic pressure: ruptured diaphragm

Seat belt injury

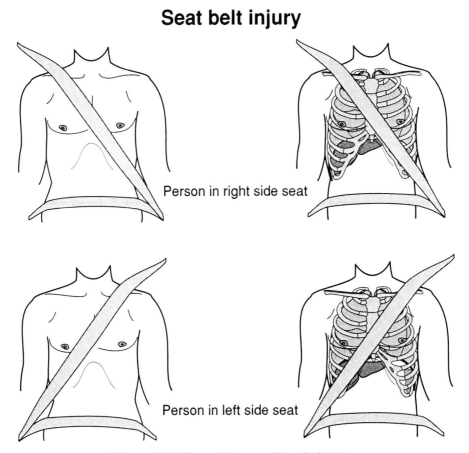

Person in right side seat

Person in left side seat

Figure 12-8 Frontal impact: Seat belt injury

Rear seat occupants
- Injuries are usually less severe than those of the front seat occupants, as rear seat occupants usually impact with the rear of the front seats after moving a relatively short distance
- Unrestrained rear seat passengers may be thrown forwards, resulting in:
    - Collision with the back of the front seats and front seat passengers, sustaining:
        - Neck injuries (hyperflexion)
        - Knee injuries
    - Collision with the windscreen and sometimes ejection through the windscreen resulting in:
        - Neck and facial injuries

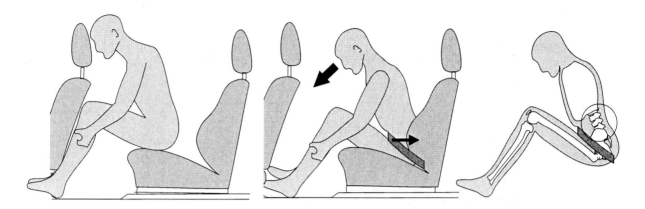

Figure 12-9 Frontal impact: unrestrained and restrained (lap belt only) rear seat passengers

- Restrained rear seat passengers using a full seat belt may sustain:
    - Facial and knee injuries (collision with the back of the front seats)
- Restrained rear seat passengers only using a lap belt, usually the centre passenger, (especially if they are involved in high speed frontal impact), will flex forward, hitting their head on the seat in front of them sustaining:
    - Injury to the lower abdominal viscera and the bladder caused by the lap belt
    - Hyperflexion injury of the cervical or upper lumbar spine (wedge fracture)
- Ejection:
    - If the casualty is ejected because he/she was either not wearing a seat belt, or it was loose:
        - Severe facial and neck injuries (see below)

Rear impact
- Occurs when a slower moving or stationary vehicle is hit from behind by a faster moving vehicle
- Results in the sudden forward acceleration of the vehicle and its occupants: the greater the difference in speed between the two vehicles, the greater the impact force transferred to the vehicle that is hit
- If the driver of the vehicle that is hit, suddenly puts on the brakes, or if the vehicle hits another vehicle in front; there will be a secondary frontal impact, and the vehicle and its occupants will experience the effects of two collisions (rear impact followed by frontal impact)

Vehicle damage
- The rear of the vehicle absorbs most of the impact energy resulting in shortening and deformity with:
- Exterior damage:
    - Shortening of the rear of the vehicle, dependent on the force of the impact
    - The boot is designed to absorb most of the impact and to collapse progressively, without involving the passenger compartment, but is less efficient at doing so than the engine compartment as it is often empty and in hatch-backs is relatively shorter
- Interior damage with:
    - Forward displacement of the contents of the boot and the rear seat:
        - Impact with rear seat occupant, pushing them forward, so that they impact with the back of the front seats, causing:
            - Damage to the back of the front seats
        - Impact with front seat occupants, pushing them forward:
            - Damage to the steering wheel, windscreen, rear view mirror and front shelf

Whiplash injury

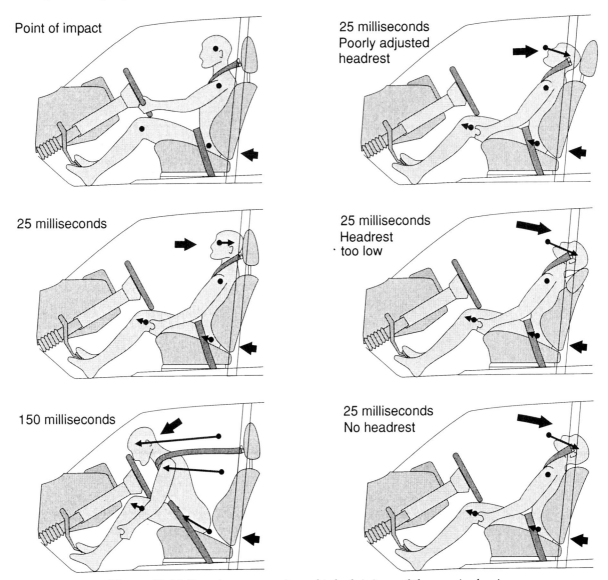

Figure 12-10 Rear impact causing whiplash injury of the cervical spine

Vehicle occupant movement
- The vehicle will be accelerated forwards, whilst the occupants will move backwards, unless they are prevented from doing so by the front of the seat back
- The head in particular will move backwards, hyper-extending the neck
- As the vehicle subsequently stops they will be accelerated forwards by the back of their seat

Restraining devices
- Head restraints:
    - These reduce the amount of backward movement of the head and minimise the amount of hyper-extension of the cervical spine
    - If wrongly positioned:
        - They may be totally ineffective
    or - They may cause even greater hyper-extension of the cervical spine, by acting as a pivot around which the head rotates (head rest too low)

Vehicle occupant injuries
- Compression injuries may include:
    - Seat belt injuries
    - Front seat occupants may have:
        - Posterior chest or spinal injuries: impact from rear seat passengers knees
    - Rear seat passengers may also have:
        - Spinal injury: rear intrusion
        - Knee/femoral injury: impact with the back of the front seat
- Shearing type injuries include:
    - Whiplash (hyperextension) injury to the cervical spine (most common injury) with tearing of the anterior cervical ligaments
    - Other shearing injuries are rare because most intra-abdominal organs are tethered to the posterior abdominal or thoracic wall, which will move forwards before impacting with the organ and carrying it forwards

Side impact
- Occurs when a vehicle is hit on one of its sides

Vehicle damage
- If the force of impact is insufficient to move the vehicle that is hit sideways:
    - All the force of the impact will be absorbed by the vehicle that is hit and will result in:
        - Exterior damage with:
            - Inward displacement of doors, dependent on the force of the impact.
            - This will be less in cars with side impact bars in their doors, but may result in more damage to the vehicle or object impacting with the door
        - Interior damage with:
            - Intrusion into the passenger compartment
- If the force of impact is sufficient to move the vehicle that is hit:
    - Some of the impact energy will be converted to movement energy and there may be less damage to the vehicle that is hit
    - Impact of vehicle occupants with the door on the side opposite the impact, may result in it opening

Vehicle occupant movement
- If no seat belt is worn:
    - The body will tend to flex towards the side of the impact, and the casualty may hit the side of their head on the window glass on the same side as the collision
    - Side intrusion may result in the casualty being pushed sideways away from the side of impact
- If a seat belt is worn:
    - It may prevent sideways movement of the hips and pelvis (but not of the thorax and head)
- If the vehicle that is hit, is pushed (accelerated) sideways by the impact, vehicle occupants will be accelerated away from the side of impact after initially moving towards it. When the vehicle stops moving sideways:
    - Vehicle occupants will continue to move sideways and may collide with other vehicle occupants on the opposite side to the collision
    - Vehicle occupants on the opposite side to that which sustains the impact may be thrown against the door opposite the impact, and if it opens they may be ejected sideways

Vehicle occupant injury
- These will sustain blunt injury resulting in lateral compression of that part of the body adjacent to the point of impact
- The injuries sustained will depend on the side of impact and the level at which it occurs:
    - Left side:
        - Mid door intrusion, e.g. caused by impact with the front of a car:
            - Left lateral flail chest and pulmonary contusion and a ruptured spleen and left kidney (the casualty's upper arm may rotate posteriorly out of the way and not be seriously damaged)
            - If the upper arm is pinned between the door and the chest, it may absorb much of the force of the impact, transferring some of it to the clavicle and the underlying thoracic wall, resulting in:
                - A fracture of the left humerus with an associated fracture of the medial third of the clavicle as it is forced upwards, and the outer aspect of the underling ribs
        - Low door intrusion, e.g. caused by impact with the front wheel of a motorcycle:
            - Femoral fractures including impaction fractures of the head of femur which is driven medially into the acetabulum
            - Left pelvic fractures as the ilium is pushed in resulting in fractures of the pubic rami anteriorly and the ischium posteriorly
        - Upper door, window or door post intrusion, e.g. caused by impact with a lorry bumper, or forced in by a mid door impact:
            - Head injuries ranging from scalp and facial lacerations to cerebral contusions, skull fractures and cerebral haemorrhage
    - Right side:
        - As the left side apart from:
            - Ruptured liver, right kidney, etc.
- If the vehicle that is hit, is rotated sideways by the impact:
    - There will be lateral flexion and rotation of the head towards the side of the impact:
        - The cervical spine has relatively good anterior/posterior stability, but is less able to resist lateral and rotational movements, especially the two combined and severe injuries to the cervical spine and its ligaments may result, including injury to the spinal cord sufficient to result in neurological deficit
    - Seat belts may reduce direct impact injury by 'pulling' the casualty away from the point of impact
    - Vehicle occupants colliding with other vehicle occupants on the opposite side to the collision may sustain impact injuries to that side of the body
- Vehicle occupants on the opposite side to that which sustains the impact:
    - May be thrown against the door opposite the impact (especially in high speed impacts), which may burst open and the casualty be ejected sideways (seat belts are designed to prevent forward movement only), sustaining:
        - Injuries to the shoulder, upper arm, and chest, caused by impact with the door
        - Ejection injuries, the severity of which depends on the force of impact, the weight of the casualty and the surface on which they land
    - May be injured on the same side as the impact by vehicle occupants thrown towards them by the impact
- If a seat belt is worn, there may be greater injury than if the body was free to move out of the way

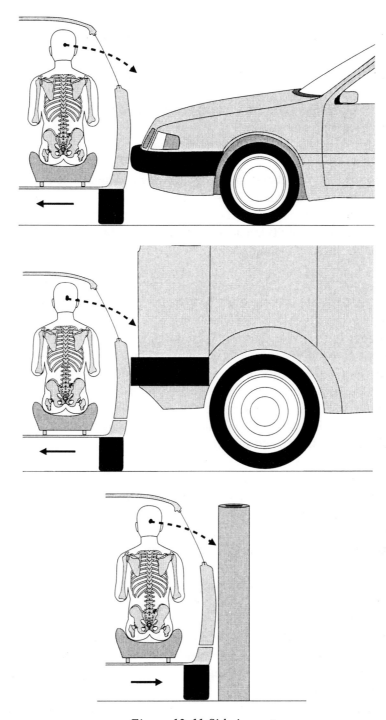

Figure 12-11 Side impacts

Injury prevention devices

Side impact bars
- These are intended to prevent/limit side intrusion into the passenger compartment, thereby preventing/ reducing injury
- Some authorities claim that side impact bars may make matters worse, as although they may limit side intrusion, when the vehicle occupant comes into contact with the side of the vehicle, there is more energy transfer, resulting in more severe chest and pelvic injuries
- Side impact bars may also act as a kind of locking bolt in frontal impacts, making it harder for the rescue services to force the door open

Side impact air bags
- These are a new development, and are now being fitted to the seats of some cars to prevent the casualty coming into direct contact with the passenger door

SIPS
- This is a system which allows the drivers/front seat passengers seat to move sideways into a collapsible centre console in the event of a side impact

Rotational impacts
- These occur when one corner of a vehicle collides with either an immovable object or a vehicle moving more slowly or in the opposite direction
- That part of the vehicle involved in the impact ceases forward movement, but the rest of the vehicle continues to move forwards until all its kinetic energy is converted to rotational movement, and so the vehicle rotates around the point of the impact

Vehicle damage
- Vehicle damage will be similar to that sustained by vehicles involved in frontal and side impacts

Vehicle occupant movement
- After the initial frontal impact of the vehicle, the vehicle occupant will continue to move forwards and may impact with the front of the interior of the vehicle, before impacting with the side of the vehicle

Vehicle occupant injury
- The injuries sustained by vehicle occupants in rotational impacts are similar to those sustained by vehicle occupants involved in frontal and side impacts

Roll over accidents
- May often occur in conjunction with some other kind of impact

Vehicle damage
- The impact is usually spread over a wide area, i.e. the whole of the side or roof of the vehicle at any point in time and is spread over a relatively large amount of time, as the vehicle rolls over and over. As a result the amount of damage done and injury resulting from the roll over component is usually relatively minor
- Vehicle exterior:
    - Deformity with buckling and inward displacement of the roof, which has little strength to resist direct force, most marked between any roll over bars
    - Inward displacement of doors and floor pan

Vehicle occupant movement
- There is a significant risk of ejection, especially of unbelted occupants:
    - Front seat occupants are most frequently ejected through a side door, window or sun roof
    - Rear seat occupants are most frequently ejected through the rear window

Vehicle occupant injury
- Injuries are usually multiple and depend on the points of impact between car and occupant:
    - Depression of the vehicle roof may result in injuries of:
        - The head
        - Cervical, thoracic and lumbar spine (as the force of impact is transmitted down the spine)
- The severity of injury varies depending on the amount of residual impact energy transferred to the casualty
- Fractures of the femur occur relatively frequently

Trucks

Vehicle damage
- The driver's cab usually sits on top of the engine compartment and there is no crumple or impact zone in front of the driver
- Impact with cars:
    - Exterior and interior damage is usually relatively minor, and rarely affects the driver's compartment
- Impact with other trucks:
    - Frontal impact is the most significant, as rear impact usually only affects the trailer
    - The whole of the vehicle front may be damaged resulting in significant intrusion into the driver's compartment
- Roll over accidents are relatively common, but rarely result in significant injury

Vehicle occupants movement
- Truck drivers do not usually wear seat belts or have airbags, and so tend to move like unrestrained front seat car occupants

Vehicle occupant injury

Frontal impacts
- Frontal or part frontal impacts cause the majority of injuries, the severity of which depends on the forces involved in the impact:
    - The steering wheel is usually larger than in cars and may help to reduce driver forward movement and prevent driver ejection (passengers may be ejected and suffer major secondary injury)
- Forward movement of the driver may result in:
    - Impact with the steering wheel may result in upper and central abdominal injury
    - Impact with the windscreen may result in facial and head injuries
- Intrusion of the front of the vehicle may cause severe lower limb injuries

Side impacts
- May result in sideways ejection if the side door is torn off

Motorcycles
- Most major injuries are due to ejection of the motorcyclist onto the road or adjacent surfaces or objects, due to the inherent instability of the vehicle and its frequent high speed
- Many injuries are caused by the motorcyclist losing control of their vehicle on adverse surfaces
- The majority of deaths occur as a result of head injury
- Lower limb injuries are particularly common, occurring in over 50% of motorcylists attending hospital, of these 50% are of the lower leg

Protection
- The severity of injury caused by impact will depend on the protection used by the motorcyclist

Crash helmets
- These provide protection for the head and face and can reduce the risk of the wearer suffering from a severe head injury by over 60% and loss of consciousness by up to 85%
- A pedal/motor cyclist's helmet should always be inspected and sent with them to hospital

Protective clothing
- Leather suits may help to protect the wearer from dermal injury, in particular friction burns
- Tight trousers may help to reduce blood loss from pelvic and lower limb fractures, by tamponade

Frontal impact
- Caused by the front wheel of the motorcycle impacting with another stationary or moving object

Motorcycle damage
- Frontal impact with a solid object will result in damage to the front wheel and rearward displacement of the front forks, the amount of displacement being dependent on the force involved
- The motorcycle will rotate forwards pivoting on the front wheel as its centre of gravity is above and behind the front axle

Motorcyclist movement
- Sudden deceleration will result in the motorcyclist being thrown forwards impacting with the petrol tank
- If the motor cycle decelerates very suddenly and pivots on the front wheel, the rider may be ejected

Motorcyclist injury
- If the motorcyclist moves forward the front of his pelvis will impact with the petrol tank resulting in pelvic fracture
- If the motorcyclist is ejected from the bike, his thighs may impact with the handlebars, especially if they are of the cow horn shape, and the impact force may be transmitted to the shafts of both femurs resulting in bilateral fractures

Ejection
- If the motorcyclist is ejected, he will continue to move through the air until he impacts with another object or the ground
- All the force of the impact will be transmitted through that part of him which impacts first, resulting in injury at that point. The impact energy will then be transmitted to the rest of the body
- The severity of any injuries sustained as a result is dependent on the speed of impact, the trajectory and angle of impact, and the surface on which the motor cyclist lands; near vertical impact on hard surfaces resulting in the most severe injuries:
    - Head, face and cervical spine, chest and abdominal injury
    - Friction burns may result from the casualty sliding at speed along the road surface

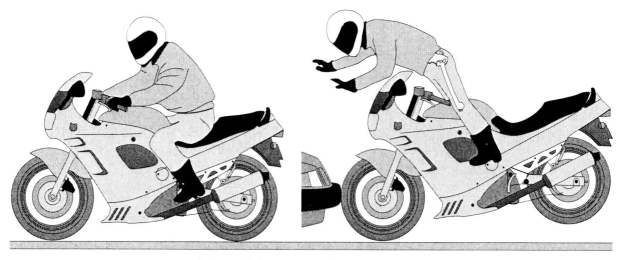

Figure 12-12 Motorcycle: frontal impact

Falling over
- Following the initial impact, if the motorcyclist is not ejected, the motorcycle may fall over onto the motorcyclist's legs, crushing them and causing a secondary injury of the upper leg, lower leg or ankle, resulting in fractures of the femoral shaft, tibia/fibula, and ankle, including dislocation, which are often open/compound

Tailgating
  - Collision with the back (tail-gating), or side of a lorry, may result in:
    - Hyperextension injury of the cervical spine and head injury
    - Decapitation

Side impacts
  - Caused by impact with another moving object, usually the front bumper or side of a car, impacting with the side of the motorcycle or the motorcycle moving sideways and colliding with an object

Motorcycle damage
  - This will result in damage to the pedals and occasionally the engine and petrol tank of the motorcycle

Motorcyclist injury
  - Usually caused by direct impact with a car:
    - Fractures of the femur (most common), lower leg and ankle
  - May result in entrapment of the lower limb between the motorbike and the other vehicle or object:
    - The upper leg is usually trapped by the petrol tank and car wing (less common)
    - The lower leg is usually trapped between the motorcycle gearbox and the front bumper or corner of the car (most common)
  - A glancing blow may cause tissue rotation, resulting in severe soft tissue damage including neuro-vascular injury
  - If the motorcyclist is thrown off the motorcycle he may land on his hands/elbows sustaining fractures of the humerus and radius/ulna

Pedal cyclists

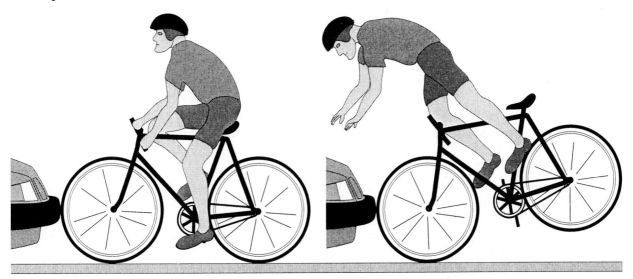

Figure 12-13 Pedal cyclist: frontal impact

  - If the pedal cyclist collides with a stationary object or slow moving vehicle, the mechanism of injury is generally similar to that of motorcyclists, but their velocity is usually considerably less, and injuries are consequently usually less severe
  - If they are hit by a fast moving car, the mechanism of injury is similar to that of pedestrians (see below), except that the pedal cyclist may be a little higher off the ground, with the pedal cyclist sustaining:
    - A scooping-up injury
  - If they are hit by a lorry, the mechanism of injury is similar to that of pedestrians, with the pedal cyclist sustaining:
    - A running-over injury

- Uniquely the skin from the lower leg may be stripped (avulsed) from the lower leg due to the limb being forced between the wheel spokes
- Most child pedal cyclists are injured after losing control and falling from their bicycle
- Head injuries are more likely if:
    - The accident occurred on hard rather than soft surfaces
    - The pedal cyclist has made contact with a moving vehicle.

Pedestrians
- Injuries occur when a pedestrian is hit by a moving vehicle
- Most pedestrians are hit from the side while crossing the road
- The type of injuries sustained depends on the age group, height and weight of the casualty
    - Adult pedestrians tend to turn away to protect themselves if they anticipate an impact, resulting in injuries due to lateral or even posterior impacts
    - Children tend to turn towards and face the oncoming vehicle

Primary injury
- The primary impact/injury is due to the initial collision with the vehicle
- The injuries caused depend on the height, weight and age of the casualty and on the velocity, size and type of vehicle

Adult pedestrian
- The car bumper usually hits the casualty first, knocking the feet out from under them and resulting in:
    - Injuries to the side (if facing the vehicle) or front of the knee/lower leg, including fractures of the tibia and fibula
- The casualty then rotates and flexes forwards impacting with the radiator grille, lamps or bonnet causing further primary injury to the thigh or hip and fractures of the upper femur and pelvis
- At low speeds, the casualty is usually knocked forwards or obliquely sideways (impacts are usually caused by impact with the front or front corner of the vehicle)
- At higher speeds, casualties may be thrown into the air on impact:
    - At fairly low speeds (20 kph), the body may be thrown violently away
    - At higher speeds (60-100 kph), the casualty may be ejected up into the air and may land on the roof of the vehicle or may travel a considerable distance before hitting the ground or other object resulting in secondary injuries, which may be more severe than the primary injury

Scooping-up injury
- This tends to occur at speeds over 25 kph (cars only):
    - The casualty has their feet knocked out from under them by the car bumper, and they are thrown up onto the bonnet of the car, resulting in their head impacting with the windscreen (sometimes going through the glass) windscreen pillar, or roof (windscreens deform fairly easily and absorb energy well):
        - Impact with the bonnet will result in:
            - Fractures of the upper femur, pelvis, ribs, and spine
            - Intra-abdominal and intra-thoracic injury
        - Impact with the windscreen may result in:
            - Injury to the head, face, and cervical spine

- Once on the bonnet, the casualty assumes the same velocity as the vehicle, but seldom stays there long before being flung:
  - Sideways onto the road, sustaining severe secondary injuries, including head and cervical spine injury and severe injuries to the side of the body on which they land, and are then at risk of being run over by passing cars
  - Forwards onto the road if the driver of the vehicle brakes suddenly
  - Over the roof of the car (at high speeds) hitting the road behind the vehicle, and sometimes the rear window before that
- If the vehicle is large (lorry or bus):
  - The primary injuries may be at a higher level: on the chest, arms, or head

Running-over injury
- This type of injury tends to occur if that part of the front of the vehicle coming into contact with the casualty is relatively high, and the centre of gravity of the casualty is relatively low:
  - More likely to occur in children who are hit by lorries
- Occurs if:
  - A wheel passes over the casualty
  - The vehicle passes over the casualty, and part of the underside of the vehicle catches on part of the casualty and results in them being dragged along the road surface
- May result in severe injury to the:
  - Head, causing gross distortion and very severe injury and immediate death
  - Chest, resulting in a flail chest with fractured ribs, sternum, spine and severe lung contusion
  - Abdomen and pelvis, causing rupture of the internal organs

Flaying injury
- Occurs where the wheel (usually from a large vehicle, e.g. lorry or bus) rotates the body on the ground ripping off the skin and subcutaneous tissue (usually of a leg, arm or the scalp)

Child pedestrian
- Children are shorter, lighter and have a relatively large, heavy head
- The impact occurs higher up the body than with adults
- The first injury (impact with the bumper) may result in fractures of the femur and pelvis
- The second impact occurs almost simultaneously with the first impact, as the front of the bonnet impacts massively with the thorax, pushing it backwards. The neck is hyperflexed and the head and face impact with the bonnet
- After this the child may be:
  - Thrown down and dragged along by the car
  - Knocked to one side and the lower limbs run over by a wheel
  - Knocked backwards, falling under the car, where they may be:
    - Hit by undercar projections
    - Dragged along after getting stuck on part of the car
    - Run over by a wheel

Injuries
- Child pedestrians often sustain serious injuries including:
  - Head injury
  - Spinal injury (especially cervical and mid-thoracic)
  - Intra-abdominal injury

Secondary injury
- This is caused by the pedestrian impacting with the ground or other objects resulting in:
    - Skidding causing "brush" abrasions
    - Head injury (most common) including scalp laceration, skull and facial fractures, resulting in meningeal haemorrhage and cerebral contusion
    - Spinal injury especially of the cervical and thoracic regions with spinal cord involvement
    - Chest and pelvic injuries
    - Fractures of the femur and tibia
- The severity of the injury depends on the weight of the casualty, the surface on which they land or the object with which they collide, their velocity at the time of impact and the angle of their trajectory

Examples of other injuries

Falls from heights
- The severity of the injury depends on:
    - The height of the fall:
        - The greater the height, the greater the velocity achieved by the body and the greater the decelerative force when the casualty impacts with the ground
        - As an approximate guide, falls from more than three times the height of the casualty, result in serious injury
    - The type of surface on which the casualty lands:
        - Impact with a non-compressible surfaces, e.g. concrete, will result in a more severe injury than an impact with a relatively compressible surface, e.g. a field of corn, which helps absorb some of the impact force
    - The part of the body which impacts with the ground
- Falls from heights onto the heels/feet:
    - Results in the whole of the impact force being transmitted through the feet, up the legs and via the pelvis to the spine and head, causing:
        - Fractured calcaneii
        - Fractured/dislocated hips
    - After the feet come into contact with the ground and stop moving, the body is forced into flexion as the head, thorax and abdomen continue to move downwards. This will result in hyper-flexion of the spine at the apex of each curve of the spine resulting in:
        - Compression fractures of lumbar, thoracic and cervical spine
    - Flexion and partial relaxation of the ankles, knees and hips prior to the impact may help to absorb part of the decelerative force/impact energy and so reduce the severity of injury
    - Extension and locking of the ankles, knees and hips prior to impact will result in the transmission of the decelerative force up the spine and increase the likelihood of significant spinal injury
    - Falls onto the hands:
        - If the casualty falls forward onto their outstretched hands to break their fall, they are likely to sustain:
            - Bilateral Colles and clavicular fractures
    - The sudden deceleration caused by a fall from a height onto a hard surface may also result in shearing injuries:
        - Rupture of the arch of the aorta
- If the casualty falls so that another part of their body impacts with the ground:
    - The part of their body impacting with the ground should be assessed first
    - The direction in which the resultant force is transmitted through the skeleton should be worked out and the likely injuries determined
- Falls onto the head with the body in line (commonly occurs when diving into shallow water):
    - Will result in the whole of the force of the impact being transmitted though the head and spine, causing a severe hyperextension injury of the cervical spine and less commonly severe head injury

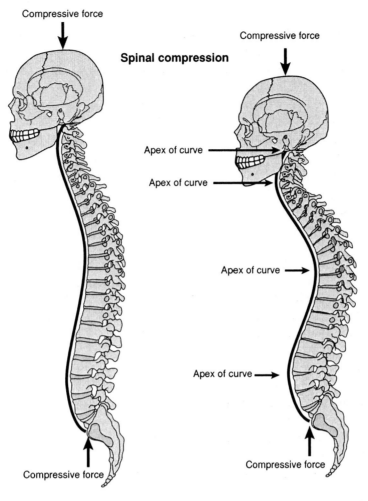

Figure 12-14 Spinal compression caused by falling from a height

Sporting injuries
- The same principles regarding the mechanism of injury also apply to sporting injuries
- Injuries may be caused as a result of:
    - Sudden severe deceleration
    - Excessive compression
    - Twisting
    - Hyperextension
    - Hyperflexion
- Other factors involved in the aetiology of injury may include:
    - Lack of proper training/inexperience/poor technique/inadequate supervision
    - Poor physical fitness
    - Lack of adequate protective clothing/equipment.
- Sports in which relatively high velocities may be achieved include:
    - Downhill skiing
    - Downhill sledging/tobogganing
    - Water skiing
    - Pedal cycling
    - Skate boarding
    - Horse riding
- If a participant in one of these sports is ejected following an initial collision, the potential injuries are similar to those following ejection from a motor vehicle

Penetrating trauma

- In penetrating trauma, injury is caused as a result of an object or missile with a small frontal area and high kinetic energy, coming into contact with skin and underlying tissues, which it penetrates entering the body
- It moves through the various tissues in its track, until its progress is either stopped by a tissue that it is so dense that it is unable to move forward, and it ceases forward movement and comes to rest, or it is deflected, or it exits the body
- As the penetrating object/missile moves through the tissues it collides with the cells in its track. With each collision there is an exchange of energy resulting in the release of heat and tissue movement, causing the penetrating object to lose some of its kinetic energy. The more kinetic energy the penetrating object/missile loses, the slower it will move
- The amount of energy lost (exchanged) from the penetrating object depends on:
    - The type of target and the density of the tissues through which the penetrating object/missile passes
    - The frontal area of the missile/object:
        - A large frontal area will result in a greater number of cells being in the track of the penetrating object, resulting in a greater energy exchange, greater tissue damage and larger cavity formation
- The frontal area of a penetrating object will depend on its:
    - Profile; bullets have a small profile, whereas bomb fragments will usually be relatively large
    - Angle of yaw/amount of tumble
    - Fragmentation

Profile

- This is the shape of the front of the penetrating object/missile, which may be pointed or blunt.
    - A penetrating object with a sharp point entering a tissue:
        - Will collide with a smaller number of cells
        - Will result in less energy transfer and less energy loss
        - Will cause less tissue damage and cavitation
    - A penetrating object with a blunt point entering a tissue:
        - Will collide with a larger number of cells
        - Will result in more energy transfer and greater energy loss
        - Will cause greater tissue damage and cavitation
    - A hollow point bullet has a sharp point as it flies through the air, losing little kinetic energy as it does so, but when it penetrates the skin and enters the tissues, its point becomes flattened or blunted and as a result of which, it collides with a lot of cells losing a lot of kinetic energy and causing a lot of tissue damage and cavitation, as it penetrates the body further

Angle of yaw

- Most missiles will tend to yaw a little from side to side as they fly through the air
- This varies during flight, and can affect the amount of kinetic energy transferred to the tissue by a factor of up to 200, depending on the angle at which the bullet strikes the skin. Thus:
    - The same weapon firing identical rounds may have different effects
    - In some circumstances a very fast bullet may produce a small energy transfer wound, whilst a slow bullet may produce a high energy transfer wound

Tumble

- If the penetrating missile/object, e.g. a bullet, is wedge shaped, it will have its centre of gravity nearer its base than its front
- If the bullet has relatively low energy, when its front collides with a tissue, it will slow rapidly. However its centre of gravity will try to continue to move forward, and the base of the bullet will try to become its leading point, resulting in an end over end cart-wheeling movement or tumble
- As it tumbles, the sides of the bullet will may become the leading edge of the bullet, impacting with a lot more cells than the front or even base of the bullet, causing much greater tissue damage and cavitation

Tumbling bullet

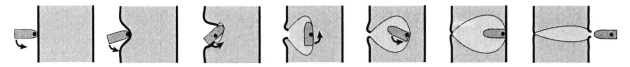

Figure 12-15 Penetrating injury: Tumbling bullet wound

Fragmentation
- If the penetrating missile/object breaks apart or separates on impact with the skin or bone, e.g. bullets with soft or hollow tips (or noses), or vertical cuts in the tip (all are called *dum-dums*) or the cupro-nickel coating of fully jacketed rounds fired by high velocity rifles, each part or fragment produced may cause significant tissue damage by itself, including multiple exit wounds; the sum of all the damage caused by all the fragments from one bullet being much greater than that caused by the bullet if it had not fragmented
- The multiple pieces of shot or pellets from a shotgun produce a similar effect

Range (the distance over which the projectile has to travel)
- Air resistance slows the passage of projectiles significantly: the greater the distance, the greater the reduction in velocity and the less the kinetic energy and the injury causing potential when the projectile penetrates the body
- The majority of shootings take place at close range, using handguns, with the result that the potential for severe injury is high

Energy levels and tissue damage
- The tissue damage likely to be caused by a penetrating object/missile can be estimated by classifying the penetrating missile/object according to its kinetic energy, and thus the amount of energy likely to be transferred to the tissues
- Firearms produce either medium or high energy projectiles; the greater the explosive power of the gunpowder in the bullet case or cartridge, the greater the velocity and kinetic energy imparted to the bullet or pellets when the weapon is fired, and the greater the tissue damage caused when those bullet/pellets impact with part of a body

Low energy weapons, e.g. knifes
- These weapons only produce tissue damage at their sharp point or cutting edge, and usually there are no secondary injuries associated with them; i.e. there is no energy transfer
- Injury only occurs along the penetration track, but there is usually some elastic recoil of the tissues after the weapon has been inserted, so penetration and tissue damage is deeper than it would appear
- If the attacker moves the weapon around inside the body, extensive tissue damage may be caused
- In stab wounds:
    - Nearly 25% of penetrating abdominal injuries also involve the thoracic cavity and its contents (the diaphragm is attached lower down posteriorly than anteriorly, has no bony protection anteriorly and descends during inspiration)
    - Penetrating wounds of the thorax below the nipple line often also involve the abdominal cavity

Practical points
- If there is one stab wound there are likely to be others
- If the penetrating object has been removed, it is important to ascertain what the object was, and in cases of assault the sex of the attacker:
    - Men tend to stab with an upward stroke, holding the blade on the same side as the thumb
    - Women tend to stab downwards holding the blade on the same side as the little finger

Low velocity bullet

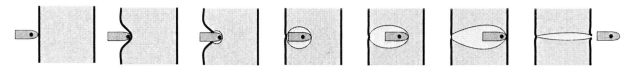

Figure 12-16 Penetrating injury: Low velocity bullet wound

Medium energy weapons, e.g. hand guns, some rifles, shotguns
- The difference between medium and high energy weapons is the size of the temporary and permanent cavities that are usually produced when their projectiles penetrate body tissues:
    - Medium energy projectiles generally cause damage to tissues on either side of their track as well as to tissues directly in their track (low energy transfer wounds)
    - As the projectile passes through the tissues, there is a build up of pressure in front of the projectile resulting in compression and stretching of the tissues as they move out of its track. As a result, there is temporary cavity formation which is usually three to six times the area of the projectile's frontal surface
    - The amount of tissue damage caused will also depend on the profile and amount of tumble and fragmentation of the projectile
    - The missile may drag in bits of clothing, etc. as it enters the body, but contamination is confined to the missile track, and does not cause gross contamination

High energy weapons, e.g. hunting rifles, assault weapons
- These generally cause much greater tissue damage than medium energy weapons (high energy transfer wounds):
    - A much larger temporary cavity is produced which extends way beyond the actual track of the projectile, resulting in much greater tissue damage and injury than may be apparent initially
    - The vacuum created behind the projectile sucks in particles of clothing, bacteria and other debris from the surrounding area into the wound, resulting in severe contamination

High velocity bullet

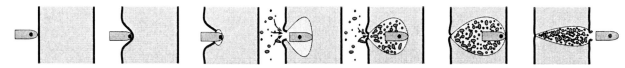

Figure 12-17 Penetrating injury: High velocity wound

13

Head injuries

Head injuries

Introduction

- Head injury is probably the most significant single injury encountered in Immediate Care, as either in isolation or in combination with other injuries; its severity affects the eventual outcome more than any other injury
- Half of all those patients who die as a result of head injury do so before they reach hospital. The skilful and aggressive pre-hospital management of these injuries is the only way that this appalling waste of (mostly young) life may be reduced
- It is the injury to the brain itself that is most significant, although it is usually associated with scalp and skull injury

Incidence

- Head injury is common in the UK:
    - Nearly 2000 patients per 100000 attend an Accident and Emergency department annually of whom approximately 250 per 100000 population require admission as a result
    - Occurs in 60-70% of all injury road traffic accidents
- Approximately 9 per 100000 population die as a result, the majority of these die within the first 24 hours following injury
- 25% of all multiply injured patients who die, do so as a result of their head injury
- Head injury is the commonest cause of death in the 15-24 age group
- Children:
    - Head injury is the commonest single cause of death in children aged over 1 year accounting for:
        - 25% of deaths in children aged 5-15 years
        - 15% of deaths in children aged 1-15 years
    - Half of all those admitted with a head injury are under 20 years old

Aetiology

- The commonest causes are:
    - Road traffic accidents
    - Assaults
    - Falls
- Other significant causes are:
    - Sporting accidents, especially golf (in children), and riding
    - Industrial accidents
- Alcohol related head injury is very common

- Commonest cause of head injury in:
    - Males: Road traffic accidents
    - Females: Domestic accidents
    - Children:
        - Road traffic accidents: 76% (most as pedestrians)
        - Falls: 13%
- Head injury resulting in unconsciousness and pulmonary aspiration of vomit is a major early cause of death (10% die before reaching hospital)

Anatomy
- Knowledge of the anatomy and physiology of the skull, its covering the scalp, and the brain is essential for an understanding of the causes and effects of head injury

Scalp
- The bony skull is covered by the scalp which has a very good blood supply and is made up of six layers:
    - Hair
    - Skin
    - Subcutaneous tissue
    - Galea aponeurotica
    - A layer of loose areolar tissue

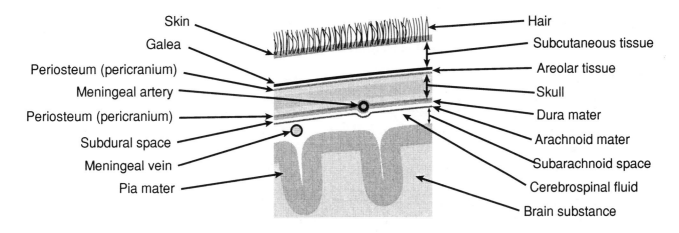

Figure 13-1 Cross section of scalp, skull and brain

Skull
- The skull has an outer and inner lining of periosteum (pericranium)
- The skull comprises:
    - The cranial vault, which is relatively thin in the temporal regions
    - The base, which is irregular and rough on its inner surface, which may cause injury when the brain impacts with it as a result of acceleration/deceleration

Meninges
- The meninges are composed of:

Dura mater
- This is a tough, fibrous membrane which is adherent to the skull's inner periosteum (pericranium)
- In some places it splits into two surfaces to form venous sinuses, that provide the major venous drainage from the brain

Arachnoid mater
- This is a thin, transparent membrane

Pia mater
- This is the membrane which covers and is attached to the cortex of the brain

Subdural space
- This is the potential space between the dura mater and the arachnoid membrane
- The subdural space is transversed by bridging veins

Subarachnoid space
- This is the space between the arachnoid membrane and the pia mater
- The subarachnoid space is filled with cerebrospinal fluid

Meningeal arteries
- The meningeal arteries lie between the inner pericranium and the dura mater

Meningeal veins
- These lie on the outer surface of the pia mater in the subarachnoid space
- There are also bridging veins which transverse the subdural space, connecting the meningeal veins to the venous sinuses

Cerebrospinal fluid (CSF)
- Cerebrospinal fluid is produced in the choroid plexus, passing into the ventricles after which it flows through the subarachnoid space, surrounding the brain

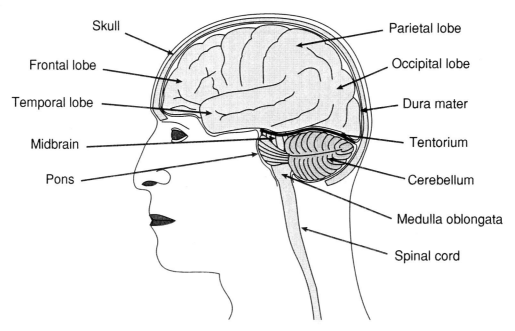

Figure 13-2 Section of through the head

Brain
- The brain is made up of the:
    - Cerebrum, composed of right and left hemispheres, separated by a reflection of dura; the falx cerebri:
        - Each hemisphere has:
            - A frontal lobe, which is involved with emotion and motor function
            - An occipital lobe, which is involved with vision
            - A parietal lobe, involved with sensory function
            - A temporal lobe, which is involved with memory, but may be relatively silent on the non-dominant side
        - In right handed people the left side of the brain is dominant, and contains the language centres; in left hand people this is reversed
    - Brain stem, composed of:
        - Midbrain ⎤ together these contain the reticular activating system,
        - Pons   ⎦ which is responsible for the 'awake' state
        - Medulla oblongata, which contains the cardiorespiratory centres
    - Cerebellum:
        - This surrounds the pons and medulla in the posterior fossa
        - The cerebellum is responsible for subconscious movement, co-ordination and balance

Tentorium
- The tentorium is a fold in the dura mater at the junction of the midbrain and cerebrum which divides the cranial cavity into the:
    - Supratentorium, composed of the anterior and middle cranial fossae, containing the cerebrum
    - Infratentorium, composed of the posterior fossa, containing the medulla and cerebellum
- The midbrain runs from the cerebrum through the opening in the tentorium, along which the third cranial (oculomotor) nerve, also passes

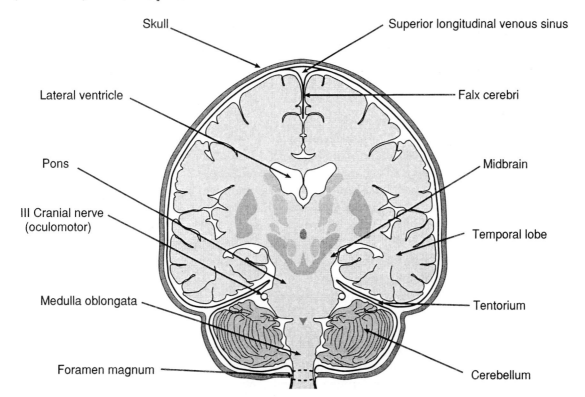

Figure 13-3 Section through the brain

Mechanisms of injury

Blunt (closed or concussional) head injuries

Incidence
- Blunt trauma is the commonest cause of brain injury in the United Kingdom
- More than one type of injury may occur following a single impact

Compression injury
- Occurs under the area of impact
- There is usually an area of diffuse tissue damage under the point of impact, the amount and severity of the damage being proportional to the amount of energy transferred from the compressing object
- A relatively minor blow may only result in cerebral concussion
- A blow of sufficient energy will result in a local fracture of the skull, and an area of cerebral contusion or even laceration under the site of the fracture, especially if the fracture is depressed
- Blows of increasing energy will progressively result in:
    - Cerebral contusion
    - Small areas of haemorrhage, resulting in prolonged unconsciousness or even death

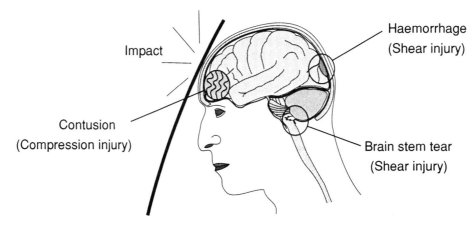

Figure 13-4 Blunt injury to the head resulting in compression injury

Acceleration, deceleration, shear injuries
- Occur when the head is subjected to sudden acceleration/deceleration often associated with rotation
- A sudden change in speed (deceleration) may result in distortion and damage of brain tissue; the actual amount of brain damage being related to the degree of stretching:
    - Cerebral contusion caused as the brain moves away from the initial point of impact and impacts with the interior of the skull furthest from the initial point of impact. This often results in a more severe cerebral contusion, than that caused by the initial impact, a 'contre-coup' injury
    - Vascular shearing injury with stretching and tearing of blood vessels resulting in:
        - Temporal or frontal lobe bruising/haematoma formation
        - Subdural haematomas
    - Shearing injury to the spinal cord or brainstem
- There is usually a period of unconsciousness
Examples:
- In road traffic accidents involving a frontal impact, the unrestrained head of a front seat occupant will continue to move forward until it impacts with the front windscreen. At the site of impact, the skull may be fractured, and there may be an underlying cerebral contusion. At the back of the skull, there may be stretching and shearing of the bridging veins, resulting in a subdural haemorrhage. If the deceleration is severe, there may also be a shearing injury of the brain stem resulting in a tear, and a 'contre coup' injury of the occipital lobes

- Patients who fall backwards, hitting the back of their head on a hard floor, e.g. concrete, are often found to have a contusion of the frontal lobes, caused by the brain moving forward and colliding with the front inside of the skull, without any skull fracture

'Contre-coup' brain injury

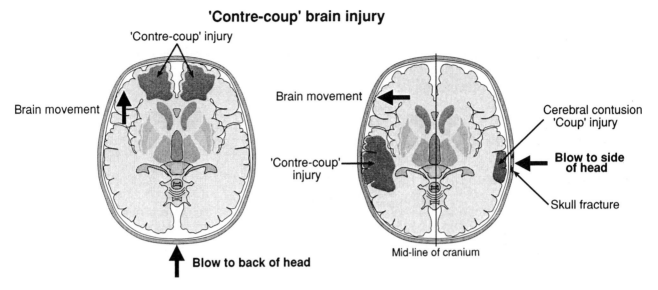

Figure 13-5 Blunt injury to the head resulting in 'contre-coup' injury

Laceration injuries
- Scalp lacerations may occur under the area of impact due to tearing and stretching
- Cerebral laceration may occur in blunt trauma if the brain impacts violently with part of the sharp irregular interior surface of the skull, e.g. the sphenoidal ridge, or as result of blunt injury resulting in a severe depressed skull fracture

Penetrating (or open) head injuries

Incidence
- Relatively rare in the United Kingdom
- More common in areas where where there is a high incidence of civil violence, firearm use or warfare

Aetiology
- The head is usually static or moving at a low velocity, and is struck by a small (relatively) high velocity, often sharp, object

Pathophysiology
- With the exception of high velocity gunshot wounds, the penetrating object is usually of relatively low velocity/energy; much of the energy is expended in penetrating the skull and there is little energy transfer to brain tissue: resulting in a relatively localised brain injury. This also applies to relatively low velocity gun-shot injuries, such as those caused by air-guns and handguns
- If the skull is penetrated by a high velocity missile, there will be massive transfer of energy to the brain tissue, which can result in an explosion of the skull and its contents
- However, even in low energy transfer wounds:
    - The outer coverings of the brain are penetrated, resulting in exposure of the intracranial contents
    - Fragments of bone, scalp, hair, clothing, vehicle and road may be carried into the brain substance; this may be both epileptogenic and act as a focus of infection resulting in meningitis, brain abscess and osteomyelitis
- There is often no history of unconsciousness
- If the injury is in a neurologically "eloquent" area of the brain, focal neurological deficits may occur

Scalp injury

Mechanism of injury

Blunt trauma
- Compression injury may result in:
    - Contusion: bruising may indicate the site of impact and thus of underlying injury
    - Avulsion: caused by a tangential force
    - Laceration as a result of splitting of the scalp under the area of impact

Penetrating injury
- Lacerations may be caused by impact with sharp objects

Pathophysiology

- The scalp has an extremely good blood supply, and haemorrhage may be considerable. If left untreated, scalp haemorrhage may result in hypovolaemic shock, especially in children and the elderly
- The loose areolar tissue, which separates the galea from the pericranium may easily be damaged or torn resulting in profuse haemorrhage, especially in:
    - Scalping injuries
    - Lacerations resulting in the formation of large flaps
    - Subgaleal haematoma formation
- Scalp lacerations may overly a skull fracture, when there may be an extracranial haematoma
- The absence of scalp injury does not preclude brain injury

Symptoms/signs
- There may be an obvious scalp laceration, abrasion or a 'boggy swelling' overlying a skull fracture
- In children there may be a subgaleal haematoma which may be very painful and is tense and fluctuant

Management

Primary survey and management
- Airway management with cervical spine stabilisation
- Breathing: ensure adequate ventilation
- Circulation with control of haemorrhage:
    - Application of direct pressure over the site of the haemorrhage with:
        - A pressure dressing:
            - Skin flaps should be restored to their anatomical position before applying any dressings, so as to avoid causing ischaemia in a creased flap
        - Clips/artery forceps:
            - If used, these should be applied to the cut edge of the galea, which should then be pulled up to compress the blood vessels between the galea and the skin (usually, just hanging the forceps over the edge of the skin flap, will produce sufficient control, by virtue of the weight of the forceps alone)
            - *No* attempt should be made to grasp the bleeding vessel itself
    - Undersewing with a quick tacking stitch (not usually possible in the pre-hospital situation)
    - Intravenous infusion with colloid to prevent/treat any hypovolaemic shock (see below)

Skull injury

Aetiology
- Skull fractures are usually caused by blunt trauma, e.g. when a deforming force such as a deceleration impact is applied to the skull
- Less commonly penetrating trauma may cause a skull fracture, which invariably also involves the brain

Mechanism of injury

Blunt trauma
- Compression injury may result in linear fractures extending away from the impact site

Penetrating injury
- Penetrating injury may result in multiple fractures around the entry wound

Pathophysiology
- The severity of any fracture is an indication of the degree of force involved/used
- Fractures usually involve the vault or less often the base of skull, or occasionally both:
    - Base of skull fractures may involve the paranasal or mastoid air sinuses, and the cranial nerves where they pass through the bone
- Skull fractures are not usually significant in themselves, but their presence indicates a greatly increased risk of:
    - Cerebrospinal fluid leakage
    - Cranial nerve damage
    - Intracranial haematoma
- Skull fractures may be:

Closed fractures

Linear fractures
- Most fractures are linear and extend from the impact site
- The length and shape of fracture lines depend on the degree of force, the area over which the deforming force is applied, and the structure and thickness of the skull at that point. The temporal region is relatively thin and therefore prone to fracture
- Linear fractures may be complicated by intracranial haemorrhage, especially the temporal region which has the middle meningeal artery running immediately underneath it
- Skull fractures in conscious and orientated patients are associated with a 1:30 risk of intracranial haemorrhage, and 1:4 patients with a skull fracture, who are not fully conscious have an intracranial haemorrhage

Depressed fractures
- Depressed fractures are often complicated by intracranial haemorrhage

Compound fractures
- Compound fractures may occur when:
    - There is a scalp laceration over the fracture; when the injury may also involve the dura or brain
    - The fracture involves the air sinuses or cribriform plate
- In compound fractures, there is a risk of the later development of infection (meningitis) and in penetrating fractures cerebral abscess

Symptoms/signs
- Simple linear fractures may be undetectable on clinical examination
- Depressed skull fractures may be palpable as an area of scalp depression surrounded by boggy scalp haematoma formation
- Compound fractures should be suspected if the patient has:
    - An overlying scalp wound
    - Mastoid bruising (Battle's sign):
        - Indicates a probable fractured base of skull (middle cranial fossa)
    - Periorbital haematoma (panda or racoon eyes):
        - In the absence of an injury to the eye itself, this may be indicative of:
            - Blow-out fracture of the orbital floor
            - Anterior (middle third) skull fracture
    - CSF rhinorrhoea or otorrhoea (see below)
    - A nasal or facial fracture

Management

Primary survey and management
- Airway care with stabilisation of the cervical spine if indicated:
    - Maintenance of adequate oxygenation
- Breathing: maintenance of adequate ventilation
- Circulation care with control of any obvious haemorrhage

Complications of skull fracture

CSF leak

Aetiology/pathophysiology
- Indicates a compound skull fracture with an associated dural tear:

Rhinorrhoea (most common cause of CSF leak) indicates:
- Anterior fossa fractures (25%), including the frontal ethmoid or sphenoid sinuses, especially the cribriform plate (50% of patients will have anosmia)
- Fracture of the petrous temporal bone (rarely)

Otorrhoea indicates:
- Fracture of base of skull (7%)
- Laceration or perforation of the eardrum

Sign: CSF may be a clear or bloodstained fluid and it may be difficult to differentiate heavily bloodstained CSF from blood alone. However, if bloodstained CSF is put on a slide, it will separate out so that the red cells concentrate in the centre of the drop; the 'Ring Test' for CSF

Aerocoele
- Due to the entry of air inside the cranial cavity

Cranial nerve palsy

Incidence
- Occurs in about 30% of patients with severe head injuries
- Commonest:
    - I: Anosmia: may occur in association with fractures of the cribriform plate, followed by:
    - VII: Facial nerve palsy
    - VIII: Deafness
- Less common (others are rare):
    - III: Traumatic mydriasis: (pupil dilation may indicate uncal herniation due to cerebral oedema)

Aetiology
- Cranial nerve palsies occur in base of skull fractures where the nerve penetrates the skull:
    - Cribriform plate: I (may also occur in mild head injury without skull fracture)
    - Orbit (apex) or cavernous sinus: II, III, IV and VI
    - Base of skull: VI (diplopia)
    - Petrous temporal bone: VII, VIII

Management
- Very little in the Immediate Care situation, other than recording any obvious motor or sensory deficit and drawing the attention of the receiving doctor to it

Brain injury
- Head injury is a dynamic situation, involving both acceleration and deceleration
- Injury often involves all three tissues: scalp, skull and brain, but the brain injury is the most significant

Incidence
- Brain injury occurs in 30 % of head injuries

Primary brain injury
- This is the injury incurred at the time of impact; it is established immediately after the initial impact and is not amenable to surgical management
- The severity of the primary brain injury may vary from minor to severe

Mechanism of injury

Blunt trauma
- Compression injury may result in:
    - Cerebral concussion
    - Cerebral contusion under the area of impact
- Acceleration, deceleration and shear injury may result in sudden movement of the brain inside the cranial cavity, resulting in:
    - Shearing of bridging veins
    - Cerebral laceration, caused by impact of the sharp interior edges of the cranial cavity

Penetrating injury
- Penetrating injury may result in very severe brain injury, depending on the amount of transferred energy

Pathophysiology

Severity of brain injury

Minor head injury
- Accounts for the majority of head injuries
- The injury is frequently trivial with minor concussion and transient loss of consciousness
    - Short initial period of unconsciousness (<6 hours)
    - Post traumatic amnesia is short (<24 hours)
    - The majority recover fully

Major head injury
- There may be prolonged or profound loss of consciousness and severe focal damage:
    - Coma lasting >6 hours
    - Post traumatic amnesia >24 hours
- The degree of eventual recovery depends on the initial brain injury, if recovery facilities are satisfactory

Types of brain injury

Cerebral concussion
- A blow to the head may result in a brief period of unconsciousness with some memory deficit, caused by an injury to the reticular activating system in the brain stem and cerebral cortex
- Usually associated with a transient physiological disturbance in brain function without any identifiable gross tissue injury

Cerebral contusion
- Cerebral contusion occurs after more violent blunt trauma resulting in:
    - Anatomical disruption of brain tissue with damage to axons and synapses, resulting in localised brain swelling
    - A more prolonged period of unconsciousness with retrograde and sometimes antegrade amnesia and vomiting

Cerebral laceration
- Cerebral laceration results in major damage to the brain and is a much more severe injury than cerebral concussion or contusion
- Cerebral laceration is often associated with severe haemorrhage, brain swelling and coma

Secondary brain injury
- This is the injury that is sustained after the impact, and is due to a variety of preventable or irreversible causes
- Although the primary brain injury may be relatively minor, the secondary injury may be life threatening

Aetiology
- Intracranial haemorrhage
- Impaired respiration resulting in hypoxia and hypercapnia
- Reduced cerebral perfusion due to hypotension secondary to major trauma

Physiology
- The brain occupies the cranial cavity, which being bony is inelastic
- Brain is a:
    - Fluid, and is therefore incompressible
    - Biological tissue and its response to injury, e.g. contusion, is swelling

- An adequate blood supply to the intracranial contents depends on:
    - Cerebral perfusion pressure (CPP), which depends on the mean arterial (blood) pressure (MAP)
    - Cerebrovascular resistance, which may be increased by:
        - Extracranial venous obstruction caused by e.g. compression of the jugular veins in the neck (which may be caused by a cervical collar, which is too tight)
        - Impeding the venous return due to putting the patient in the head down position
- A rise in intracranial pressure (ICP), which is not accompanied by a compensatory rise in systemic blood pressure, will result in reduced cerebral perfusion and a reduction in venous outflow, thus further increasing cerebral oedema and intracranial pressure (worse if there is CO_2 retention)
- Cerebral perfusion is all important, and depends on there being an adequate blood pressure and blood oxygenation:
    - *Cerebral perfusion pressure (CPP) = mean arterial pressure (MAP) - intracranial pressure (ICP)*
- A cerebral perfusion pressure below 40 mmHg will result in a critical reduction in cerebral blood supply

Effect of changes in arterial $PaCO_2$ on cerebral blood-flow

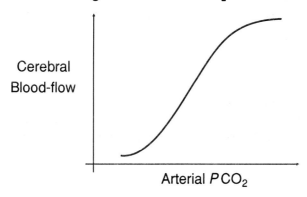

Figure 13-6 Effect of changes in PaCO₂ on cerebral blood flow

$PaCO_2$
- The $PaCO_2$ has a significant effect on intracranial pressure because the cerebral arterioles react to changes in $PaCO_2$:
    - A rise in $PaCO_2$ results in the cerebral arterioles dilating:
        - An increase in the $PaCO_2$ from 40 to 80 mmHg, results in a doubling of cerebral blood-flow
        - A rise in the $PaCO_2$ due to impaired ventilation in a head injured patient will result in a rise in the intracranial pressure and impaired cerebral perfusion
    - A fall in $PaCO_2$ results in the cerebral arterioles constricting
        - An decrease in the $PaCO_2$ from 40 to 20 mmHg, results in a halving of cerebral blood-flow
        - A reduction in the $PaCO_2$ due to hyperventilation in a head injured patient will result in a reduction in the intracranial pressure

Relationship of intracranial pressure to blood volume

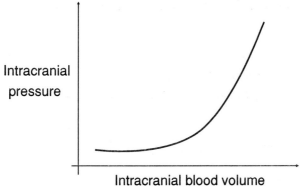

Figure 13-7 Relationship of intracranial pressure to blood volume

Cerebrovascular autoregulation
- Cerebral blood-flow is usually regulated by the arterioles of the cerebral circulation:
  - In healthy patients a constant cerebral blood-flow is maintained by:
    - Arteriolar dilation, when the systemic systolic blood-pressure falls, even as low as 60 mmHg
    - Arteriolar constriction when the systemic systolic blood-pressure rises, even up to 160 mmHg
- Brain injury results in impairment of this autoregulatory system, and a reduction in arterial blood pressure may result in reduced cerebral blood-flow/perfusion, thus hypovolaemic shock will exacerbate any reduced cerebral perfusion due to a brain injury

Increasing intracranial pressure
- An increase in intracranial pressure after a head injury is caused by one or a combination of the following factors:
  - Diffuse brain swelling due to:
    - Cerebral oedema secondary to injury
    - An increase in the cerebral blood volume
  - Intracranial haematoma formation
  - CSF or venous outflow obstruction
- Initially an increase in the volume of the contents of the cranial cavity, e.g. cerebral swelling, results in minimal rise in the intracranial pressure (ICP), until the critical point when no more CSF or venous blood can be absorbed or squeezed out of the cranial cavity is reached, after which the intracranial pressure rises rapidly as the volume of the intracranial contents increases
- A continuing rise in intracranial pressure above the tentorium will eventually result in:
  - Downward (caudal) displacement of the brain
  - The medial components of the temporal lobes herniate through the tentorial hiatus, stretching the ipsilateral oculomotor nerve, resulting in pupil dilation and eventually failure to react to light
  - Compression of the upper brain stem
  - Herniation/impaction of the medulla through the foramen magnum, resulting in ischaemic damage to the respiratory centres (coning)
  - Reduction in the level of consciousness
  - Deterioration of respiratory and cardiac function
  - Untreated (untreatable) herniation results in secondary brain stem infarction and death

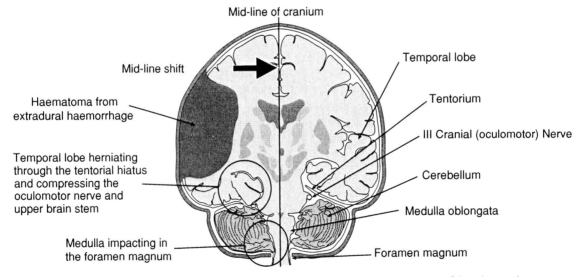

Figure 13-8 Increasing intracranial pressure due to haematoma, resulting in coning

Cushing reflex
- A rise in the intracranial pressure results in a reflex increase in blood pressure and an early reduction in pulse rate, followed later by an increase in pulse rate and widening of the pulse pressure

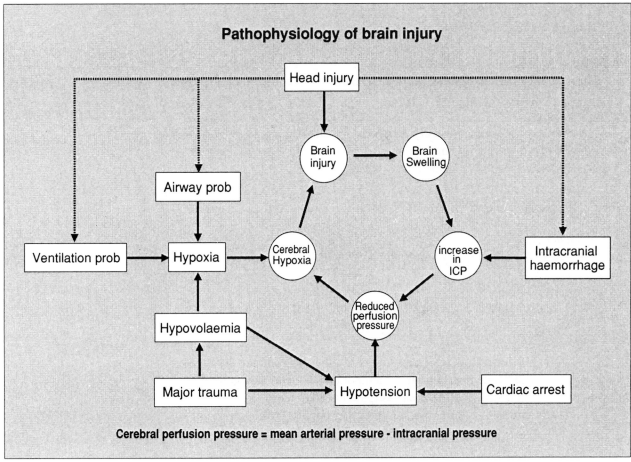

Figure 13-9 Pathophysiology of brain injury

Physiological effects of increasing intracranial pressure
- The physiological effects of increasing intracranial pressure progress rapidly:
    - The initial effect of raised ICP on the cerebral cortex and brain stem results in:
        - A rise in blood pressure
        - Slowing of the pulse rate
        - Slight pupil constriction, but the pupils react to light
        - Cheyne-Stokes respiration due to a fall in PaO_2 and a rise in $PaCO_2$
        - Cerebral irritability; the patient will attempt to localise and remove painful stimuli. As intracranial pressure increases they will only withdraw from painful stimuli and later will show decorticate posturing with flexion of the upper extremities and rigid extension of the lower limb extremities
    - Later as intracranial pressure continues to rise and there is more brainstem compression, there is:
        - A further rise in blood pressure
        - Slowing of the pulse rate
        - Fixation of the pupils or a sluggish pupil reaction
        - A tachypnoea with a fast, shallow respiratory pattern
        - Decerebrate posturing with extension of the upper extremities, torso and legs
    - Finally there is irreversible lower brain stem compression resulting in:
        - A fall in blood pressure
        - A rapid and irregular pulse
        - Dilation and fixation of one or both pupils
        - Ataxic breathing (irregular with no rhythm) or apnoea
        - Flaccidity and an absence of any response to painful stimuli, followed by death

Intracranial haemorrhage
- This is a major cause of preventable early death following head injury

Mechanism of injury
- Intracranial haemorrhage may occur as a result of blunt or penetrating trauma

Pathophysiology
- Intracranial haemorrhage usually occurs as a result of trauma to blood vessels:
    - Within the skull, e.g. middle meningeal artery
    - Adjacent to bone, e.g. the major dural sinuses

Extradural (epidural) haemorrhage

Incidence
- <2% of all head injury admissions

Aetiology
- Usually associated with skull fracture, as a result of blunt trauma

Pathophysiology
- Arterial haemorrhage (bleeding) between the skull and the dura mater:
    - Middle meningeal arteries: temporal or parietal haematoma
    - Dural sinuses: frontal or occipital haematoma
- Rapid arterial bleeding results in the development of a large haematoma, which causes cerebral compression and eventually coning

Symptoms/signs
- There is usually an initial loss of consciousness
- This is followed by apparently full recovery
- The patient may later become aggressive due to cerebral irritability, increasingly drowsy and complain of a headache, before losing consciousness as the intracranial pressure rises, with:
    - A motor weakness on the opposite side to the injury
    - A fixed and dilated pupil on the same side as the injury
    - The patient may become progressively more unconscious

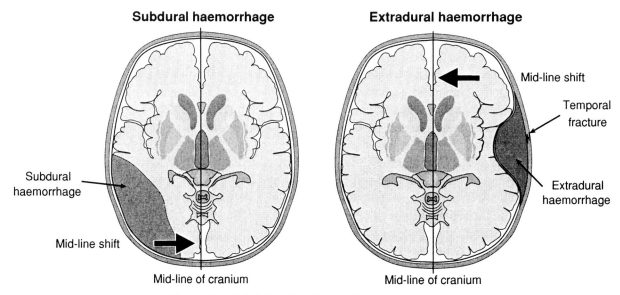

Figure 13-10 Subdural and extradural haemorrhage

Subdural haemorrhage

Mechanism of injury
- Usually occurs as a result of rapid deceleration causing a shear injury

Pathophysiology
- Venous haemorrhage occurs as a result of rupture of the bridging veins from the cortex to the dural sinuses in the subdural space

Intracerebral haemorrhage

Mechanism of injury
- Blunt trauma resulting in cerebral laceration or contre-coup injury
- Penetrating trauma (more rarely)

Pathophysiology
- Bleeding into the brain substance itself, resulting in diffuse brain injury and swelling

Assessment

History
- Obtaining and providing an accurate history is probably more important in the head injured patient than in any other type of injury, as the patient's hospital management depends on exactly what has happened to him. It is up to those at the scene of the accident to obtain and provide it
- The history should include:
    - The time of injury
    - The type of injury
    - The estimated speed of impact/amount of deceleration
    - The mechanism of injury, especially if there is any indication of associated injury to the cervical spine, e.g. hyperextension of the neck
    - Whether or not the head injury was secondary to some other event: syncope, AMI or fit
    - Whether or not a crash helmet, seat belt, etc. was worn
    - Whether or not alcohol was involved (alcohol may also alter the level of consciousness, by inducing hypoglycaemia)
    - The patient's condition immediately after the injury and any changes in that condition
    - Any periods of altered consciousness: If so when ? how long ?
    - Amnesia:
        - Retrograde amnesia
        - Post-traumatic amnesia

Practical point: If the casualty was wearing a crash helmet of any type, it should be sent with them to hospital as careful examination of it may give a very good idea as to the mechanism of injury/impact, the amount of force involved, and the degree of brain injury that can be predicted

Symptoms/signs
- The objective of head injury assessment is to identify the primary injury and to recognise (and therefore prevent) any further deterioration or potential deterioration, before or as it arises
- It is therefore extremely important in head injured patients to record the patients's symptoms, and obtain and record serial observations of their vital signs

Primary assessment

Airway
- Assess the airway; impaired consciousness can result in airway obstruction by tongue, dentures, or vomit

Breathing
- Assess the adequacy of ventilation
- Look for:
    - An increased respiratory rate
    - Irregularity of respiration
- Measure the oxygen saturation:
    - A reduced saturation indicates reduced ventilatory efficiency, and the cause should be looked for and managed appropriately

Circulation
- Look for obvious signs of haemorrhage and apply direct pressure to any bleeding scalp wounds
- Measure:
    - Blood pressure
    - Pulse: rate, volume, regularity
- *Never* assume that hypotension is caused by head injury

Disability (neurological state)
- Assess the state of the higher functions:
    - Confusion, unconsciousness
    - Irritability (indicates hypoxia)
- Is there evidence of:
    - "Vegetative" disorders: vomiting
    - Hypersecretion: bronchus, saliva
    - Motor dysfunction: decerebration
    - Fits
    - Pupil abnormalities:
        - Pupil size changes are usually a late and serious sign, and are unlikely in the alert patient
        - Unilateral pupil dilation:
            - Indicates an uncal herniation with oculomotor lobe dysfunction
            - Associated brain stem compression and may indicate a developing space occupying lesion, e.g. an expanding haematoma due to arterial bleeding
        - Bilateral dilation and loss of reactivity indicates secondary brain stem compression, with a risk of brain stem infarction, increasing brain stem injury progressing to irreversible damage
- Temperature elevation

Initial neurological assessment
- This is especially important in head injuries, and is useful both as a prognostic indicator, and as a guide to further management
- Measure/establish the base lines (including temperature if possible/practicable)
- Compare these with the history
- Record them for future reference

AVPU scale
A: Alert
V: Responds to verbal stimuli
P: Responds to painful stimuli
U: Unresponsive

Primary management
- The objective of head injury management is the prevention and treatment of secondary brain injury
- The first priority is to reduce any cerebral hypoxia and hypercapnia and to preserve the vital functions

Airway care
- Airway protection:
    - From obstruction: position, airway
    - From aspiration (a major cause of mortality after head injury), especially if there is a history of alcohol ingestion: intubation
- Oxygen (vital) in as high a concentration as possible, as even slight hypoxia results in an increase in brain swelling and intracranial pressure
- Cervical spine immobilisation, if indicated, with a semi-rigid cervical collar (avoid compressing the jugular veins which may cause obstruction of the venous return of the brain and a rise in intracerebral pressure)

Note: It must be assumed that the unconscious head injured patient has a cervical spine injury until proven otherwise; they must be handled accordingly, and the neck immobilised in a semi-rigid cervical collar

Breathing: ventilation care
- Ventilation
    - Ventilation should be considered especially if the patient has an associated chest injury, depressed respiration or a compromised airway necessitating intubation
    - If there is evidence of inadequate ventilation, the patient should be intubated and ventilated
    - Consideration should be given to hyperventilating the patient to reduce brain swelling and increase oxygenation, but be aware that prolonged hyperventilation may cause hypocapnia, resulting in cerebral arteriolar constriction, cerebral hypoxia and may exacerbate brain swelling
    - In children intubation should be considered due to the high risk of gastric aspiration

Note: 1. Chest injury is often (in up to 40% of patients) associated with serious head injury, and exacerbates any hypoxia (the prognosis is much worse)
    2. Head injured patients tolerate hypoxia badly, so it is very important to treat any chest injury impairing efficient respiration, e.g. pneumothorax, flail chest, early

- Sedation
    - The commonest cause of cerebral irritability is hypoxia, which requires immediate treatment
    - Cerebral irritability may result in inappropriate muscular action, and exacerbates hypoxia, by diverting the circulation to the skeletal muscles, which metabolise the already scarce oxygen
    - Sedation may be appropriate in the confused hypoxic and violent patient in whom airway and respiratory care to correct their hypoxia is not possible because of the difficulty experienced in restraining them and preventing them from removing airway devices, e.g. oxygen mask, airway
    - The drugs of choice are midazolam or propofol, titrated to the patient's response (for dosage, see chapters on Pain management and Airway care)
- Fitting
    - This usually indicates severe cerebral injury with focal injury or increased intracranial pressure
    - It may result in impairment of oxygenation and ventilation, making efficient management of the patient difficult, and will exacerbate hypoxia
    - The treatment is administration of midazolam or diazepam (see above)
- Vomiting
    - This may result in:
        - Pulmonary aspiration of gastric contents
        - An increase in intracranial pressure

Cardiovascular care

- Hypotension is *not* caused by head injury (patients with a head injury do not regulate their blood pressure when there is coexistent blood loss)
- If hypotension is present, it *must* be due to hypovolaemia, which if not treated will exacerbate hypoxia

Management

- Establish an intravenous infusion which will help to reduce hypoxia if the patient is hypovolaemic
- Colloids are preferred to crystalloids, as they are less likely to cause cerebral oedema
- Treatment of the cause of the hypovolaemia, if appropriate, e.g. splinting of fractures

---

Discussion point: Infusion of patients with a head (brain) injury and hypovolaemic shock

Concerns

- Controlled hypotension is designed to provide adequate tissue perfusion of vital organs in the patient with hypovolaemia due to multiple trauma, without raising the systolic pressure to the level at which blood loss increases (see chapter on Circulation care: shock)
- The prime objective of cardiovascular care of the brain injured patient however is to maintain cerebral oxygenation and perfusion, which necessitates maintaining an adequate cerebral perfusion pressure: which may be difficult in the presence of increasing intracranial pressure and hypovolaemic shock, and will necessitate raising the systolic pressure well above that used for controlled hypotension
- An inadequate cerebral perfusion pressure will result in cerebral hypoxia, increased brain swelling and ultimately death
- Overtransfusion, especially with crystalloid will increase cerebral oedema and intracranial pressure

Conclusion

- Controlled hypotension is therefore not appropriate in the severely head injured patient, and the systolic blood pressure should be kept at the usual level (or even slightly above) for that patient

---

Analgesia

- Pain relief is important especially if the patient is restless and in pain, as pain itself may result in a rise in intracranial pressure
- It is mandatory to record the patient's neurological status before and after administration of analgesics, especially opiates, which may cause a change in the patient's pupil size, level of consciousness and respiratory state, together with the time the drug was administered
- The patient's response to treatment should be carefully monitored (see below)

General care

- Treat other injuries:
    - Dress lacerations/abrasions
    - Splint fractures

Associated problems affecting management

- Alcohol:
    - Coma will be present with blood alcohol levels >400 mg/100 mL
    - Intoxication is usually evident at 100 mg/100 mL
- Illegal drugs:
    - If the patient has pinpoint pupils: administration of naloxone intravenously may be beneficial
- Hypoglycaemia:
    - All patients with impaired consciousness should have their capillary blood sugar level checked. If hypoglycaemia is found, intravenous glucose or glucagon should be administered (it can do little harm and may be beneficial)

Transportation
- If the patient has a significant head injury, he should be transported to a Neurosurgical Unit, if circumstances and local geography permit

Monitoring

Secondary neurological assessment
- It is very important to carry out serial observations of all the vital signs, at regular intervals so as to detect any changes or "trends" in the patient's condition
- Should be performed in the pre-hospital situation *only* if it will not cause unnecessary delay in evacuation of the patient

Glasgow coma scale
- This is based on the best eye opening response, best verbal and best motor responses and is a practical method of monitoring changes in the patient's condition and level of consciousness
- Head injuries may be classified according to their Glasgow coma scale score (GCS):
    - GCS: 13-15   Minor head injury
    - GCS: 9-12   Moderate head injury
    - GCS: <8   Severe head injury

PRACTICAL POINT:- The coma scale may be expressed as: E1, M1, V1, etc. (this may be useful when communicating by radio, especially as neurosurgeons prefer to know the value of each component, not just the total score)

Glasgow coma scale

Eye opening	Spontaneously		4
	To verbal command		3
	To pain		2
	No response		1
Best motor response	To verbal command:	Obeys	6
	To painful stimulus:	Localises pain	5
		Flexion/withdrawal	4
		Flexion decorticate	3
		Extension decerebrate	2
		None	1
Best verbal response	Orientated/converses		5
	Disorientated/confused		4
	Inappropriate words		3
	Incomprehensible sounds		2
	Nil		1
	Total	**(3-15)** _____	

Figure 13-11 Glasgow coma scale

Head/skull
- Examination of the patient's head for:
    - Abrasion or laceration to the scalp
    - Scalp haematoma formation
    - Depressed fracture
    - CSF rhinorrhoea or otorrhoea
    - Bleeding from the ear
    - Mastoid bruising

Sensation
- A brief examination of the patient's ability to feel light touch and pain

Motor power
- A brief examination of the patient's motor system; the ability to move parts of their body on request

Reflexes
- Deep tendon reflexes (including plantar responses)

Prognosis
- Factors associated with poor prognosis include:
    - Increasing age
    - Abnormal motor signs
    - Pupil abnormalities
    - Massive lesions
    - Diffuse bilateral CT lesions
    - Multiple injuries resulting in hypovolaemia
    - Increasing intracerebral pressure

Guidelines for the management of patients with a recent head injury

Criteria for admission after a recent head injury
- The presence of one or more of the following:
    - Confusion or any other depression in the level of consciousness at the time of admission
    - Open skull fracture
    - Neurological signs or severe headache or persistent vomiting
    - Difficulty in assessing the patient, e.g. due to alcohol, in the young, in epilepsy
    - Other medical conditions, e.g. haemophilia, epilepsy (due to risk of a secondary injury during a fit)
    - The patient's social conditions or lack of a responsible adult or relative

    Note: Post-traumatic amnesia with full recovery is not an indication for admission

Criteria for consultation with a neurosurgical unit
- The presence of one or more of the following:
    - A fractured skull in combination with:
        - *Either:* Confusion or other depression of the level of consciousness
            or: Focal neurological signs
            or: Fits
    - Confusion or other neurological disturbance persisting >12 hours, even if there is no skull fracture
    - Coma continuing after resuscitation
    - Suspected open fracture of the vault or the base of skull
    - Depressed fracture of the skull
    - Deterioration in the patient's condition

14

Facial injuries

Facial injuries

Introduction

- Facial injuries may occur in isolation or may be associated with other trauma especially to the head, neck and chest
- Facial injuries are not usually in themselves life-threatening, but may become so if they result in airway obstruction or severe haemorrhage

Incidence
- Severe facial injuries are relatively uncommon

Aetiology
- In the UK facial injuries are commonly caused by:
    - Road traffic accidents (less so since the introduction of compulsory seat belt wearing)
    - Assaults (especially in young males in whom alcohol is often a contributing factor) and violent crime (incidence is increasing)
    - Sporting accidents, notably rugby, boxing, cricket, ice hockey and small ball sports (eye injuries)
- Isolated injury usually occurs as a result of assault: blows to the face
- May occur in association with multiple trauma; 2% of cases are associated with cervical spine injury
- In road traffic accidents, facial injury is often associated with head, chest and abdominal injury

Anatomy
- The facial skeleton is composed of the:

Maxilla
- The maxilla contains the air-filled maxillary sinus, and forms the medial part of the lower orbit and supports the teeth in the dentoalveolar bone

Nasal bones
- The nasal complex is composed of the nasal bones which are connected to the frontal bone, maxilla and the thin ethmoid bones which form the medial wall of the orbit

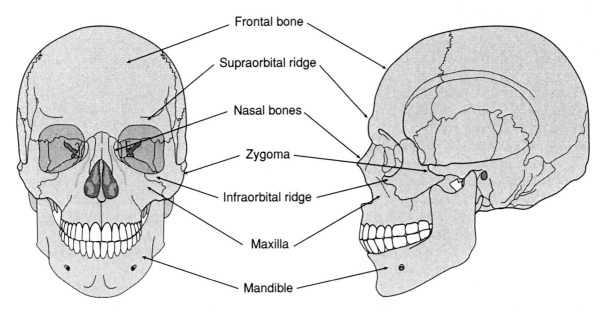

Figure 14-1 The bony skull

Orbit and zygoma
- The zygoma forms the lateral part of the floor and the lateral rim of the orbit and the lateral cheek prominence
- The orbit has a floor, roof and medial and lateral walls:
    - The frontal bone forms the upper rim
    - The zygoma forms the lateral wall and the lateral part of the floor
    - The maxilla and ethmoid bones form the medial part of the floor

Eyes
- The eyes are retained within the bony orbit, together with the extraocular muscles and periorbital fat

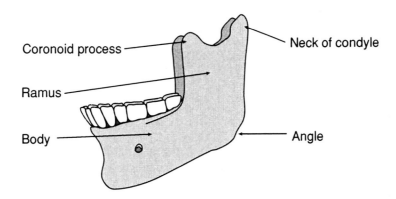

Figure 14-2 The mandible

Mandible
- The mandible holds the lower teeth, and articulates with the skull at the temporomandibular joint
- It is composed of the body, in which are inserted the teeth, the ramus and the thin neck of the condyle

Mechanism of injury

Blunt trauma

Compression
- Facial injury usually occurs as a result of blunt trauma to the face
- The impact force may be:
    - Localised, e.g. when a fist or squash ball impacts with the eye and orbital rim resulting in injury to the eye and a blowout fracture of the orbit
    - Generalised, when the impact force is spread out over the whole of the face, e.g.: extensive fractures of the mandible, maxilla and nasal bones may occur:
        - When there is high velocity frontal impact resulting in facial contact with the steering wheel in the seat-belted driver with no airbag
        - When an unrestrained front seat passenger is ejected in a frontal impact and lands head (face) first in the road, resulting in flattening of the facial contour

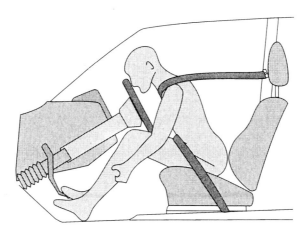

Figure 14-3 Face impacting with steering wheel in frontal impact

Penetrating trauma
- Penetrating trauma to the face is rare in the UK, but is most commonly due to airgun pellets and assault with sharp weapons

Pathophysiology

- The airway may become blocked by vomit, blood, local oedema, fractured teeth, or dentures, displaced tongue, bones or debris, which must be recognised early, especially in the unconscious patient
- Circulation:
    - The facial soft tissues have a good blood supply and tend to swell easily and bleed profusely

Symptoms/signs

- Facial deformity: swelling, oedema, and facial flattening
- Epistaxis and/or haemorrhage from the mouth
- Inability to close/clench the teeth properly (an anterior open bite indicates a middle third fracture)
- Abnormal phonation or snoring (in the unconscious patient)
- In facial fractures, there is usually surprisingly little pain, except on movements of the fracture site

Management

Primary survey
- Facial injuries may not require immediate management themselves, but if they result in airway obstruction or severe haemorrhage, they should be managed during the primary survey

Airway care
- Remove any debris, e.g. fractured teeth, dentures, from the mouth by gentle sweeping movements with a slightly flexed index finger or with McGill forceps and suction. Keep any fragments of teeth or broken dentures so that the possibility of inhaled fragments can be excluded by reconstruction
- Use a Yankauer sucker to remove any blood in the pharynx as a result of a fractured base of skull or facial bones, or tongue and mouth lacerations
- Effective airway care is especially important in the unconscious patient with a facial injury, as they may have an injury resulting in airway obstruction:
    - Posterior displacement of a fractured maxilla: hook two fingers up behind the hard palate and pull forwards and upwards (see below)
    - Posterior displacement of the tongue due to laceration/mandibular fracture: pull the tongue forward
- If there is a severe epistaxis, consider nasal packing or insertion of a balloon catheter
- Insert a device to maintain the airway if indicated:
    - Oropharyngeal or nasopharyngeal airway (but *not* the latter, if there is an associated fractured base of skull)
    - Tracheal tube; especially if there is:
        - Grossly impacted maxilla which it it not possible to disimpact
        - An unconscious patient with an absent gag reflex
        - Profuse nasal haemorrhage
        - A major head injury
        - An associated chest injury impairing ventilation, e.g. flail chest
    - Cricothyrotomy; if there is difficulty with tracheal intubation due to distorted anatomy/swelling
- If evacuation is likely to be delayed, and examination of the mechanism of injury indicates that a cervical spine injury is unlikely; place the patient in the lateral position, this:
    - Prevents the tongue causing obstruction of the airway
    - Allows blood, etc. to drain out of the mouth
- Administer oxygen if there is an associated head or chest injury or hypovolaemia

Note: Always beware of the possibility of a cervical spine injury, and take appropriate care moving the patient

Breathing
- Consider ventilation, especially if the patient:
    - Is unconscious
    - Has a major head injury
    - Has any respiratory impairment

Circulation care
- Apply firm direct pressure with a dressing over any bleeding facial lacerations
- If haemorrhage is severe; set up up an intravenous infusion

Disability
- Most facial trauma is associated with significant head injury:
    - Assess the patient's neurological status
    - Examine the skull for lacerations and CSF leakage from the nose or ears
- Examine the eyes for evidence of direct injury

Soft tissue injury of the face

Pharynx

Incidence
- Severe pharyngeal injury is rare

Pathophysiology
- The pharynx may become swollen from retropharyngeal haemorrhage and oedema, and filled with blood from a fractured base of skull, fractured facial bones, or tongue and mouth lacerations

Symptoms/signs
- Blood in the mouth
- Difficulty with breathing and swallowing
- Associated injury: fractured teeth or dentures

Management
- Gently suction away any debris, under direct vision (may not be easy with a conscious patient)
- Consider tracheal intubation or cricothyrotomy

Tongue

Incidence
- Minor tongue lacerations are relatively common. especially when caused by assault and RTAs

Aetiology
- Lacerations:
    - These are usually caused by the teeth, typically by a blow to the underside of the jaw
    - May also be caused by the patient's dentures, which may be intact or fractured

Pathophysiology
- The tongue:
    - Has a good vascular supply and tends to bleed profusely
    - May swell considerably if traumatised
- Injury may cause major problems with airway maintenance, especially if there is a transverse laceration or a fractured mandible involving the lingual blood vessels, resulting in profuse haemorrhage
- Bilateral fracture of the mandible may result in an unstable anterior segment, which may be displaced backwards together with the tongue and compromise the airway further

Symptoms/signs
- Bleeding from the mouth

Management
- Insert a suture in the tongue to pull it forward

Method
- Insert a curved needle transversely into the dorsum of the middle third of the tongue
- Tie the suture and pull the tongue forward

PRACTICAL POINT: *If a suture is not available, a safety pin and tape or string may be utilised instead*
If this is not possible, e.g. in severe transverse laceration of the tongue and intubation is not possible, consider performing a cricothyrotomy.

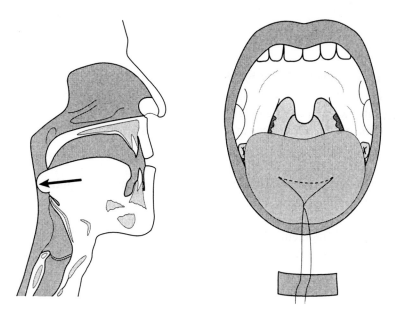

Figure 14-4 Securing the displaced tongue

Larynx/hyoid

Aetiology
- This is a very uncommon injury
- May be caused by incorrectly adjusted seat belt, or by hanging

Mechanism of injury
- Blunt trauma resulting in compression of the larynx

Pathophysiology
- May result in airway obstruction

Symptoms/signs
- Local swelling and tenderness
- Dyspnoea

Management
- If intubation is not possible due to laryngeal disruption, consider:
    - Cricothyrotomy
    - Tracheotomy

Eye

Incidence
- Ocular trauma is responsible for 5% of blind eyes in pre-school and school children
- Eye injuries are more common in males due to sporting, shooting, industrial and DIY activities, drunkenness and subsequent assault and RTAs
- One third of domestic eye injuries occur in children under 16

Aetiology
- Eye injury is now relatively uncommon in road traffic accidents, as a result of the law making the wearing of seat belts compulsory
- In industry, corneal foreign bodies are the commonest form of ocular injury (25-80%), with 60% caused by hammer/chisel fragments
- Chemical splash injury is also fairly common, especially in the manufacturing and building industries

Mechanisms of injury

Blunt trauma
- Usually caused by a direct blow
- Bruising of the eye and lids
    - This often occurs as a result of assault, or sometimes in sporting activities, especially ball games, e.g. squash, badminton, cricket and football:
        - Squash balls are hard, travel very fast (over 100 mph) and fit the eye socket exactly
        - Badminton quoits may also cause a surprisingly severe degree of injury
        - Accidental blows from the edge of sports raquets, and elbows can also cause severe injury

Penetrating trauma
- Penetrating trauma may be caused by:
    - Penetration by windscreen and spectacle glass in road traffic accidents
    - Penetration by small metallic foreign bodies created from hammer/chisel fragments

Chemical injury
- Chemical splash

Pathophysiology

Blunt trauma
- Blunt trauma of the eye seldom results in severe damage to the eye itself, but may result in dilation (traumatic mydriasis) and irregularity of the pupil, haemorrhage into the anterior or posterior chambers, retinal tears, and a blow out fracture of the floor of the orbit

Penetrating injury
- Where there is a perforation of the eye, any rise in extraocular pressure may result in extrusion of part of the intraocular contents, especially the iris

Chemical burns
- The severity of the injury is related to the duration of contact, and the concentration and pH of the chemical involved:
    - Alkalis, including cement and building lime react to form soluble compounds which penetrate the cornea almost immediately, and usually cause severe tissue damage resulting in permanent visual problems including blindness
    - Weak acids have much more limited tissue penetration

Symptoms/signs

Blunt injury
- Lid swelling and bruising with subconjunctival haemorrhage (sign of zygomatic complex fracture)
- Unilateral dilated pupil;'traumatic mydriasis'
- Distortion of the pupil:
    - This is due to splits in the iris or to the root of the iris being torn away in one area (iridodonesis)
- Hyphaema:
    - Blood in the anterior chamber, with blurred vision
- Vitreous haemorrhage:
    - The patient complains of floaters and blurred vision
- Retinal tears:
    - The patient may complain initially of flashing lights (photopsia), new floaters or visual impairment, including dense shadows in the vision or visual field loss

Penetrating injury
- Usually there is obvious damage to the cornea, with accompanying lacerations of the face and eyelids and with deformity of the pupil and sometimes prolapse of the iris or vitreous, the presence of uveal tissue in the wound, and sub-conjunctival haemorrhage

High velocity penetration
- Penetration by small metallic foreign bodies may not be obvious in the Immediate Care situation
- *Any patient who has felt something go into the eye whilst striking one piece of metal with another, especially a hammer and cold chisel, must be assumed to have sustained a penetrating eye injury until this has been excluded by a full ophthalmological examination including suitable X-rays of the globe*
- Penetrating injuries of this type are frequently absolutely pain free, seldom cause infection, and visual loss may not occur for days, weeks or even months after the original injury. Failure to recognise one may result in permanent visual loss for the patient and medico-legal proceedings against the doctor concerned
- *If a penetrating eye injury is suspected urgent ophthalmological follow up is mandatory*
- Can result in brain injury (common cause of death from airgun pellets, due to penetration via the orbit)

Chemical injury
- Severe conjunctival injection with profuse lacrimation and pain

Management
- Pad the eye

Prevent complications
- Avoidance of coughing, sneezing, straining, struggling or anything else which might raise either the intraocular or extraocular pressure

Chemical burn
- Immediate prolonged copious irrigation with tap water or a buffered solution, if available, is vital
- The patient's eye may need to be held open by an assistant during irrigation
- All solid matter, such as particles of cement should be removed with cotton wool buds, if conditions permit, however painful this may be for the patient (consider using amethocaine as a local anaesthetic)
- In severe cases irrigation should be continued for at least 30 minutes

PRACTICAL POINT: In the pre-hospital situation an infusion of N-Saline or Hartmann's solution attached to a giving set may be used to irrigate the eye, until the patient reaches hospital

Fractures of the facial bones

General
- Maxillofacial injury is rarely life threatening, unless it results in airway obstruction or severe blood loss
- Maxillofacial injury is often associated with severe head and cervical spine injury (unconscious patients with facial bone fractures should be assumed to have a cervical spine injury until proven otherwise)

Mechanism of injury

Blunt trauma
- Fractures of the facial bones are usually caused by compressive blunt trauma

Penetrating trauma
- Penetrating trauma of the facial bones is rare, but may occur due to missile injuries or stabbing

Symptoms/signs
- Facial fractures are not always obvious
- If a facial fracture is suspected, the facial contours and teeth should be carefully examined, together with palpation for surgical emphysema, which may occur when the para-nasal sinuses have been fractured

Management
- Airway care with stabilisation of the cervical spine if indicated
- Circulation care with management of haemorrhage from cancellous bone exposed at the fracture sites (rare if the bony fragments are adequately stabilised)

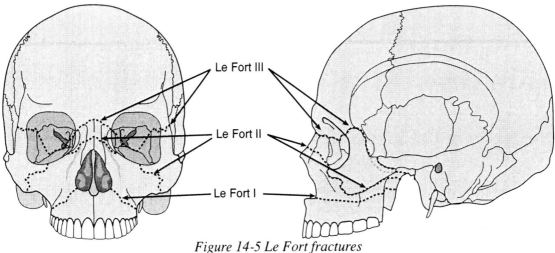

Figure 14-5 Le Fort fractures

Maxilla

Incidence
- Fractures of facial bones are relatively common (especially zygomatic complex fractures), accounting for about 30% of all bony injuries
- May be associated with head and cervical spine injuries

Aetiology
- Maxillary fractures are usually caused by:
    - Road traffic accidents (injuries are likely to be more severe)
    - Assaults
    - Sport, especially rugby, football and cricket
    - Industrial accidents

Mechanism of injury
- Usually caused by a direct high energy blunt trauma, usually a blow to the face:
    - In RTAs impact with the steering wheel in frontal impacts, and with the ground if ejected

Pathophysiology
- The maxilla may be displaced backwards and downwards causing/aggravating obstruction of the airway

Symptoms/signs
- Swelling (which may be considerable in Le Fort II and III fractures), deformity and flattening of the face around the mouth, nose and eyes "dish or long face", and bruising around the eyes, "panda or raccoon eyes"
- There may be obvious mobility of the maxilla and associated fractures of the teeth, which may be ascertained by gripping the upper teeth and adjoining gums and trying to move them. Any movement of the teeth and adjoining gum suggests a Le Fort fracture
- Cerebrospinal fluid rhinorrhoea
- Anaesthesia in the area of the infraorbital nerve is often present
- Irregularities of the dentition, dental malocclusion or an open bite may suggest a maxillary or Le Fort fracture

Management
- If the maxilla is mobile or obstructing the airway, stabilise it:

Method:
- Place the index and middle fingers into the mouth (behind and above the soft palate, if they are long enough, or in the arch of the palate) and grasping the maxilla by the alveolar margin, lift it upwards and forwards, to try to stabilise it

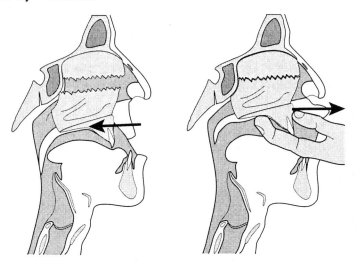

Figure 14-6 Stabilisation of the maxilla

- If manual disimpaction is unsuccessful, and there is gross displacement and the back of the soft palate is causing airway obstruction (this usually occurs only if there is an associated mandibular fracture):
    - Intubate and ventilate the patient
    - Perform a cricothyrotomy if intubation is not possible
- If there is haemorrhage (which may be profuse):
    - Set up an intravenous infusion

Note: If a maxillary fracture is suspected the patient should not blow the nose, as this may result in surgical emphysema of the soft tissues of the skin if the fracture connects with the nasal cavity or an air sinus

Nasal bones

Incidence
- Fractures of the nasal bones are a relatively common injury

Aetiology
- Injury to the nasal bones often occurs as a result of assault

Mechanism of injury
- Usually arises as a result of blunt trauma; a direct blow to the nose from the front or side
- Fractures of the nasal bones are sometimes associated with significant head injury

Pathophysiology
- Buckling of the nasal septum or depressed fractures may cause nasal obstruction
- Associated nasal haemorrhage (which may be severe) and local oedema of the nasal passages may result in nasal obstruction, and if severe, obstruction of the nasopharynx and airway obstruction
- If there is any associated obstruction of the oropharyngeal airway, the patient will rapidly asphyxiate
- Severe blunt trauma of the mid face may result in disruption of the ethmoid bones, resulting in flattening of the bridge of the nose and an increase in the distance between the eyes; 'hypertelorism'

Symptoms/signs
- Nasal deformity reflecting the direction of injury (ascertain if there is a history of previous fracture)
- Nasal obstruction: on one or both sides
- Epistaxis

Management

Airway
- If there is no possibility of a cervical spine injury; position the patient in the lateral position so that blood can drain out of the nose
- Airway management in the unconscious patient, with care of the cervical spine:
    - Oropharyngeal airway
    - Intubation
- If in any doubt, hold the teeth apart with your hands

Note: Do *not* hold the jaw forward as this may occlude the oropharyngeal airway

Haemorrhage
- Apply local pressure (with a cold pack or ice if available)
- Consider inserting a nasal catheter or nasopharyngeal airway
- Institute an intravenous infusion if the haemorrhage is profuse
- If haemorrhage is uncontrollable and intubation impossible, consider cricothyrotomy

Orbit and zygoma

Orbital fracture

Incidence
- This is the most common facial fracture
- Fractures of the inferior orbital floor 'blow-out fractures' are the most common, followed by fractures of the medial orbital wall

Aetiology
- Orbital fracture usually occurs as a result of assault or sport; especially squash

Mechanism of injury

Blunt trauma
- Blunt trauma; a direct blow to the orbit or cheek, by a fist or squash ball may cause an orbital fracture
- There is usually, but by no means always, an associated injury to the eye

Penetrating injury
- Penetrating injury may cause severe disruption of the contents of the orbit and possibly cerebral injury

Pathophysiology
- The contents of the orbit may herniate through the inferior orbital floor resulting in a "blow-out fracture"
- In particular, the inferior rectus muscle may be trapped and anchored producing total inability to elevate the eye on the injured side

Symptoms/signs
- Conjunctival/subconjunctival injection or haematoma
- Periorbital swelling and tenderness
- Restricted eye movement, especially on attempted upgaze, with double vision
- Paraesthesiae or anaesthesia over the area supplied by the inferior orbital nerve
- Fractures of the zygoma will often result in a triangular shaped lateral sub-conjunctival haemorrhage and numbness over the cheek
- If surgical emphysema is present, there must be paranasal sinus involvement, even if the patient is asymptomatic

Management
- Pad the affected eye, and do not allow the patient to blow their nose

Zygomatic arch

Incidence
- Fractures of the zygoma are relatively common

Aetiology
- Zygomatic fractures are usually caused by assault

Mechanism of injury
- Fractures of the zygomatic arch are usually caused by blunt trauma; a blow to the side of the face

Symptoms/signs
- Swelling and tenderness over the zygoma
- Zygomatic arch fracture may cause difficulty in opening the mouth if the masticatory muscles are involved in the fracture

Management
- None immediately

Mandible

Incidence
- Mandibular injury is relatively common

Aetiology
- Most mandibular fractures are caused by assault
- Other common causes include road traffic accidents, sports injuries, falls and industrial accidents

Mechanism of injury

Blunt trauma
- Mandibular fractures are usually caused by blunt trauma
- The commonest fracture is through the extracapsular part of the condylar neck, and is usually caused by a blow to the chin. It may be unilateral or bilateral
- A fracture through the angle and body of the mandible is also common, usually caused by a direct blow to the mandible from the side

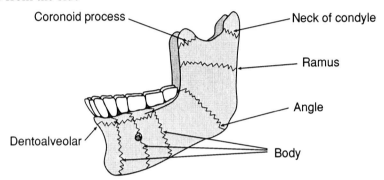

Coronoid process — Neck of condyle
Ramus
Angle
Dentoalveolar — Body

Figure 14-7 Common sites of mandibular fracture

Pathophysiology
- The common sites of fracture are:
    - The neck of the mandible
    - The body of the mandible
    - The angle of the mandible
    - The ramus of the mandible
- There is often more than one fracture, so after finding one, others should be looked for
- Fractures through both sides of the jaw may result in posterior displacement of the tongue and airway obstruction
- If the blow to the mandible is forceful enough, it may be sufficient to drive the condyle of the mandible backwards, resulting in fracture of the squamous temporal bone and result in cerebrospinal fluid leak and haemorrhage from the external auditory meatus
- Most mandibular fractures are compound and should be managed as such

Symptoms/signs
- Localised pain
- Swelling and deformity of the jaw
- Associated fractures of the teeth
- Loss of bite, malocclusion of teeth, often producing a lateral crossbite
- Bleeding and lacerated gum margins with ecchymosis on the lingual gingivae
- Anaesthesia of one half of the lower lip and chin due to trauma to the inferior dental nerve
- Absence of forward movement of the condylar head on opening the mouth
- Difficulty with swallowing, breathing and speech
- Mobility of the fractured segment of mandible

Management
  - Airway obstruction:-
    - Maintain a patent airway by pulling the tongue forward (as described above)
  - Breathing
  - Circulation:
    - Control/treat any haemorrhage
    - Obtain intravenous access and provide fluid replacement of major blood loss

Temporomandibular joint subluxation

Incidence
  - This is relatively rarely encountered in Immediate Care

Aetiology
  - May occur spontaneously (usually by yawning) or as a result of a blow to the open mouth e.g. a punch or kick

Mechanism of injury
  - Blunt trauma to the mandible results in forward subluxation of the condyle out of the glenoid fossa, whilst still remaining within the joint capsule
  - Very rarely there may be posterior subluxation (see above)
  - Subluxations may be unilateral or bilateral

Symptoms/signs
  - The patient with a bilateral subluxation will have an anterior open bite with forward jaw protrusion

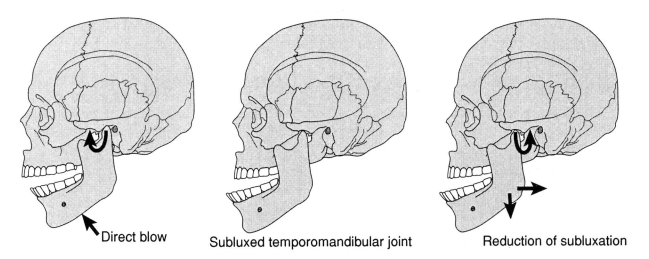

Direct blow   Subluxed temporomandibular joint   Reduction of subluxation

Figure 14-8 Mandibular subluxation and reduction

Management
  - Immediate reduction may be possible, if necessary using nitrous oxide/oxygen anaesthesia
  - The patient should be advised not to yawn or open their mouth wide for at least 24 hours after reduction

Method
  - Stand in front of the patient, insert the thumb of both hands into the mouth, grasp the angle of the jaw and apply pressure to the lower molar teeth angle of the jaw pushing the jaw downwards and backwards, and at the same time tilting the chin upwards

Teeth

Incidence
- 25% of children suffer some form of injury to their front teeth

Aetiology
- The teeth are often damaged in facial injuries due to assault, road traffic accidents, sporting or industrial accidents

Mechanism of injury
- Blunt trauma to the face is the usual cause of damage to the teeth
- Children usually injure their front teeth as result of falling onto their face

Pathophysiology
- Teeth may be displaced, fractured or dislodged from their sockets
- If displaced teeth are not reinserted rapidly; the peridontal cells dry out and then die. After 24 hours the chances of a displaced tooth being successfully retained after reimplation is minimal
- The premature loss of an anterior adult tooth can be particularly disfiguring, as the bone around the edge of the socket becomes resorbed, if the tooth is no longer in place. Once this has occurred, it is not reversible and the bone loss will impair restorative dental care, e.g. bridge work

Symptoms/signs
- Displacement of teeth and haemorrhage from the gums

Management
- The sooner any displaced adult teeth are reimplanted, the greater the chance that they will be retained
- If a tooth is only partially avulsed or if only one or two teeth are avulsed, they should cleaned in N-saline, Hartmann's solution or milk, and reinserted into the socket(s) as soon as possible. Do *not* use disinfectant or tap water
- If this is not possible, any loose whole teeth displaced from the mouth should be collected, put in milk, Normal saline, or Hartmann's solution and sent with the patient to hospital for later reimplantation
- If the patient is fully conscious the teeth may be held in the buccal cavity between the cheeks and jaw
- Milk teeth should *not* be reimplanted, as to do so may result in damage to the developing adult tooth underneath

15

Chest injuries

Chest injuries

Introduction
- Chest injuries are the primary cause of death in 25% of fatal trauma cases and are a contributing factor in up to half of the remainder
- Chest injuries in conjunction with other major injuries, especially head injuries are a major cause of death following road traffic accidents
- The correct immediate management of chest injuries has a major beneficial effect on the mortality and morbidity following major trauma

Incidence
- Chest injuries are common in high speed road traffic accidents, especially in those:
    - Unrestrained by seat belts
    - Ejected from vehicles
    - Injured when there is significant side intrusion into the vehicle of which they are an occupant
    - Motorcyclists who part with their bicycles at high speed
- Chest injuries are often associated with head and abdominal injury

Aetiology
- Road traffic accidents are the major cause of major chest injuries in the UK
- Penetrating injury due to gunshot wounds, missile injuries and stabbing are relatively rare

Anatomy

Thoracic cage
- The thoracic cage is composed of:
    - The sternum anteriorly, which is composed of the manubrium, body and xiphisternum
    - The thoracic/dorsal spine posteriorly
    - Twelve pairs of ribs:
        - Posteriorly each rib articulates with the thoracic/dorsal spine
        - Anteriorly:
            - The first ten ribs articulate with costal cartilages; the last four of which are connected to each other, which articulate with the sternum
            - The last two pairs of ribs are loose
    - In between each rib are the intercostal muscles

Diaphragm
- This is the large dome shaped muscle which is situated at the base of the thorax

Lungs
- The two lungs lie inside the thoracic cage, in the thoracic cavity, one on each side of the body
- The inner surface of the thoracic cavity is lined by the parietal pleura, and the outer surface of the lungs is lined by visceral pleura. Between the two is a small quantity of serous fluid, which helps the two surfaces to move separately from each other. The two pleural surfaces are held together by surface tension, which acts in a similar way to a vacuum

Mediastinum
- The mediastinum lies between the two halves of the thoracic cavity and contains the heart, the great vessels, the trachea and bronchi, and the oesophagus

Note: The liver, spleen and stomach are situated within the dome of the diaphragm, together with parts of the kidneys and colon (the splenic and hepatic flexures and the transverse colon), and may be considered to be situated within the thorax

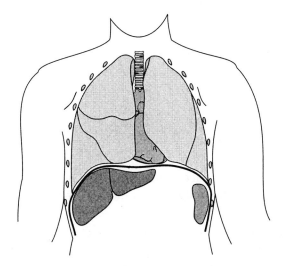

Chest: thoracic cage: front view

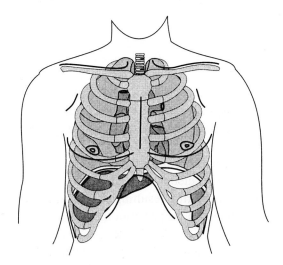

Chest: thoracic cage: back view

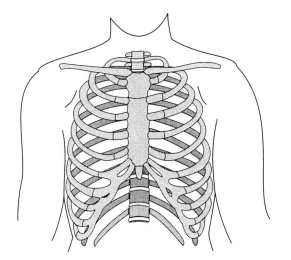

Chest: front view: internal organs

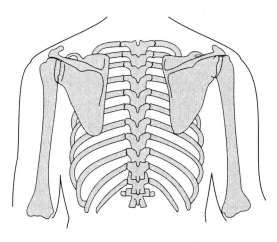

Chest: front view: surface anatomy

Figure 15-1: Anatomy of the thorax

Physiology

- Physiologically the heart and lungs may be considered to be a single unit; the lungs extract oxygen from the air breathed in, which enters the circulatory system and is pumped by the heart around the body in the arterial system to the tissues. In the tissues oxygen enters the cells in exchange for carbon dioxide, which then returns to the heart via the venous system, before being pumped to the lungs, where it is exchanged for oxygen
- The lungs draw in air by expanding their volume, due to the effect of the intercostal muscles which increase the volume of the thoracic cage and its contents, and/or the diaphragm, which contracts resulting in downward movement of its dome

Mechanism of injury

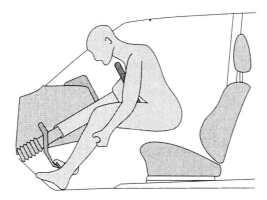

Figure 15-2: Thorax impacting with the steering wheel in an unrestrained driver

Blunt trauma

Compression injury
- Compression of the anterior chest wall may result in fractures of the underlying ribs and sternum, together with contusion of the lung beneath the area of impact
- If compression occurs suddenly, and the victim holds their breath at the moment of impact, the lungs may burst, rather like a paper bag filled with air that is then suddenly compressed
- In road traffic accidents chest injuries may be caused by:
    - Unrestrained vehicle drivers impacting with the steering wheel in frontal collisions, resulting in compression of the thorax and fractured ribs or a fracture or dislocation of the sternum. Very severe frontal impact may also result in cardiac compression and wedge fractures of the thoracic vertebrae, due to hyperflexion
    - Seat belts, if the vehicle occupant is wearing a three point seat belt, especially if there is high speed deceleration, resulting in compression and fracturing of the underlying bones, including clavicles, sternum and ribs, and damage of the underlying structures
    - Side door intrusion may result in rib and clavicle fractures
    - Collision with other vehicle occupants

Acceleration, deceleration, shear injury
- Massive deceleration may result the heart moving forward and impacting with the inner surface of the sternum and ribs, resulting in myocardial contusion, and shearing of the arch of the aorta, near its attachment to the posterior thoracic wall

Penetrating trauma
- Penetrating chest injuries may be caused by missile and bullet wounds

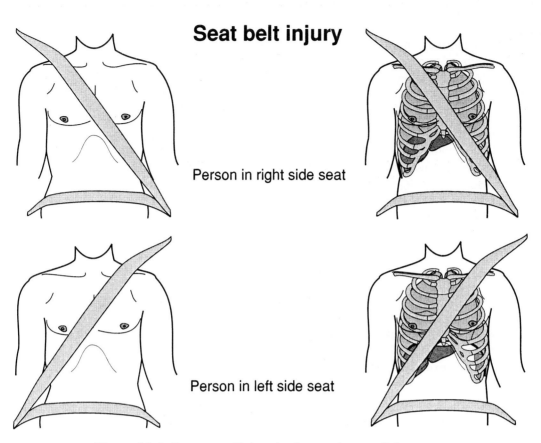

Seat belt injury

Person in right side seat

Person in left side seat

Figure 15-3: Patterns of injury in three point seat belt wearers

Pathophysiology
- Any structure in the chest may be damaged by trauma, including:
    - Skin
    - Ribs, sternum
    - Pleura
    - Lungs
    - Heart and mediastinum
    - Liver and spleen within the bony thorax

Ventilation-perfusion mismatch
- This occurs when there is perfusion of non-ventilated lung, resulting in intrapulmonary shunting
- Even a small amount of intrapulmonary shunting may significantly reduce the benefit of administering high concentration oxygen in the inspired air, and will cause persistent arterial hypoxaemia (increasing the oxygen concentration in inspired air will only increase the arterial concentration, if there is gaseous exchange in ventilated areas of lung)
- Causes of ventilation-perfusion mismatch include:
    - Pulmonary contusion (commonest), with:
        - Damage of the lung tissue with associated haemorrhage, oedema and an increase in pulmonary permeability
    - Pulmonary aspiration
    - Simple pneumothorax
    - Inhalation burns
- Chest injuries, e.g. rib and sternal fractures, causing pain on breathing may inhibit respiration and significantly reduce tidal volume
- Rib fractures which cause disruption of the integrity of the thoracic cage, e.g. flail chest, result in failure of the normal process of lung expansion, and are often associated with pulmonary contusion

Hypovolaemia
- Significant haemorrhage may be caused by laceration of the intercostal and internal mammary arteries, resulting in severe hypovolaemia and haemothorax
- Laceration of lung parenchyma alone may not result in significant haemorrhage, because low-pressure blood vessels alone may be involved, and any bleeding is usually self-limiting

Mechanical problem
- Tension pneumothorax may cause impairment of the mechanism of ventilation
- Cardiac tamponade caused by haemorrhage into the pericardial space may cause reduction of cardiac output by reducing ventricular filling
- Expanding mediastinal haematomas may cause compression of the vena cava, resulting in impairment of the venous return and reducing cardiac output

Symptoms/signs
- Chest injuries may be difficult to assess especially if the patient is unconscious due to an associated head injury
- Chest injury should always be positively searched for in these circumstances, especially if an examination of the mechanism of injury indicates that a significant chest injury is likely to have been sustained
- Always remember to examine the back of the chest as well as the front

Pain
- Especially on inspiration or coughing

Dyspnoea
- Difficulty with breathing, feeling of chest tightness

Inspection
- Inspection of the neck and chest should be carried out with good lighting if possible, look for:
    - Obvious bruising, external wounds
    - Paradoxical chest movement
    - Increased/reduced respiratory rate
    - Raised jugular venous pressure on examination of the neck veins
    - Respiratory distress
    - Surgical emphysema
- After inspecting the neck, immobilise it with a semi-rigid collar

Palpation
- Feel the trachea and ribs, to identify:
    - Tracheal deviation (a late sign)
    - The crackling sensation of surgical emphysema
    - Pain over fracture site produced by springing the ribs
    - Clunking sensation over fractured ribs/sternum

Percussion
- Percussion of the chest is usually difficult due to the high ambient noise levels usually encountered in the pre-hospital situation
- Percuss at the top and bottom of both axillae
- There may be hyper-resonance over a pneumothorax
- The percussion note may be dull over a haemothorax or pulmonary contusion

Auscultation
- Listen at the top of the chest and in both axillae for reduced air entry over a pneumothorax or haemothorax

ECG
- Damage to coronary vessels or myocardial contusion may produce ECG changes suggestive of AMI

Pulse oximetry
- Hypoxia may be indicated by a reduced oxygen saturation (SpO_2)

Management

Primary survey
- All patients with a chest injury have an increased requirement for oxygen, which should be administered via a high concentration oxygen mask, and at a high flow rate (12-15 litres per minute)

Priorities
- Airway with cervical spine stabilisation:
    - Upper airway obstruction:
        - Maintain the correct neck position
        - Use an oro- or nasopharyngeal airway
        - Consider tracheal intubation
- Breathing:
    - Tension pneumothorax:
        - Decompress with a needle
        - Insert a chest drain
    - Seal any open chest wound
    - Flail chest:
        - Stabilise
        - Support respiration by ventilating the patient
- Circulation with control of haemorrhage:
    - Monitor the pulse and blood pressure, and even if there is evidence of hypovolaemia, infuse sparingly (pulmonary oedema may be aggravated by use of intravenous fluid replacement)
- Disability
- Exposure with control of the environment
- Relieve any pain which may be impairing respiration:
    - Intravenous analgesia
    - Local anaesthetic nerve block

Note: Nitrous oxide/oxygen (*Entonox®, Nitronox®*) are contraindicated in chest injuries, due to the potential risk of causing a tension pneumothorax (see chapter on Pain management)

Secondary survey
- If time and circumstances permit, carry out a head to toe survey of the patient and treat any problems as appropriate:
    - Assess the quality of ventilation
    - Carefully inspect the chest wall for evidence of bruising, asymmetrical chest wall movement and wounds
    - Palpate the sternum and each rib looking for tenderness, bony crepitus and subcutaneous emphysema, and the trachea to make certain that it is not deviated to one side or the other
    - Listen to the chest for abnormal breath sounds

Open chest wounds

Incidence
- These are relatively rare in the UK

Aetiology
- A stab wound is one cause

Mechanism of injury

Blunt trauma
- Blunt trauma does not usually cause an open chest injury, unless there is a severe abrasion of the chest wall, resulting in exposure of the ribs and underlying lung

Penetrating injury
- Penetrating injury will nearly always result in an open chest wound

Pathophysiology
- The depth of penetration/damage may be deeper than may be immediately apparent
- There is nearly always some degree of lung damage and a risk of developing a pneumothorax/tension pneumothorax

Management
- Close the wound to prevent the development of a tension pneumothorax with:
    - An airtight/waterproof occlusive dressing, with one edge left free to form a one way valve
    - An *Asherman*^{TM} chest seal
- Consider insertion of a chest drain
- If there is a knife in the chest, do *not* remove it

Rib fractures

Incidence
- This is a relatively common injury
- In road traffic accidents it is often found in those patients who are not restrained by seat belts

Aetiology
- Fractures of the ribs and sternum usually occur as a result of blunt trauma:
    - Road traffic accidents
    - Falls onto sharp objects, e.g. the corner of a table
- Rib fractures as a result of penetrating trauma are relatively rare

Mechanism of injury

Blunt trauma

Compression
- Compressive blunt trauma is the usual mechanism of injury causing fractured ribs
- If the compressive force is applied over a relatively small area, the rib(s) under that area will fracture
- If the compressive force is applied over a large area, the ribs will bow and may fracture at the apex of their curve, or sublux/dislocate at the costochondral joint
- If the compressive force results in a large transfer of energy, there may be considerable disruption of the underlying ribs and associated organs and structures

- In road traffic accidents, rib injuries may be caused by:
    - Impact with the steering wheel
    - Restraint by seat belts in high speed collisions
    - Side door intrusion
    - Collision with other vehicle occupants

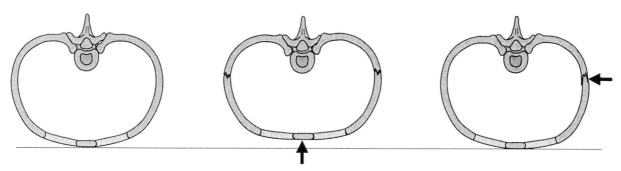

Figure 15-4: Mechanism of rib fracture

Penetrating injury
- Penetrating injury will result in a rib fracture, if the the rib is at or very close to the site of penetration, and there is a major transfer of energy. The underlying fracture is likely to be comminuted and bone fragments may fly off in various directions, causing additional internal thoracic injury

Pathophysiology
- The severity of rib fractures and their location may indicate the amount of energy transferred on impact:
    - The upper ribs are relatively well protected by the scapula, shoulder complex, and upper arm; fractures of these ribs are therefore associated with major energy transfer and are associated with damage to the aorta and great vessels, the trachea and bronchial tree, and the brachial plexus
    - Fractures of the lower ribs (9th, 10th and 11th) are often associated with damage to the liver/spleen
- The young have a relatively elastic thoracic cage, that may be able to withstand considerable compressive forces without the ribs fracturing
- The elderly have a rather rigid/brittle thoracic cage and may fracture their ribs/sternum on minor impact
- Fractured ribs, with the exception of very low energy impacts, are invariably associated with:
    - Significant haemorrhage (up to 150 mL per rib) due to damage to the intercostal and internal mammary blood vessels, which may result in haemothorax and impair ventilation further
    - Considerable underlying pulmonary contusion
- Blunt trauma of the chest may result in:
    - An isolated rib fracture
    - Multiple unilateral fractures
    - A flail chest:
        - Occurs when the integrity of the thoracic cage is breached in two places, and one part is able to move independently of the rest. As the patient inspires, the segment will move inwards, and as they expire the segment will move outwards (paradoxical respiration)
        - Will impair respiration because expansion of the underlying lung does not occur and there is a reduction in tidal volume, resulting in hypoventilation, hypoxaemia, intrapulmonary shunting and a reduction in cardiac output
    - A flail chest may be:
        - Unilateral flail segment affecting only one side of the chest
        - Bilateral with flail segments affecting both sides of the chest (this is a very serious injury, as respiration is severely impaired)
        - A flail sternum which occurs when the ribs on both sides of the sternum are fractured
        - Posterior, with a flail segment that is often relatively stable (rarely causes problems)
        - Lateral or anterior, which often results in severe respiratory distress

- The extent to which the flail segment compromises effective respiration depends on its size, and the severity of the underlying lung injury (it is the pulmonary contusion that is most significant)
- A flail chest may be complicated by the development of a pneumothorax

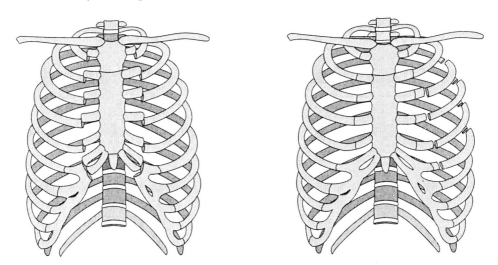

Figure 15-5 Flail sternum and flail segment

Symptoms/signs
- Rib fractures may be difficult to recognise immediately in the pre-hospital situation if the patient is unconscious; but should be positively sought for if an examination of the mechanism of injury indicates that a significant chest injury is likely to have been sustained
- Localised pain on inspiration/expiration, aggravated by coughing or sneezing, resulting in a reluctance to breathe in deeply, loss of chest movement on the affected side and impaired ventilation
- Dyspnoea, respiratory distress, an abnormal respiratory rate (usually a tachypnoea) and cyanosis when breathing air alone
- Tenderness and bony crepitus over the fracture site
- Surgical emphysema
- Reduced oxygen saturation (SpO_2)
- In flail chests there may be paradoxical movement (in the opposite direction to the rest of the thorax) of the flail segment (this may be masked initially due to spasm of the surrounding muscles, but may become more obvious later as the patient's condition deteriorates)

Management
- Oxygen:
    - This should be administered in as high a concentration as possible
- Assisted ventilation:
    - Intubation and ventilation should be considered if there is any respiratory distress due to ineffective chest expansion, but beware of a pneumothorax as this may become a tension pneumothorax with intermittent positive pressure ventilation
- Stabilisation of the thorax with appropriate care of the cervical spine, if indicated:
    - With a firm pad and bandage (flail chest only)
    - Consider lying the patient with the injured side over a sandbag (unilateral flail chest only)
    - Position/turn onto the affected side during transport
- Pain relief:
    - This is very important and is often overlooked, as chest expansion may be greatly reduced by pain
    - Be cautious with:
        - Respiratory depressants
        - Nitrous oxide/oxygen (may aggravate/exacerbate, *but not cause,* a tension pneumothorax)
    - Consider an intercostal nerve block

Sternum

Incidence
- Fractures and dislocations of the sternum are relatively rare, occurring more often in the elderly in whom the sternum is more rigid and the manubriosternal joint is ankylosed

Aetiology
- Injuries of the sternum are most commonly found in road traffic accidents

Mechanism of injury

Blunt trauma
- Direct impact is the usual mechanism of injury for sternal injury, typically occurring due to impact with the steering wheel in high speed frontal impacts, involving rapid deceleration. They have become less common since the obligatory wearing of seat belts, and rare if an air bag is deployed

Pathophysiology
- The sternum may fracture or dislocate at the manubriosternal joint
- Sternal fracture may be associated with underlying myocardial contusion, and with other chest injuries

Symptoms/signs
- The patient will have pain over the front of the chest aggravated by movement, especially deep breathing, coughing, sneezing etc.
- There may be pattern bruising over the anterior chest wall
- Localised tenderness on palpation
- If the fracture is displaced or there is a manubriosternal joint dislocation or subluxation, there may be a step deformity

Management
- Administer high flow oxygen via a high concentration mask
- Establish intravenous access for administration of fluid replacement, analgesia or cardiac drugs
- Administer appropriate analgesia, especially if pain is impairing ventilation
- Constantly monitor the pulse, blood pressure, oxygen saturation, respiratory rate and ECG tracing, in case of myocardial contusion

Pneumothorax

Incidence
- Pneumothorax occurs in up to 50% of patients with blunt thoracic trauma, and in nearly all those with penetrating thoracic injury

Aetiology
- In blunt thoracic trauma pneumothorax is nearly always associated with an overlying rib fracture, but also occurs spontaneously due to rupture of a bulla (usually a previous history) or acute severe asthma

Mechanism of injury

Blunt trauma
- In blunt trauma rib fractures are the usual cause of pneumothorax

Penetrating trauma
- Penetrating chest trauma invariably results in a pneumothorax

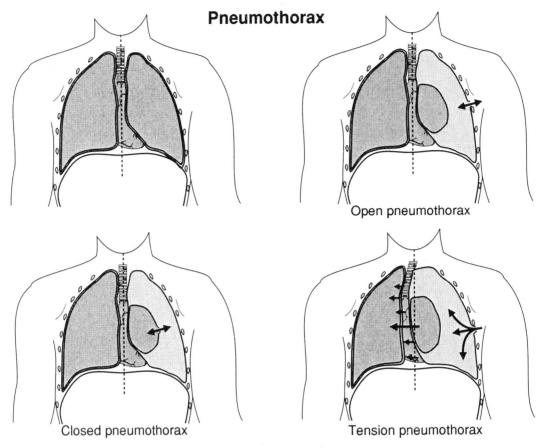

Figure 15-6 Pneumothorax

Pathophysiology

- A pneumothorax occurs when air, either from the outside or from within the lungs, enters the pleural space between the parietal and visceral pleura, resulting in partial collapse of the underlying lung
- A pneumothorax may be:
    - Partial: occurs when underlying disease tethers part of the pleura together
    - Complete: resulting in total collapse of one lung
    - Tension (see below)
    - Bilateral; occurring on both sides
    - Combined with a haemothorax, resulting in a haemopneumothorax

Symptoms/signs

- Pain, which may be central or pleuritic
- Increasing dyspnoea, respiratory distress, and cyanosis with a reducing SpO_2
- Chest movement; may be reduced or unequal
- Surgical emphysema
- Percussion note will be hyper-resonant over the pneumothorax (also found in patients with emphysema)

Management

- Oxygen
- Consider needle thoracocentesis to confirm the diagnosis if the patient's condition is deteriorating, followed by chest drain insertion
- Monitor the patient's condition carefully, in case a tension pneumothorax develops

Tension pneumothorax

Incidence
- Occurs rarely, but is rapidly life-threatening and eminently treatable

Pathophysiology
- Air enters the pleural cavity during inspiration, via a tear in the lung or chest wall, which acts as a one way flap valve, but cannot go out, resulting in a pneumothorax
- With each inspiratory breath, more air is drawn into the pleural space; and so the pneumothorax enlarges
- As the pneumothorax gets larger:
    - The lung on the same side collapses progressively, resulting in hypoxia
    - The mediastinum is progressively displaced away from the pneumothorax resulting in compression of the vena cava which may dramatically reduce the venous return and cardiac filling and cause a reduction in cardiac output. This may be disastrous in the already hypoxic and hypovolaemic patient and will eventually result in cardiorespiratory arrest and death

Symptoms/signs
- A developing tension pneumothorax can be difficult to detect in the pre-hospital situation, but inspection of the mechanism of injury and a high index of suspicion, will help avoid it being left undetected
- Tracheal deviation (a late sign) and mediastinal shift towards the unaffected side (displacement of the apex beat)
- Respiratory embarrassment:
    - Increasing dyspnoea
    - Tachypnoea
    - Expiratory grunting
    - Raised jugular venous pressure and distension of the neck veins (if there is no hypovolaemia)
    - Possible cyanosis (a late sign)
    - Hypoxia with a reduced SpO_2
- Hyper-resonance to percussion and reduced air entry (breath sounds) on auscultation on the affected side
- Tachycardia
- A decreasing level of consciousness

Management
- This depends on the clinical condition of the patient, but may be life saving; it may include:
    - Oxygen
    - Needle decompression to provide immediate relief and confirm the diagnosis
    - Chest tube drainage with a Heimlich valve or chest drainage bag
    - Pain relief

Needle decompression
- Needle decompression may be performed to:
    - Establish the diagnosis
    - Relieve the symptoms while a chest drain is prepared for insertion

Method
- Administer high flow oxygen via a mask or airway
- Identify the site for insertion: the second intercostal space in the mid-clavicular line
- Clean the site with antiseptic, and infiltrate with local anaesthetic down to the pleura:
    - Lidocaine 1% (with or without epinephrine)
- Use a wide bore (14, 16g) intravenous cannula with a 10-30 mL syringe
- Penetrate the parietal pleura and aspirate air (if unsuccessful, seal the puncture site and observe the patient for the possible development of a pneumothorax)
- Proceed to chest drain insertion (see below)

Complications
- Local cellulitis
- Local haematoma
- Pleural infection
- May cause a pneumothorax, if one is not already present

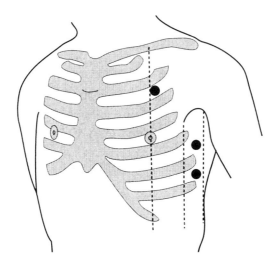

Figure 15-7 Chest tube drainage: sites for insertion

Chest tube drainage

Indications
- Life threatening tension pneumothorax
- Chest injury, requiring positive pressure ventilation or air transportation

Sites
- Lateral (*best*):
    - Over the fourth or fifth intercostal space, anterior to the mid axillary line
- Posterior:
    - In the auscultatory triangle, just below the tip of the scapula with the arms abducted
- Anterior (*not often used now*):
    - Over the second intercostal space, 2.5 cm lateral to the mid-clavicular line. Insert the drain outwards and upwards

Chest drain insertion

Method
- Make a generous (2-3 cm) cut with a sharp ended scalpel, parallel to the ribs. Be careful not to go too near the inferior border of the ribs (risk of damage to the intercostal nerve and artery)
- Insert blunt artery forceps, and spread them out in the middle of the space
- Put a gloved index finger through the chest wall and into pleural space, and perform a finger sweep to identify adhesions, blood clots, etc.
- Remove the trochar of the chest drain, and attach artery forceps to the distal end of the chest drain
- Insert the drain with the forceps, using your finger as a guide aiming towards the apex of the lung (if there is surgical emphysema, be careful to insert the drain far enough)
- Look for "fogging" of the chest tube with expiration, or listen for air movement out of the tube (often difficult in the pre-hospital situation)
- Attach the end of the tube to a one way Heimlich valve or drainage bag/valve and secure it in place with a strong (0/00) string suture

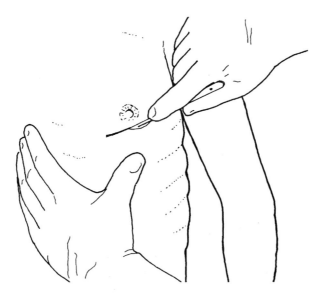

Figure 15-8 Chest drain insertion: Making the incision

- If necessary use a single purse string suture to close the incision (this should be cut and *not* tied)
- Apply a dressing and airtight tape around the tube and tape the tube to the chest
- Following the procedure, check the patient and sit them up at 45°

Complications
- Allergic reaction to the surgical skin preparation or anaesthetic (unlikely in Immediate Care as there is usually little time for surgical preparation)
- Damage to the intercostal nerve, artery or vein:
    - May convert pneumothorax into haemopneumothorax
    - May cause intercostal neuralgia/neuritis later
- Damage to the internal mammary vessels if anterior puncture is too medial, resulting in a haemopneumothorax and major blood loss
- Damage to intrathoracic or intra-abdominal organs (this can be avoided by using the finger technique before inserting the tube)
- Subcutaneous emphysema at insertion site
- Incorrect tube positioning
- Persistent pneumothorax due to:
    - Air leak
    - Failure of apparatus due to tube kinking or blood clogging or freezing the Heimlich valve

Note: Always try to obtain adequate venous access prior to chest drain insertion, in case of haemorrhage

Drainage
- This may be direct by Heimlich valve or chest drainage bag

Haemothorax

Incidence
- Haemothorax is a relatively common injury in severe blunt and penetrating thoracic trauma

Aetiology
- Thoracic trauma resulting in damage to the bony thorax (even a single rib fracture may result in the loss of 150 mL of blood into the pleural cavity)

Pathophysiology
- A haemothorax is caused by haemorrhage from the intercostal, internal mammary and pulmonary arteries and veins or their branches and may result in the loss of a considerable volume of blood into the pleural space, resulting in profound hypovolaemia and shock
- A haemothorax will cause an increase in intrathoracic pressure and collapse of some of the lung on the same side, resulting in impaired ventilation and cardiac function

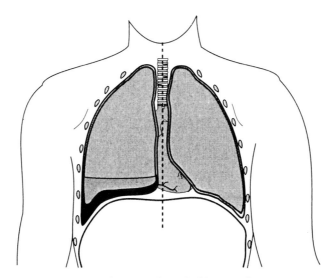

Figure 15-9 Right sided haemothorax

Symptoms/signs
- Evidence of a chest injury
- Profound shock
- Dullness to percussion in the dependant areas of the chest (may be difficult to elicit if the patient is supine, especially in the pre-hospital situation)

Management
- Oxygen administration
- Any patient with a chest injury and signs of significant hypovolaemia, needs fluid replacement and treatment of hypovolaemic shock with an intravenous infusion of colloid or crystalloid
- Insertion of chest drain
- Tracheal intubation and assisted ventilation

Trachea and main bronchus

Incidence
- Rare

Aetiology
- Usually associated with other major injuries
- In road traffic accidents may be caused by the steering wheel rim impacting with the upper part of the front of the chest: resulting in ruptured bronchus, trachea and larynx

Mechanism of injury

Blunt trauma

Compression
- Compression may cause rupturing or tears of the trachea and bronchial tree (most occur near the carina)

Penetrating injury
- Penetrating injury may result in a defect in the wall of the trachea and bronchial tree

Pathophysiology
- A tear or defect in the wall of the trachea or bronchial tree may allow air to enter the pleural space or mediastinum, resulting in surgical emphysema and/or a pneumothorax, which fails to respond to decompression (a complete transection of the bronchial tree is usually rapidly fatal)
- If decompression is attempted, there will be a steady flow of air out of the drainage tube, rather than the initial rush of air
- Tracheal intubation and assisted ventilation may make matters worse

Symptoms/signs
- Evidence of a high thoracic compression or penetrating injury
- Respiratory distress
- Surgical emphysema
- Haemoptysis
- Pneumothorax

Management
- Oxygen
- If there is surgical emphysema: be very careful about intubating the patient (see above)
- If there is absolute tracheal obstruction: consider performing a cricothyrotomy

The great vessels (aorta)
- Injury of the aorta has a high mortality; occurring in 15-20% of all those killed in road traffic accidents and is often associated with severe thoracic and extrathoracic injuries

Incidence
- Aortic injury is rare, but is relatively common in accidents involving high speed deceleration

Aetiology
- Partial or complete rupture of the thoracic aorta is a relatively common injury in:
    - High velocity frontal impact road traffic accidents, especially in the young
    - Falls from a considerable height

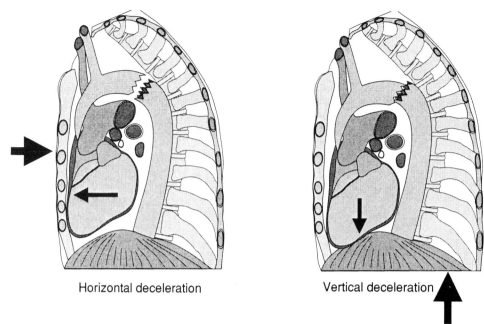

Horizontal deceleration   Vertical deceleration

Figure 15-10 Rupture of the arch of the aorta

Mechanism of injury

Blunt trauma

Compression
- Compression injury alone rarely results in significant aortic damage

Acceleration, deceleration, shear
- Severe aortic injury (rupture or partial rupture) is usually caused by:
    - High velocity frontal impact, resulting in massive horizontal deceleration
    - Falls from great heights, resulting in massive vertical deceleration
- The descending aorta is firmly tethered to the posterior thoracic wall and thoracic vertebrae, but the arch of the aorta and heart are not and are relatively free to move.
- In sudden severe frontal (horizontal) deceleration of the thorax, the heart will continue to move forward until it impacts with the sternum. This may result in tearing or shearing of the arch of aorta restraining the heart, where the mobile arch of aorta joins the tethered descending aorta
- Sudden severe vertical deceleration may result in a similar injury to horizontal deceleration as the heart continues to move downwards until it impacts with the diaphragm, with shearing of the arch of the aorta

Penetrating injury
- Penetrating injury may occur due to deeply penetrating missile injuries or stab wounds

Pathophysiology

Aortic rupture
- Partial rupture:
    - In about 10% of cases there may only be a partial tear, involving the inner walls of the aorta, the 'intima' and 'adventitia', resulting in a traumatic aneurism of the aorta. These patients will only lose about 500 mL of blood into the aneurism initially
    - The aneurism may slowly enlarge and extend, due to the maintenance of a high systolic pressure, until the outer wall of the aorta, the 'adventitia' gives way, making the tear complete and resulting in aortic rupture

- Patients with a traumatic aortic aneurism may survive for several hours before going rapidly into profound shock, as the rupture becomes complete
- Survival rates following early surgical management of acute traumatic aneurism may be >80%
- Complete rupture:
  - Death usually occurs immediately from exsanguination, but may be delayed in 10-20% of cases, which may be long enough for surgical repair, provided that a rapid and accurate diagnosis is made, followed by active resuscitation and transfer of the patient to the operating theatre

Symptoms/signs
- Between one third and half of those patients with a ruptured aorta have no external evidence of thoracic injury at the time of their initial examination
- There may be:
  - Central chest pain, especially radiating through to the back
  - Hoarseness of the voice, due to pressure on the recurrent laryngeal nerve by expanding haematoma
  - Pulse differences between upper and lower limbs, and between limbs on different sides of the body
  - Blood pressure differences between upper and lower limbs with that in the upper limb being higher, and between limbs on different sides of the body
- Evidence of rapidly developing hypovolaemic shock/exsanguination (if the aneurism suddenly ruptures)

Management
- Administer oxygen
- Infuse cautiously, being careful not to push the systolic pressure >100 mmHg, as this may cause further haemorrhage
- Consider applying a pneumatic anti-shock garment (PASG)
- Monitor the patient's haemodynamic state carefully

The heart
- Cardiac injuries are potentially fatal and require immediate recognition and appropriate management

Incidence
- Significant blunt injury to the heart is relatively rarely encountered in the UK
- Penetrating trauma of the heart is rare in the UK, but the incidence of stab wounds is increasing

Aetiology
- Common cause of myocardial injury include:
  - Stab wounds due to assault
  - High velocity frontal road traffic accidents
- Myocardial injury is often associated with fractures of the sternum and thoracic vertebrae

Mechanism of injury

Blunt trauma
- In high velocity frontal impacts, the vehicle occupants will continue to move forward until their chests impact with the interior of the vehicle, usually the steering wheel of front fascia, or are restrained by their seat belts, both of which may cause significant injury

Compression
- Sudden severe compression of the heart may occur, as the heart is trapped and squeezed between the front and back of the inside of the thoracic cage, after it has already impacted with the front of the interior wall of the thoracic cage

Acceleration, deceleration, shear
- In high speed frontal vehicle impacts, the heart will continue to move forward until it impacts with the inside of the front of the thoracic cage resulting in myocardial contusion, usually of the left ventricle

Penetrating trauma
- Penetrating trauma of the heart will result in injury to the pericardium and myocardium

Pathophysiology

Blunt trauma
- Blunt injury may result in:
    - Myocardial contusion with bleeding into the cardiac muscle, which may vary from partial to full thickness (with myocardial infarction and cell death) depending on the amount of energy transferred, and may result in minimal up to severe impairment of cardiac function
    - Disruption of the cardiac conducting system resulting in arrhythmias (usually after an anterior chest wall injury), most commonly ventricular tachycardia, PVCs and atrial fibrillation/flutter
    - Myocardial or septal rupture (rapidly fatal)
    - Rupture of the aortic, mitral or tricuspid valves, due to sudden severe cardiac compression
- Penetrating myocardial injury may result in cardiac tamponade:
    - This is due to the collection of blood in the pericardial space from haemorrhage into it from the coronary vessels or one of the chambers of the heart
    - This results in increasingly severe impairment of cardiac contraction as more and more blood is drawn into the pericardium

Note: Penetrating injury of the right ventricle is the most common, but as it is thin walled, continued haemorrhage may occur in the absence of tamponade; injury of the the left ventricle is the next most common, but its thick muscular wall may often close off the wound initially

Symptoms/Signs
- Evidence of a mechanism of injury likely to result in cardiac injury:
    - Severe frontal impact with deformity of the steering wheel, and an anterior chest wall injury
    - Stab wound of the thorax or upper abdomen

Myocardial contusion
- Chest pain
- ECG changes (injury pattern):
    - Non-specific ST-T wave changes
    - Widened QRS complex
    - Ventricular tachycardia
    - PVCs
    - Atrial fibrillation/flutter

Cardiac tamponade
- Increasing dyspnoea
- Cyanosis
- *Distension of the neck veins with a raised jugular venous pressure (JVP)*
- *Tamponade: muffled heart sounds* ⎫
- *Hypovolaemic shock with tachycardia and a rapidly falling blood pressure* ⎬ *Beck's triad (rarely seen)*
- A narrow pulse pressure
- Kussmaul's sign: a rise in venous pressure with inspiration indicates tamponade

Note: If the patient is severely hypovolaemic, the neck veins may *not* be distended

Management
- Oxygen
- Intravenous infusion if there is any evidence of hypovolaemic shock
- Careful monitoring of the pulse rate, blood pressure, etc.
- Analgesia
- Pericardiocentesis if there is evidence of cardiac tamponade (it is usually best to convey the patient rapidly to hospital as this procedure may buy only a few minutes extra time; open surgery is required)

Pericardiocentesis (pericardial aspiration)

Indications
- Cardiac tamponade (stab wound where there is no evidence of a pneumothorax and no improvement in the patient's condition with oxygen)

Monitoring
- This procedure should be performed only with careful monitoring of the patient's vital signs and ECG before, during and after the procedure

Method
- The patient should be on oxygen and have a large bore intravenous infusion in place
- Obtain a long (15 cm), wide bore (16-18 SWG) intravenous cannula and attach it to a 20 mL syringe, ideally with a three way tap
- Insert the needle into the left costo-xiphoid angle 1-2 cm below and to the left of the xiphisternum)
- Puncture the skin and aim the needle cephalad towards the middle of the left clavicle, so as to avoid the superior epigastric vessels, at an angle of about 45° to the skin
- Insert the needle about 4-6 cm, withdrawing the plunger until the syringe fills with blood
- If the needle is advanced too far (into the myocardium), an injury pattern will show on the ECG tracing

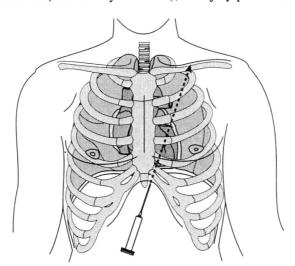

Figure 15-11 Pericardiocentesis

- Withdraw as much non clotted blood as possible
- During aspiration, as blood is removed from the pericardial sac, the tip of the needle may come into contact with the inner pericardial surface overlying the myocardium. This will show as an injury pattern on the ECG monitor and the needle should be withdrawn a little
- If the injury pattern persists or if there is no further aspirate, cease aspiration and withdraw the needle completely, keeping the cannula in place
- Attach a three way tap and secure the cannula, so that further aspiration can take place if cardiac tamponade persists or reoccurs

Oesophagus

Incidence
- Blunt oesophageal injury is rare
- Penetrating oesophageal injury is more common

Aetiology
- There may be spontaneous rupture
- Rupture may also be caused by:
    - External blunt trauma
    - Penetrating injury
    - Iatrogenic instrumental perforation

Mechanism of injury

Blunt trauma

Compression
- Sudden severe compression of the epigastrium, may result in squeezing of the stomach, forcing gastric contents into the lower oesophagus, resulting in its rupture

Penetrating trauma
- Penetrating trauma may cause rupture of the oesophagus at any level, and is likely to be associated with injury to nearby structures

Pathophysiology
- Oesophageal rupture may result in the leakage of oesophageal contents, causing mediastinitis

Symptoms/signs
- Severe retrosternal chest pain, out of proportion to the patient's apparent injuries
- Mediastinal and subcutaneous emphysema of the neck and upper chest

Note: The presence of a left sided pneumothorax or pleural effusion in the absence of left sided chest trauma or fractured left ribs may indicate the presence of a ruptured oesophagus

Management
- Treatment of shock

Diaphragm (see chapter on Abdominal and pelvic injuries)

Thoraco-abdominal injuries
- Consider injury to the liver, spleen, stomach, duodenum, etc. (see chapter on Abdominal and pelvic injuries)

16

Abdominal and pelvic injuries

Abdominal and pelvic injuries

Abdominal injuries

Incidence
- Major intra-abdominal injuries are relatively rarely encountered in Immediate Care, accounting for only 1% of hospital admissions for trauma, and is often not recognised and poorly managed
- In the UK:
    - The majority of abdominal injuries are caused by road traffic accidents, and are usually associated with significant injury to other areas, e.g. head, chest, pelvis and limbs
    - Blunt trauma is much more common than penetrating injury, although penetrating trauma due to assault is increasing, especially in some inner city areas

Aetiology
- Blunt abdominal injury may occur as a result of:
    - Rapid severe increase in intra-abdominal pressure:
        - Direct blow
        - Restraint, e.g. car seat belt
    - Direct compression of organs
    - Rapid deceleration or acceleration
    - Ejection
    - Crush
- Penetrating abdominal injury occurs as a result of:
    - Stabbing
    - Shooting
    - Explosions: producing high velocity fragments
    - Impalement

Anatomy
- The abdomen has three regions:

The peritoneal cavity
- The peritoneal cavity may be divided into two compartments:

The intrathoracic compartment
- The intrathoracic compartment is that part of the peritoneal cavity enclosed by the lower ribs, it contains:
    - Diaphragm
    - Liver
    - Spleen
    - Stomach
    - Transverse colon
- The intrathoracic compartment varies in its size depending on the phase of respiration; on full expiration it may rise up as far as the 4th intercostal space

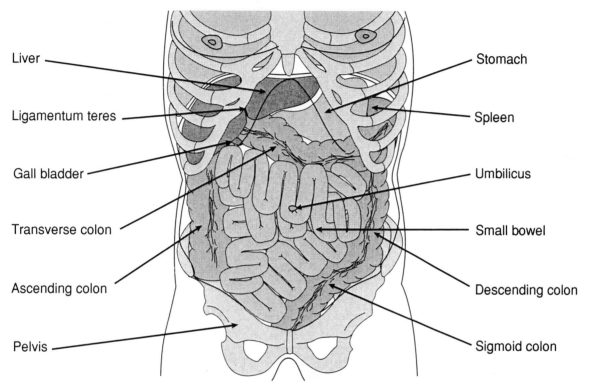

Figure 16-1 Anatomy of the abdomen: anterior view of the peritoneal cavity

The Abdominal compartment
- The abdominal compartment is surrounded anteriorly and laterally by the muscular abdominal wall, and posteriorly by the spine and retroperitoneum, and contains:
    - The small bowel
    - The ascending colon, including the caecum
    - The descending colon

The retroperitoneum
- The retroperitoneum lies behind the abdominal compartment of the peritoneal cavity and contains the:
    - Major blood vessels, including the aorta, inferior vena cava and renal and iliac blood vessels
    - Pancreas
    - Kidneys and ureters
    - Parts of the duodenum and colon

The pelvis
- The pelvis is the area enclosed by the bony pelvis and contains the:
    - Rectum and bladder
    - Major blood vessels
    - Reproductive organs: vagina and uterus in the female, prostate in the male

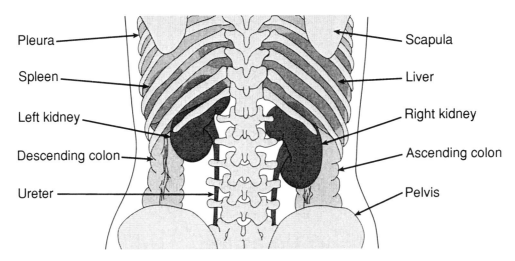

Figure 16-2 Anatomy of the abdomen: posterior view

Mechanism of injury

Blunt trauma

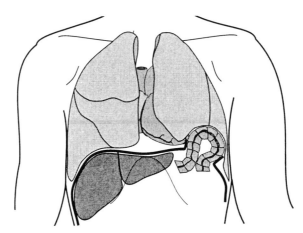

Figure 16-3 Blunt abdominal trauma: compression

Compression injury
- Sudden severe compression of the abdomen may result in:
    - Damage to the underlying viscera caused by direct impact spread over a relatively small area
    - Compression of organs, e.g. the liver, pancreas and retroperitoneal duodenum, between the compressing force and the vertebral column (e.g. car seat belt injury)
    - A sudden rise in intra-abdominal pressure resulting in a rupture through the wall of the abdominal cavity at its weakest points, e.g. the left side of the diaphragm, or rupture of a loop of bowel

Acceleration, deceleration, shear injury
- Sudden severe frontal deceleration will result in:
    - The more massive intra-abdominal organs, e.g. the liver and spleen, colliding with the anterior abdominal wall, sustaining a compression injury. In addition the liver may be transected by the firm ligamentum teres as it does so
    - Extreme forward movement also results in shearing or tearing forces (proportional to the mass and mobility of the organ) of the more massive organs, e.g. the liver, spleen, kidneys and small bowel mesenteries, which take their vascular supply from blood vessels firmly tethered to the posterior abdominal wall resulting in their being torn

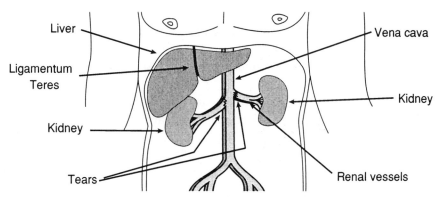

Figure 16-4 Blunt abdominal trauma: deceleration, shear injury

Note: In high speed frontal impacts the seat belt may cause a combination of compression and deceleration/ shear injury. The incidence of injury increases with incorrect usage

Penetrating trauma
- In penetrating abdominal wounds the nature and extent of injury depends on the type of weapon used and the amount of energy transferred to the tissues:
    - Stab wounds from broken glasses, knives, etc. usually only result in local tissue injury and are only immediately life threatening if they involve major blood vessels
    - High velocity missiles from rifles may result in high energy transfer wounds with severe massive injury to many intra-abdominal structures due to cavitation, fragmentation and ricocheting
- Penetrating trauma of the chest below the 4th rib may involve intra-abdominal structures

Pathophysiology
- Injury to solid organs and blood vessels will result in haemorrhage with an early risk of hypovolaemia
- Injury to hollow organs will result in leakage of their contents with a delayed risk of peritonitis
- More than one mechanism of injury may be involved in abdominal trauma

Blunt abdominal injury
- May occur as a result of several different mechanisms acting alone or together

Compression injury
- Compression of solid organs, e.g. the liver, kidneys and spleen will result in local tissue damage with tears extending away from the point of impact and haemorrhage within the organ
- Compression of hollow organs, e.g. stomach, ileum and large bowel may have little effect, unless massive forces are applied over a small area, when the local effect will be the same as for solid organs

Acceleration, deceleration and shear injury
- Blood vessels injury can result in severe haemorrhage, and ischaemic injury of the organ they supply

Penetrating abdominal injury

Stab wound
- There is a 25% chance of damage to major viscera
- Adjacent structures (including intrathoracic organs) are often involved

Shooting/explosion injury
- There is a 75% chance of damage to major viscera, usually: bowel, liver and diaphragm
- Many non adjacent organs may be damaged

Assessment

- Evidence of abdominal injury is often overshadowed by other more obvious injuries, e.g. head injury, or may be masked by alcohol
- Up to 25% of those with serious intra-abdominal injuries will show no evidence of these injuries on initial examination
- Any examination therefore should include assessment of the mechanism of injury and any patient sustaining a significant deceleration injury or a penetrating abdominal wound should be assumed to have an abdominal visceral injury

History

- It is important to obtain a clear history as to the mechanism of injury if possible, e.g. in road traffic accidents, including:
    - Time of accident
    - Mechanism of vehicle impact and patient injury
    - Use of seat belts
    - Injuries to other vehicle occupants
- It is also important to obtain the nature and time of any recent meal, and when urine was last passed, as distended organs are more liable to rupture than empty ones
- In penetrating injury it is important to ascertain the type of weapon used and whether it is likely to produce a high or low energy transfer wound

Symptoms/signs

- In abdominal injury any symptoms/signs are often unreliable in the pre-hospital situation: up to 25% of significant injuries may be missed initially (50% if the patient is unconscious)
- The severity of any injury depends on the structure involved
- Consider any abdominal injury in conjunction with injuries to associated areas: chest, pelvis, spine
- Positively look for intra-abdominal injury if:
    - The patient appears to be more shocked than would be expected from their other obvious injuries
    - Examination of the mechanism of injury leads one to suspect an intra-abdominal injury even if one is not apparent

Examination

- If appropriate in the circumstances:
    - Undress the patient and examine the abdomen rapidly, but thoroughly
    - Examine the back as well as the front of the patient, log rolling them as necessary

Pain
- Abdominal pain or discomfort with localised tenderness and guarding is the most reliable indicator of abdominal injury:
- Shoulder tip pain indicates diaphragmatic irritation

Inspection
- Look for pattern bruising (usually indicates significant injury even if physical examination is unremarkable)
- Look for loss of normal abdominal wall contour if lighting conditions permit

Palpation
- Palpate for localised tenderness and guarding

Auscultation
  - Even if it is possible to listen for the presence or absence of bowel sounds in the Immediate Care situation, they are an unreliable indicator of abdominal injury

Pulse, blood pressure
  - Look for evidence of hypovolaemic shock: especially if there are indications of splenic or hepatic injury

Management

Primary survey
  - Airway with cervical spine stabilisation:
  - **B**reathing
  - **C**irculation with control of haemorrhage
  - **D**isability
  - **E**xposure
  - Relieve any pain

Secondary survey
  - Head injury
  - Chest injury
  - Abdominal injury
  - Extremity injury
  - Spinal injury

Open abdominal wounds
  - These are usually visually impressive and distracting, but are rarely immediately life threatening

Aetiology
  - Open abdominal wounds are usually caused by laceration with a sharp knife or similar weapon

Incidence
  - Open abdominal wounds are rarely encountered

Mechanism of injury
  - Penetrating injury

Pathophysiology
  - The omentum and/or small bowel will usually prolapse through the defect in the abdominal wall

Management
  - Cover the extruded bowel and omentum with clingfilm or clean towels soaked in N-saline or Hartmanns, solution, to prevent it becoming dry and necrotic, and to reduce the risk of infection/contamination

Diaphragmatic injury

Incidence
- Rupture of the diaphragm is a relatively common injury, occurring in 5% of patients suffering blunt trauma of the chest or abdomen, and is often overlooked
- Associated with a relatively high mortality if not recognised early

Aetiology
- Injury to the diaphragm may occur due to road traffic accidents and assault with a sharp weapon

Mechanism of injury

Blunt trauma
- Sudden severe compression of the abdomen, e.g. due to abdominal compression by the steering wheel may result in the herniation of abdominal contents including bowel, stomach, spleen, liver or kidney, most often through the left postero-lateral hemi-diaphragm (the diaphragm's weakest point, and on the right it may be protected by the liver)

Penetrating trauma
- Penetrating injury, e.g. stab injury of the lower thorax may result in injury of the diaphragm (usually on the left side, as the majority of assailants hold the knife with their right hand)

Pathophysiology
- Diaphragmatic rupture impairs the use of the diaphragm as a muscle of respiration and the presence of bowel, etc. in the thoracic cavity will cause some lung compression and impair ventilation
- Herniation of stomach and bowel through the diaphragm may result in their obstruction and strangulation, and herniation of the spleen, liver or kidney may result in impairment of their blood supply

Symptoms/signs
- Dyspnoea with evidence of impaired ventilation
- Profound shock
- Bowel sounds may occasionally be heard in the left side of the chest

Management
- Oxygen
- Assisted ventilation
- Intravenous infusion

Duodenum

Incidence
- Duodenal injury is unusual

Aetiology
- Classically encountered in the unrestrained intoxicated car driver involved in a frontal impact, or the cyclist involved in a severe frontal impact, resulting in the handlebars being displaced backwards and impacting with the upper abdomen

Mechanism of injury
- Blunt trauma in which the retroperitoneal duodenum is compressed between the anterior abdominal wall and the lumbar spine, e.g. severe frontal impacts in pedal cyclists when there is massive backwards displacement of the handlebars, which impact over a small area with the upper abdomen

Pathophysiology
- Severe compression of the duodenum may result in rupture, with haemorrhage into the lumen of the duodenum and leakage of its contents into the retroperitoneal space

Symptoms/signs
- Bloody nasogastric aspirate

Liver

Incidence
- The liver is the most commonly affected organ in severe blunt abdominal trauma

Aetiology
- Usually caused by severe blunt trauma, especially in road traffic accidents

Mechanism of injury

Blunt trauma
- Compression injury:
    - Sudden severe compression of the right hypochondrium, lower right ribs, and the right loin, caused by e.g. the seat belt in the front seat passenger in severe frontal impacts, and by right side intrusion, may result in severe hepatic injury
- Acceleration, deceleration, shear injury:
    - Sudden high speed frontal deceleration may result in:
        - The anterior surface of the liver impacting with the anterior abdominal wall under the ribs/costal margin resulting in a hepatic contusion
        - Transection of the liver by the ligamentum teres
        - Shearing injury of some of the hepatic blood supply resulting in haemorrhage

Penetrating trauma
- Low energy penetrating trauma of the liver will result in local haemorrhage, which may be severe especially if the weapon used is then twisted
- High energy penetrating trauma of the liver may result in severe hepatic disruption and catastrophic haemorrhage

Pathophysiology
- The liver is a highly vascular solid organ with a very good blood supply
- Injury of the liver may result in severe haemorrhage, and cause significant hypovolaemia and shock
- There may be an associated injury of the right lower ribs and lung

Symptoms/signs
- Pattern bruising over the right side of the chest, anteriorly, laterally or posteriorly
- Localised tenderness
- Fractures of the right lower ribs
- Evidence of hypovolaemic shock

Spleen

Incidence
- The spleen is relatively commonly injured

Aetiology
- Usually caused by severe blunt trauma, especially in road traffic accidents

Mechanism of injury

Blunt trauma
- Compression injury:
    - Sudden severe compression of the left hypochondrium, lower left ribs, and the left loin, caused by e.g. the seat belt in the driver in severe frontal impacts, and by left side vehicle intrusion, may result in splenic injury
- Acceleration, deceleration, shear injury:
    - Sudden high speed frontal deceleration may result in:
        - The anterior surface of the spleen impacting with the anterior abdominal wall under the ribs/costal margin resulting in splenic contusion
        - Shearing injury of some of the splenic blood supply resulting in haemorrhage

Penetrating trauma
- Low energy penetrating trauma of the spleen will result in local haemorrhage, which may be severe especially if the weapon used is then twisted
- High energy penetrating trauma of the spleen may result in severe splenic disruption and haemorrhage

Pathophysiology
- Injury of the spleen may result in severe haemorrhage, and cause significant hypovolaemia, but this may be delayed as initial haemorrhage may be controlled by tamponade within the splenic capsule
- There may be an associated injury of the left lower ribs, lung and heart

Symptoms/signs
- Pattern bruising
- Localised pain/tenderness
- Hypovolaemic shock, which may not develop immediately

Pancreas

Incidence
- Injury of the pancreas is a relatively unusual injury

Aetiology
- Pancreatic injury may occur due to road traffic accidents and assault

Mechanism of injury

Blunt trauma
- Pancreatic injury most often results from a direct epigastric blow, compressing the pancreas against the vertebral column

Kidneys

Incidence
- Damage to the kidneys is a fairly common injury, but one that is usually not obvious initially

Aetiology
- Renal damage may be caused by sporting accidents, road traffic accidents and assaults

Mechanism of injury

Blunt trauma:
- Compression
  - Usually caused by a severe blow to the loin or lower ribs posteriorly (usually severe enough to result in a fracture)
- Acceleration, deceleration, shear
  - Sudden severe frontal deceleration may result in the kidney shearing off part of its blood supply, near where it is attached to the posterior abdominal wall, resulting in severe haemorrhage
- Penetrating injury:
  - Renal injury may be caused by penetrating trauma of the loin

Symptoms/signs
- Localised pain/tenderness
- Fractured lower ribs
- Haematuria

Bowel

Incidence
- Bowel injury is relatively rare

Aetiology
- Bowel injury may occur due to injuries in road traffic accidents and assaults with a sharp weapon

Mechanism of injury

Blunt trauma
- Severe compression may result in contusion and perforation of the bowel

Penetrating trauma
- Low energy transfer penetrating trauma of the bowel may result in a small defect in the bowel wall
- High energy transfer penetrating trauma of the bowel may result in severe disruption of the bowel and adjacent abdominal structures

Pathophysiology
- Perforation of the bowel will result in leakage of bowel contents into the peritoneal space, resulting in the gradual development of peritonitis, which is not immediately life threatening
- Damage to the mesentery may result in significant intra-abdominal haemorrhage

Symptoms and signs
- Pattern bruising of the abdomen
- A mechanism of injury suggestive of severe blunt or penetrating injury of the abdomen
- Abdominal tenderness and guarding

Pelvic injury

Pelvic fractures

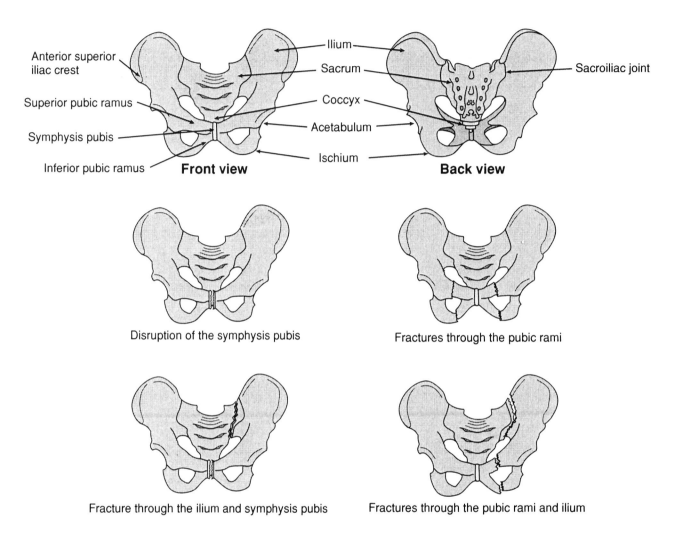

Front view

- Anterior superior iliac crest
- Superior pubic ramus
- Symphysis pubis
- Inferior pubic ramus
- Ilium
- Sacrum
- Coccyx
- Acetabulum
- Ischium

Back view

- Sacroiliac joint

Disruption of the symphysis pubis

Fractures through the pubic rami

Fracture through the ilium and symphysis pubis

Fractures through the pubic rami and ilium

Figure 16-4 Pelvic anatomy and common types of fracture

Incidence
- Pelvic fractures:
    - Are relatively commonly encountered in accidents resulting in major injuries, and are associated with severe head, chest and abdominal trauma
    - Have a significant morbidity and mortality (open pelvic injuries have a mortality rate of more than 50%)

Aetiology
- Pelvic fractures may be trivial or complicated
- Minor pelvic fractures may be caused by falls, especially in the elderly
- Most severe pelvic injuries are associated with high velocity accidents or those involving massive forces, e.g. car-pedestrian, motorcycle or high fall accidents

Mechanism of injury

Blunt trauma
Compression
- Pelvic fractures are usually caused by blunt trauma; direct compression or by forces transmitted along the femur:
    - Antero-posterior compression may result in disruption of the symphysis pubis or in the creation of a butterfly segment due to bilateral fractures of the pubic rami
    - Lateral compression, caused when, e.g. pedestrians are hit by a car, may result in 'bucket handle' displacement of one half of the pelvis, with severe disruption of one of the sacroiliac joints and symphysis pubis or pubic rami on one side
    - Falls onto the hip, especially in the elderly may result in a lateral compressive force causing a fracture of one or both pubic rami on the affected side
    - Acetabular fracture may arise due to severe compressive forces from the femur, e.g. fall from a height, when the acetabulum may be driven into the pelvis, or due to posterior dislocation of the hip, when a posterior fragment may be sheared off

Acceleration, deceleration, shear
- Falls from a height may cause a vertical shear injury with severe displacement of one half of the pelvis, with severe disruption of one of the sacroiliac joints and pubic rami on one side

Penetrating trauma
- Penetrating trauma may result in fractures of the bony pelvis
- High energy transfer wounds may result in bony fragments flying off and causing secondary damage to intrapelvic structures

Pathophysiology
- Isolated fractures:
    - Any part of the pelvis may be affected especially the pubic rami
- Unstable fractures are caused by:
    - Two or more fractures with loss of the integrity of the pelvic ring, and is likely to be associated with major blood loss and injury to the intrapelvic organs

Complications
- Vascular injury:
    - The common iliac artery and associated blood vessels lie close to the anterior surface of the sacroiliac joint and may be damaged if the sacroiliac joint is disrupted, resulting in severe haemorrhage
    - Pelvic fractures may result in haemorrhage into the retroperitoneal space, which is very difficult to control, and blood loss may be very considerable (6-10 units of blood), sometimes resulting in exsanguination
- Neurological injury:
    - Common where there has been major pelvic disruption, resulting in sciatic nerve damage
- Visceral injury:
    - 20% of pelvic fractures are associated with abdominal/visceral injury
- Bladder injury:
    - Disruption of the symphysis pubis, or penetration by a bony spike

Symptoms/signs
- A history of an accident with a mechanism of injury likely to result in pelvic fracture
- Pain at the site of the fracture or sometimes in the groin/hip (fractures of the pubic rami in the elderly)
- Apparent shortening of one leg if there is a vertical shear fracture
- Evidence of an unstable pelvis:
    - Examine the pelvis to see if it feels firm or is there bony crepitus? (pain on pelvic springing by itself is not a good predictor of pelvic fractures)
- Urethral bleeding
- Rectal bleeding
- Evidence of hypovolaemia

Management
- Follow the usual guidelines:
    - **Primary survey/initial management:**
        - Airway with stabilisation of the cervical spine
        - Breathing:
            - Consider tracheal intubation and assisted ventilation if there is impaired ventilation, due to, e.g. a ruptured diaphragm
        - Circulation:
            - If there is evidence of hypovolaemia:
                - Secure two intravenous lines with wide bore intravenous cannulae
                - Infuse cautiously with careful continuous haemodynamic monitoring
                - Stabilise the pelvis to reduce internal bleeding with:
                    - Triangular bandages
                    - *Frac-Straps®*
                    - PASG
                    - Spinal board strapping
                    - Extrication device and strapping
                - If the anticipated blood loss is considerable, then consider application of a PASG
            - If there is obvious external bleeding:
                - Control with direct pressure
        - Disability
        - Exposure with control of the environment
    - **Secondary survey/management:**
        - Head injury
        - Chest injury
        - Abdominal injury:
            - Exposed or prolapsed viscera:
                - Cover with clingfilm or saline soaked towels (Hartmann's solution will do)

Bladder rupture

Incidence
- Bladder rupture is a relatively rare injury, usually occurring in accidents involving severe force

Aetiology
- Bladder rupture may be caused by blunt compression (especially common when the patient is drunk and the bladder is distended) or penetrating injury

Mechanism of injury

Blunt trauma
- Sudden severe compression will result in rupture of a full bladder

Penetrating trauma
- Rupture by a bony spike from a pelvic fracture
- Penetration of the bladder by a low or high energy missile

Pathophysiology
- Compression injury :
    - Sudden severe abdominal compression of the bladder may cause a tear along the peritonealised posterior wall, resulting in intraperitoneal extravasation of urine
- Pelvic disruption/bony penetration may result in:
    - An anterolateral tear of the bladder wall, resulting in extraperitoneal extravasation of urine

Symptoms/signs
- If the rupture is intraperitoneal, these may be delayed
- Lower abdominal and pelvic pain and associated tenderness
- Loss of desire to micturate and inability or pain on attempting to void
- Associated hypovolaemic shock

Urethral rupture

Incidence
- Occurs in approximately 10% of pelvic fractures, more commonly in males than females because of the greater length of the male urethra
- In females urethral rupture may be associated with other pelvic and perineal injuries

Aetiology
- Urethral rupture may be caused by road traffic accidents or falls

Mechanism of injury
- *Blunt trauma:*
    - Urethral rupture is usually caused by compression, e.g. a direct blow to the perineum, with damage to the bulbar urethra in particular resulting from straddle injuries, i.e. falling astride
    - Urethral rupture is common in disruption of the symphysis pubis

Symptoms/signs
- Inability to void or pain on attempted voiding
- Blood at the urethral meatus (not always)
- In 20% of injuries of the posterior urethra, there is an associated pelvic fracture
- In females there may be vaginal bleeding/laceration
- In males there may be a high riding prostate on rectal examination (not usually appropriate in the Immediate Care situation)

External genitalia

Incidence
- Injury is uncommon

Aetiology
- Blunt trauma:
    - Kick or sporting injury
- Lacerations
- The most severe injuries occur as a result of missile or blast trauma

Mechanism of injury

Blunt trauma
- Compression injury

Penetrating trauma
- Local penetration by a low energy transfer missile/weapon
- Severe disruption caused by a high energy transfer missile

Pathophysiology
- There may be considerable haemorrhage if large blood vessels are damaged

Symptoms/signs
- Pain, swelling and obvious blood loss

Management
- Apply a dressing with direct pressure to reduce blood loss
- Set up an intravenous infusion with wide bore cannulae if blood loss has been severe, or it is not possible to stop haemorrhage

17

Extremity injuries

Extremity injuries

Introduction

- Skeletal injuries are probably the commonest significant type of injury encountered in Immediate Care, and their management is something with which all those involved in Immediate Care should be fully competent and experienced in managing
- It should not be forgotten, however, that they are rarely immediately life threatening, and that assessment and management of the airway, breathing, circulation and abdominal and pelvic injuries, head, and facial injuries come first

Incidence

Age

- Fractures are encountered at all ages but:
  - The very young have very flexible bones, so fractures are unusual except where very considerable force is used
  - Children are very active and liable to injury. Their bones are still relatively supple and so they may only sustain a "green stick" fracture where the bone is buckled, or there is an incomplete break in the bone cortex
  - The elderly have relatively brittle bones which are relatively easily fractured

Sex

- Boys are usually more adventurous than girls and are more liable to injury
- Post-menopausal women, and sometimes older men may suffer from osteoporosis, which results in thinning of the bony cortex and their bones are more susceptible to fractures especially of the hip and wrist

Aetiology

- Fractures are caused as a result of bones being exposed to abnormal forces or because the bones are unable to withstand normal forces because they themselves are weak, e.g. in osteoporosis

Anatomy

- The human skeleton is composed of over 200 bones and is the framework on which 'hangs' the rest of the body
- Bones are joined to each other by joints, and may articulate with each other with the aid of muscles
- Bones have a relatively thin outer layer; the cortex, which is covered by the periosteum, which can manufacture new bone
- The inner core of the bone is called the medulla and consists of a matrix of trabeculae, containing fat and in some bones; the bone marrow

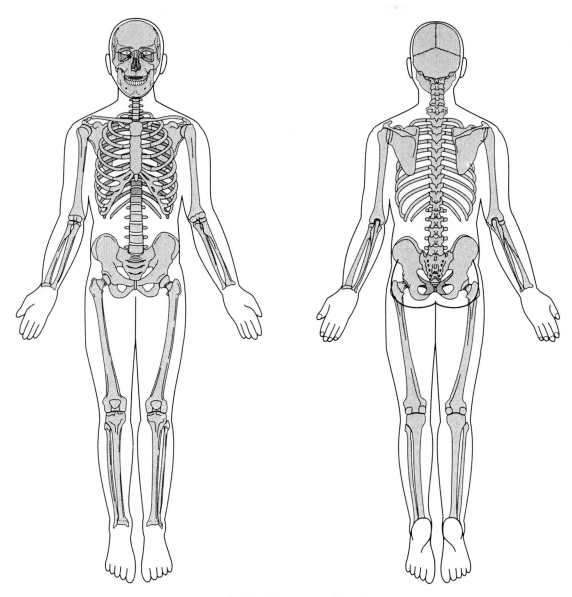

Figure 17-1 Skeleton: back and front

Mechanism of injury

- Bones fracture when the force applied to them is greater than their tensile or compressive strength
- Bones may be weakened by:
    - Osteoporosis which results in a relative loss of calcium and thinning of the trabeculae
    - Cysts or tumour

Blunt trauma

Compression

- The forces causing a fracture may be:
    - Direct, resulting in
        - A transverse or oblique (if the force is applied at an angle) fracture of the bone, in which the fracture line extends away from the point of impact
        - Considerable soft tissue injury between the point of impact and the bone due to compression
        - An open fracture, if the force of impact is sufficient to produce a fissure in the skin and tissues under the point of impact extending to the fracture itself, or it forces part of the fractured bone through the skin opposite the point of impact

- Indirect/transmitted, resulting in:
    - Spiral fracture due to a shearing/twisting force
    - Compression fracture (typically seen in vertebrae) due to, e.g. falls from a height

Long bone fractures: mechanism of injury

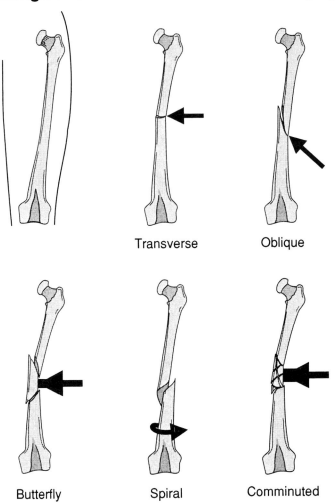

Transverse   Oblique

Butterfly   Spiral   Comminuted

Figure 17-2 Mechanism of injury: force applied and type of fracture

Pathophysiology

Fractures

- Fractures may be:
    - Open/compound:
        - Where the bone penetrates the skin
    - Closed/simple:
        - Where there is no skin penetration
        - Closed fractures may cause pressure on the skin, resulting in ischaemic damage
    - Complicated, involving:
        - Blood vessels resulting in vascular injury
        - Nerves
        - Viscera
    - Comminuted:
        - Multiple fractures at the same site
- Blood loss following bony injury may be considerable (see chapter on Circulation care: shock)

Long bone fractures: types of fracture

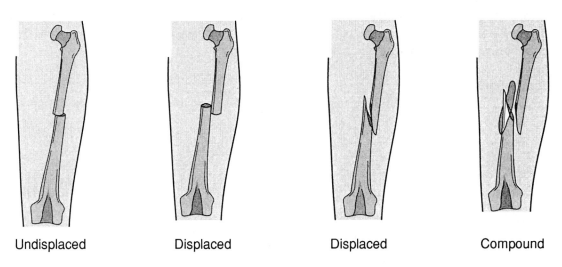

| Undisplaced | Displaced | Displaced | Compound |

Figure 17-3 Fractures: results of compression injury

Fractures in children

Greenstick fractures
- Children have softer bones than adults, as a result of which they are more flexible and less likely to fracture completely than adults' bones, but may buckle or there may only be a partial break in the bony cortex:
    - A Greenstick fracture occurs where one cortex and the underlying medullary bone is fractured, but the other cortex is only buckled and not fractured
    - A Torus fracture occurs where the bony cortex is buckled, but not broken

Fractures in children

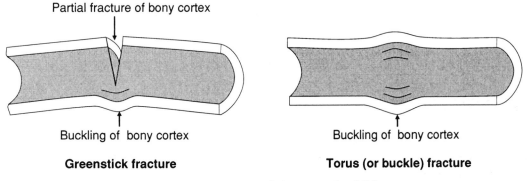

Partial fracture of bony cortex

Buckling of bony cortex   Buckling of bony cortex

Greenstick fracture   **Torus (or buckle) fracture**

Figure 17-4 Greenstick fractures in children

Epiphyseal fractures
- Children's bones are still growing; the increase in length occurring due to growth at the epiphyses or growth plates, formed of cartilage. This is potentially a weak spot in the bone, and is subject to damage by shearing forces

Dislocations
- Dislocations occur when forces similar to those causing fractures in bones, are applied to joints, resulting in disruption of the joint capsule and displacement of one of the bones
- Dislocations may occur in isolation or in combination with a fracture

Assessment

The history/mechanism of injury
- This may or may not be obtainable, but the experienced Immediate Care doctor should be able to read the wreckage, predict the likely injuries, and seek them out

Symptoms/signs
- The examination of bones and joints to assess if there is any possible injury should be systematic:
  - Look
  - Feel
  - Move
- Pain/loss of function:
  - In the pre-hospital situation the patient may not or cannot complain of quite significant injuries
- Suspect a fracture, if there is:
  - Deformity
  - Swelling
  - Visible bruising
- There is a definite fracture if there is:
  - Gross deformity
  - Bony crepitus
  - Abnormal mobility
- Suspect vascular damage if there is:
  - Skin discolouration: looks pale, blue
  - Reduced skin temperature: feels cold
  - Reduced capillary return
  - Poor or absent peripheral pulses
  - Reduced peripheral SpO_2
- Suspect nerve injury if there is reduced or absent sensation or voluntary movement

Management
- Depending on the effects of extremity injury, it may be appropriate to manage extremity injury during the primary survey, especially to reduce haemorrhage and relieve pain, and to facilitate extrication and movement of the patient prior to transport
- Extremity injuries may appear visually dramatic, and the rescuer should be careful not to be diverted by them from attending to lifesaving but less obviously necessary procedures
- Follow the usual guidelines:

  - **Primary survey/initial management:**
    - Airway with stabilisation of the cervical spine;
      - Administer oxygen to all patients with a suspected long bone fracture
    - Breathing:
      - Consider tracheal intubation and assisted ventilation if there is impaired ventilation, due to, e.g. a ruptured diaphragm
    - Circulation:
      - Evidence of hypovolaemia:
        - Secure two intravenous lines with wide bore cannulae and infuse sparingly
        - If the anticipated blood loss is considerable, then consider application of a PASG
      - Internal bleeding:
        - Control by reduction and application of suitable splinting
      - Obvious external bleeding:
        - Control with direct pressure

- **D**isability
- Exposure with control of the environment

- **Secondary survey/management:**
    - Head injury
    - Chest injury
    - Abdominal injury
    - Extremity injury
    - Spinal injury

Extremity injury

- Expose and thoroughly examine the affected limb
- If there is:
    - Exposed bone:
        - Take a *Polaroid*® photograph, cover with a sterile dressing soaked in N-Saline (or aqueous iodine solution or spray with an antiseptic spray, e.g. povidone iodine, if there is likely to be a long delay before the patient is likely to reach hospital), and then seal with clingfilm
    - Exposed or prolapsed viscera:
        - Cover with clingfilm or saline soaked towels (Hartmann's solution will do)
- Immobilisation:
    - Immobilise the affected limb with a sling or splint
- Traction:
    - Consider applying traction to lower limb fractures using a traction splint. This is a modified version of the Thomas splint with its own self-contained method of applying traction (usually to a hitch attached to the ankle)
- Reduce any easily reduced or skin threatening fractures:
    - Depending on the type and location of the fracture, this may be possible and will minimise the complications and tissue damage following a fracture
    - Immediate reduction is specifically indicated where there is impaired circulation or sensation, distal to the fracture or when the skin is at risk.
    - Take *Polaroid*® photographs before and after reduction
    - Monitor the peripheral pulses, peripheral SpO_2, sensation and movement before and after fracture reduction
    - The patient should be given adequate analgesia (although sometimes none is necessary, especially if reduction is carried out almost immediately after the injury) with:
        - Nitrous oxide/oxygen mixture, e.g. *Entonox*®, *Nitronox*®, but not if there is a chest injury with the potential for a pneumothorax
        - Local nerve block
        - Intravenous opiate
- Try to prevent complications, e.g. haemorrhage, vascular and nerve injury by careful handling
- Skin injury:
    - Preserve as much skin as possible
    - In compound or degloving injuries:
        - Cover the wound with a sterile dressing soaked in N-Saline (or aqueous iodine solution or spray with an antiseptic spray, e.g. povidone iodine, if there is likely to be a long delay before the patient is likely to reach hospital), and then seal with, clingfilm, after first taking *Polaroid*® photographs
- Bone loss:
    - Collect any large extruded bone fragments, wrap them up in a sterile dressing soaked in N-saline, and send them with the patient to hospital

Splinting/immobilisation

Triangular bandages
- A triangular bandage used as a sling is the method of choice for supporting most upper limb injuries
- Triangular bandages may be folded to make ties suitable for immobilising the lower limb

Splints

Inflatable splints
- Used to provide immobilisation and support for fractures of the forearm and wrist, and upper and lower limb

Mode of action
- Immobilisation
- Reduction of haemorrhage by tamponade

Disadvantages
- May produce impairment of the distal circulation and cause a compartmental syndrome
- May be punctured easily

CONCLUSION: Only used if no better splint is available

Box splints
- Used to provide support and splintage for lower limb injuries from (and including) the knee to the foot
- May also be used to immobilise upper limb injuries

Advantages
- Quick and easy to apply
- Effective

Disadvantages
- Do not apply traction

CONCLUSION: Splint of choice for lower limb injuries when traction splintage is contraindicated or inappropriate

Traction splints
- Developed from the Thomas splint for splinting femoral shaft fractures

Aims
- To reduce blood loss
- Minimise pain
- Prevent fracture movement, usually by fracture reduction
- To reduce neurovascular complications

Mode of action
- Reduce and immobilise the fracture
- With a fractured femur:
    - The splinting effect of the bone is lost and the muscle bunches up causing the fractured bony ends to override
    - This increases the local diameter of the muscle and initially allows a greater space into which blood can escape
    - Further extensive blood loss may result in a compartmental syndrome with an increase in the intra-compartmental pressure eventually resulting in:
        - Pressure necrosis of nerves
        - Tamponade of the arterial blood supply and muscle necrosis
        - Impairment of the venous return
- Reduction results in restoration of the normal anatomical configuration and hence prevents this initial blood loss

Indications
- Closed/simple fracture of the femoral shaft
- Closed/simple fracture of the tibia/fibula (except undisplaced fractures of the proximal shaft of fibula)
- Open/compound fractures of the femoral shaft, tibia and fibula
- With minimal traction:
    - Dislocation of the hip
    - Fractures around the knee

Contraindications
- Fracture dislocation of the knee
- Ankle fractures

Method of application
- Administer analgesia:
    - Nitrous oxide/oxygen mixture, e.g. *Entonox®, Nitronox®*, but not if there is a chest injury with the potential for a pneumothorax
    - Femoral nerve block
    - Intravenous opiate
- Expose the whole of the injured leg from groin to toes by removing clothing
- Examine the whole leg especially for peripheral pulses, colour, temperature, SpO_2, sensation, and motor power distal to the fracture
- Prepare the splint
- Apply a dressing to any wounds (if the fracture is open, this *must* be recorded on the patient report form)
- Apply gentle manual traction to the ankle, warning the patient before you do so
- Attach the ankle hitch to the ankle
- Position the splint and attach the ankle hitch to the traction device hook
- Position padding as necessary and gently apply traction (up to 7 kg (15 lbs) for an adult male) until the deformity disappears or the leg is the same length as the other one
- Re-examine the limb distal to the fracture, paying attention to the peripheral pulses, colour, temperature, SpO_2, sensation, and motor power distal to the fracture

CONCLUSION: Method of choice for the management of most lower limb injuries

Upper limb injuries

Fracture of the clavicle

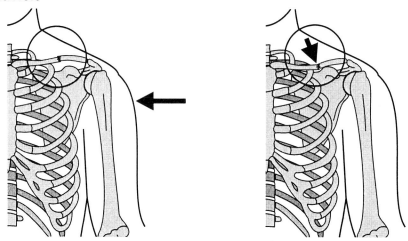

Figure 17-5 Mechanism of injury: fracture of the clavicle

Incidence
- A relatively common injury in teenagers

Aetiology
- In adolescents a fractured clavicle is often caused by falls from a tree, bicycle or horse
- In adults a fractured clavicle is often caused by a fall from a motorcycle or by side impacts in vehicle road traffic accidents, resulting in side intrusion

Mechanism of injury

Blunt trauma
- A direct blow to the clavicle
- A severe blow to or fall onto the shoulder or less commonly a fall onto the outstretched hand, which results in the impact force being transmitted to the clavicle, which fractures at its weakest point

Pathophysiology/complications
- The clavicle is the only bony connection between the upper limb and the rest of the bony skeleton
- Most clavicular fractures occur at the junction of the medial (inner) two thirds and distal (outer) third
- Severely displaced fractures of the clavicle may cause:
    - Pressure on the subclavian or innominate arteries and veins, especially if the fracture is caused by a direct blow resulting in depression
    - Pressure on the trachea, which can be life threatening and necessitating urgent reduction
    - Penetration of the pleura and/or lung resulting in pneumo- or haemothorax

Symptoms/signs
- The patient will tend to clutch the elbow on the same side as the fracture to try to reduce movement
- Localised swelling and bruising and rarely a local wound

Management
- Check the pulses on the same side as the injury
- A broad arm sling
- If there is severe posterior displacement:
    - Reduce the fracture immediately by applying backward traction to the shoulder/arm

Sternoclavicular joint dislocation

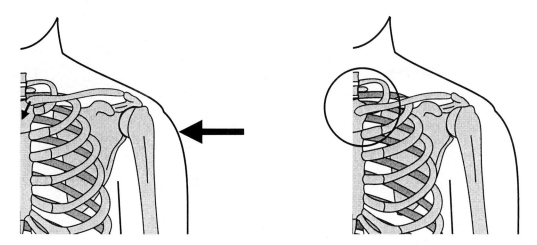

Figure 17-6 Mechanism of injury: dislocation of the sternoclavicular joint

Incidence
- Dislocation of the sternoclavicular joint is a relatively rare injury

Aetiology
- Usually caused by a fall

Mechanism of injury

Blunt trauma
- Usually caused by a direct blow to the anterior of the shoulder joint or a fall onto the laterally outstretched hand which results in the clavicle dislocating medially and inferiorly

Pathophysiology
- Severe posterior dislocation of the clavicle at the sternoclavicular joint may result in:
  - Pressure on the subclavian or innominate arteries and veins
  - Pressure on the trachea, which can be life threatening and necessitating urgent reduction
  - Penetration of the pleura and/or lung resulting in pneumo- or haemothorax

Symptoms/signs
- Pain and localised tenderness over the affected joint, aggravated by movement of the arm on the same side as the injury

Management
- Check the pulses on the same side as the injury
- A broad arm sling
- Always admit to hospital due the risk of complications

Acromioclavicular joint dislocation

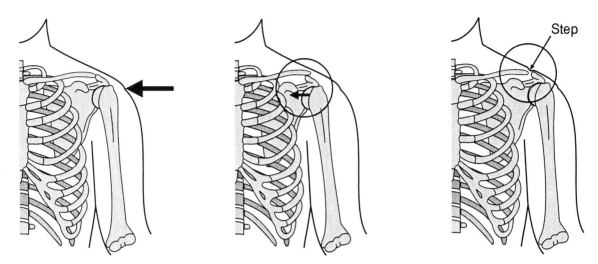

Figure 17-7 Mechanism of injury: dislocation of the acromioclavicular joint

Incidence
- Acromioclavicular joint dislocation is a relatively rare injury

Aetiology
- Acromioclavicular joint dislocation may occur due to road traffic accidents and sport; it is a relatively common injury in rugby players who fall onto the shoulder

Mechanism of injury

Blunt trauma
- Acromioclavicular joint dislocation is usually caused by a direct blow to the point of the shoulder

Pathophysiology
- There is medial movement of the scapula with disruption of the acromioclavicular joint and its ligaments and in some severe cases tearing of the coraco-clavicular ligament or even an avulsion fracture of the coracoid process of the clavicle
- There is a risk of damage to the brachial plexus
- There may be an associated injury of the cervical spine

Symptoms/signs
- May be very painful with localised tenderness
- A step may be palpable between the end of the clavicle and the acromion process

Management
- Check the pulses on the same side as the injury
- A broad arm sling

Scapular fracture

Incidence
- This is a relatively rare injury

Aetiology
- Usually caused by:
    - A fall from a motorcycle
    - An accidental blow with an implement during sporting events, e.g. a cricket bat or a hockey stick
    - Assault with e.g a baseball bat, club or police baton

Mechanism of injury

Blunt trauma
- Fractures of the scapula are usually caused by a severe localised compressive force, as the scapula is covered by several layers of protective muscle

Pathophysiology
- Often associated with fractures of the underlying ribs

Symptoms/signs
- A fracture of the scapula may be very painful, made worse by shoulder movement
- Localised tenderness

Management
- Analgesia, as required
- immobilisation in a broad arm sling

Shoulder injuries

Anterior dislocation of the shoulder

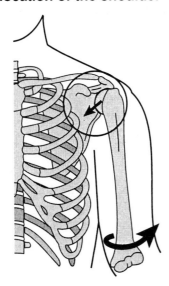 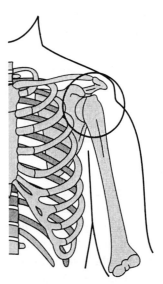

Figure 17-8 Mechanism of injury: anterior dislocation of the shoulder

Incidence
- Anterior dislocation is the most common dislocation of the shoulder

Aetiology
- Usually caused by a fall, sport (rugby) or arm wrestling

Mechanism of injury

Blunt trauma
- Anterior shoulder dislocation is caused by forced external rotation of the humerus at the glenohumeral joint, usually as a result of the lower forearm/wrist being forced laterally, whilst the elbow is held flexed close to the trunk

Pathophysiology/complications
- Dislocation of the head of the humerus results in a tear of the anterior part of the shoulder joint capsule caused by anterior and inferior displacement of the humeral head
- The axillary nerve may be damaged, resulting in deltoid paralysis, and occasionally the axillary artery
- After an anterior dislocation there will be a persistent weakness in the anterior part of the shoulder joint capsule if the patient continues to use the shoulder before it has healed (and sometimes even if they have), which will leave the shoulder vulnerable to being repeatedly dislocated. Patients with this condition may be able to dislocate their shoulders at will

Symptoms/signs
- The shoulder is usually very painful (there is usually protective spasm of the deltoid muscle), and the patient will usually hold their forearm with the elbow flexed
- There will be loss of the shoulder contour, and the lateral margin of the scapula may appear to be unusually prominent
- There may be paraesthesiae/numbness in the distribution of the axillary nerve

Management
- Immobilisation with a broad arm sling
- Analgesia
- Reduction (reduces the amount of local damage caused by the dislocation)

Reduction of anterior shoulder dislocation
- This procedure should only be carried out in the pre-hospital situation by experienced personnel, after a careful examination of the patient and the mechanism of injury, as a fracture dislocation of the shoulder may appear very similar
- Pain relief may be required, but in general the sooner reduction is performed, the less likely it is to be very painful, as severe muscle spasm may not have developed
- Polaroid photographs should be taken before and after reduction
- There are various methods of reduction, but Kocher's method is probably the most suitable for the pre-hospital situation

Kocher's method:
- With the elbow flexed to a right angle, apply steady downwards traction in the line of the humerus
- Rotate the arm laterally
- Adduct the arm by moving the elbow across the body towards the midline
- Rotate the arm medially, so that the hand lies across the opposite side of the chest
- As you do so the dislocation should reduce with a slight clunk, accompanied by a reduction in the pain experienced by the patient
- Examine the shoulder to make certain that the shoulder contour has returned to normal
- If reduction is not successful, it is probably best not to try again
- After successful reduction, apply a broad arm sling together with a triangular bandage folded and tied across the affected arm and chest to prevent any shoulder movement

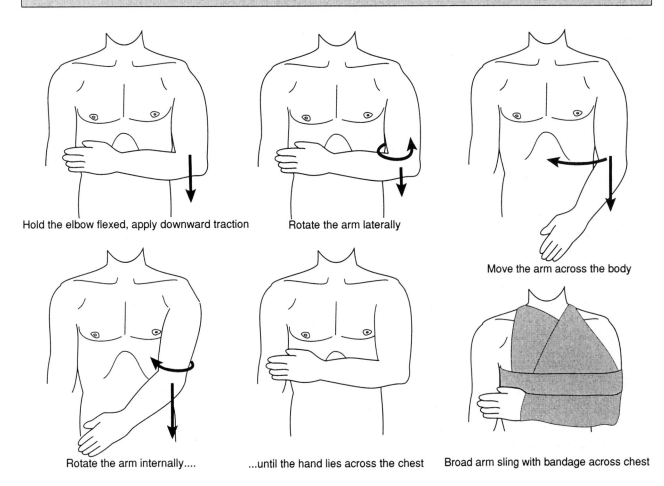

Hold the elbow flexed, apply downward traction

Rotate the arm laterally

Move the arm across the body

Rotate the arm internally....

...until the hand lies across the chest

Broad arm sling with bandage across chest

Figure 17-9 Kocher method of reducing an anterior dislocation of the shoulder

Posterior dislocation of the shoulder

Incidence
-   Posterior dislocation of the shoulder is relatively rare

Aetiology
-   Caused by a direct blow to the shoulder, electric shock or epileptic fit

Mechanism of injury
-   A direct blow to the front of the top of the shoulder, accompanied by forced lateral flexion of the head in the opposite direction
-   A fall onto the outstretched hand whilst the arm is internally rotated

Pathophysiology/complications
-   May result in a brachial plexus injury due to the posterior displacement of the head of humerus

Symptoms/signs
-   May not be obvious and is often missed
-   Pain, swelling and local deformity with some change on the normal contour of the shoulder

Management
-   Immobilisation with a broad arm sling
-   Immediate reduction is not indicated in the Immediate Care situation
-   Analgesia as appropriate

Inferior dislocation of the shoulder

Incidence
- Inferior dislocation of the shoulder is very rare

Aetiology
- Caused by an electric shock or violent epileptic fit

Mechanism of injury
- Violent muscular contractions of the muscles of the shoulder girdle result in inferior displacement of the humeral head

Symptoms/signs
- The arm is held extended above the head
- Inferior shoulder dislocation may be extremely painful

Management
- Analgesia as appropriate
- Fitting the patient onto a stretcher or into the ambulance may be difficult

Humerus

Neck of humerus fractures

Incidence
- Fractures of the neck of humerus usually occur in the elderly, but may occur in the young in violent accidents

Aetiology
- Fractures of the neck of humerus are usually caused by accidental falls

Mechanism of injury

Blunt trauma
- Fractures of the neck of humerus are usually caused by:
    - A fall onto the upper arm or a direct blow resulting in a transverse fracture
    - A fall onto the outstretched hand, when the impact force is transmitted up the humerus resulting in impaction

Symptoms/signs
- The patient will experience pain over the fracture site and will tend to hold the elbow of the injured arm
- In impaction fractures of the neck of humerus there may be some function and not a lot of pain
- In transverse fractures there may be deformity over the fracture site with local swelling and bruising

Pathophysiology
- There is often considerable muscle injury resulting in extensive bruising
- Fractures of the neck of humerus may sometimes involve the axillary nerve

Management
- A collar and cuff, unless it is too painful, then apply a broad arm sling

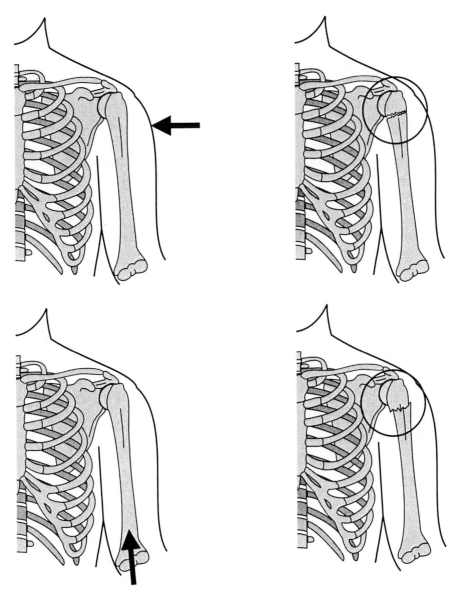

Figure 17-10 Mechanism of injury of fractures of the proximal humerus

Shaft of humerus fractures

Incidence
- Fractures of the shaft of humerus are relatively common, especially in the elderly

Aetiology
- Fractures of the humeral shaft are usually caused by as a result of a side impact, e.g in a fall or road traffic accident, which may be relatively minor if the humerus is weakened by secondary tumour deposit

Mechanism of injury

Blunt trauma
- Direct force will result in a transverse, oblique or comminuted fracture
- A fall onto the outstretched hand, resulting in internal or external rotation at the shoulder and a twisting force which causes a spiral fracture of the humeral shaft

Pathophysiology

- Usually the middle third of the humerus is involved (a common place for secondary tumour deposits)
- The radial nerve runs down a groove on the posterior of the humerus, and is easily damaged if the humerus is fractured (usually resulting in a contusion; rarely a complete division) or a compartmental syndrome develops
- Radial nerve damage will result in a wrist drop on the affected side (the patient will be unable to extend the wrist) with impaired sensation on the radial side of the back of the hand
- A fracture of the shaft of humerus may also result in damage to the brachial artery, which is the main artery supplying the upper limb (a compartmental syndrome may compress this artery and impair the blood supply to the upper limb by applying a constricting pressure)
- Fractures of the shaft of humerus are often associated with injury of the underlying ribs and lung

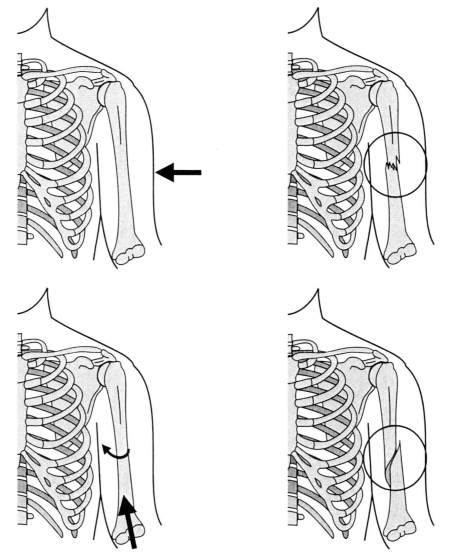

Figure 17-11 Mechanism of injury of fractures of the shaft of humerus

Symptoms/signs

- The patient will be in pain and will tend to support the affected arm at the elbow with the opposite hand
- There may be obvious swelling and deformity over the fracture site, but any rotation may not be obvious

Management

- Management of any associated chest injury
- Immobilisation with a broad arm sling

Elbow

Supracondylar fracture

Incidence
- Commonly occurs in children/adolescents, rare in adults

Aetiology
- Caused by a fall

Mechanism of injury

Blunt trauma
- A fall onto the outstretched arm, with the elbow flexed resulting in the transmission of the impact force to the elbow

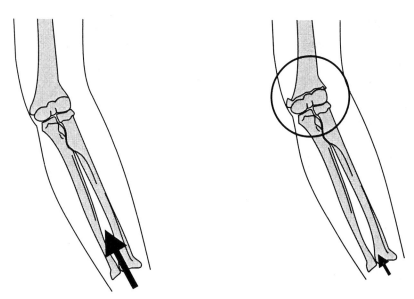

Figure 17-12 Mechanism of injury of supracondylar fracture

Pathophysiology
- Fractures may range from undisplaced crack fractures to severely displaced fractures with vascular and neurological damage
- The most important complication arising from supracondylar fracture is brachial artery injury, caused by trapping or kinking of the artery between bone ends or direct injury: which can result in avascular necrosis of the forearm muscles (Volkmann's contracture) and a permanent deformity/disability

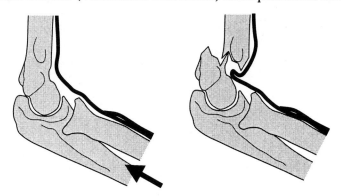

Figure 17-13 Mechanism of injury: brachial artery injury in supracondylar fracture

Symptoms/signs
- The child will tend to support the injured elbow with their hand
- Pain and swelling over the fracture site
- An absent or weak radial pulse; *always* check the radial pulse if this injury is suspected

Management
- Check for the radial pulse:
    - If the radial pulse is absent: attempt to straighten the elbow, with careful monitoring of the radial pulse or peripheral circulation with a pulse oximeter
    - If the radial pulse is present: immobilise the arm using a broad arm sling with the angle between the upper arm and forearm at the elbow greater than 90°, then recheck the pulse again

Condylar fractures

Incidence
- Uncommon, usually occurs in children
- The lateral epicondyle is most usually fractured

Aetiology
- Caused by a fall onto the outstretched hand

Mechanism of injury

Blunt trauma
- The impact force is transmitted up the forearm to the elbow and via the radius to the lateral epicondyle

Pathophysiology
- The lateral condyle is fractured much more commonly than the medial
- The fracture involves the joint surface and extends obliquely upwards and laterally
- Displacement is rarely severe, the importance of these fractures is that they involve the joint surface and are prone to non union, resulting in osteoarthritis

Symptoms/signs
- Pain and swelling around the elbow, made worse by attempted movement

Management
- Immobilisation with a broad arm sling

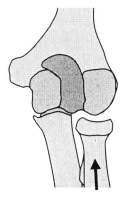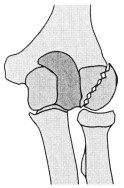

Figure 17-14 Mechanism of injury: fracture of the lateral humeral condyle

Epicondylar fracture

Incidence
- Uncommon, occurs more often in children than adults

Aetiology
- Usually caused by a fall

Mechanism of injury

Blunt trauma
- May be caused by:
    - Avulsion: the epicondyle may be pulled off by the forearm flexor muscles that are attached to it typically due to a fall onto the outstretched hand (avulsion)
    - A direct compressive impact

Pathophysiology
- Usually the medial epicondyle is fractured, which may result in damage to the ulnar nerve

Symptoms/signs
- Pain and swelling over the elbow
- Ulnar nerve injury:
    - Inability to extend the fingers fully
    - Tingling/loss of sensation in the little and ring fingers

Management
- Immobilisation in a broad arm sling

Elbow dislocation

Incidence
- Common both in children and adults

Aetiology
- Caused by a fall onto the outstretched hand

Mechanism of injury

Blunt trauma
- The force of impact is transmitted up the ulna to the elbow joint forcing the ulna backwards resulting in its dislocation

Pathophysiology
- The dislocation is usually posterior, but may also be anterior
- There may be an associated fracture (usually minor) of the coronoid process, or of the head of radius or medial epicondyle
- Rarely the brachial artery may be damaged due to swelling or the ulnar nerve due to stretching

Symptoms/signs
- The patient may be in a lot of pain
- Obvious deformity with considerable swelling
- There is usually pain on any attempted elbow movement

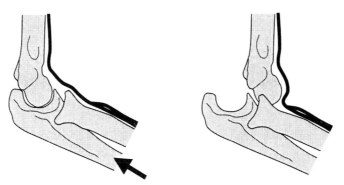

Figure 17-15 Mechanism of injury: dislocation of the elbow

Management
- Assess and monitor the radial pulse and motor power and sensation in the hand/fingers
- Reduction may be considered by the experienced Immediate Care Doctor
- The elbow should be immobilised in a broad arm sling or other splint in the position of greatest comfort

Reduction of elbow dislocation

Method:
- Provide adequate analgesia with nitrous oxide/oxygen and opiates if necessary (may require a GA)
- Pull on the forearm with the elbow semi-flexed
- At the same time apply forward pressure behind the olecranon process

Olecranon process

Incidence
- Usually found in adults

Aetiology
- Caused by a fall onto the point of the elbow

Mechanism of injury

Blunt trauma
- The force of impact results in fracture of the olecranon

Pathophysiology
- The fracture nearly always involves the middle of the joint and -may be:
    - A crack fracture without displacement
    - A fracture with separation of the two fragments
    - A comminuted fracture

Symptoms/signs
- Pain and swelling of the elbow joint with inability to extend the elbow without considerable pain

Management
- Immobilisation with a broad arm sling

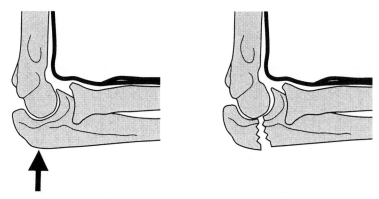

Figure 17-16 Mechanism of injury: fracture of the olecranon process

Radial head fracture

Incidence
- Fracture of the radial head is common in adults, usually the young

Aetiology
- Caused by a fall onto the outstretched hand

Mechanism of injury

Blunt trauma
- The force of impact is transmitted up the radius resulting in an impaction fracture

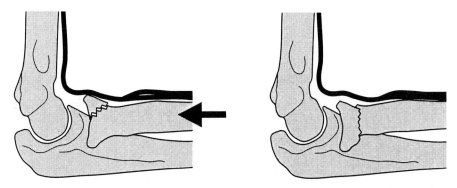

Figure 17-17 Mechanism of injury: fracture of the head and neck of radius

Pathophysiology
- The fracture may be undisplaced in over 50%
- In most of the rest a segment of the radial head breaks off and is depressed below the line of the articular cartilage
- In a small number of cases there may be severe comminution of the radial head
- The cartilage lining the radial head and the capitulum is usually severely contused

Symptoms/signs
- Pain and swelling over the radial head
- Reduced elbow flexion with reduced wrist pronation/supination

Management
- Place the arm in a broad arm sling or collar and cuff

Radius/ulna shaft fractures

Incidence
- Fractures of the shafts of the radius and ulna are a relatively common injury

Aetiology
- Caused by assault or a fall

Mechanism of injury

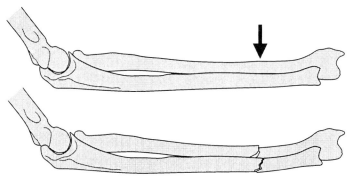

Figure 17-18 Mechanism of injury: fracture of the radius and ulna due to direct blunt trauma

Blunt trauma
- Forearm fractures may be caused by
  - A direct blow
  - Transmitted force from, e.g. a fall onto the outstretched hand, or from the steering wheel in a severe frontal impact

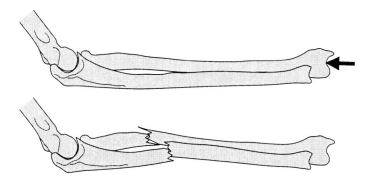

Figure 17-19 Mechanism of injury: fracture of the radius and ulna due to indirect blunt trauma

Pathophysiology
- Both the radius and ulna are usually fractured, but sometimes one bone only may be fractured, when there is usually an associated dislocation at the elbow (Monteggia fracture) or wrist (Galeazzi fracture)
- There may be (rarely) an associated neurovascular injury
- If there is significant angulation, there may be pressure on the skin, which will result in skin necrosis if it continues for any length of time
- In children the fracture is usually a greenstick fracture of the midshaft, or may involve the growth plates at the epiphyses

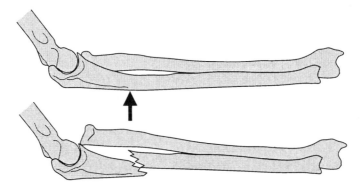

Figure 17-20 Mechanism of injury: (Monteggia) fracture of the ulna alone with dislocation of the head of radius typically caused by a fall associated with forced pronation or a direct blow

Symptoms/signs
- The patient will be in pain and will usually support the injured limb, by holding it
- There may be obvious deformity with angulation

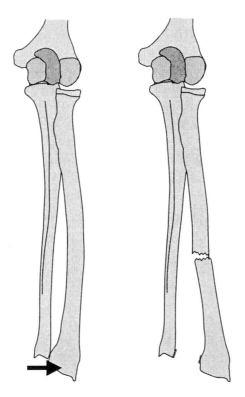

Figure 17-21 Mechanism of injury: (Galeazzi) fracture of the radius alone, caused by a fall onto the hand

Management
- Assess the forearm/wrist/hand for evidence of:
  - Impaired circulation: check the radial pulse
  - Neurological deficit: ask the patient to move their fingers and check for any numbness
  - Severe angulation with pressure on the skin from a fractured bone end: consider reduction
- Immobilise the arm in a broad arm sling or small box splint

Lower end of radius (Colles and Smith's) fractures

Incidence
- This is the most common type of wrist fracture
- Very common in:
    - Those over 65 and female (especially if there is associated osteoporosis)
    - The winter months: snow and ice

Aetiology
- Nearly always caused by a fall onto the outstretched hand (Colles fracture) or back of the wrist (Smith's fracture)

Mechanism of injury

Blunt trauma
- The impact energy from a fall onto the outstretched hand with the palm down, is transmitted to the wrist forcing it dorsally, resulting in the classical Colles fracture
- In Smith's fracture the fall is onto the back of the wrist whilst the wrist supinated, resulting in the impact force being transmitted to the wrist and forcing it ventrally

Pathophysiology
- There may be associated injury to:
    - The median nerve which passes through the carpal tunnel in the wrist and is relatively easily involved in Colles fractures. It supplies motor power to the small muscles of the thumb and sensation to the palm of the hand and the palmar surface of the thumb, index and middle fingers
    - The ulnar nerve (relatively rarely); it supplies motor power to the small muscles of the hand and sensation to the palmar aspects of the ring and little fingers
    - Children may sustain a fracture of the distal radius but this is usually a greenstick fracture or epiphyseal injury, and is associated with the application of considerable force

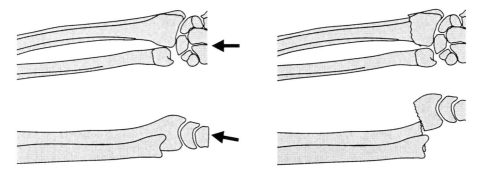

Figure 17-22 Mechanism of injury: Colles fracture

Symptoms/signs
- The will be pain and swelling of the wrist
- There may be the classic dinner fork deformity (this may be reversed in a Smith's fracture)
- Sometimes there may be impaired sensation in the palm of the hand and rarely in the ring and little fingers

Management
- Remove any rings from the fingers
- Immediate reduction and splinting if circumstances permit, and there are no life threatening injuries
- Apply a broad arm sling
- Monitor the peripheral circulation and neurological status in the hand

Carpal fractures

Incidence
- The scaphoid is the most commonly fractured carpal and usually occurs in young adults, but rarely in children or in those >35 years old

Aetiology
- A scaphoid fracture is usually caused by a fall onto the outstretched hand

Mechanism of injury

Blunt trauma
- A fall onto the outstretched hand with the palm down, forcing the wrist into hyperextension and resulting in the compression force being transmitted to the scaphoid which is compressed and fractures

Pathophysiology
- The scaphoid usually fractures across its middle

Symptoms/signs
- A characteristic history
- Pain in the wrist with tenderness in the anatomical snuff box

Management
- Remove any rings from the fingers
- Immobilisation in a broad arm sling

Metacarpal fractures

Incidence
- Metacarpal fractures are fairly common, usually occurring in adults

Aetiology
- The metacarpals are usually injured due to assault or a fall

Mechanism of injury

Blunt trauma
- Metacarpals may be fractured due to direct or indirect compression trauma:
    - The head/distal shaft of the fifth metacarpal may be fractured by using a clenched fist to hit a hard object
    - The base of the first metacarpal may be fractured by a direct blow

Pathophysiology
- The fracture may be transverse or oblique and may involve the shaft, base or neck of the metacarpal

Symptoms/signs
- Pain and swelling over the site of the fracture

Management
- Remove any rings from the fingers
- Immobilisation in a high arm sling

Finger (phalangeal) injuries

Incidence
- Fractures:
  - Not very common
- Dislocations:
  - More common

Aetiology
- Phalangeal injuries are commonly caused by sport, industrial accidents and assault

Mechanism of injury

Blunt trauma
- Compressive blunt trauma may cause fractures of the phalanges by direct pressure, usually over the mid shaft of the phalanx, resulting in a fracture that may be transverse, oblique or comminuted, if the applied pressure is very high
- Phalangeal dislocations are usually caused by forced hyperextension, with the distal fragment being displaced backwards

Pathophysiology
- The fracture may be transverse or oblique and may involve the shaft, base or neck of the carpal
- A displaced phalangeal fracture or dislocation may cause pressure damage to the skin

Symptoms/signs
- Pain and swelling over the injury
- There may be obvious deformity

Management
- Remove any rings

Fractures
- Immediate reduction is usually possible, and will reduce the amount of soft tissue injury

Method:
- Pull on the affected finger
- Apply pressure over the proximal end of the fracture and manipulate it into its natural alignment
- Apply neighbour strapping

Dislocation
- Immediate reduction

Method:
- Pull on the affected finger
- Apply direct pressure over the base of the displaced phalanx at the same time
- Apply neighbour strapping

Lower limb injuries

Hip: posterior dislocation

Incidence
- Posterior dislocation is the commonest hip dislocation

Aetiology
- Posterior dislocation of the hip is usually caused by road traffic accidents and falls, and is often associated with other major trauma, including major fractures of the contralateral limb

Mechanism of injury

Blunt trauma
- Posterior dislocation of the hip is usually caused by severe indirect compression, usually a blow to the knee whilst the hip is flexed or semi-flexed, causing the impact force to be transmitted along the femoral shaft to the hip forcing it backwards, e.g. from the front fascia of a car involved in a frontal impact

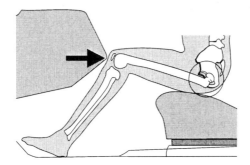

Figure 17-23 Mechanism of injury: Posterior dislocation of the hip

Pathophysiology
- The femoral head is driven backwards out of the acetabulum, often (in 50% of cases) fracturing the posterior acetabular wall and taking part of the wall with it, resulting in severe local tissue trauma and haemorrhage
- Posterior dislocation of the hip may cause:
    - Damage or disruption of the blood supply of the femoral head, sometimes (in 15-20% of cases) resulting in avascular necrosis of the femoral head, if it is not treated as soon as possible
    - Damage to the articular surface of the femoral head, later resulting in osteoarthritis
    - Sciatic nerve injury

Symptoms/signs
- The patient will be in a great deal of pain, which will be made worse by any attempted hip movement
- Hip and knee flexion with slight apparent shortening of the femur, and internal rotation of the ankle
- Sciatic nerve injury:
    - Distal sensory loss with pain radiating down the leg to the foot from the buttock
    - Foot drop (detect by asking the patient to dorsiflex the foot)

Management
- Administer high flow oxygen via a high concentration mask
- Set up an intravenous infusion with two wide bore cannulae and infuse cautiously monitoring the patient's haemodynamic state continuously
- Support the affected hip in flexion (do *not* attempt to reduce the dislocation or apply traction splintage)
- Provide adequate analgesia (the patient may require very strong pain relief)

Hip: anterior dislocation

Incidence
- Rare

Aetiology
- Road traffic and aircraft accidents

Mechanism of injury

Blunt trauma
- Anterior dislocation of the hip usually occurs as a result of very forceful abduction and then lateral rotation of the leg

Pathophysiology
- The femoral head is driven forwards out of the acetabulum, resulting in local tissue damage and damage to the blood supply of the femoral head via the ligamentum teres, which may result in avascular necrosis
- The acetabulum is not usually damaged

Symptoms/signs
- The hip is usually held in marked lateral rotation

Management
- Administer high flow oxygen via a high concentration mask
- Set up an intravenous infusion with two wide bore cannulae and infuse cautiously, monitoring the patient's haemodynamic state continuously
- Apply gentle traction
- Provide adequate analgesia

Hip: central fracture/dislocation

Incidence
- Rare

Aetiology
- Falls from a height

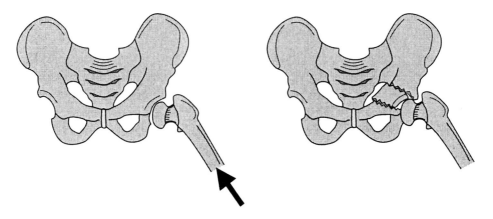

Figure 17-24 Mechanism of injury: Central fracture/dislocation of the hip

Mechanism of injury

Blunt trauma
- Central fracture dislocation of the hip usually occurs as a result of a very severe lateral blow to the femur, or a severe longtitudinal force being applied to the femur via the knee, whilst the hip is abducted
- The amount of displacement will depend on the amount of compressive force applied

Pathophysiology
- The femoral head is driven into the acetabulum, which may result in damage to the ligamentum teres (its blood supply), which may later result in avascular necrosis. The joint capsule is not usually damaged
- The medial wall of the acetabulum (innominate bone of the pelvis) may be pushed inwards and extensively fractured, the severity of the damage caused depending on the amount of force used
- There may be significant blood loss resulting in hypovolaemic shock

Symptoms/signs
- The hip is usually held in marked lateral rotation

Management
- Administer high flow oxygen via a high concentration mask
- Set up an intravenous infusion with two wide bore cannulae and infuse cautiously, monitoring the patient's haemodynamic state continuously
- Apply gentle traction
- Provide adequate analgesia (the patient may require very strong pain relief)

Femoral neck and trochanteric fractures

Incidence
- Femoral neck and trochanteric fractures are a very common type of injury, affecting up to 46,000 people per year in England and Wales
- They are common in the elderly and female (with osteoporosis) of whom about 25% die as a result

Aetiology
- Usually caused by an accidental fall

Mechanism of injury

Blunt trauma
- Femoral neck and trochanteric fractures are usually caused by compression injury due to:
    - A direct blow to the greater trochanter caused by a fall onto the hip
    - A transmitted rotational shearing force caused by tripping and twisting of the lower leg

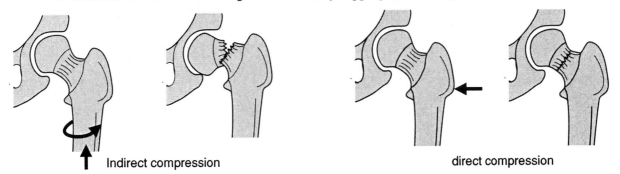

Indirect compression   direct compression

Figure 17-25 Mechanism of injury: Femoral neck fractures caused by indirect and direct compression

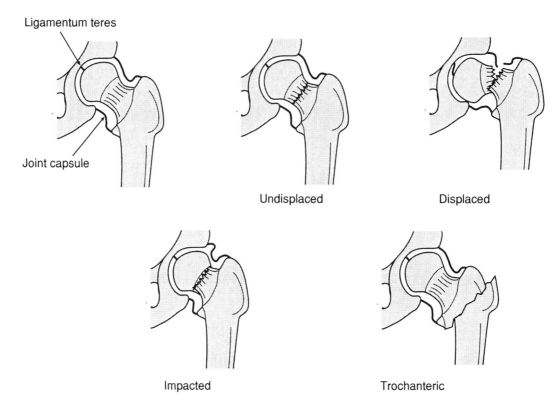

Figure 17-26 Types of femoral neck and trochanteric fractures

Pathophysiology

Femoral neck
- Fractures of the neck of femur may be:
    - Impacted
    - Undisplaced
    - Displaced
- The most important possibly preventable complication from a fracture of the neck of femur is damage to the blood supply to the femoral head, which usually only occurs if the fracture is displaced and may result in avascular necrosis, depending on the amount of damage and the severity of displacement:
    - Blood is supplied to the head of the femur by three routes:
        - Blood vessels in the ligamentum teres which is attached to the femoral head itself
        - Blood vessels in the capsule of the hip joint
        - Nutrient blood vessels in the femur
    - In displaced femoral neck fractures, the blood supply via the nutrient vessels is cut off and that via the capsular vessels may be severely damaged, only leaving the blood supply in the ligamentum teres intact, which is usually inadequate by itself.
- Displaced femoral neck fractures usually require arthroplasty although minimal displacement can often be treated by internal fixation

Trochanteric fractures
- Trochanteric fractures may be undisplaced or displaced, but usually heal well as there is no impairment of the blood supply

Slipped epiphyses
- This injury may occur in children with minimal trauma

Symptoms/signs
- The elderly are often unable to get up after the fall, and may not be found for sometime; if the weather is cold or they are only wearing night clothes, they may be suffering from hypothermia as well as the fracture
- Pain in the hip and sometimes the knee, aggravated by attempts to move the hip or weight bear (impacted fractures may be almost pain free)
- Shortening of the femur with external rotation of the ankle (the wider the displacement the greater the degree of rotation)

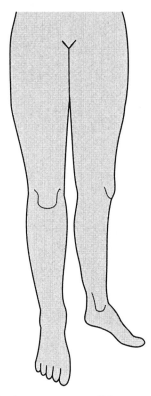

Figure 17-27 Typical appearance of fractured left neck of femur

Management
- Administer oxygen
- Set up an intravenous infusion and infuse cautiously monitoring the patient's haemodynamic state carefully as you do so
- Manage any hypothermia: make the patient warm and comfortable
- Administer appropriate analgesia
- Manage the fracture:
    - The object of management is to prevent any further damage to the vascular supply to the femoral head
    - Tie both feet together with a figure of eight bandage, to prevent further external rotation and vascular injury

Femoral shaft fractures

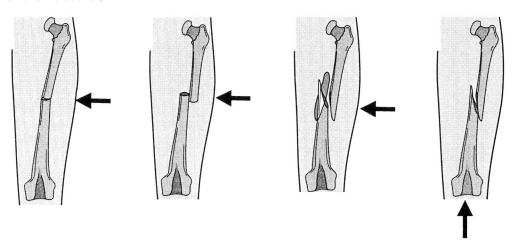

Figure 17-28 Mechanism of injury of fractures of the femoral shaft

Incidence
- Common injury in the young, especially motorcyclists

Aetiology
- Commonly found in high impact frontal road traffic accident impacts; front and side vehicle collisions and motor cycle side impacts, and falls from a height

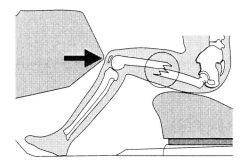

Figure 17-29 Mechanism of injury of fractures of the femoral shaft in frontal vehicle impact

Mechanism of injury

Blunt injury
- The femoral shaft is usually fractured due to severe direct or indirect compressive blunt injury to the femoral shaft or knee, when the compressive force is transmitted along the femur

Pathophysiology
- Fractures of the femur may occur at any site: upper, middle or lower shaft, and may be transverse, oblique, spiral, comminuted or (in children) greenstick
- There is often marked displacement of the fragments, due to muscle spasm, and extensive local tissue injury and haemorrhage
- Fractures of the lower third of the femur may involve the popliteal artery
- Blood loss due to intramuscular haemorrhage may be considerable (up to three units of blood if the fracture is simple, double this if the fracture is compound)

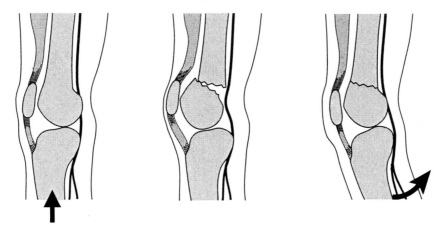

Figure 17-30 Rotation of the distal fragment in supracondylar fracture and effect of knee flexion

Supracondylar and condylar fractures
- In supracondylar fractures the distal femoral fragment may be rotated by gastrocnemius, which is attached to the distal femur
- In both supracondylar and condylar fractures of the femur there is a (small) risk of damage to the popliteal artery

Symptoms/signs
- The patient will be in considerable pain
- There will be local swelling and tenderness over the fracture site and the patient will be unable to weight bear or walk with the affected leg
- The femur on the affected side may be shortened and there is usually some angular or rotational deformity
- Rarely there may be impairment of the distal pulses, and motor and sensory impairment due to pressure on the femoral nerve

Management
- Administer high flow oxygen via a high concentration oxygen mask
- Set up an intravenous infusion and infuse cautiously monitoring the patient's haemodynamic state carefully as you do so
- Tight trousers may be left on the patient as they may reduce the amount of intramuscular haemorrhage by tamponade (but may make full evaluation of the injury difficult)
- Manage the fracture by splinting:
    - Traction splinting is the method of choice
        - If the fracture is near the knee, the distal fragment is usually tilted posteriorly and may impinge on the popliteal vessels, when traction is applied
        - If a supracondylar or condylar fracture is suspected, traction may be applied with the knee semi-flexed, and with constant monitoring of the distal pulse
    - If traction splinting is not available; immobilisation with a box splint or series of triangular bandages is appropriate
- Provide adequate analgesia, especially if the fracture is comminuted:
    - Inhalational analgesia: nitrous oxide/oxygen mixture
    - Intravenous analgesia
    - Regional anaesthesia (femoral nerve block)

Patellar injuries

Incidence
- Fracture of the patella is a relatively rare injury
- Dislocation of the patella is most commonly seen in adolescent girls

Aetiology
- Fractures of the patella may occur due to road traffic accidents or falls
- Dislocations may occur due to sporting injuries

Mechanism of injury

Fracture
- Fractures of the patella are usually caused by blunt trauma: direct compression, e.g. impact with the front fascia of the vehicle in high speed frontal collisions, falls onto a hard floor landing directly on the patella or sudden violent contraction of the quadriceps muscle

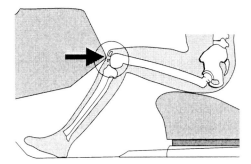

Figure 17-31 Mechanism of injury of fracture of the patella due to impact with the front fascia

Dislocation
- Usually caused by indirect twisting pressure, e.g. in football, resulting in the patella dislocating laterally

Pathophysiology

Fracture
- The patellar fracture may be transverse or comminuted
    - Muscular contraction usually causes a transverse fracture
    - A direct blow usually causes a crack or a comminuted fracture

Dislocation
- Some patients are particularly at risk of dislocating their patellae because they have slight laxity of the prepatellar ligament, the groove holding the patella in place is rather shallow, the lateral condyle is underdeveloped, they have a rather small high lying patella or they are knock kneed and when the quadriceps muscle contracts, the patella is pulled laterally
- Dislocation of the patella will result in damage to the medial patellofemoral ligament and make subsequent dislocations more likely

Symptoms/signs

Fracture
- There will usually be an abrasion or laceration over the knee, caused by the impact
- Pain and swelling over the knee, with increased pain on attempting to extend the knee
- It may be possible to feel a gap between the ends of the patella, if they have separated widely

Dislocation
- The knee will be acutely painful
- The patella is displaced laterally

Management

Fracture
- Assess both lower limbs for other associated injuries, e.g. femoral fractures
- Immobilise the knee in a long leg box splint

Dislocation
- Reduce the subluxation/dislocation immediately, using inhaled analgesia
- If the subluxation has occurred with the knee flexed, the knee must be extended as the patella is pushed back medially (otherwise reduction is very difficult to perform!)

Knee dislocation

Incidence
- Dislocation of the knee is a relatively rare injury

Aetiology
- May be caused in a road traffic accident or sporting injury

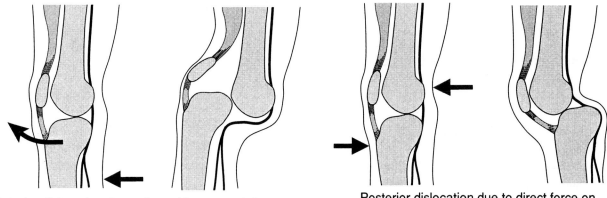

Anterior dislocation due to forced hyperextension

Posterior dislocation due to direct force on the lower thigh or front of the lower leg

Figure 17-32 Mechanism of injury of dislocation of the knee

Mechanism of injury

Blunt trauma:
- A dislocation of the knee may be caused by:
    - Forced hyperextension of the knee due to a direct compressive force below the back of the knee
    - A severe direct compressive force applied to the upper part of the lower leg or lower thigh:
        - Intrusion of wheel arch, front shelf in a severe frontal vehicle impact or collision whilst skiing

Pathophysiology
- The knee joint is stabilised by its strong ligaments, the medial and lateral ligaments, the anterior and posterior cruciate ligaments and the joint capsule. To cause a dislocation requires considerable force and may result in:
    - Disruption of the knee ligaments
    - Popliteal nerve injury
    - Vascular injury: popliteal artery

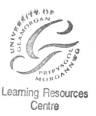

Learning Resources
Centre

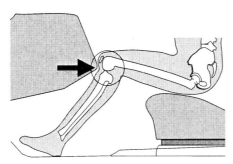

Figure 17-33 Dislocation of the knee due to impact with the front fascia

Symptoms/signs
- Pain and swelling of the knee with inability to weight bear on the affected leg
- Angular deformity of the knee joint (not always present as the knee joint may have returned to its normal alignment due to the elastic recoil of the soft tissues around the knee)
- An effusion and instability of the knee joint
- Impaired peripheral circulation, motor power and sensation

Management
- Handle the knee with care, being careful not to cause any (further) damage to the popliteal vessels or nerves
- Check the distal circulation and neurological status
- Immobilise the knee in a long leg box splint, supporting the knee in its normal anatomical alignment as you do so

Ligament and soft tissue injuries of the knee

Incidence
- Injuries to the ligaments and menisci are common

Aetiology
- Damage to the ligaments and menisci are often caused by sporting activities, including football, rugby and skiing

Mechanism of injury
- Injuries to the ligaments and soft tissues of the knee are usually caused by blunt trauma:
    - Damage to the ligaments usually occurs due to indirect pressure (varus or valgus strain), resulting in tears of the medial and lateral ligaments, or direct pressure on the tibia just below the knee resulting in injury of the cruciate ligaments
    - Meniscal damage, usually a tear, usually occurs due to twisting of the knee
- Often injury to the the ligaments and soft tissues is caused by a combination of different forces, which may result in injury to both ligaments and menisci

Pathophysiology
- Severe disruption of the knee ligaments may result in instability of the knee joint and may result in dislocation of the knee joint

Symptoms/signs
- Pain and swelling of the knee

Management
- Immobilise the knee in a long leg box splint

Tibial plateau fractures

Incidence
- Tibial plateau fractures are relatively rare

Aetiology
- May occur when a pedestrian is hit by a car or due to skiing accidents when a skier falls, but the ski binding fails to release

Mechanism of injury

Blunt trauma
- Tibial plateau fractures usually occur due to indirect force; pressure on the lower leg or ankle forcing varus (towards the midline) or valgus (away from the midline) movement of the tibia at the knee

Pathophysiology
- There will be a crush type fracture of the lateral or medial (very rare) tibial plateau

Symptoms/signs
- Pain and swelling of the knee, with inability to weight bear on the affected leg

Management
- Immobilise the knee in a long leg box splint

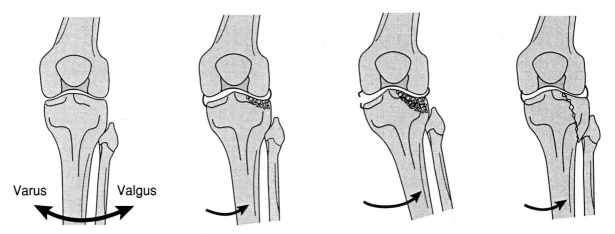

Figure 17-34 Mechanism of injury of tibial plateau fractures

Tibia/fibula shaft fractures

Incidence
- This is a common injury in motor cyclists and front seat car occupants, where there has been a significant amount of wheel arch intrusion
- Also commonly seen in car drivers where the feet/ankles have become trapped by the control pedals

Aetiology
- Usually caused by road traffic accidents or sport

Mechanism of injury

Blunt trauma
- Direct compression on the shafts of the tibia and/or fibula
- Indirect compression of the tibia/fibula due to longitudinal compression
- Indirect rotational compression due to twisting of the ankle or the upper body while the ankle is fixed
- Often the mechanism of injury will involve more than one destructive force

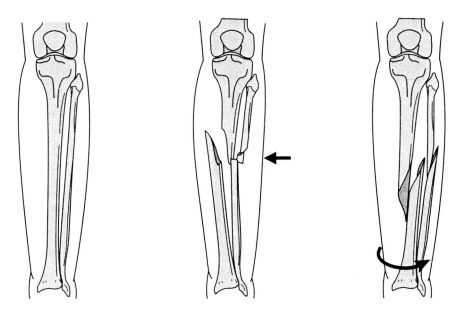

Figure 17-35 Mechanism of injury of fracture of the shafts of tibia and fibula

Pathophysiology
- Direct compression usually results in a transverse or oblique fracture, but there may be a comminuted or butterfly fracture if the force is applied over a large area, especially of the fibula
- Indirect compression usually results in oblique fractures
- Indirect rotational compression may result in a spiral fracture of one or both bones
- Grossly displaced fractures may cause pressure on the skin and compromise its viability
- Vascular damage, resulting in haemorrhage and impaired distal circulation may occur at the bifurcation of the popliteal artery or posterior tibial vessels in:
    - Fractures of the upper tibia in adults
    - Fractures of the mid-shaft of the tibia
    - Injury to the upper tibial epiphysis in children
- Fractures of the tibia and fibula are often associated with considerable local tissue trauma, and haemorrhage, even if no major blood vessels are damaged
- Nerve damage:
    - The common peroneal nerve or tibial nerve just below the knee may be damaged due to fractures of the upper tibia
    - The tibial nerve may be damaged in fractures of the lower quarter of the tibia
- Compound fractures of the lower leg are relatively common

Symptoms/signs
- Localised pain, tenderness, swelling and deformity over the fracture site
- The casualty will be unable to stand on the affected leg
- There may be impairment of the distal circulation
- There may be neurological damage resulting in impaired distal sensation and motor power

Management
- Administer high flow oxygen via a high concentration oxygen mask
- Set up an intravenous infusion with a wide bore cannula and infuse cautiously, monitoring the patient's haemodynamic state as you do so
- Assess the peripheral circulation and neurological status
- Reduce the fracture if it is displaced:
    - Administer inhalational anaesthesia
    - Exert longitudinal traction on the distal fragment and manipulate it into its normal alignment
    - Monitor the peripheral pulses and neurological status before and after reduction
    - Take a *Polaroid*® photograph, before and after reduction

Ankle fractures and dislocations

Incidence
- Injuries to the ankle are very common

Aetiology
- Found relatively often in all types of accident:
    - Tripping up, falls
    - Sport
    - Road traffic accidents

Mechanism of injury

Blunt trauma
- The usual mechanism of injury is indirect blunt trauma:
    - Inversion or eversion of the ankle, or a fall onto the ankle
- May occur due to direct blunt trauma, e. g. in road traffic accidents due to footwell intrusion when the ankle is trapped between the foot pedals and motor cyclist hit on the ankle by a side impact

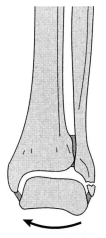
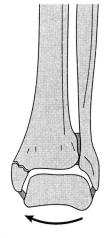
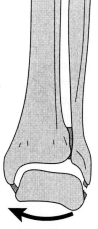
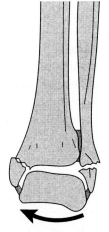

| Avulsion fracture of lateral malleolus | Compression fracture of medial malleolus | Tear of lateral ligament | Avulsion fracture of lateral malleolus and shear fracture of medial malleolus |

Figure 17-36 Mechanism of injury of fracture of the ankle: inversion

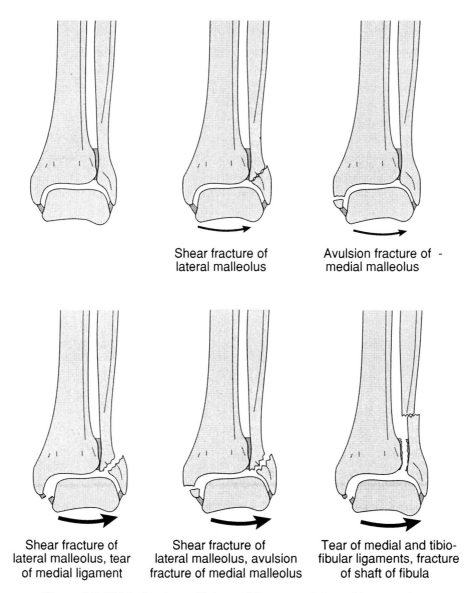

Shear fracture of
lateral malleolus

Avulsion fracture of -
medial malleolus

Shear fracture of
lateral malleolus, tear
of medial ligament

Shear fracture of
lateral malleolus, avulsion
fracture of medial malleolus

Tear of medial and tibio-
fibular ligaments, fracture
of shaft of fibula

Figure 17-37 Mechanism of injury of fracture of the ankle: eversion

Pathophysiology
- The fracture may be simple or compound
- The severity of injury is usually dependent on the amount of energy involved
- There may be avascular damage to the skin, especially in bimalleolar fractures over the medial malleolus due to fragment displacement, subluxation or dislocation
- Injuries may involve both a fracture and ligament damage

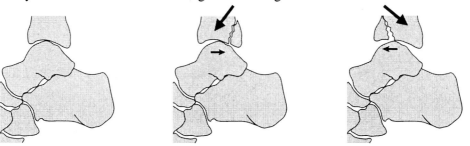

Fracture of posterior malleolus   Fracture of anterior malleolus

Figure 17-38 Mechanism of injury of fracture of the anterior and posterior malleoli due to oblique force

Symptoms/signs
- Pain, tenderness and swelling over the fracture site, with deformity if there is any degree of displacement, suluxation, or dislocation
- Inability to full weight bear on the affected foot
- Signs of impaired circulation and neurological status distal to the fracture

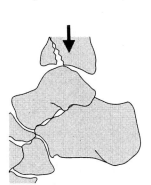 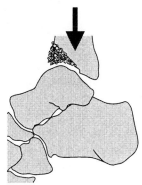 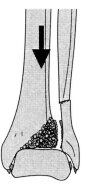

Vertical compression: moderate force   vertical compression: severe force

Figure 17-39 Mechanism of injury of fracture of the distal tibia due to vertical compression

Management
- Reduce the fracture/subluxation/dislocation as soon as possible after the injury, as this will minimise vascular and skin problems:
  - Administer inhalational anaesthesia
  - Exert longitudinal traction on the distal fragment and manipulate it into its normal alignment
  - Monitor the peripheral pulses and neurological status before and after reduction
  - Take *Polaroid®* photographs before and after reduction
- Immobilise the injured limb in a lower leg box splint

Calcaneal and talar fractures

Incidence
- Injury to the os calcis is a relatively common injury but talar fractures are rare

Aetiology
- Usually caused by falls from a height or in motorcycle road traffic accidents

Mechanism of injury

Blunt trauma
- Fractures of the os calcis and talus are usually caused by a direct compressive force to the heel, vertically due to a fall from a height or laterally due to side impact to a motorcyclist's heel, which is compressed between the compressive force and the foot pedal

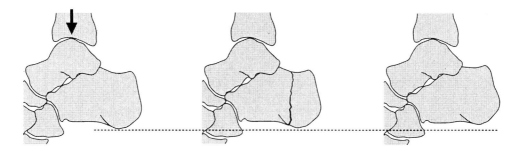

Figure 17-40 Mechanism of injury of fracture of the os calcis

Pathophysiology
- Vertical force will usually be transmitted down through the talus to the top of the os calcis, and if severe will result in compression and flattening of the os calcis, the talus itself rarely fractures
- The severity of the damage to the os calcis depends on the amount of force involved and will range from an isolated crack or fracture without any displacement to a severe comminuted compression injury
- Falls from a height may also result in fractures of the femoral neck, acetabulum, upper lumbar spine and upper cervical vertebrae
- Often both heels are involved

Symptoms/signs
- The patient will complain of pain around the heel, aggravated by attempted weight bearing
- There will be some swelling around the ankle, with flattening and broadening of the heel
- There may be obvious deformity if the injury is associated with ankle or forefoot dislocations

Management
- Assess the circulatory and neurological status of the foot
- Immobilise and elevate the affected lower leg and foot in a well padded box splint

Midfoot (tarsometatarsal) dislocations

Incidence
- Midfoot dislocations are rare

Aetiology
- Dislocations of the midfoot usually occur due to a fall from a height

Mechanism of injury

Blunt trauma
- Direct compressive trauma due to landing heavily on the foot with the toes turned inwards or outwards

Pathophysiology
- Dislocation of the forefoot usually result in considerable soft tissue swelling
- There may be an associated neurovascular injury

Symptoms/signs
- The patient will be in considerable pain and will not be able to weight bear on the affected foot
- Deformity (which may not be obvious if the casualty is wearing a boot), with considerable swelling, which will increase as times goes on

Management
- Reduce the dislocation as soon as possible after the injury:
    - Use adequate analgesia (inspired analgesia (oxygen/nitrous oxide mix is probably the best, provided that there are no contraindications to its use))
    - Monitor the neurovascular status of the foot carefully as you do so
- After reduction, or if you are unable to reduce the dislocation, immobilise the lower leg in a box splint

Metatarsal and toe fractures

Incidence
- Injuries to the metatarsals and toes are relatively common

Aetiology
- May be caused by falls and domestic, industrial or sporting accidents

Mechanism of injury
- Blunt trauma:
    - Direct compression, e.g. a heavy blow
    - An indirect blow, e.g. stubbing the big toe, or a valgus force applied to the little toe
    - Indirect shearing force, e.g. ankle inversion may cause avulsion of the base of the fifth metatarsal

Pathophysiology
- The fracture may be transverse, oblique or comminuted, and may involve the shaft or either end of the bone. Displacement is rarely severe

Symptoms/signs
- Pain and swelling over the dorsum of the foot with pain on weight bearing

Management
- Elevation and splinting, if appropriate

Notes

18

Spinal injuries

Spinal injury

Introduction

- Although spinal injuries are relatively rare (17 new cases per week in the United Kingdom); it is very important that those involved in Immediate Care are fully competent in their management, as early recognition and appropriate treatment is vital, if aggravation of severe injuries and possibly even death due to incorrect initial management, is to be avoided

Incidence

- Spinal injuries are relatively common in certain accident situations:
    - Motorcycle accidents
    - Horse riding accidents
    - Falls from heights
    - Ejection from military aircraft (less common with newer ejection seats and may be asymptomatic)
    - Diving into shallow water
- Cervical spine injury is the most common cause of damage to the spinal cord, as the cervical spine is the most vulnerable to injury
- Injuries of the thoracic and lumbar spine are relatively uncommon

Aetiology

- The major problem following a vertebral column injury is due to spinal cord injury
- The major causes of spinal cord injury are:
    - Road traffic accidents (50%):
        - Ejection
        - Sudden deceleration (whiplash injury)
        - Collision with another (unrestrained) vehicle occupant
        - Motor or pedal cycle accidents (25%)
        - There is a strong association between spinal injury and:
            - Chest injury
            - Sternal injury
    - Falls from a height onto the feet:
        - Accidental
        - Deliberate:
            - Suicide attempt
            - Under the influence of alcohol
    - Falls onto the head:
        - Down stairs
    - Sporting accidents:
        - Gymnastics and trampolining

- Rugby football:
  - Scrum collapse
  - Due to tackling or being tackled
- Riding and hunting on horseback
- Skiing:
  - Collision between skiers
- Hang gliding.
- Diving, especially under the influence of alcohol:
  - Into shallow pools
- Dysbarism induced spinal cord injury
- Industrial accidents:
  - Heavy objects falling onto the back
- Cervical spine injury occurs most often in unseated motorcyclists, pedal cyclists and horse riders and results in the most severe disability
- Fractures of the thoracic spine are usually caused by a direct blow to the back, e.g. as a result of a fall onto a bar, impact from behind or a heavy object falling onto the back
- Fractures of the lumbar spine may be caused by falls from a height or road traffic accidents

Anatomy

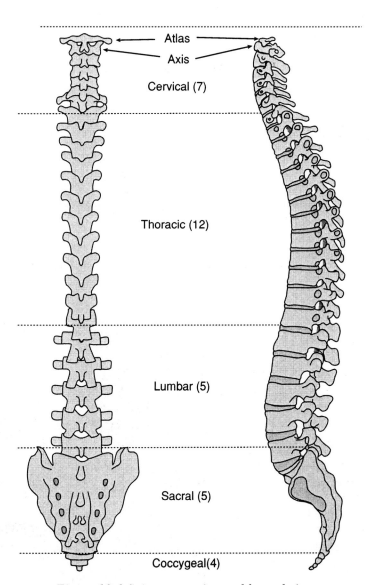

Atlas
Axis
Cervical (7)

Thoracic (12)

Lumbar (5)

Sacral (5)

Coccygeal(4)

Figure 18-1 Spine: posterior and lateral views

The spine

- The spine is composed of 33 vertebrae:
    - 7 Cervical vertebrae:
        - The first cervical vertebra is called the atlas, and articulates with the skull above it, allowing flexion and extension
        - The second cervical vertebra is called the axis, and articulates with the atlas above it allowing rotation
    - 12 Thoracic vertebrae which articulate with the ribs
    - 5 Lumbar vertebrae
    - 5 Sacral vertebrae which are fused to form the sacrum
    - 4 Coccygeal vertebrae which articulate in the young, but fuse with age

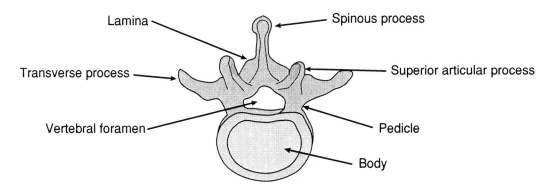

Figure 18-2 Spine: view of a lumbar vertebra from above

- The bodies of the vertebrae are separated from each other by the intervertebral discs
- Each vertebra articulates with the vertebrae above and below it at its superior and inferior articular processes which interlock
- The vertebrae are held together by strong ligaments anteriorly (the anterior longitudinal ligament) and posteriorly (the posterior longitudinal and interspinous ligaments), which prevent forward movement of one vertebral body on another

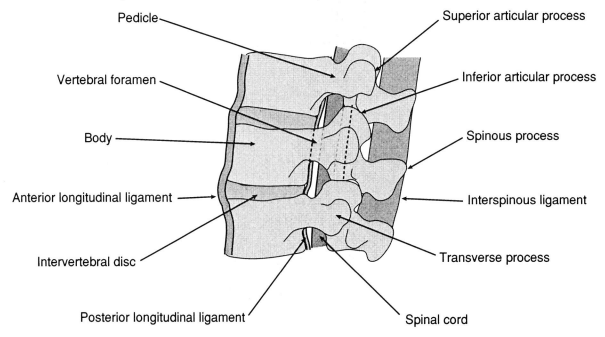

Figure 18-3 Spine: view of lumbar vertebrae from the side

Spinal cord

- The spinal cord runs from the foramen magnum at the base of the skull down to the level of L1 in adults and L3 in children
- Below the spinal cord a mass of nerve roots, called the cauda equina runs down from the spinal cord and terminates at the filum terminale
- Nerve roots below the level of L1 are enclosed in a sac called the theca, which contains cerebrospinal fluid
- Motor nerve fibres leave the spinal cord to form the anterior nerve roots
- Sensory nerve fibres leave the spinal cord to form the posterior nerve fibres, and are enlarged to form the dorsal root ganglia
- The anterior and posterior nerve fibres merge to form the spinal nerves, which contain a mixture of motor and sensory nerve fibres
- The spinal nerves divide to form the anterior and posterior rami of mixed nerves, and sympathetic nerves which run to the sympathetic nerve chain

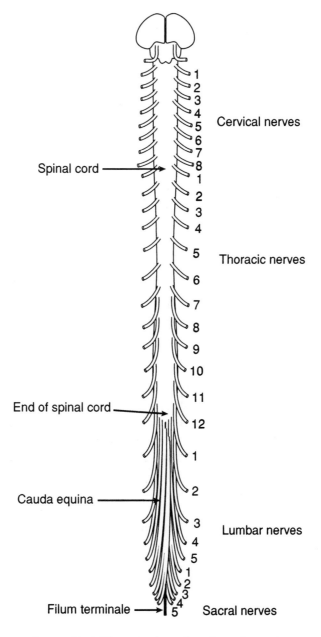

Figure 18-4 The spinal cord and cauda equina

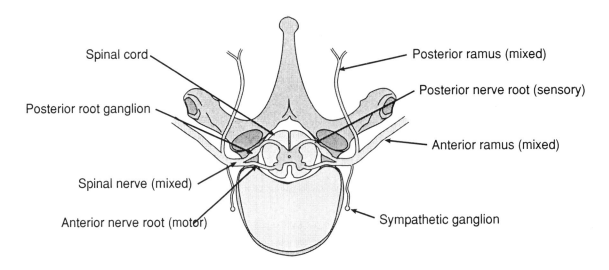

Figure 18-5 Section through a vertebra and spinal cord

Mechanism of injury

Blunt trauma
- Nearly all spinal injury is caused by blunt trauma

Compression:
- Vertical compression, caused by, e.g. a fall from a height, ejection from a motor cycle resulting in impact with another object, or a severe blow to the top of the head will result in forced flexion of the spine
- Forced flexion of the spine will result in injury to the vertebrae at the apex of the spine's curves, where the associated muscles may be weaker, and where movement is greatest at the cervico-thoracic and thoraco-lumbar junctions
- Horizontal compression, caused by e.g. a heavy weight falling onto the back, a severe compressive force applied to the front of the chest, will have different effects depending on where the force is applied, and on whether the result is forced flexion, extension or rotation of the spine:
    - The thoracic vertebrae which are connected to the thoracic cage from which the impact force may be transmitted are particularly vulnerable to injury

Cervical spine
- Compression injury of the cervical spine may be caused by:
    - An indirect vertical compressive force, resulting in forced flexion of the cervical spine, as a result of e.g.:
        - A severe blow to the top of the head
        - Ejection from a motor cycle and the subsequent impact with the ground or another object
        - An unrestrained front seat occupant in a vehicle involved in a frontal or side impact may be ejected through the windscreen or sideways through a door bursting open, landing on their head
        - An unrestrained rear seat passenger in a car involved in a frontal impact being ejected forwards and hitting the windscreen
    - An indirect horizontal compressive force, e.g. running under injury in motorcyclists/front seat car occupants running under the back or into the side of a lorry, resulting in severe hyperextension of the cervical spine

Thoracic and lumbar spine
- Indirect vertical compression of the spine may result in forced flexion of the thoracic spine and extension of the lumbar spine
- Indirect horizontal compression of the thoracic spine may be caused by a severe compressive force applied to the sternum and front of the chest
- Direct horizontal compression of the thoracic and lumbar spine may be caused by a severe blow to the back

Spinal compression (vertical)

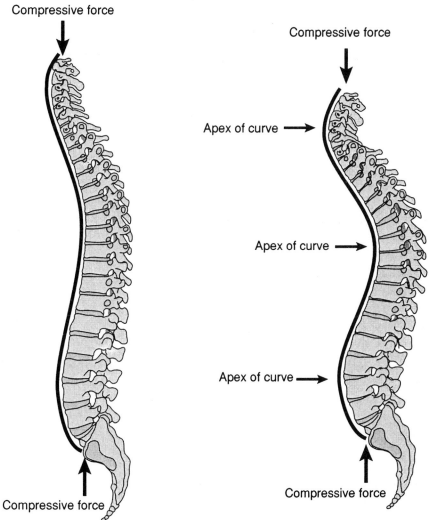

Figure 18-6 Spinal injuries: vertical compression

Acceleration, deceleration, shear
- The effect of these injuries too will depend on whether the result on the spine is forced flexion, extension or rotation

Cervical spine
- The neck is very vulnerable to this type of injury, because it connects the heavy head to the even heavier trunk. If the moving trunk accelerates or decelerates suddenly, due to an impact, the unrestrained head will continue to move until restrained by the neck, resulting initially in flexion/extension and distraction followed by movement of the head in the opposite direction once the limit of movement has been reached

Whiplash injury

- Whiplash injury is a very common injury in road traffic accidents, when vehicles are hit from behind, due to sudden extension of the neck followed by forward flexion.
- The initial cervical extension will be worse if either no head restraint is fitted or the head restraint is set too low to prevent backwards movement/extension

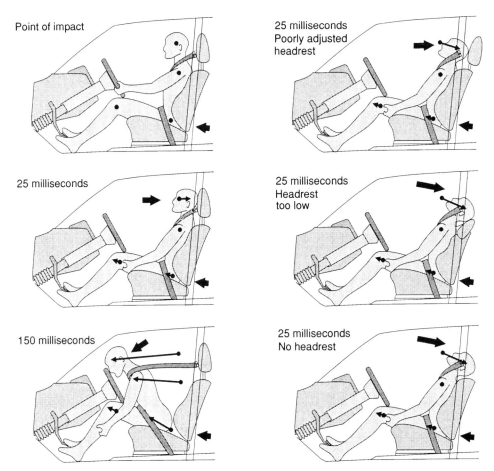

Figure 18-7 Whiplash injury: with/without head restraint and with poorly set head restraint

Thoracic and lumbar spine

- Sudden severe deceleration as may occur in a frontal vehicle impact may result in sudden forward flexion of the spine in unrestrained or partially restrained vehicle occupants. This may be worse if the patient is only wearing a lap belt which restrains the pelvis, but not the rest of the torso from flexing forwards, as a result of which the degree of flexion is even greater and may result in a wedge fracture of the lumbar vertebrae

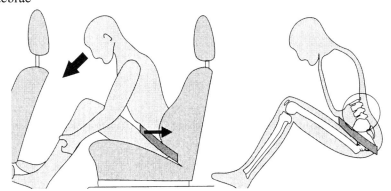

Figure 18-8 Wedge fracture of the lumbar spine due to lap belt restraint in frontal impact

Pathophysiology

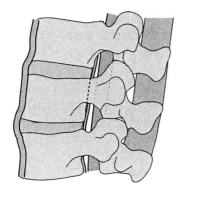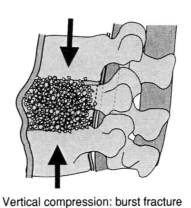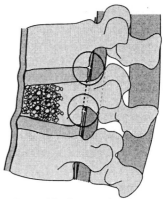

Vertical compression: burst fracture

Forced flexion: wedge fracture & posterior ligament tear

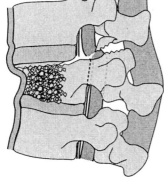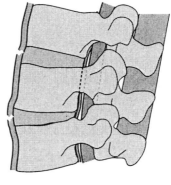

Severe forced flexion: fracture dislocation

Forced extension: anterior ligament tear

Figure 18-9 Bony injuries of the vertebral body

Bony injury

- Spinal fractures may involve:
  - The vertebral bodies and the anterior longitudinal ligament, and may be caused by:
    - Vertical compression resulting in a burst fracture, which may extend backwards to involve the spinal cord
    - Flexion resulting in a wedge fracture, or in severe cases a fracture dislocation with damage to the spinal cord
    - Extension resulting in rupture of the anterior longitudinal ligament
    - Twisting (rotational) forces, which may result in a variety of bony and ligamentous injuries
  - The neural arch and transverse and spinous processes and are caused by direct compressive blunt injury

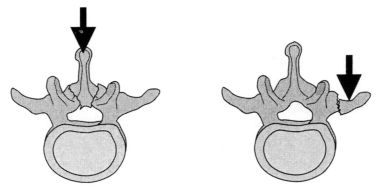

Figure 18-10 Bony injuries of the neural arch and spinous process due to horizontal compression

Ligament injury
- Forced spinal flexion:
    - May result in rupture of the posterior ligaments of the spine; the posterior longitudinal and interspinous ligaments, which may allow the higher vertebra to move forwards on the lower vertebra
- Forced spinal extension:
    - May result in rupture of the anterior longitudinal ligament, allowing the lower vertebra to move forwards on the vertebra above it
- A tear of both anterior and posterior ligaments (which is fortunately rare) may make the spine unstable and is likely to result in injury to the spinal cord

Cervical spine
- Injury of the cervical spine and its ligaments may be caused by excessive movement in any direction:
    - Flexion
    - Extension
    - Lateral flexion
    - Rotation (often a combination of these)
- The cervical spine is least likely to be damaged by forced forward flexion, and most likely to be damaged by forced lateral flexion or lateral flexion/rotation
- Forced flexion alone may result in:
    - Wedge compression fracture
    - Posterior ligament/interspinous ligament rupture, allowing the vertebra above it to move forward
- Hyperextension may result in:
    - Fracture of the neural arch, especially of the atlas or axis
    - Fracture of the odontoid peg of the axis
    - May rupture the anterior longitudinal ligament and the annulus fibrosus, forcing the vertebrae apart anteriorly (extension subluxation)
    - Damage to the facets of the intervertebral joints
- Acute neck sprain (whiplash injury) rarely results in a bony injury, but there is usually a soft tissue injury to the muscles and ligaments of the cervical spine
- Flexion/rotation may result in:
    - Subluxation, dislocation or fracture dislocation (this is the most common cause of spinal cord injury resulting in paralysis)
    - This may also cause massive displacement of an intervertebral disc without any bony injury
- Vertical compression:
    - This may cause a fracture of the atlas (if the pressure is applied downwards from the skull)
    - May result in a burst fracture of the vertebral body
- Movement of one vertebra on another will result in narrowing of the vertebral canal and spinal cord damage

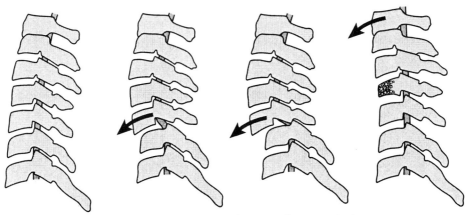

Figure 18-11 Cervical spine: flexion injuries

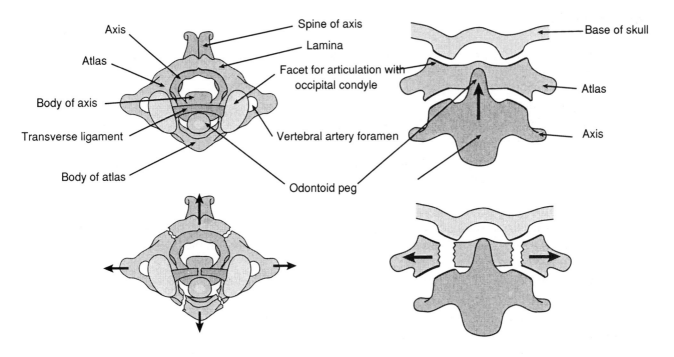

Figure 18-12 Cervical spine: compression fracture of the atlas

Fractures of the atlas/axis
- Fractures of the atlas/axis are usually caused by vertical compression and result in widening of the spinal canal
- If the odontoid peg is fractured together with rupture of the ligaments attaching it to the atlas, it may become free and there is a major risk of it causing spinal cord damage

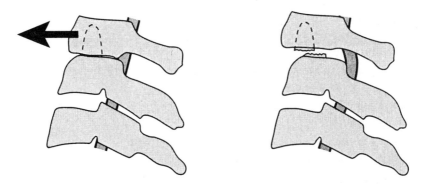

Figure 18-13 Odontoid peg fracture due to forward movement of atlas on axis

Thoracic and lumbar spine
- Fractures of the thoracic and lumbar spine may occur due to:
    - Flexion (the major cause), resulting in:
        - Burst fracture
        - Wedge fracture
        - Shear fracture
    - Flexion/rotation:
        - Dislocation of the intervertebral joint, with forward displacement of the upper vertebra on the lower, resulting in spinal cord injury

Spinal cord injury

Primary injury
- Partial (<60%) or complete transection of the cord, is usually caused by injury resulting in movement of one of the components of the spinal column on another
- Spinal cord damage results in:
    - Impaired distal motor function
    - Impaired distal sensation
    - Impaired distal autonomic (sympathetic) function resulting in:
        - The parasympathetic nervous system being unopposed. The effect of this is that the stimulus required to induce bradycardia and asystole is much less than would normally be the case. This effect may be aggravated by hypoxia and hypothermia.
        - Generalised vasodilation which will exacerbate the effects of any hypovolaemia due to associated trauma or produce hypovolaemia on its own due to the relative increase in vascular volume
- The higher up the spinal cord, the greater the resulting disability and risk to life

Cervical spine
- Spinal cord is most vulnerable to injury in the neck because the spinal canal is relatively narrow
- Spinal cord damage is more likely in arthritic cervical vertebrae, in which the spinal canal is already narrowed by osteophytes

Thoracic and lumbar spine
- The spinal cord ends at the level of L1, so below this the spinal cord becomes the cauda equina, injury to which carries a much better prognosis than injury to the spinal cord itself

Secondary injury
- Mechanical injury:
    - Mechanical displacement of the cord between vertebrae
    - Movement of bony fragments of vertebrae impinging on the cord
    - Usually caused by movement of the patient in the vertical position
    - Unlikely to be caused by careful movement of the patient in the horizontal position
- Non-mechanical injury of the spinal cord may occur due to:
    - Hypoxia as a result of:
        - Airway obstruction
        - Ventilatory problems: chest injury, splinted diaphragm
    - Underperfusion due to:
        - Hypovolaemia, occurring as a result of major trauma
        - Underperfusion may be exacerbated by orthostatic hypotension as a result of cord injury with autonomic dysfunction

Symptoms/signs
- It is essential to recognise that a spinal injury may be present following certain types of injury, and one should be positively sought for in those circumstances
- The symptoms and signs due to a spinal injury will depend on which structures have been damaged and at what level
- If the patient is unconscious (10-15% will have some kind of spinal injury), it will not be possible to examine them fully. In this instance a careful examination of the mechanism of injury should give an indication as to whether a spinal injury is likely or not, and the relevant signs sought for
- *A cervical spine injury in the unconscious patient following trauma should be presumed until proven otherwise*

Spine
- Pain especially if there is dislocation or a fracture, but this may be masked if there is a more painful/severe injury
- Swelling
- Tenderness on palpation
- Irregularity on palpation of the spine with a step deformity (only present in 10% of spinal fractures)

Spinal cord
- Try to assess initially whether the cord lesion is complete or incomplete. It may be possible to establish the level of motor and sensory change, which may itself alter
- The initial symptoms may be bizarre, and should not be dismissed as being due to hysteria/intoxication:
  - Sensory:
    - Burning pain in both the arms and lower limbs
    - Pins and needles
  - Proprioception:
    - A feeling that the present position of the body is still that in which it was prior to the accident, despite it clearly being in another
- The classical signs are:
  - Local tenderness
  - Total sensory loss below the injury
  - Motor loss below the injury
- Hemisection of the cord (Brown-Séquard syndrome), which may be caused by a stab wound or a rotational/side swipe injury, will result in:
  - Reduction/absence of power, but relatively normal pain and temperature sensation on the same side as the injury
  - Loss of pain, temperature and touch (pin prick), on the opposite side to the loss of power
- In the unconscious patient, spinal injury may be indicated by:
  - Hypotension with bradycardia
  - Diaphragmatic ventilation
  - Differential pain responses
  - Flaccid tone
  - Priapism
  - Loss of sphincter control

Cervical spine
- Neck pain and/or tenderness
- Spasm of the neck muscles
- There may be a boggy swelling along the dorsum of the cervical spine
- Irregular breathing
- In the conscious patient there may be:
  - Reduced or absent motor power distal to the injury in the trunk or limb muscles
  - Reduced, altered or absent sensation distal to the injury over the trunk or limb

Thoracic and lumbar spine
- Local pain and/or tenderness
- Prominent spinous process, tenderness, or step in the normal contour (may be the only sign in the unconscious patient)
- Painful limitation of movement
- Reduced or absent power distal to the injury
- Reduced or absent sensation distal to the injury

Management

Aim
- The aim of specific management of spinal injury is to prevent any secondary injury to the spinal cord:
    - Attempt to prevent death or disability from associated injuries
    - Handle carefully, to prevent further mechanical injury to the spinal cord
    - Ventilate adequately to maintain oxygenation of the spinal cord
    - Maintain adequate tissue perfusion. This must be controlled carefully as:
        - Any fall in arterial pressure caused by, e.g. sitting or standing up, will aggravate spinal hypoxia
        - Any major rise in perfusion pressure caused by, e.g. excessive volume replacement, may result in a haemorrhagic infarct of the cord
- Position
    - Leave the patient supine in a neutral position
    - Do not allow the patient to get up
    - Move the patient as little as possible

Primary survey
- The first priority is to perform a primary assessment and perform initial life saving procedures

Airway "Think spinal, do airway"
- Care of the airway and cervical spine has the first priority in the initial management of the injured patient, as it can be difficult to provide good airway care in the presence of a cervical spine injury, which itself may be a life threatening injury
- Adequate airway maintenance is vital
- Move the head into a neutral position and apply a jaw thrust (*avoid* chin lifts):
    - Do not move the patient's cervical spine any more than the absolute minimum amount necessary to achieve a clear airway
- Avoid suctioning in the tetraplegic patient, as this may stimulate the vagal reflex resulting in worsening of any pre-existing bradycardia or may even occasionally precipitate cardiac arrest
- It is not usually possible to tell whether or not a fracture is stable or unstable initially (only 1 in 300 deceleration victims who are unconscious have biomechanical instability), so any suspected neck injury should be immobilised in a neutral position, in a cervical splint such as the *Hines*®, or a semi-rigid cervical collar of the correct size such as the *Stiffneck*®, *Neclok*® or *Vertebrace*®, until it can be X-rayed

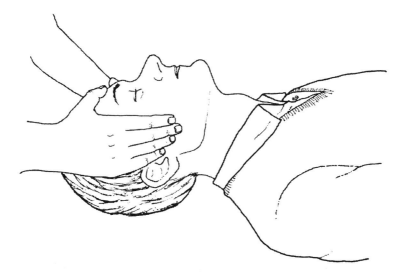

Figure 18-14 Immobilisation of the neck with gentle in-line cervical stabilisation

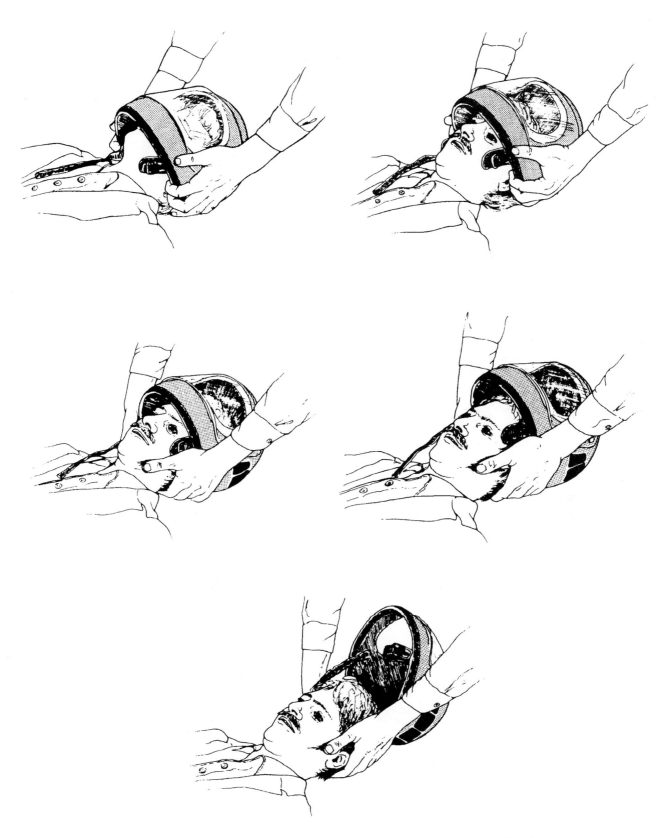

Figure 18-15 Helmet removal maintaining in-line cervical stabilisation: Single rescuer

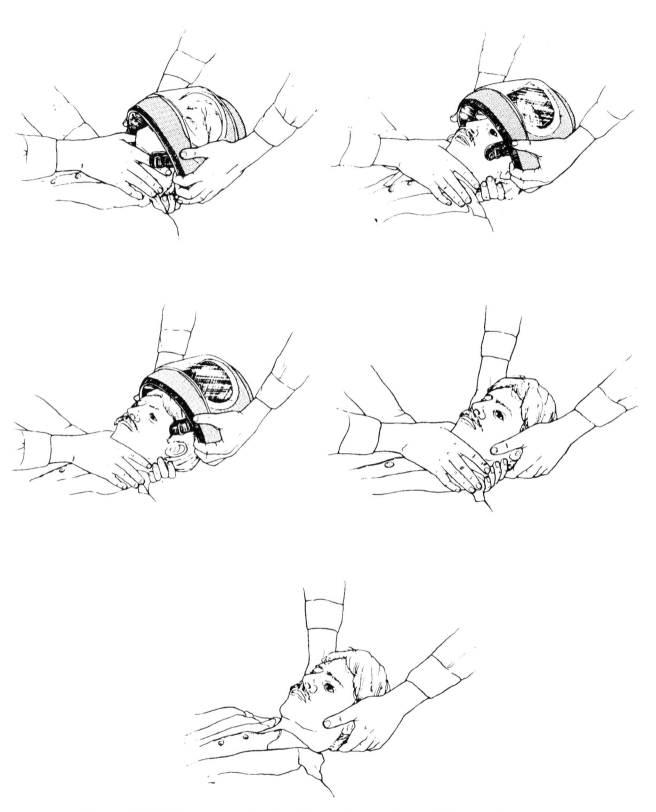

Figure 18-16 Helmet removal maintaining in-line cervical stabilisation: Two rescuers

Semi-rigid cervical collars

Description
- There are various different makes and designs of cervical collars
- They may be:
    - One piece, adjustable or non-adjustable:
        - Adjustable semi-rigid collars are a fairly recent development, and mean that a smaller number of collars need be carried to fit every size and shape of patient
        - Have an aperture in the front for access to the trachea
    - Two piece non-adjustable:
        - These probably provide better immobilisation than one piece collars, but are bulkier, take up more storage space and are more difficult to fit

Note: The *Hines*® cervical splint is a two piece semi-rigid splint with a long back extension

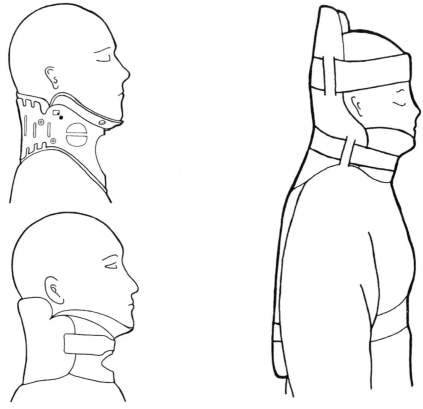

Figure 18-17 Rigid cervical collars and cervical splint

Indications
- When immobilisation of the cervical spine is indicated (see above)
- Application of a cervical collar and spinal board may *not* be necessary for car occupants when the following circumstances coexist (although if in doubt apply the collar and board):
    - Low impact velocity
    - Minimal vehicle damage
    - The patient is young and usually fit
    - The patient does not complain of neck pain
    - There is no neck spasm or spinal tenderness
    - There is no distracting pain
    - The patient is able to appreciate pain, i.e. they are fully conscious, on no drugs and have no coexisting disease that might cause confusion

Advantages
- Semi-rigid cervical collars are light and relatively easy to apply
- Prevent cervical flexion, extension and lateral flexion
- Help to signal the fact that a patient may have a possible cervical spine injury

Disadvantages
- A correctly sized and applied semi-rigid cervical collar will prevent cervical flexion, extension and lateral flexion, but will not prevent rotation, so they should always be used in conjunction with manual in-line cervical stabilisation or together with head blocks, a long spinal board and body straps
- Incorrect application of a cervical collar may result in airway obstruction
- Prolonged wearing of cervical collars may result in an increase in intracranial pressure from venous obstruction (a cervical collar applied at the scene should be removed, especially in cases of severe head injury (or a Glasgow coma score of 8 or less) as soon as feasible, e.g. once the patient has reached hospital)

Method of application
- This requires two people to be performed satisfactorily
- The head and neck should be stabilised/supported by one person with gentle in-line manual stabilisation in a neutral position throughout the procedure
- Any applied traction should be minimal, as excessive force can cause a traction injury to the spinal cord in high cervical injuries
- Any helmet should be carefully removed first, together with any tie (if the patient is wearing one), and any shirt buttons undone around the neck. Any clothing around the back of the neck should be removed
- The collar should be sized and then carefully applied and done up (the person stabilising the head and neck should transfer their hands from the patient's head and neck to the head and collar)
- Once the collar has been applied, check that the patient is comfortable, unable to move their neck, that it has not pinched the patient's ears and that it has not been applied over any clothing
- If the collar does not fit well, it should be replaced immediately
- *If in doubt immobilise the entire spine*
- After fitting the collar the cervical spine should be fully immobilised by the application of a spinal board and blocks with straps or tapes

CONCLUSION
- Semi-rigid cervical collars have a valuable role in the management of the patient with a possible cervical spine injury, but they tend to be over used (for patients in whom a significant neck injury is unlikely), and at the same time there is a lack of appreciation of their limitations (there is too much confidence placed in their ability to completely immobilise and stabilise the cervical spine)

Breathing/ventilation
- Oxygen (important to reduce any cord hypoxia to the minimum)
- Maintenance of effective ventilation
- If this is inadequate and the patient has a bradycardia (less than 45 bpm):
    - Consider the administration of atropine 0.5 mg intravenously, prior to the insertion of an airway, suctioning or intubation to prevent inducing asystole
- Intubate the patient if they are in danger of aspirating (nasotracheal intubation is preferred by many)

Circulation
- If the patient has a bradycardia (less than 45 bpm):
    - Consider prophylactic atropine as even a trivial stimulus may cause asystole due to unopposed vagal activity (see above)
- Set up an intravenous infusion and infuse cautiously (the hypotension due to increased vagal tone will exacerbate the effects of hypovolaemia)

- An isolated cord lesion requires little in the way of fluid replacement:
    - 500 mL is usually sufficient to restore the systolic blood pressure to 90 mmHg
    - Unless other injuries dictate otherwise, fluid replacement should not exceed 1500 mL
    - Colloid is preferred to crystalloid (which may cause cord oedema)

Disability
- Rapidly assess the patient's central (brain) and peripheral (spinal cord) neurological status:
    - Central nervous system:
        - AVPU scale:
            - **A** - Alert
            - **V** - Responds to verbal stimuli
            - **P** - Responds to pain
            - **U** - Unresponsive/unconscious
        - Assess the pupils: size, equality and reactivity
        - Ask the patient to put their tongue out
    - Peripheral nervous system:
        - Ask the patient if they can feel their:
            - Fingers
            - Toes
    - Ask the patient to:
        - Squeeze your hand with their fingers
        - Wriggle their toes

Exposure with control of the environment
- Keep patients with a spinal injury warm as they are especially vulnerable to hypothermia due to their inability to appreciate temperature changes and are not able to to shiver or sweat, and are vasodilated

Secondary survey
- Examine the whole body in the following order:
    - **H**ead (including neurological status) and **N**eck
    - **C**hest
    - **A**bdomen and **P**elvis
    - **E**xtremities
    - **S**pine and **B**ack

Spine and back
- If spinal injury is suspected:
    - Do *not* move the patient unnecessarily:
- If movement *is* necessary, move the patient with great care, in the horizontal axis only
- Look for:
    - Sensory deficit
    - Motor deficit
    - Abnormal reflexes
    - Priapism
- Log roll the patient, but with great care, if a spinal injury is suspected, and examine the back for:
    - Bruising
    - Lacerations/open wounds
- Auscultate the back of the chest
- Examine the spine for:
    - Tenderness or muscular spasm
    - Bogginess
    - Irregularity (step deformity) of the contour of the spinous processes

Pain control
- Avoid opioid analgesics in cervical and upper thoracic spine injuries, especially if ventilation is impaired, due to their ability to cause respiratory depression
- If pain is not controlled adequately with nitrous oxide/oxygen (*Entonox®*, *Nitronox®*), try:
    - Intravenous non-steroidal anti-inflammatory drugs (NSAIDs), e.g. diclofenac, ketoprofen.
    - Small doses of opioids carefully titrated to patient response and avoiding respiratory depression.
- Avoid using buprenorphine, because its effects are only partially reversed by naloxone, if respiratory depression develops

Moving the spinal patient
- The patient with a possible spinal injury should be moved as little as possible initially, and then only:
    - Away from danger to a place of relative safety
    - If needed to manage other serious injuries
- The injured spine should be immobilised with gentle manual in-line stabilisation before *any* movement is attempted
- If the patient is wearing a helmet, this should be removed carefully whilst still maintaining manual in-line stabilisation of the cervical spine

Note: There is no urgency to extricate or move the patient with an isolated spinal injury

Loading and transportation
- Loading, transportation and conveyance should be carried out with the minimum of unnecessary movement
- A long spinal board, or if unavailable a scoop stretcher or Donway lifting frame should be used for transferring the patient onto the ambulance trolley (which ideally should have a vacuum mattress on it), and then from the ambulance trolley onto the hospital examination couch
- Consideration should be given to the patient with a spinal injury being conveyed to hospital by helicopter, which offers a more stable ride and lower chance of further cord injury, especially in the patient with an unstable spine, than land ambulance

Spinal immobilisation
- The patient with a suspected spinal injury should have their entire spine immobilised with a correctly applied semi-rigid cervical collar, spinal board with head blocks (or a similar head immobilisation device and tape or strapping, to firmly secure the head to the board) and a spider harness or body straps to firmly secure the rest of the body to the board, before any movement is attempted
- In children, there is no method, at present, that reliably achieves immobilisation of the spine in a neutral position. A padded board (to raise the torso a little), together with a correctly applied semi-rigid cervical collar and straps is probably the best method currently available

Indications
- Spinal immobilisation should always be applied when:
    - An examination of the mechanism of injury raises the possibility of spinal injury/damage
    - There is pain and tenderness over the spine
    - There is neurological evidence of a neurological injury
    - The patient has an altered level of consciousness, is intoxicated or has other distracting injuries
    - There is a history of pre-existing spinal injury

Position
- The conscious patient with a potential spinal injury should always be transported on their back, so as to avoid any respiratory embarrassment caused by splinting of the diaphragm by gas, air, or blood from any thoraco-abdominal trauma. If they are in any other position they should be turned onto their back
- The patient should *not* at any time be stood or sat up

Turning the patient
- The object is to turn the patient with a potential spinal injury, to inspect their back for any injury and/or to apply a longboard, whilst maintaining the spine and head in alignment. This involves stabilising the cervical spine and moving them with the head, neck, shoulders, thorax and pelvis in the same plane at all times, in order to ensure no further spinal injury

Log roll method
- If the patient needs turning, this may be done using the "log roll" method

Method:
- This method requires a minimum of four people to perform it satisfactorily, but more may be better
- Place the patient's arms by their side with the palms turned inwards against the legs
- Before turning the patient, remove any keys, coins, etc. from their pockets, and make certain that there is no debris or folded clothes under him, as denervated skin may be easily damaged
- One person (the team leader, who will control the turn) should kneel by the patient's head and apply gentle in-line manual stabilisation of the cervical spine
- All the other members of the team should kneel down on the same side of the patient, facing the patient:
    - The next person down from the patient's head should kneel holding the patient's shoulder furthest from them with one hand and the arm on the same side just above the elbow with the other
    - The third person down should kneel and hold the patient's forearm and pelvis furthest from them
    - The fourth person (if available) should kneel down holding and controlling the patient's legs
- The patient should be rolled over as far as necessary, by the whole team working in unison, on the spoken command of the team leader, keeping the spine in a straight line the whole time
- A fifth person (if available) should inspect the patient's back, and apply a long spinal board if one is going to be used, after which the patient should be rolled back onto their back

Note: If there is a shortage of trained persons (as often happens in the pre-hospital situation); bystanders or members of the other emergency services may be used
  On some occasions it may be necessary to perform the manoeuvre with a team of only three, in which case one team member should hold the shoulder and arm and the other the pelvis/upper leg and lower leg

Turning the spinal patient over
- This may be necessary if the patient with a possible spinal injury is lying prone (on their front)

Two scoop method
  Method:
- This method involves using two orthopaedic "scoop" stretchers
- Place one scoop stretcher under the patient and the other scoop stretcher upside down on top of them, so that they form a sandwich with the patient in the middle
- Tie the two stretchers together using triangular bandages or similar along their lengths
- Lift and rotate the patient before lowering them, and remove the scoop stretchers

Turning the patient onto their side
- It may occasionally be necessary to turn the patient with a possible spinal injury onto their side, as long as their breathing is adequate, to prevent an aspiration pneumonitis
    - The patient's head and neck must always be under the control of a skilled operator, and a semi-rigid cervical collar of the correct size used as an adjunct
    - The turn is effected, keeping the head in neutral, with the neck and back in a straight line, and providing three point stability at the shoulder, pelvis and knee
    - One hemidiaphragm should be kept clear of the ground so as to allow adequate ventilation (chest expansion)

Method:
- Before turning the patient, make sure that keys, coins, etc. have been removed from his pockets, and that there is no debris or folded clothes under him, as denervated skin may be easily damaged
- Kneel on one side of the patient and your assistant on the other
- Place the patient's arm nearest your assistant at a right angle to their body, putting the other arm across the chest and bending the furthest knee to a right angle.
- Support the patient's head with your nearest hand, grasp the patient's body at the hip and roll him towards your assistant, who should be positioned kneeling close to the patient
- The uppermost knee should then be adjusted for stability, and the hand providing head support, is carefully substituted for the other hand, taking care to leave the hand nearest the patient's abducted arm free to adjust it
- The elbow of this arm is then bent, bringing the hand close to the patient's chin or even under his head
- The patient's other arm is then adjusted to interlock in the triangle formed between the lower arm and the head and neck

Orthopaedic "scoop stretcher"

Description
- The scoop stretcher is made of aluminium, and comprises two halves which can be clipped together longitudinally:
    - Each half has a tubular frame and thin wedge shaped lifting extensions, which almost but not quite meet those from the opposite side when the stretcher is assembled, and handgrips down each side
    - The bottom can be extended to fit the the length of the patient
    - There is a head cushion which is attached to the top end
- It is designed to lift a patient up from the ground with minimal movement

Advantages
- Relatively lightweight, and easy to apply with only minimal movement of the patient

Disadvantages
- May bend/deform under the weight of very heavy patients, and not suitable for carrying patients on over any distance
- May cause pressure sores if the patient is transported on it for any length of time (probably >20-30 minutes)
- Propensity to trap the rescuer's fingers

Method of application:
- If the patient has a possible suspected cervical spine injury, the head and neck should be immobilised in a semi-rigid cervical collar and stabilised with gentle in-line manual stabilisation throughout most of the procedure
- Lay the stretcher beside the patient, and split the stretcher
- Extend the lower half of each side to accommodate the whole length of the patient

- Slide first one side under the patient from the side, rolling the patient a little as you do so, and then the other
- Bring the two sides of the stretcher together, being careful not to pinch the patient as you do so, and lock together each end
- Gently place the head cushion under the patient's head and attach it to each side, whilst still maintaining gentle in-line manual stabilisation, if the patient has a suspected cervical spine injury, and apply head tapes
- Apply body straps if the patient has a suspected spinal injury or is going to be carried any distance across rough ground, down stairs, etc. to minimise any patient movement
- If the patient has been transferred to an ambulance trolley, the scoop stretcher should be removed, unless the travelling time to hospital is short, and removing the stretcher would take too long in the time critical patient
- Remove the stretcher by unclipping each end and remove one side and then the other, rolling the patient a little if necessary

Long spinal boards

Description
- A spinal board is a long board, constructed of radiolucent reinforced plastic or fibreglass, which tapers towards the leg end, and has a row of hand grips down each side
- Both surfaces are smooth, the under surface usually having two reinforcing rails running from one end to the other
- Long spinal boards are used together with:
    - Head blocks and straps for securing and stabilising the head
    - Body straps for securing the body

Indications
- To aid extrication of road traffic accident casualties, although there is some evidence that an extrication device might provide better spinal immobilisation
- For general rescue purposes:
    - As a lifting aid
    - As an extrication device for lifting uninjured patients that are in a difficult position
    - For lifting patients with a fractured neck of femur out of an armchair
    - In patients with a cardiac arrest it may provide a firm base for closed chest cardiac compression, and be used to help remove them from an upstairs room and down narrow stairs

Advantages
- Provides satisfactory spinal immobilisation
- Easy and quick to apply (but requires training and practice in its use)
- Allows ambulance service personnel to lift heavy patients safely and without damaging their own backs

Disadvantages
- Patients with a spinal injury may develop pressure sores after only 45 minutes on a long spinal board (if the ambulance journey is likely to be more than about 30 minutes, the patient should be transferred to a vacuum mattress using an orthopaedic "scoop" stretcher)
- Long spinal boards are not ideal if the patient is already lying supine on the ground, because application of the long board requires a partial log-roll to be performed, which needs four trained people for it to be carried out properly, and is not a technique without risk:
    - An orthopaedic "scoop stretcher" may be preferred for lifting a patient with a suspected spinal injury who is already lying supine on the ground
    - An alternative method is to slide the board down under the patient's head and then sliding the rest of the patient onto the board in the usual way

Method of application:
- *Assuming that the roof has been removed and the vertical method of extrication is being used (if the patient is upright, the 'take down' method may be used*
- Apply and maintain gentle manual in-line immobilisation and stabilisation
- Apply a correctly sized semi-rigid collar
- Slide the long board down behind the patient from the head end
- Apply head blocks and body straps to immobilise the head and body:
    - The straps should be applied to the chest, abdomen, and thighs before applying the head restraint
    - Straps across the chest should not be so tight that they restrict chest expansion/ventilation
- Rolls of blanket may be placed on both sides of smaller patients to stabilise their position
- Lift the immobilised patient and board and place it on the ambulance trolley, and secure with straps

CONCLUSION
- The device of choice for extrication of the trapped patient, and useful for routine extrication

Vacuum mattress

Description
- A tough reinforced plastic mattress shaped bag filled with polystyrene beads with a nozzle and valve for the extraction of air from the bag
- Air can be sucked out from around the beads which stay in position moulding themselves around the body
- Once most of the air has been removed the mattress will become rigid, supporting and splinting the body

Indications
- The transport of patients with a spinal injury to hospital or between hospitals

Advantages
- Provides a comfortable, rigid support for the whole body
- Suitable for a patient with a spinal injury to lie on for several hours as it supports the whole body evenly and is much less likely to cause pressure sores than any other device

Disadvantages
- Vacuum mattresses cannot be used for extrication or rescue purposes
- Vulnerable to damage by sharp objects, e.g. glass, metal spikes
- Vacuum mattresses are not rigid and should be used with an ambulance trolley or spinal board to move the patient
- Take up a lot of space in the ambulance, even when folded
- Vacuum mattresses are only used rarely, and require special training for their application

Method of application
- Lay out the device on the ambulance trolley
- Gently place the patient (or limb) on the mattress, and secure them with body straps
- Actively mould the mattress around the patient, especially around the head and neck, applying gentle manual stabilisation of the spine as you do so
- Apply suction to the nozzle, removing the air from around the beads
- Remove the pump, securing the valve as you do so

CONCLUSION:
- The spinal immobilisation device of choice for the patient with a spinal injury who will have to remain on it for more than about 30 minutes

Extrication devices

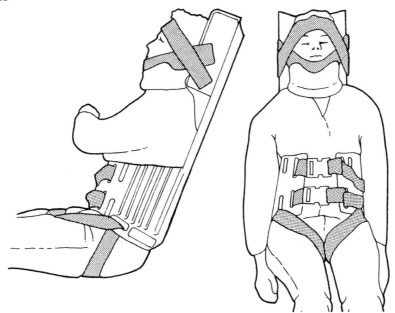

Figure 18-18 Patient immobilised in an extrication device and cervical collar

Description
- There are several different types of extrication device available, and currently in use:
  - KED: the *Kendrick Extrication Device*®
  - RED: the *Russell Extrication Device*®
  - *ED2000*®
- These all have a similar design, are made of reinforced radiolucent plastic or similar and consist of:
  - A back piece to which are attached two small wings to go on either side of the head and two larger wings to go round each side of the body, and grab handles
  - There are moulded head blocks to fit behind the head and neck, with *Velcro*® head straps, colour coded straps for attaching to the body wings, which fasten together and colour coded leg straps for holding the legs

Advantages
- Provide immobilisation and stabilisation of the head, neck and torso of the patient who is trapped sitting up in a car or other vehicle and for lifting them out of the vehicle

Disadvantages
- These devices are tall, and the roof of the car often has to be removed before attempting to apply one
- Rather fiddly and time consuming to apply, not suitable for rapid extrication (a spinal board is better), especially for the time critical patient
- Require training and practice in their use to ensure speedy application

Method of application
- Assess the patient and immobilise their cervical spine with a semi-rigid cervical collar and manual in-line stabilisation
- Slide the device down behind the patient, making certain that none of its straps entangle on anything
- Position the device correctly in relationship to the patient's head and shoulders
- Draw in the wings of the device and then fasten and tighten the chest straps, ensuring that they are not so tight that the patient has difficulty breathing or that they make the patient uncomfortable
- Pass the leg straps under the patient's legs and then back through the device before fastening and tightening them

- Place the shoulder straps across the body and fasten them to the other side of the device, ensuring that they do not overlap the cervical collar
- Fill in the space behind the head with the blocks supplied, and apply and fasten the head straps, ensuring that the head is totally immobilised. Once this has been done the person holding the head may release it
- Check all the straps to ensure that they are tight, and that the patient is held centrally in the device
- The patient may then be lifted out of the vehicle and laid on an ambulance trolley, vacuum mattress, etc.
- Loosen the leg straps, so that the patient can straighten their legs, and check that the cervical immobilisation does not need readjusting

CONCLUSION
- Extrication devices are the best devices for stabilising and immobilising the spine and extricating patients, who do not need rapid removal from a vehicle

Scoop chair

Description
- This device is a modification of the "scoop" stretcher
- It is about two thirds the length of the stretcher, and has an adjustable hinge on each side so that the angle between the shorter seat and longer backrest can be adjusted and then locked
- It can be split into four parts, vertically and on each side just above the hinge
- A headpiece clips onto the top of the frame to which padding and headstraps can be attached for immobilising the head. There are also body straps

Advantages
- Provides more support to the buttocks and thighs than an extrication device
- Easier to remove from the patient, without undue movement, once they have been placed on an ambulance trolley or vacuum mattress than an extrication device

Disadvantages
- More rigid than an extrication device, which makes it harder to apply. The seat scoops are inclined to dig into the vehicle seat, preventing joining of the two seat pieces
- Does not immobilise and stabilise the head, neck or torso as well as an extrication device

Method of application
- Assess the patient and immobilise their cervical spine with a semi-rigid cervical collar and manual in-line stabilisation
- Break the device down into its constituent pieces
- Slide the two seat sections under the patient (it may be necessary to lift each leg in turn to do this) and fasten the two halves together so that they form a seat
- Slide the two halves of the backrest down behind the patient's back and fasten them together at the top
- Adjust the hinge so that the seat and backrest sections can be fastened together, and then lock the hinge
- Fit the headpiece, and then apply the padding and headstraps
- Pass one body strap behind and then round the front of the patient at the level of the hinge, so that the two halves of the device are held together at this point (otherwise there is a risk that the back of the seat will splay apart and the patient fall though it
- Secure the patient's body with the rest of the body straps
- The patient may then be lifted out of the vehicle and laid on an ambulance trolley, vacuum mattress, etc.
- Unlock the hinge, so that the patient can straighten their legs, remove the head and body straps and gently un-fasten the two halves of the chair and remove it

CONCLUSION
- Superseded by extrication devices

19

Penetrating injuries

Penetrating injuries

Introduction

- Penetrating injuries are relatively rarely encountered in pre-hospital care, but when they do so, the pre-hospital practitioner must be able to respond appropriately immediately especially in life threatening injury
- The tissue damage likely to be caused by a penetrating object/missile can be estimated by classifying the penetrating missile/object according to its kinetic energy, and thus the amount of energy likely to be transferred to the tissues:
    - Low energy device/weapon:
        - No energy transfer wounds
    - Medium energy weapon:
        - Low energy transfer wounds
    - High energy weapon:
        - High energy transfer wounds

Low energy device injuries

- The importance, significance, and severity of penetrating and impaling injuries caused by low energy weapons and other objects may not be appreciated initially, especially by the inexperienced pre-hospital practitioner
- Penetrating and impaling injuries require aggressive and effective Immediate Care, if the high morbidity and mortality associated with these injuries is to be reduced

Incidence

- Penetrating and impaling injuries are relatively uncommon

Aetiology

- Low energy penetrating injuries may occur due to:
    - Stabbing with a knife or other similar object
    - Falls onto sharp objects
    - Entrapment in road traffic accidents
    - Entrapment in moving machinery
- Impaling injury may occur in:
    - Road traffic accidents due to:
        - The vehicle running through roadside fencing, which penetrates the passenger compartment
        - Penetration of the passenger compartment by part of a (lorry) load
        - High energy impact resulting in penetration by part of vehicle

Pathophysiology

- Low energy devices only produce tissue damage at their sharp point or cutting edge, and usually there are no secondary injuries associated with them; i.e. there is no energy transfer
- Injury only occurs along the penetration track, but there is usually some elastic recoil of the tissues after the weapon has been inserted, so penetration and tissue damage is deeper than it would appear
- If the attacker moves the weapon around inside the body, extensive tissue damage may be caused
- The penetrating injury is most serious if it involves the:
    - Head
    - Neck
    - Thoracic/abdominal cavities
- In road traffic accidents patients with penetrating/impaling injuries often have other significant injuries
- In stab wounds:
    - Nearly 25% of penetrating abdominal injuries also involve the thoracic cavity and its contents (the diaphragm is attached lower down posteriorly than anteriorly, has no bony protection anteriorly and descends during inspiration)
    - Penetrating wounds of the thorax below the nipple line often also involve the abdominal cavity

Signs/symptoms

- There may be little obvious haemorrhage initially, due to the initial arterial spasm of the transected blood vessels, but as the spasm wears off haemorrhage may be severe
- If the object has penetrated one of the body cavities, haemorrhage may not be apparent (hidden) initially
- Young men in particular may compensate very well for considerable blood loss initially and then go into profound hypovolaemic shock

Management

Primary survey
- Initial care and management of the:
    - Airway, with care of the cervical spine if indicated
    - Breathing:
        - If the penetrating injury involves the chest:
            - The patient may need ventilating
            - The entry and exit wounds should be sealed and a chest drain with a valve inserted
    - Circulation:
        - Intravenous access should be established as early as possible; preferably with two lines and large bore cannulae, and the patient's haemodynamic status continuously monitored
        - If there is evidence of hypovolaemia, either suspected from the type and location of the injury, or apparent, the patient should be transfused aggressively with careful haemodynamic monitoring to maintain an adequate blood pressure
        - Use of a PASG may be considered:
            - It may be wise to put the patient in a non-inflated PASG prior to transport, and then it is ready to be inflated should the need arise
    - Disability
    - Exposure

Practical point
- If there is one stab wound there is likely to be more
- If the penetrating object has been removed, it is important to ascertain what the object was, and in cases of assault the sex of the attacker:
    - Men tend to stab with an upward stroke, holding the blade on the same side as the thumb
    - Women tend to stab downwards holding the blade on the same side as the little finger

Secondary survey

Impalement
- In general *no* attempt should be made to remove the impaling object, and great care should be taken not to move it any more than necessary either in transit or if it requires division to release the casualty
- Blind removal will cause further trauma to the surrounding tissues, which may result in more serious injury, and may precipitate fatal haemorrhage
- Removal is best carried out in an operating theatre, with full resuscitation facilities, and where the track of the penetrating object will be obvious and can be fully explored

Analgesia
- Intravenous analgesia is usually required during release of the casualty, or while the impaling object is divided to facilitate transportation
- Impaled limbs may require regional anaesthesia

Medium and high energy device injuries: blast and gunshot injuries

Introduction
- Whilst gunshot and blast injuries are relatively rarely seen in the civilian practice of Immediate Care, their incidence is increasing due to terrorism and crime, and their effective management forms a major part of the role in which those practising military Immediate Care are trained

Missile injuries

Incidence
- Rare:
    - In rural areas, accidental shotgun injuries do occasionally happen, and there is a regrettable increase in the tendency to use firearms by the criminal fraternity
    - Unfortunately, there has also been an increase in the type of incident, when a large number of innocent civilians are shot at random as occurred at Hungerford and Dunblane

Aetiology
- The missiles may be bullets, or fragments from an explosive device such as a bomb
- Bullets are aerodynamically far more stable, and have higher kinetic energy than bomb fragments and therefore travel further and can be aimed

Pathophysiology
- The effect is the same regardless of whether the missile penetrating the skin is a bullet, pellet or a bomb fragment
- In missile injuries there will always be some tissue damage of some extent along the wound track
- If the damage is confined to this track, it is classified as being a *low energy transfer wound*
- In some wounds, however, there is tissue damage outside the track caused by the transfer of excess kinetic energy from the missile: this injury is classified as being a *high energy transfer wound*
- The kinetic energy of a missile is proportional to the product of its mass and the square of its velocity
- In general bullets from:
    - Rifles and machine guns (high kinetic energy weapons) have a high initial velocity (often up to three or four times the speed of sound), and usually cause *high energy transfer wounds*
    - Hand guns (medium kinetic energy weapons) and most bomb fragments have subsonic velocities and as a result cause *low energy transfer wounds*

- The amount of energy transferred for any given bullet will depend on:
  - Its position in flight or angle of yaw:
    - This varies during flight, and can affect the amount of kinetic energy transferred to the tissue by a factor of up to 200, depending on the angle at which the bullet strikes the skin. Thus:
      - The same weapon firing identical rounds may have different effects
      - In some circumstances a very fast bullet may produce a small energy transfer wound, whilst a slow bullet may produce a high energy transfer wound.
  - The weapon firing it
  - The type of target struck
- High energy transfer wounds are characterised by:
  - A very severe amount of tissue damage/loss around the missile track
  - Massive wound contamination with a large amount of foreign material which is sucked into both the entry and exit wounds and broken into small fragments and disseminated widely. This is caused by the negative pressure occurring behind the wave of high pressure within the soft tissues and which sucks in debris from outside
- Low energy transfer wounds are characterised by a moderate amount of tissue damage and although the missile may drag bits of clothing into the wound as it passes, this is confined to its track and does not cause gross wound contamination

Note: Irrespective of velocity or energy potential, any missile which penetrates the skin, may kill if its path passes through vital organs or structures

Specific injuries
- All the above factors will have specific effects on different parts of the body

Head
- Once the projectile penetrates the skull, it must dissipate its kinetic energy within an enclosed space. Tissues moving away from the track of the projectile, come into contact with the bony skull, which unlike other body tissues is inelastic and unyielding. This results in brain tissue being compressed against the skull, producing more injury than if the tissues could move freely. If the kinetic energy of the missile is high enough, the rise in pressure within the skull may result in it exploding/shattering
- If a projectile enters the skull at an angle, and lacks sufficient energy to exit through the skull, e.g. a bullet fired from a medium energy weapon, it may be deflected each time it comes into contact with the inside of the skull, resulting in it following the curvature of the inside of the skull, resulting in very severe brain tissue damage

Thorax
- There are three important different types of tissue in the thorax:

Lung
- This is less dense than the other tissues in the thorax, and as a result a penetrating projectile will do less damage to it than other tissues. Because it is less dense, there are fewer cells with which it will collide, resulting in less energy transfer and less tissue damage

Vascular tissue
- Small elastic blood vessels may move out of the way of the penetrating object, but larger vessels such as the aorta and vena cava, which are less mobile, are more susceptible to damage
- The myocardium which is thick muscle, stretches initially before the penetrating object passes through it, and then contracts again afterwards leaving the entrance wound smaller. If the penetrating object has a small frontal area and relatively low kinetic energy, e.g. a knife or a low velocity bullet, the cardiac muscle may contract enough to close up the wound and prevent immediate severe blood loss from inside the heart, allowing sufficient time for the patient to get to hospital

Gastrointestinal tract
- Part of the abdominal cavity including the oesophagus, stomach and colon may be penetrated by a missile entering the lower thorax, and their contents may subsequently leak into the thoracic cavity
- Evidence of this contamination may be delayed for some time after the initial injury

Note: In addition to the above, penetrating missiles entering the thorax may be deflected from their initial course as they leave the thorax by coming into contact with the ribs, and re-enter the lungs, causing further tissue damage

Abdomen
- The abdomen includes tissues of three different types:
    - Hollow, filled with air and/or some fluid:
        - Stomach
        - Small bowel
        - Colon
        - Bladder
    - Solid:
        - Liver
        - Kidneys
        - Pancreas
    - Bone
- Penetration of the abdomen by:
    - A low energy missile may not cause a significant injury
    - A medium energy missile will usually cause some significant injury (85-90% will require surgical repair)
- The tissue damage caused by medium and low energy missiles depends on which organs they impact with, and in many cases will not result in immediate death, allowing time for the patient to be conveyed to hospital for definitive treatment, after appropriate pre-hospital resuscitation
- Contamination with intestinal contents tends to occur and is a major problem, especially with high energy transfer wounds, if there is either delayed rescue or prolonged transportation to hospital

Extremities
- Penetrating injury of the extremities may involve:

Bone
- Bone may fragment when the missile impacts with it, and part of the kinetic energy will be transferred to these bony fragments, which become secondary missiles which in turn may cause further damage to the surrounding tissues

Muscle
- Muscles may stretch initially, resulting in tearing of muscles fibres and blood vessels, and when the missile enters the muscle itself further damage to muscle fibre and blood vessels will occur

Blood vessels
- These are relatively elastic and initially will tend to stretch before actual damage occurs
- If a missile comes into direct contact with a blood vessel, the blood vessel may be:
    - Severed, resulting in:
        - Arteriolar spasm of the severed ends, and no initial haemorrhage
        - Venous haemorrhage
    - Partially severed resulting in haemorrhage
    - Partially damaged with disruption of the vessel wall resulting in blood clotting within the vessel and obstruction of the blood flow

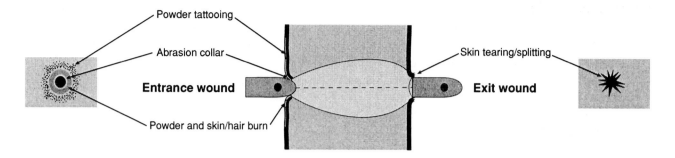

Figure 19-1 Penetrating injury: bullets; entry and exit wounds

Entrance and exit wounds
- Evaluation of the entrance and exit wounds may provide valuable information about the possible injuries that the casualty may be suffering from

Entrance wounds
- As the projectile enters the skin it pushes the skin against the underlying tissues, resulting in a circular wound
- If the projectile is spinning, e.g. a rifle bullet, it will cause a small area of abrasion (1-2 mm in size), which is usually black
- If the muzzle of a weapon is held directly against the skin when it is fired, the expanding gases produced will enter the skin and produce subcutaneous emphysema resulting in crepitus on examination (palpation)
- If the muzzle of a weapon is held within 5-7 cm of the skin when it is fired, hot gases will burn the skin
- If the muzzle of a weapon is held within 5-15 cm of the skin when it is fired, the smoke will stick to the skin
- If the muzzle of a weapon is held within 25 cm of the skin when it is fired, burning particles of cordite will tattoo the skin with small (1-2 mm) burnt areas

Exit wound
- The exit wound is caused by stretching, tearing and splitting of the skin as the projectile leaves the body

Signs/symptoms
- Patients are often unaware of their injuries initially
- The entry wound may be surprisingly small

Management
- Whilst an understanding of the pathophysiology of injury is important, it does not usually affect the Immediate Care of the patient, unless evacuation is very prolonged.
- Initial care and management of the:
    - Airway, with care of the cervical spine if indicated
    - Breathing
    - Circulation
    - Disability
    - Exposure
- If chest penetration is suspected, look for a possible tension pneumothorax
- If abdominal injury is suspected administer antibiotics and tetanus prophylaxis early:
    - If hospital admission is delayed, systemic antibiotics, e.g. benzyl penicillin administered intravenously, should be started (because of the high risk of infection with organisms such as *Clostridium tetani* and *Clostridium welchii*)

Explosives: blast injuries

Aetiology
- Explosives account for the majority of terrorist incidents
- Urban bombing may result in up to several hundred people being injured on one occasion

Types of explosive
- Low explosive:
    - Gunpowder:
        - Needs to be confined in an enclosed space to be explosive
- High explosive:
    - Does not rely on burning
    - Explodes immediately, but needs more power to set it off, i.e. a detonator

Explosive methods
- Point explosion
- Cloud explosion:
    - May occur with a chemical or gas explosion

Physical effects
- The explosive blast in a conventional explosion occurs when a large volume of gas is suddenly produced at very high pressure and temperature
- The explosion may propel missiles, but also has three primary effects:
    - The formation of a *blast shock wave:*
        - This is a wave (or front) of very high pressure, which spreads out very rapidly from the centre of the explosion (rather like the ripples on a pond, when a stone is dropped in to it), travelling at just over the speed of sound in air
    - The release of radiant heat
    - The blast shock wave is followed by a wave of swirling turbulent air, *the blast wind*, formed of rapidly moving columns of gas and debris
- In explosions, injuries may be caused by:
    - The blast shock wave
    - The radiant heat, which may cause burns
    - The blast wind which may cause injuries by bodies and debris being thrown into the air
    - Missiles from the exploding device

Pathophysiology
- Explosions may cause a variety of injuries which can be categorised according to their aetiology:

Blast shock wave: primary injury
- On hitting a human target, some of the blast shock wave is reflected, some is deflected, but the majority enters the casualty's tissues
- Before the shock wave enters the casualty's tissues, it is dammed up and increases in strength until it is sufficiently powerful to break down the resistance of the skin and pass through it
- The shock wave then passes through the tissues as a pressure wave producing its greatest effect/damage where there is a change in tissue density
- Most tissue damage occurs where there is a tissue/gas interface, causing the rupture and avulsion of small blood vessels and membranes in the gas containing organs of the body (cavitation), e.g. the lungs, *blast lung*, ears (tympanic membrane) and gastrointestinal system, resulting in pulmonary haemorrhage, pneumothorax, air emboli, and perforation of gastrointestinal organs, including the stomach, duodenum, small bowel and colon

- The tympanic membrane is the most susceptible part of the body to damage from high pressure waves, and rupture is a very common injury following exposure to an explosive force, (and is a useful indicator that a significant explosion has occurred)
- There may also be nervous system injury including anosmia due to damage to the olfactory nerve endings in the air containing nasal passages
- Serious injury and even death may occur as a result, without there being any external signs on the casualty
- Primary injury is easy to miss and should always be suspected in casualties involved in an explosion, especially if they have secondary or tertiary injuries

Note: The power of the high pressure wave may be increased many times when it is reflected from solid objects such as walls, and it therefore causes much more serious injuries when it hits people in an enclosed space

Tympanic membrane rupture

Incidence
- This is a very common injury following exposure to an explosive force

Pathophysiology
- The tympanic membrane is the most susceptible part of the body to damage from high pressure waves (and is a useful indicator that a significant explosion has occurred)
- Unfortunately the converse is not true:
    - The absence of such an injury does *not* exclude exposure to a serious blast wave/over pressure, as the main determinant is the incident angle at which the shock wave hits the tympanic membrane
- The resultant perforation usually heals spontaneously
- Higher levels of overpressure may result in additional direct sensineural damage to the cochlea, resulting in deafness similar to that produced by severe acoustic barotrauma

Symptoms/signs
- Impaired hearing
- *Always examine the tympanic membranes of anyone who has been near an explosion*

Olfactory nerve injury
- There may be damage to the olfactory nerve endings in the nasal air passages, resulting in anosmia

Lung damage: "blast lung"

Incidence
- May occur in up to 5% of those injured in explosions

Pathophysiology
- The high pressure wave may cause pulmonary contusion with:
    - Alveolar and alveolar membrane rupture with intra-alveolar haemorrhage:
        - This haemorrhage causes acute respiratory failure, and produces features similar to the adult respiratory distress syndrome (ARDS)
        - This may result:
            - Immediately in severe respiratory failure: massive contusion
            - After up to 48 hours in diffuse, but less severe lung damage
    - Even moderate exercise may have an adverse effect

- Pulmonary AV shunt damage with air entry into the pulmonary circulation, producing small arterial emboli, which may in turn produce secondary damage:
  - Multiple air emboli may cause occlusion and infarction in the:
    - Coronary circulation resulting in cardiac arrest
    - Cerebral circulation resulting in bizarre neurological symptoms/signs
  - Pulmonary air emboli:
    - May also result in pneumothoraces with or without tension

Symptoms/signs
- The lung damage presents clinically in two ways:
  - Sudden, usually fatal, respiratory failure (with no evidence of external injury)
  - Symptoms may be delayed for up to 48 hours; casualties may develop symptoms similar to those in the adult respiratory distress syndrome:
    - Increasing respiratory failure
- Air emboli:
  - Sudden cardiac arrest (due to coronary artery air emboli)
  - Symptoms similar to stroke
  - Air in the retinal vessels on fundoscopy
  - Pneumothorax

Management
- If the casualty requires ventilation:
  - Intermittent positive pressure ventilation should be avoided if possible, and positive end expiratory pressure (PEEP) should not be used, due to the danger of causing micro air emboli

Abdominal injury

Incidence
- Uncommon when the blast occurs in air, but commonly found in those exposed to underwater explosions

Pathophysiology
- Massive damage to abdominal organs may occur, but is rarely seen in the survivors of blast injury
- The most common injuries seen in survivors are:
  - Multiple contusions, with haemorrhage
  - Intestinal perforation due to necrosis secondary to ischaemia at the site of the haematomas. This may be acute or delayed (up to 5 days)

Symptoms/signs
- Diffuse abdominal pain and tenderness

Fragment injury: secondary injury
- This occurs when the casualty is hit by fragments or other objects, produced by the explosion itself, e.g. parts of the bomb casing or exploding object, and/or carried by the blast shock wave, e.g. flying glass, falling masonry and other debris from the explosion
- The severity of injury depends on the mass, velocity and nature (elasticity) of the object hitting the casualty and may range from minor lacerations and fractures to severe crush injury and death

Incidence
- More often cause injuries than the bomb explosion itself (blast shock wave)

Pathophysiology
- Fragments from the explosive device travel at high speed and may be:
  - Pieces of bomb casing
  - Fragments from near the device
  - Buckshot from a shotgun
  - Bullets from small firearms
- This is a major cause of injuries, as each fragment acts like a independent missile
- May cause multiple penetrating missile injuries

Symptoms/signs
- Casualties may be unaware of their injuries initially

Blast wind: tertiary injury
- This occurs when the casualty is picked up or thrown into the air and carried by the blast wind, and may collide with other objects before later falling to the ground, sustaining severe injuries similar to those occurring in ejection from vehicles or falls from significant heights
- The severity of any injuries depends on the mass, velocity and nature (elasticity) of the object with which the casualty collides or lands on
- Blast winds are often channelled by surrounding features, e.g. furniture, and as a result injuries may be bizarre and unpredictable, ranging from very severe to none:
  - Close to the blast:
    - Total destruction and atomisation may occur with victims being literally torn apart
  - On the periphery:
    - Traumatic amputations often occur, with different tissues and structures being avulsed at different levels
    - Nerves are often avulsed at a much higher level than other tissues

Management
- A tourniquet may be life-saving
- Remove any non-viable tissue

Flash burns: burn injury

Aetiology
- Flash burns may be caused by the radiant heat carried by the shock wave coming into direct contact with the casualty:
  - Depending on the type of explosive, the sudden release of energy may release a wave of hot gas, which may be hot enough to cause flash burns and smoke inhalation injury in those nearby
- Casualties may also be burnt by contact with fire caused by the explosion

Pathophysiology
- Injuries may include superficial burns to the hands and face
- Smoke inhalation injury may result in delayed symptoms
- The casualty's condition may get worse if he is allowed to exercise

Management
- All casualties should be admitted to hospital
- All casualties must rest
- Administer oxygen if smoke inhalation injury is suspected
- Because of the possibility of the delayed onset of respiratory failure due to either blast lung or smoke inhalation and systemic microemboli, a high index of suspicion is required and a conservative attitude adopted to the early discharge of victims home

Psychological injury

Incidence
- Over 40% of those involved in an incident involving an explosion suffer from psychological sequelae

Management
- Critical stress debriefing (see chapter on Counselling accident and disaster victims)

General management

Approach
- Be very careful with your approach to the injured:
    - There may be more explosives around
    - In a terrorist situation, there may be armed security personnel around
    - Beware of a secondary device; therefore *do not go near the incident until you are told that it is all clear, and do NOT use your radio!* (may trigger off the device)
- Do *not* touch or move anything except that necessary to provide care of the injured
- Do *not* disturb any dead bodies except the minimum necessary required to confirm death
- Be aware of the risk of:
    - Secondary panic: hysteria; myocardial infarction, etc.
    - Terrorists may attempt to kill the survivors later, e.g. in the Intensive Care Unit

Primary survey
- Initial care and management of the:
    - Airway, with care of the cervical spine if indicated
    - Breathing
    - Circulation
    - Disability
    - Exposure with control of the environment

Secondary survey: specific injuries

Head
- Note the casualty's neurological state, and their response to the injury
- Often casualties with a significant injury may *not* be unconscious
- The prognosis for penetrating injuries of the brain caused by missiles is far more accurately related to the neurological status after the injury, than in closed injury: unconsciousness is a grave sign and carries a very poor prognosis

Thorax/Thoracic cavity
- Very good at deflecting bullets
- Beware of tension pneumothorax
- Close any open wound after first inserting a chest drain
- Monitor respiratory state continuously

20

Impalement, crush injuries and amputation

Impalement, crush injuries and amputation

Introduction
- The importance, significance, and severity of impaling and crush injuries may not be appreciated initially, especially by the inexperienced pre-hospital practitioner; they require aggressive and effective Immediate Care, if the high morbidity and mortality associated with them is to be reduced
- Traumatic amputation is rarely encountered, but may be difficult to deal with both practically and emotionally; effective treatment may not only save the life of the patient, but may also be limb-saving

Impalement

Incidence
- An uncommon, but serious injury, often but not always a complication of entrapment

Aetiology
- Impalement is most serious if it involves:
    - Head
    - Neck
    - Thoracic cavity
    - Abdominal cavity
- In road traffic accidents impalement is most often caused by:
    - Vehicle running through a roadside fence which penetrates the vehicle
    - Penetration of the passenger compartment by part of (lorry) load
    - Penetration by part of vehicle
- May also be caused by:
    - Fall onto a sharp object
    - Entrapment in moving machinery
- Patients often have other significant injuries

Pathophysiology
- In general injury to underlying structures is often more severe than may be suspected at first due to elasticity of the body tissues
- There may be little obvious haemorrhage initially, due to arterial spasm, but as the spasm wears off haemorrhage may be severe
- If the object has penetrated one of the body cavities, haemorrhage may be hidden (not apparent) initially.
- Young men in particular may compensate very well for considerable blood loss initially and then go into profound hypovolaemic shock

Management

Primary survey
- Assessment and management of the patient's:
  - Airway, with care of the cervical spine
  - Breathing
  - Circulation:
    - Intravenous access should be established as early as possible; preferably with two lines and large bore intravenous cannulae, and the patient infused cautiously, with continuous monitoring of their haemodynamic status
    - If there is evidence of significant hypovolaemia, or if severe internal haemorrhage is suspected from the type and location of the injury, prepare to infuse the patient aggressively
  - Disability
  - Exposure

Pneumatic anti-shock garment (PASG)
- Use of a PASG may be considered
- It may be wise to put patient in a non-inflated PASG prior to transport, and then it is ready to be inflated should the need arise

Secondary survey

Analgesia
- Intravenous analgesia is usually required during release of the casualty, or while the impaling object is divided to facilitate transportation
- Impaled limbs may require regional anaesthesia

Removal of the impaling object
- In general *no* attempt should be made to remove the offending object, and great care should be taken not to move it any more than necessary either in transit or if it requires division to release the casualty
- Blind removal may cause further trauma to the surrounding tissues, which may result in more serious injury, and may precipitate fatal haemorrhage
- Removal is best carried out in an operating theatre, with full resuscitation facilities, and where the track of the penetrating object will be obvious and can be fully explored

Crush injuries

Incidence
- Crush injuries are relatively rarely encountered in Immediate Care, but their correct management is vital, if patients are going to survive what may be a very serious injury

Aetiology
- Significant limb compression may occur:
  - When accidents produce prolonged entrapment, e.g.:
    - Inside or under a motor vehicle
    - Beneath fallen masonry following building collapse due to gas, terrorist activity, earthquake
    - Industrial accidents when limbs are trapped in machinery
  - When there is prolonged unconsciousness following:
    - Overdosage
    - Cerebrovascular accident
  - Overinflation of a PASG

Crush injury

Pathophysiology
- Local compression causes:
    - Muscle necrosis due to direct pressure injury and ischaemia
    - Vascular injury resulting from:
        - Blunt trauma to the limb causing:
            - A rise in pressure in the limb compartments causing external compression of the blood vessels supplying the limb
        - The muscle damage results in oedema, which in turn raises the intracompartmental pressure, causing embarrassment of the venous return
        - This results in increased swelling and a further rise in compartmental pressure and so a vicious cycle develops
        - Later, the intracompartmental pressure may be so high that the arterial supply to the compartment is compromised, resulting in further ischaemia and necrosis
    - Direct arterial injury with intimal vessel injury, which may result in occlusion of the vessel by flaps of the intima or by reactive thrombus formation

Symptoms/signs
- Petechial haemorrhages: especially of the face and chest
- Swelling: this is usually severe with tense, shiny skin
- Significant injury may not always be apparent
- Absent/reduced peripheral pulses (the presence of a distal pulse does *not* exclude a dangerously high intracompartmental pressure)
- Skin mottling:
    - This is a bad prognostic sign, but if capillary blanching on direct pressure is present, the outlook may not be so gloomy
- Pallor, cold skin
- Sensory changes:
    - Reduced sensation/anaesthesia; this may be patchy unless a nerve is damaged
- Muscle weakness
- Severe pain on passive stretching of the affected muscles

Crush syndrome

Pathophysiology
- Death and necrosis of muscle cells results in the release of toxic intracellular constituents into the circulation, after the trapped limb is released, causing:
    - Myoglobinaemia which results in:
        - Myoglobinuria, which causes renal failure (this occurs in 50 % of patients with a crush injury; 100% of those who receive inadequate early fluid replacement)
    - Hyperkalaemia:
        - Arrhythmias and cardiac arrest
    - An increase in plasma uric acid
    - An increase in plasma phosphate
    - An increase in plasma creatinine phosphokinase
    - A decrease in plasma calcium
    - A metabolic acidosis
- Hypovolaemia: due to capillary leakage

Symptoms/signs
- Neuropsychiatric disturbance: behavioural problems
- Respiratory distress: Adult Respiratory Distress Syndrome
- Hypovolaemic shock
- Acute renal failure: oliguria
- Disseminated Intravascular Coagulation
- Stress induced upper gastrointestinal tract ulceration

Management

Primary survey
- Initial care and management of the:
    - Airway support and oxygen, with care of the cervical spine if indicated
    - **Breathing**: ventilatory support
    - **Circulation**:
        - Aggressive intravenous fluid infusion:
            - Crystalloid is preferred as it helps to produce a diuresis, which may prevent the distal tubules of the kidneys from being damaged by absorbed toxin
    - **Disability**
    - **Exposure** with control of the environment

Secondary survey:
- Analgesia:
    - Nitrous oxide/oxygen
    - Opiates
- Consider amputation:
    - *Only* if the limb is non viable, or to expedite release from a hazardous environment:
        - Fire, toxic fumes, rising water level, collapsing building, etc.
    - The best anaesthetic is probably ketamine
- Sedation: diazepam/midazolam
- Apply adequate splintage

Amputation

Introduction
- Both traumatic amputation, and the need for field amputation are situations which most of those involved in Immediate Care dread, but, thankfully, only experience rarely.
- Effective management may not only save the patient's life, but may be limb-saving as well, as appropriate handling of the amputated part may allow it to be replanted thanks to modern microsurgical techniques

Traumatic amputation/avulsion

Incidence
- This is a relatively rare injury

Aetiology
- May result from road traffic accidents, industrial accidents, etc.
- Is usually associated with other severe injury, except in industrial accidents, when partial or complete amputation may be the only injury

Pathophysiology
- Immediately after amputation/avulsion there may be little blood loss due to arterial spasm. As this wears off there may be profuse haemorrhage
- Owing to advances in microsurgical techniques, it may be possible for the severed limb, etc. to be replanted. This depends on the:
    - Level of the amputation
    - Duration of ischaemia
    - Type of injury:
        - Amount of bone and tissue loss
    - Age of patient: fitness to undergo surgery and ability to rehabilitate
    - Patient's occupation: how important is the severed limb to their job
    - Severity of associated injuries
    - Fitness to undergo prolonged surgery

Management

The patient
- Assessment and management of the patient's:
    - Airway, with care of the cervical spine
    - Breathing
    - Circulation:
        - Prevention of haemorrhage:
            - Tourniquet, arterial clamps
        - Treatment of hypovolaemic shock:
            - Intravenous infusion of colloid: aggressive fluid replacement may be indicated
            - It may be possible to cannulate a major vein, which has been left exposed directly
        - Consider application of a PASG

The severed limb, etc.
- Should be placed in a clean dry plastic bag, put inside another bag, and kept cool with an instant cool pack, etc. in the outer bag (prolongs ischaemic life)
- If the patient is trapped: the severed part should be sent immediately to the hospital to which the patient will be sent, so that it can be further cooled and prepared for replantation

Emergency amputation

Incidence
- Emergency amputation very rarely has to be performed at the scene of an accident

Management
- Unless other dangers dictate the need for immediate rescue, it is best performed by a surgical team from the appropriate district hospital
- The decision to amputate should never be taken lightly and is best made by two doctors
- If there is a need for immediate amputation, it is also best performed by two doctors:
    - One to provide analgesia/anaesthesia
    - One to perform the amputation

Method
- Establish an intravenous infusion, preferably with two lines and large bore cannulae
- Administer analgesia, consider:
    - Intravenous opiates
    - Regional anaesthesia
    - Ketamine anaesthesia
- Consider sedation:
    - Midazolam, diazepam
- Apply a tourniquet and amputate as low as possible with all tissues being divided in the same plane
- If possible tie off all bleeding vessels
- Apply a pressure dressing, and elevate the limb (it should then be possible to remove the tourniquet)

Note: Minimum desirable equipment:
    - 6 inch amputation knife
    - 4 inch finger saw
    - Artery forceps and sutures

Elective dismemberment

Incidence
- Very rarely has to be performed

Aetiology
- May be necessary:
    - To facilitate the release of other live but trapped casualties
    - To allow removal of the deceased

Management
- To facilitate the release of live trapped casualties:
    - Establish an intravenous infusion, if not already done:
        - For management of haemorrhage
        - For administration of drugs
    - Appropriate anaesthesia should be provided:
        - Ketamine
        - Local/regional anaesthesia
- To allow removal of the deceased:
    - Death should always be confirmed first
    - If possible, local guidelines should be discussed with the local Coroner and senior police officers (preferably before the event!)
    - If there is any suggestion of foul play, then if time permits, a forensic pathologist, or if he is not available the local police surgeon, should be called in for his opinion
    - If possible a photographic record of the circumstances should also be kept (if time permits, the police will call in a Scenes of Crimes Officer (SOCO) to photograph events)
- Disarticulation through the appropriate joint using an amputation knife, scalpel, etc. is the preferred method

Notes

21

Burns

Burns

Introduction

- Severe burns are relatively rarely encountered in Immediate Care, but they can be amongst the most severe injuries encountered, and require appropriate and effective Immediate Care if patients are going to survive them

Incidence

- Severe burns are most common in the very young and the elderly (nearly 25% of all deaths in house fires are in people aged over 75 years old)
- Burns caused by house fires account for about 10% of all accidental deaths and are the second most common cause of accidental death in children in the UK
- Account for 10,000 hospital admissions per year in England and Wales, of whom 1000 (>10% of children and >15% of adults) suffer from hypovolaemic shock. Of these up to 30% can be expected to have an inhalational injury
- Many accidental house fires are alcohol related. Victims over the age of 65 are less likely to have alcohol in their blood than younger victims, but the fire is more likely to be due to electrical faults, especially with electric blankets, and smoking

Aetiology

- Usually hot liquids under the age of 3 years
- Careless smoking and hot liquids in the elderly
- Accidents with flammable liquids: adults
- RTAs and house fires: adults

Pathophysiology

The insult
- The insult causing damage to the skin may be:
    - Heat/cold/friction
    - Electricity:
        - There may be associated cardiorespiratory arrest/cardiac arrhythmias
        - Electrical burns are usually full thickness, with considerable underlying tissue damage
    - Chemicals:
        - Acids
        - Alkalis
    - Radiation

Burn oedema
- Shortly after the burn, plasma begins to pool beneath the damaged area, as a result of the altered capillary permeability, and there is fluid (plasma) shift from the intravascular space to the extravascular space
- There is a rise in haematocrit, as more plasma is lost from the intravascular to the extravascular space
- If more than 15% of the body surface is burnt, progressive fluid loss from the circulation will result in hypovolaemic shock:
    - Critical % levels:
        - Child: >10%
        - Adult: >20%
        - Elderly: >10%

Depth of burn
- This is determined by:
    - The nature of the agent: temperature, concentration
    - The length of contact
    - The tissues' resistance to injury:
        - Skin: vascularity, thickness

Classification of burns

Superficial
- Involves the epidermis only

Partial thickness
- Involving the epidermis and the superficial dermis
- Often caused by flash burns, scalds in adults

Full thickness
- Damage extending through the dermis to the subcutaneous tissues
- Caused by flames, burning clothing and scalds in young children
- Usually there is a combination of both full and partial thickness burns

Symptoms/signs

Superficial and partial thickness burn
- Pain, erythema, blistering
- Tenderness, blanching with applied pressure

Full thickness burn
- Dull red, grey-white
- Painless, insensitive, does not blanch with pressure

Assessment of area of burn
- This is done roughly using the "rule of nines" (but not for children):
    - The body is divided up into eleven areas, each representing 9% of the total body surface
- A Lund & Browder chart gives a more accurate assessment

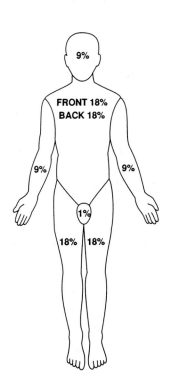

Figure 21-1 Rule of nines

Initial management

Heat burns
- Remove the casualty from the source of the danger:
    - Fire, heat, etc.
- Lie the casualty down, and smother any flames (flames travel upwards, and may cause burns of the face and head)
- If there is smoke or toxic fumes:
    - Remove the patient into fresh air
- Clothing:
    - If it is still smouldering: douse with water
    - If it is saturated with hot liquids: remove or cool with water
    - Other than this, especially if clothing is adherent to skin: leave it on

Chemical burns
- Remove the chemicals:
    - Usually by applying copious fluids, especially to the eyes and face, and continue applying for as long as possible
- Remove any contaminated clothing
- Note the identity of the chemical

Electrical burns
- Domestic:
    - Unplug the appliance involved and/or if possible switch off the mains electricity
    - Remove the patient from the source of electricity, with a non conducting object
- Begin Basic Life Support immediately, and defibrillate if appropriate
- Treat the dermal injury (see below)

Specific injuries

The airway

General
- Oxygen:
    - Put the patient in a respirable atmosphere, especially when they have been exposed to smoke and noxious gases
- If unconscious:
    - Make sure that the patient has an adequate airway
    - In electrical burns/electric shock, be prepared to begin expired air ventilation

Upper airway injury: laryngeal oedema

Aetiology
- May be caused by:
    - Burns
    - Scalds to the face
    - Inhalation of flame, hot gases or steam

Pathophysiology
- Acute tissue injury resulting in oedema and swelling, which may eventually obstruct the airway
- The more severe the thermal injury, the earlier obstruction will be apparent

Symptoms/signs
- Facial burns especially around mouth, nose and neck
- Soot in the nostrils
- Singed nasal hairs
- Carbonaceous sputum
- Pharyngeal oedema
- Laryngeal oedema:
    - Hoarseness
    - Stridor

Management
- Airway:
    - Maintain a satisfactory position for the head/neck
    - Administer humidified air or oxygen if available (consider using a nebuliser)
    - Tracheal intubation:
        - Should be performed on a conscious patient using a local anaesthetic (lidocaine) spray
        - Perform early, using a smaller tube than usual, as intubation may be difficult later due to laryngeal oedema
    - Cricothyrotomy:
        - For severe facial injury
        - If tracheal intubation is not possible
- Inhaled beclomethasone may help reduce inflammation and make the patient more comfortable

Lower airway injury

Aetiology
- Injury may be caused by
    - Fire in an enclosed space
    - Facial burns
    - Inhalation of smoke or steam (may cause a severe thermal injury)
    - Noxious gases:
        - Hydrogen cyanide
        - Isocyanates
        - Isocyanides
        - Nitrogen dioxide
        - Sulphur dioxide
        - Hydrogen chloride ⎤ given off when
        - Phosgene ⎦ PVC burns
        - Phenol
        - Toluene
        - Carbon monoxide

Pathophysiology
- Damage to the lung parenchyma is due to a combination of:
    - Poor tissue perfusion of the lungs, secondary to hypovolaemia
    - The corrosive effect of chemicals, rather than heat (with the exception of steam)

Symptoms/signs
- Perioral burns/soot in the nostrils
- Pharyngeal oedema
- Hoarseness/loss of voice/stridor
- Wheezing
- Soot in the sputum
- Bronchorrhoea
- A reduced peak flow
- A reduced SpO_2, but beware of over optimistic readings, as a pulse oximeter probe is unable to distinguish carboxyhaemoglobin from oxyhaemoglobin
- Altered level of consciousness

Management

Airway (see above)

Breathing: ventilation
- Intermittent positive pressure ventilation
- Bronchospasm:
    - Nebulised β_2 agonists (salbutamol)
    - Steroids are of no immediate value
- If circumferential burns of the chest are interfering with effective ventilation by restricting chest expansion, consider:
    - Escharotomy

Circulation
- Cardiac arrest:
    - Begin external chest compressions immediately
- Fluid replacement:
    - Aggressive fluid replacement should be started as soon as possible:
        - Rate of infusion in the first hour post burn: 1 mL/%burn/10 kg body weight
    - Use two large bore cannulae: 12/14/16 gauge
    - The best veins for this are:
        - Antecubital fossa veins
        - Forearm veins
        - Jugular veins
    - An intravenous cutdown may be necessary, but may not require local analgesia due to damage to the sensory nerve endings (there may also be damage to the superficial veins)
    - Blood samples should be obtained if possible
    - Crystalloid is preferable to colloid initially
- Keep the patient warm

Note:- Sites distal to the burn may be shut down, and those under the burn may be thermally coagulated

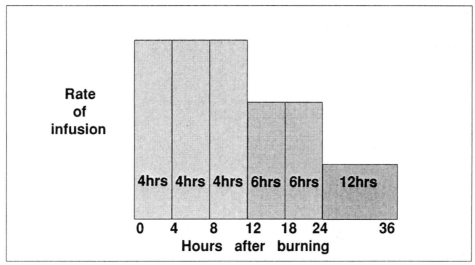

Figure 21-2 Infusion for burns using the Muir and Barclay formula: each block represents an equal volume of plasma. The volume of plasma to be infused in each block is 0.5 mL/kg/% burn.

Pain

- There may be less pain than expected in full thickness burns
- Analgesia:
    - Nitrous oxide/oxygen mixture (*Entonox®, Nitronox®*)
    - Morphine, preferably combined with an antiemetic
- Sedation of the burnt patient:
    - Consider chlorpromazine:
        - Potentiates narcotics
        - Antiemetic
        - Sedative
        - (Also long acting)

Dermal injury

Assessment of the severity of burns
- Nature
- Depth
- Area: "rule of nines" or calculated from Lund and Browder chart

Management

Dressings
- Cover the burns with sterile dressings:
    - Cling film (ideal)
    - Polythene bags
- If the travelling time to hospital is more than 1 hour consider using Roehampton burns dressings or similar
- Minor/small injury:
    - Cooling with water may be very useful

Note: Do not burst blisters
Do not apply cream, e.g. *Flamazine®*, as this can make subsequent assessment of the burn difficult

Infection
- Avoidance of unnecessary contamination
- Antibiotics:
    - Erythromycin
    - Flucloxacillin
    - May not be practical in the Immediate Care situation and should only be used if the travelling time to hospital is very prolonged or delayed

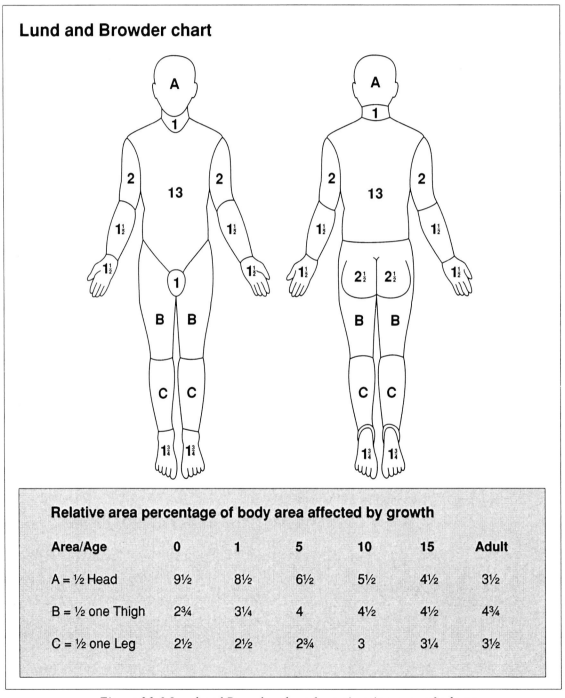

Lund and Browder chart

Relative area percentage of body area affected by growth

Area/Age	0	1	5	10	15	Adult
A = ½ Head	9½	8½	6½	5½	4½	3½
B = ½ one Thigh	2¾	3¼	4	4½	4½	4¾
C = ½ one Leg	2½	2½	2¾	3	3¼	3½

Figure 21-3 Lund and Browder chart for estimating area of a burn

Electrical burns

Incidence
- One third of all victims of electrical injuries are children, of whom about 20% die as a result

Aetiology
- Over 90% involve generated electricity (rather than lightning strike)

Pathophysiology

Flash burns
- These are probably caused by a wave of heat from a remote electrical flash; no current actually flows through or around the body

Arc burns
- These are caused by high voltage electrical currents short-circuiting outside the body, often causing very high temperatures

Direct burns
- These are caused by electricity flowing through the body
- The severity of injury sustained depends on:
    - The type of current:
        - Alternating current (AC) causes cardiac arrest at lower voltages than direct current (DC), and may cause tetanic muscle spasm making it difficult for the victim to let go of the source of the electricity
    - The size of the current:
        - High voltage electrocution, e.g. from high voltage electric power cables and lightning cause more tissue damage than lower voltage current, e.g. from car batteries, mains electricity
    - Contact time:
        - The length of time that the current passes through the body tissues
- The amount of electrical resistance of the various tissues of the body determines the path of the electrical current through the body, current flows through the tissues with least resistance and greatest cross sectional area:
    - Electric current tends to flow more easily through nerves, blood vessels and muscle than through skin, tendon, fat or bone
- AC shock may cause ventricular fibrillation
- There will be an entry and an exit burn (exit burns are often more severe than entry burns)
- There may be severe muscular spasm, resulting in fractures, dislocations or muscle tearing
- The amount/severity of tissue damage is always more extensive than it may appear to be on initial examination

Lightning strike
- Lightning may strike the body directly causing severe tissue damage as all the current flows through the body
- Lightning may act like a massive DC shock, and may depolarise the myocardium resulting in asystole, respiratory arrest and immediate death
- Lightning may also arc around the body resulting in more widespread burns

Secondary injury
- In addition the the electrical injury the casualty may sustain other injuries including:
    - Burns from clothing catching fire
    - Exposure to fire and smoke
    - Major injuries, including cervical spine injury, if the casualty is thrown some distance by the electric shock
    - Falls from heights
    - Blast injury

Symptoms/signs
- Flash burns:
    - Usually the face and exposed parts of the body will be burnt superficially, but the heat may also cause ignition of the casualty's clothing resulting in more serious burns
- Arc burns
    - The victim may be thrown some distance by the arc, often resulting in secondary injury
- Lightning strike:
    - Superficial burns on the head and lower limbs, and hair scorching
    - Feather-like burn patterns may be seen on the thorax
- AC shock
    - Ventricular fibrillation with unconsciousness
- Small deep burns

Management

Primary assessment
- Assess the scene:
    - Always make sure that you are safe, and do not risk getting electrocuted yourself
    - *Always make certain that the electric power source is turned off before you approach the victim;* if this is not possible, and *only* where low voltage currents are involved, try to remove the casualty from the power source using something that does not conduct electricity e.g. a wooden pole

CAUTION: *High voltage currents can jump considerable distances. DO NOT go near until the current has been switched off*

    - In lightning injury:
        - Get out of the open and to a place of safety, e.g. a building or vehicle, and *not* under a tree, with the casualty as soon as possible as lightning can strike twice in the same place!

- Airway management with cervical spine stabilisation, especially if the patient is unconscious or has been thrown or fallen any distance
- Breathing: ensure adequate ventilation
- Circulation:
    - Defibrillate immediately if the patient has no pulse and is in VF
    - If the patient has extensive burns:
        - Administer intravenous or intraosseous fluids
- Disability:
    - It is important to ascertain if there has been any significant nerve or muscle injury
- Exposure:
    - Assess the severity and degree of burns and dress them as appropriate
- Analgesia:
    - Provide adequate analgesia

22

Care in pregnancy

Care in pregnancy

Introduction

- When the pregnant patient is seriously ill or injured, two lives are at risk: the mother and the fetus
- Efficient and effective Immediate Care may make all the difference between saving or losing one or two patients. In rare circumstances a decision may have to be made as to which life has the higher priority. This may place an almost intolerable burden on those involved in their Immediate Care
- The management of the seriously ill or injured pregnant patient is essentially the same as that for any patient but should take into consideration differences in anatomy and physiology

Incidence

- Cardiac arrest in late pregnancy is rare (and recovery even rarer) occurring in about 1:30,000 pregnancies
- Trauma occurring during pregnancy is much more common

Aetiology

- Acute causes of maternal death in pregnancy include (in descending order of frequency):
    - Haemorrhage :
        - Uteroplacental
        - Cerebrovascular secondary to eclampsia
    - Embolism:
        - Pulmonary
        - Amniotic fluid
    - Cardiac
    - Status epilepticus

Pathophysiology

- In pregnancy both the anatomy and the physiology of the mother change, especially towards the end of the pregnancy
- These changes have a significant effect both on the mother's response to life threatening conditions and on the techniques required for successful resuscitation

Anatomical changes in pregnancy

Heart
- Increases in size and may be displaced slightly upwards and to the left as the uterus enlarges

Uterus
- In the first trimester of pregnancy the uterus is thick walled and is protected by the bony pelvis
- During the course of the pregnancy the uterus grows out of the pelvis and becomes an intra-abdominal organ. As such it is also more susceptible to injury
- In later pregnancy the wall of the uterus becomes progressively thinner, and there is relatively less amniotic fluid offering less protection for the fetus
- The placenta, because of its lack of elastic tissue, is particularly vulnerable to shearing forces, especially those caused by blunt injury, which may result in placental abruption

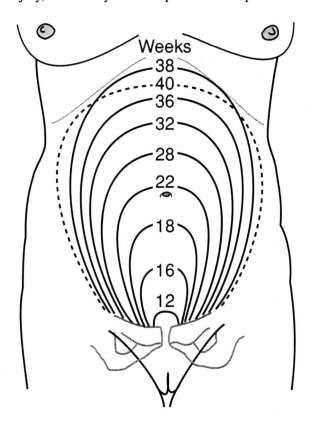

Figure 22-1 Uterine enlargement in pregnancy

Physiological changes in pregnancy

Airway
- There is relaxation of the gastro-oesophageal junction and delayed gastric emptying which results in an increased risk of oesophageal reflux and aspiration of gastric contents
- Intubation is therefore advisable in the unconscious pregnant patient

Respiratory system
- Increased oxygen requirement
- Increased ventilation:
    - The tidal volume is increased by 40%, without an increase in respiratory rate
    - There is a relative respiratory alkalosis
- Reduced chest compliance
- Reduced functional residual capacity

Cardiovascular system
- *Cardiac output:*
  - Increased by 30% (40% at term)
- *Plasma volume:*
  - This is increased by up to 50%, without a corresponding increase in total oxygen carrying capacity (red blood cells)
  - This results in a relatively low haemoglobin level (true anaemia is also common)
- *Pulse rate:*
  - The resting pulse rate increases: 84-92 bpm
- *Blood pressure:*
  - The systolic and diastolic blood pressure falls by 5-15 mmHg
- *Hypovolaemia:*
  - The pregnant patient is able to tolerate greater blood and plasma loss than the non pregnant patient before showing signs of hypovolaemia (see chapter on Shock), but this is at the cost of shunting blood away from the uterus and placenta
- *The Supine Hypotension syndrome:*
  - The gravid uterus may cause pressure on the inferior vena cava when the pregnant patient is supine, resulting in impairment of the venous return and a fall in the cardiac output of up to 40%. This in turn can result in a fall in blood pressure

Neurological system
- There is a risk of eclampsia in the third trimester. This may mimic the fits due to severe head injury and should always be borne in mind especially if hyper-reflexia is present

Skeletal system
- The sacro-iliac and pubic ligaments relax

Gastrointestinal system
- Incompetent gastro-oesophageal (cardiac) sphincter
- Increased intra-abdominal pressure, leading to increased intragastric pressure

  } results in an increased risk of gastric aspiration

Features predisposing to difficult resuscitation management

Intubation
  - Full dentition
  - Oedema or obesity of the neck
  - Supraglottic oedema

Ventilation
  - Greater oxygen requirement
  - Reduced chest compliance
  - More difficult to observe the rise and fall of the chest with ventilations

Chest compressions
  - Enlarged breasts
  - Vena caval compression by gravid uterus
  - Flared rib cage
  - Raised diaphragm

Assessment of the pregnant patient

The mother
- This should be the same as for the non pregnant adult and should be as rapid as possible
- Hypotension may be due to placental abruption

The fetus
- This should *only* take place after the mother has been assessed *and resuscitated* if necessary
- Determine the date of the mother's last menstrual period and calculate the duration of the pregnancy
- Measure the fundal height and see if this corresponds with the dates. If it is higher than expected, this may indicate placental abruption
- Examine the uterus looking for:
    - Uterine contractions
    - Uterine tenderness
    - Fetal movement
    - Fetal parts abnormally palpable:
        - Indicates uterine rupture
- Monitor the fetal heart rate (if possible). This depends on the age of the fetus and the monitoring aids available:
    - Pinard fetal stethoscope
    - Doppler ultrasound device
        - Normal heart rate: 120-160 bpm
        - Fetal distress: Bradycardia: <110 bpm
- Look for vaginal loss of blood or fluid (do *not* perform a vaginal examination)

Management of the pregnant patient
- The prime objective in managing the seriously ill or injured pregnant patient is to assess, manage and stabilise the mother first, and then the fetus
- Only in exceptional circumstances, e.g. when the mother is about to die or has just died should the assessment and management of the fetus come first
- The outcome of resuscitation following serious illness or injury is more favourable after delivery of the fetus (immediate surgical delivery should be considered if feasible, if there is no improvement in the condition of the moribund pregnant patient within 5 minutes)

Basic life support in pregnancy

Airway
- Maintain the airway (with cervical spine stabilisation in trauma)
- Apply cricoid pressure if the patient is unconscious, because of the increased risk of gastric regurgitation

Breathing
- Effective ventilation may be relatively difficult because of the patient's:
    - Increased oxygen requirement
    - Reduced chest compliance
    - Rib flaring and diaphragmatic splinting
- In pregnancy, it may also be more difficult to see if the patient's chest is expanding during ventilation

Circulation

Position
- The pregnant patient should be placed on her left side so as to reduce the effects of the Supine Hypotension syndrome

Method
- If there is *no possibility of cervical spine injury:*
    - With the patient lying on her back, elevate the right hip, flex the right knee, and displace the right leg to the left and put the patient into the left lateral position
    - Displace the uterus manually to the left
- If there *is a possibility of cervical spine injury:*
    - Immobilise the cervical spine by applying in-line cervical stabilisation
    - Elevate the right hip by putting a pillow under the right buttock (being careful not to move the cervical spine)
    - Manually displace the uterus to the left

Cardiac arrest
- This may be more difficult in the pregnant patient due to the flared ribs, raised diaphragm, enlarged breasts, and obesity
- Vena caval compression *must* be relieved by positioning the patiently correctly, *otherwise all attempts at effective resuscitation will be futile*

Hypovolaemia
- If a PASG is applied, only inflate the leg compartments

Advanced life support in pregnancy

Airway

Oxygen
- Administer high flow oxygen: important due to the increased oxygen requirement of mother and fetus

Intubation
- This should be performed early if the patient is unconscious because of the increased risk of aspiration
- This may be more difficult in the pregnant patient
    - In particular laryngoscope insertion may be more difficult if the patient has a short obese neck and large full breasts

Circulation

Arrhythmia management
- This is as for non-pregnant adults, except that bretylium should be used before lidocaine

Hypovolaemia (this a major cause of fetal death)
- Establish intravenous access using two large bore intravenous cannulae if the patient has suffered major trauma
- Rapid fluid replacement should be started using colloid initially

Obstetric emergencies

Introduction
- A knowledge of the Immediate Care of obstetric emergencies is a prerequisite for those in General Practice involved in Immediate Care, especially with the recent run down of obstetric flying squads, and the current proposals that the ambulance service, supported by pre-hospital physicians, take over this role

Antenatal problems

Vaginal bleeding in pregnancy

Miscarriage

Incidence
- Approximately 10-15% of confirmed pregnancies end in miscarriage/spontaneous abortion.
- Most often occurs at about 8 weeks and again at about 12 weeks from the first day of the last menstrual period
- Less commonly, it may occur later in pregnancy, i.e. up to 28 weeks due to:
    - Cervical incompetence
    - Rarely:
        - Congenital uterine abnormality
        - Severe maternal illness

Aetiology
- The precise cause for most miscarriages is unknown, but may include:
    - Fetal abnormality
    - Failure of implantation and malimplantation "placenta praevia"
    - Cervical incompetence
    - Uterine abnormality
    - Maternal illness
- Many threatened miscarriages may progress to an established pregnancy and the successful delivery of a normal infant

Pathophysiology

Threatened miscarriage/abortion
- There is some vaginal bleeding, which may or may not be retroplacental
- The pregnancy may continue to term

Inevitable miscarriage/abortion
- Complete:
    - More likely after 16 weeks
    - This occurs when the cervix dilates and the products of conception are extruded into the cervical canal
    - The uterus expels its contents completely and the cervical os is open
- Incomplete:
    - More likely before 16 weeks
    - The blood loss may be considerable
    - The cervix is open and the uterus contracts, expelling some, but not all, of its contents. Some decidua is retained, so the miscarriage is incomplete

Septic abortion
- This occurs following an incomplete or induced abortion, when, due to non-sterile conditions, pathogenic organisms ascend from the vagina into the uterus
- The commonest organisms involved are *E. coli* and *Streptococcus faecalis,* which may cause septic shock due to endotoxin release

Symptoms/signs
- Known to be pregnant or late with a period
- History of a recent spontaneous miscarriage
- Vaginal blood loss:
    - This may be either light or heavy
    - Will be offensive in septic abortion
- Lower abdominal pain:
    - There may be no pain initially, or there may be colicky lower abdominal pain similar to dysmenorrhoea (it may be less or more severe)
- Hypovolaemic shock
- Toxic shock

Management
- If the blood loss is:

Minor (threatened miscarriage/abortion)
- Bed rest for 48 hrs
- Consider sedation
- If the vaginal loss continues:
    - Consider performing a speculum examination of the cervix to exclude:
        - Cervical polyps
        - Severe cervical erosion
        - Carcinoma of the cervix
- Arrange an urgent outpatient assessment:
    - For probable ultrasound scan
Note: Digital vaginal examination is not advisable

Moderate
- Set up a precautionary intravenous infusion
- Arrange immediate hospital admission (there is little justification for examination)

Severe (indicates an inevitable abortion)
- Set up an intravenous infusion of colloid
- Examine the patient vaginally:
    - Remove any products of conception from the cervical os
    - Evacuate the vagina (send all fetal material to the hospital with the patient if possible)
- Administer:
    - Ergometrine and oxytocin (*Syntometrine*®) intramuscularly or intravenously
- Transfer to hospital immediately

Septic shock
- See chapter on Circulation Care: Septic shock

Hydatidiform mole

Incidence
- Occurs in approximately 1:2-3000 pregnancies

Pathophysiology
- Chromosomal changes in the fertilised oocyte lead to degeneration of the blood vessels in the villi in very early pregnancy, resulting in vesicles being formed inside the uterus (usually no fetus is found)
- 10% progress to become an invasive mole or choriocarcinoma

Symptoms/signs
- May present at 8-10 weeks with symptoms similar to a threatened miscarriage
- The uterine size is usually larger than the dates would suggest
- Vomiting may be severe
- The signs of pre-eclampsia may develop with hypertension and proteinuria
- No fetal heart is heard and no fetal parts are palpable

Management
- Treatment of complications, e.g. vomiting, eclampsia
- Hospital admission

Pain in pregnancy

Differential diagnosis
- Abruption: see above
- Renal colic:
    - Acute loin pain radiating to the groin, haematuria
- Fibroids:
    - Torsion
    - Red degeneration: acute pain, vomiting, tenderness, pyrexia at 24-30 weeks
- Ovarian cysts:
    - Torsion: acute pain, tenderness, vomiting and often pyrexia
- Uterine rupture:
    - Rupture of old LSCS, myomectomy or hysterotomy scar: obvious on palpation
    - In high parity
- Aortic aneurysm:
    - Rupture
- Appendicitis:
    - The point of tenderness is usually higher than normal
    - Nausea
    - There is a reduced response to inflammation
- Cholecystitis:
    - Tenderness in the right hypochondrium
- Toxaemia: may also present as abdominal pain (see below)

Ectopic/extrauterine pregnancy

Incidence
- Ectopic and extrauterine pregnancy occurs in 1% of all pregnancies in the UK and is increasing
- Ectopic pregnancy is the most important cause of maternal death in early pregnancy, accounting for about 30% of maternal deaths in the first trimester, and 10% of all maternal deaths, although this is falling, due to increased awareness and improved early diagnostic facilities
- Deaths usually occur due to a delay in diagnosis and poor early management
- Occurs most commonly in women aged 25-34 years

Aetiology
- Most often occurs due to tubal damage caused by previous:
    - Infection; salpingitis and pelvic inflammatory disease
    - Sterilisation and tubal surgery
- Other precipitating factors include:
    - Endometriosis
    - IUCD use
    - Use of the progesterone-only oral contraceptive pill
    - History of infertility/attempts at IVF

Pathophysiology
- An ectopic pregnancy occurs when a fertilised ovum implants in a site other than the endometrial cavity; most (95%) occur in the fallopian tube

Tubal ectopic pregnancy
- Once established, the trophoblast may abort or continue to invade the wall of the tube, resulting in:
    - Bleeding and eventually rupture of the pregnancy through the tubal wall, with brisk intra-peritoneal haemorrhage *or*
    - Leakage of a little blood from the fimbrial end of the tube, which causes irritation of the peritoneum in the pouch of Douglas

Symptoms/signs
- Diagnosis may be difficult: 40% are missed by the first doctor
- There are two distinct presentations:
    - Tubal rupture:
        - Sudden severe lower abdominal pain with hypovolaemic shock and collapse (10%)
    - Subacute presentation in which the pregnancy has not ruptured, but has been leaking chronically:
        - Lower abdominal pain with brown vaginal loss
- Lower abdominal pain in either iliac fossae (present in 97% of cases) which may be referred to the shoulder:
    - Stabbing, colicky, cramping
    - Usually precedes the vaginal loss (other causes usually result in vaginal loss followed by the onset of pain)
- Syncope or hypovolaemic collapse (unusual as the initial presentation)
- Symptoms of early pregnancy (present in 30% of cases):
    - Frequency
    - Breast tenderness
- History of;
    - Irregular/abnormal vaginal bleeding (present in 85% of cases):
        - May be scanty, dark brown (like prune juice)
    - Menstrual disturbance (typically 6-8 weeks amenorrhoea; 60% of cases)
    - Current IUCD or progesterone-only oral contraceptive pill usage
    - Previous pelvic surgery or old pelvic inflammatory disease

- Evidence of hypovolaemic shock
- Localised lower abdominal tenderness with the signs of peritonism (only if the pregnancy has ruptured):
    - Guarding
    - Shifting dullness
    - Evidence of infective shock
    - Pyrexia
- On vaginal examination (should be very gentle, so as to avoid rupturing the pregnancy):
    - Cervical excitability is characteristic
    - Tenderness in either adnexa with the presence of a tender mass (40%), or in the pouch of Douglas
- Anaemia: there may have been blood loss for some time

Differential diagnosis
- Incomplete spontaneous abortion:
    - The vaginal loss is usually more profuse, with fresh blood
- Salpingitis:
    - Swelling, bilateral lower abdominal pain, pyrexia and a vaginal discharge
- Appendicitis:
    - The area of tenderness is usually higher
- Torsion, rupture or haemorrhage of an ovarian cyst

Management
- Initial resuscitation, if there is evidence of hypovolaemic shock:
    - Administration of high flow oxygen via a high concentration oxygen mask
    - Set up an intravenous infusion(s) of colloid using two wide bore cannulae
- Monitor the pulse and blood pressure.
- Consider:
    - Application of a PASG
    - Calling for the assistance of a flying squad, or another Immediate Care doctor, if they can be on the scene very rapidly
- Arrange for immediate admission

Cyst accidents

Incidence
- Rare

Aetiology
- Torsion of an ovary containing a functional, e.g. luteal, or neoplastic cyst

Symptoms/signs
- Collapse
- Vomiting
- Pain in the region of the sacro-iliac joint or iliac fossa

Differential diagnosis
- Tubal pregnancy (very difficult to distinguish from this)
- Renal colic
- Infection
- Appendicitis
- (Dysmenorrhoea)

Management
- Treat symptomatically and admit to hospital

Antepartum haemorrhage (bleeding after 24 weeks of pregnancy)

Incidence
- Occurs in 3% of pregnancies
- Haemorrhage due to placenta praevia and placental abruption together account for over 10% of all perinatal deaths, and 10% of all maternal deaths, and has also been shown to result in excessively high rates of pre-term delivery, low birthweight, still birth and neonatal death

Pathophysiology
- Placenta praevia and placental abruption occur when the placenta separates before delivery, resulting in profuse bleeding from the denuded placental bed
- The amount of placental separation and its effects varies from small and relatively insignificant, to large, when the placental circulation may be compromised and fetal death may ensue

  Placental abruption
    - Occurs when the placenta is situated in the upper uterus
    - The blood from the placental bed is confined initially between the placenta and the uterine wall, concealing the haemorrhage
  Placenta praevia
    - Occurs when the placenta is in the lower segment
    - The blood from the placental bed is released into the vagina

Aetiology
- Bleeding from the cervix due to:
    - Cervical erosion, polyps or carcinoma
- Retroplacental bleeding: placenta praevia and placental abruption:
    - Grand multiparity, non-singleton pregnancies, uterine scarring, uterine tumours, cigarette smoking

Symptoms/signs
- Assessment must be rapid: rely on the physical signs:
    - General maternal appearance with evidence of hypovolaemic shock
    - Vaginal bleeding; *do not perform a vaginal examination* (minimal examination only is indicated)
    - Uterine irritability with abdominal pain/tenderness
    - Increasing fundal height
    - Evidence of fetal distress (fetal heart rate slow or very fast)

Management
- The urgency with which the patient should be managed depends on:
    - The amount of blood loss (which may be covert)
    - Whether or not maternal resuscitation is needed first
    - Whether there is evidence of fetal distress
  Minor blood loss
    - Put up an intravenous infusion of colloid or crystalloid
    - Transfer the patient to hospital
  Major blood loss with evidence of hypovolaemic shock:
    - Administer high flow oxygen via a high concentration oxygen mask
    - Set up a infusion of colloid in both arms, using wide bore cannulae (14/16 SWG)
    - Take blood for group (if not already done), cross match and clotting factors
    - Infuse rapidly monitoring the patient's haemodynamic state as you do so
    - Provide adequate pain relief; there may be little or no pain with a placenta praevia, but placental abruption may result in very severe pain; requiring intravenous opiates for its relief
    - Monitor the fetal heart
    - Transfer the patient quickly to hospital (an accurate diagnosis is irrelevant)

Pre-eclamptic toxaemia/eclampsia
- Pre-eclampsia is the most dangerous of the common complications of pregnancy, a leading cause of maternal death and a major contributor to perinatal mortality
- More likely to be fatal outside hospital due to poor recognition and the earlier it occurs in pregnancy

Pre-eclamptic toxaemia

Incidence
- Commonest major problem in pregnancy affecting up to 10% of all pregnancies (20% first pregnancies)
- More likely to develop into eclampsia in concealed pregnancy due to failure to recognise the significance of the symptoms
- Usually occurs in the third trimester, but may occur as early as 20 weeks or a few days after delivery
- Pregnancy-induced hypertension is the most common cause of iatrogenic prematurity, being responsible for 25% of cases of low and very low birth-weight babies

Aetiology
- The precise cause is unknown, but predisposing risk factors include:
    - Maternal: *Chance of pre-eclampsia*
        - First pregnancy 5%
        - Family history 10%
        - Age below 16 or over 40 years 5-10%
        - Previous history of severe, early onset eclampsia 20%
        - Renal disease 10-60%
        - Diabetes mellitus 10-30%
        - Short stature, pre-existing/pregnancy induced hypertension, obesity and lower social class
    - Fetal:
        - Multiple pregnancy 10-30%
        - Hydatidiform mole 10-30%
        - Hydrops 10-30%
        - Trisomy 13 5-10%

Pathophysiology
- The underlying pathophysiology is not fully understood, but pre-eclampsia is primarily a placental disorder associated with poor placental perfusion:
    - There is abnormal invasion of the uterus by the trophoblast, with absence of the second phase in which the trophoblast usually invades the spiral arteries. As a result, the spiral arteries retain their muscular coat and their responsiveness to myotonic stimuli
    - There is abnormal fibrin deposition in the placenta with acute atheroma deposition
    - Vascular endothelial damage activates the coagulation cascade resulting in increased platelet aggregation
    - There is a failure of adequate dilation of the maternal spiral arteries feeding the placenta, resulting in placental ischaemia, and maternal and fetal illness
    - Severe arteriolar constriction results in:
        - Cerebral haemorrhage (the cause of most of the maternal mortality associated with eclampsia)
        - Eclampsia with fitting and cerebral oedema
        - Secondary pulmonary oedema and the Adult Respiratory Distress Syndrome (ARDS)
        - Cortical blindness
        - HELLP syndrome (haemoptysis, elevated liver enzymes, low platelets)
        - Hepatic oedema and rupture with liver failure
        - Acute renal failure
        - Disseminated intravascular coagulation
        - Intrauterine growth retardation, fetal hypoxia resulting in fetal distress and intrauterine death
        - Placental abruption

Symptoms/signs
- Pre-eclampsia is diagnosed when a pregnant woman of 20 or more weeks' gestation has a blood pressure greater than 140/90 mmHg, and she has proteinuria +, or more, on dipstick testing
- Headache, vomiting and itching in the mask area of the face
- Visual disturbance:
    - Spots in front of the eyes
    - Angular flashes at the periphery of the visual fields
    - Loss of vision in some areas
- May be jittery, hyperreactive/hyper-reflexic before the onset of fits
- Upper abdominal pain (usually epigastric or right sided), with hepatic tenderness:
    - Due to sub-capsular hepatic haemorrhage or peritoneal stretching over an oedematous liver
- Oedema, involving the face and hands and recent rapid weight gain
- Hypertensive retinopathy (in a few cases)

Management
- If not fitting:
    - Admit those women with hypertension and proteinuria the same day
    - Admit women with additional features immediately
- If there appears to be imminent risk of fitting (jittery, hyper-reflexic):
    - Establish intravenous access
    - Sedate with intravenous or rectal diazepam *(Stesolid®)*
    - Arrange immediate hospital admission
    - Carry out continuous monitoring of the patient's condition before and during transfer to hospital
- Consider administration of a hypotensive, e.g. methyldopa or a β-blocker (labetalol)

Eclampsia

Incidence
- Occurs in about 1:1,500 deliveries, but less common now than it used to be because of improvements in antenatal care
- Major cause of maternal mortality in the UK resulting in the death of about 10 women (over 15% of all perinatal maternal deaths) and 1000 babies each year in the UK. Most maternal deaths (80%) are associated with suboptimal care
- Nearly 40% of cases occur antepartum, most before 37 weeks' gestation

Symptoms/signs
- It is very difficult to predict all those women who will progress from having pre-eclampsia to eclampsia as only about 60% of women have significant warning symptoms and both hypertension and proteinuria

Management (delivery is the definitive treatment for eclampsia)
- Manage as for epilepsy:
    - Stop fitting (intravenous magnesium sulphate is the drug of choice for the prevention of further fits in eclampsia, but currently is not used in the pre-hospital situation):
        - Diazepam: 10-40 mg, administered intravenously/rectally (consider a diazepam infusion)
        - Midazolam: 5-10 mg administered intravenously
    - Airway maintenance
        - Position the patient on their left side
        - Consider intubation to protect the airway from the risk of gastric aspiration (a common cause of maternal death).
    - Administer oxygen
    - Prevent self injury during fits
- Monitor the fetal heart
- Transfer the patient to hospital immediately

Problems during labour

Labour at home

Aetiology
- May be:
    - Unplanned: concealed pregnancy
    - Early labour
    - Rapid labour
    - Complicated delivery

Assessment
- History
- Is the patient:
    - In labour?
    - Bleeding?
- Is the blood pressure elevated or depressed?
- Is the fetal heart rate satisfactory?

Management
- Decide whether patient should:
    - Stay at home
    - Be transferred to hospital

Uncomplicated
- Medical practitioners may deliver the baby and then transfer mother and baby to hospital

Complicated delivery
- Delay in the second stage:
    - Admit to hospital
- Fetal distress:
    - Medical practitioners may deliver rapidly or if this is not possible arrange immediate admission to hospital
- Cord prolapse:
    - If there is *no* detectable fetal heart:
        - Allow the patient to deliver
    - If there *is* a good fetal heartbeat:
        - Consider an attempt to reduce the cord back into the vagina with a pack, as this will keep it warm and moist, and will reduce the risk of cord spasm and avoids any unnecessary handling
        - Put the patient in the knee elbow position with elevation of the buttocks
        - Convey to hospital for probable LSCS
- Breech presentation:
    - If in the second stage:
        - Control delivery with the patient in the lithotomy position using an effective episiotomy.
        - Maintain jaw flexion, exert gentle shoulder traction to the aftercoming head, allowing controlled delivery
- Shoulder dystocia:
    - Deliver with the patient lying on her left side with a large episiotomy
    - Pull the head back to allow the anterior shoulder to escape beneath the symphysis pubis

Note: Whilst medical practitioners may consider delivering the patient, paramedics and other should convey the patient rapidly to hospital, providing care of the ABC as appropriate

Pulmonary embolism of amniotic fluid

Incidence
- This is very rare, with an incidence of 1:60,000 pregnancies, and accounts for about 10% of all perinatal maternal deaths in the UK
- It usually occurs as a complication of surgical induction, and is therefore almost unknown outside hospital
- It is usually fatal (20% survive if treated appropriately immediately); often the diagnosis is only made at postmortem
- If the patient survives the initial shock, a coagulation defect is inevitable

Aetiology
- May occur as a result of:
    - Surgical induction
    - Placental abruption
    - Multiple pregnancy
    - Polyhydramnios

Pathophysiology
- Amniotic fluid or trophoblast tissue enters the maternal circulation, where the thromboplastins provoke disseminated intravascular coagulation, which leads to depletion of plasma fibrinogen

Symptoms/signs
- May occur immediately after amniotomy, but is usually preceded by strong uterine contractions
- Pulmonary embolism: intense dyspnoea, followed by loss of consciousness
- Severe shock with total circulatory collapse
- If caused by abruption, there may be loss of fetal movement and heartbeat

Management
- Treat shock aggressively:
    - Oxygen
    - Administer intravenous fluids
    - Consider application of PASG
- Arrange for immediate conveyance to hospital

Post-partum problems

Post partum haemorrhage

Incidence
- Uncommon outside hospital, but increasing due to early discharge policies

Aetiology

Primary
- Retained placenta
- Atonic uterus

Secondary
- Retained placenta (more likely to happen at home with the current vogue for early discharge)
- Post LSCS: infected placental site or incision site
- Uterine inversion
- Infection

Management
- Assess the blood loss (it is easy to over estimate this)
- Establish an intravenous infusion
- Administer intravenous oxytocics: ergometrine
- Treat the cause:
    - Haemorrhage:
        - Stop the bleeding by applying bimanual uterine pressure after first emptying the bladder (if possible)
    - Uterine inversion:
        - Needs to be corrected immediately, as this condition may be fatal very rapidly due to irreversible shock
    - Retained placenta:
        - Attempt removal (empty the bladder first)
- Apply controlled cord traction
- Transfer the patient to hospital immediately

Obstetric pharmacology

Introduction
- The drugs used in obstetrics are smooth muscle stimulants, and cause uterine contraction
- Those involved in Immediate Care should carry one drug rather than the whole range of drugs

Ergometrine maleate

Indications
- Active management of the third stage of labour, post-partum haemorrhage

Contraindications
- 1st and 2nd stages of labour
- Vascular disease
- Impaired pulmonary, hepatic or renal function

Cautions
- Toxaemia
- Cardiac disease
- Hypertension
- Sepsis

Side effects
- Nausea, vomiting
- Transient hypertension
- Peripheral vasoconstriction

Presentation
- Ergometrine 500 μg per mL: 1 mL ampoule

Dosage
- Intramuscularly: 200-500 μg: (onset 5-7 minutes, duration about 45 minutes)
- Intravenously (emergency control of haemorrhage): 100-500 μg (onset 1 minute)

CONCLUSION: The oxytocic of choice for the management of post-partum haemorrhage

Oxytocin *(Syntocinon®)*

Indications
- Induction and augmentation of labour
- Management of incomplete and missed abortion

Contraindications
- Severe toxaemia
- Predisposition to amniotic fluid embolism

Cautions
- Hypertension
- High parity

Side effects
- Violent uterine contractions
- Maternal hypertension and subsequent subarachnoid haemorrhage
- Cardiac arrhythmias
- Water intoxication

Presentation
- Oxytocin: 5 units/mL: 1 mL ampoules
            10 units/mL: 1 mL ampoules

Dosage
- Missed abortion:
    - 10-20 units/500 mL given at a rate of 15 drops per minute and adjusted according to response

Ergometrine maleate/oxytocin (*Syntometrine®*)

Action
- Combines the rapid action of oxytocin with the more sustained action of ergometrine, both of which cause uterine contraction

Indications
- The active management of the third stage of labour
- The prevention of post-partum haemorrhage, following delivery of the placenta
- To control post-partum haemorrhage

Presentation
- Ergometrine 500 µg/5 units oxytocin per 1 mL: 1 mL ampoule

Dosage
- 1 mL intramuscularly or 0.5-1.0 mL intravenously (if there is a high risk of post-partum haemorrhage)

CONCLUSION: The oxytocic of choice for the active management of the third stage of labour and controlling haemorrhage due to incomplete abortion (ergometrine and oxytocin may be used alone for the management of haemorrhage due to incomplete abortion, but have less effect on the early pregnant uterus). It is the drug most commonly used in the pre-hospital situation

Trauma in pregnancy

Blunt trauma in pregnancy

Aetiology
- The most common causes of blunt trauma in pregnancy are:
    - Road traffic accidents: seat belt injury, abdominal trauma
    - Falls
    - Assaults

Placental abruption
- A common cause of fetal death
- May occur up to 48 hrs after injury
- May be associated with seat belt use

Signs
- Vaginal bleeding
- Uterine irritability
- Abdominal tenderness
- Increasing fundal height
- Maternal hypovolaemic shock
- Fetal distress

Traumatic uterine rupture
- Occurs in late pregnancy

Signs
- May range from massive haemorrhage and hypovolaemic shock to minimal symptoms/signs
- A separately palpable uterus and fetus is pathognomonic

Pelvic trauma
- Associated with a high incidence of fetal intracranial trauma, resulting in skull fracture and intracranial haemorrhage

Penetrating trauma in pregnancy
- As the uterus enlarges it becomes increasingly vulnerable to penetrating trauma, when its presence can protect the other intra-abdominal organs from injury
- Gunshot and stab wounds often result in fetal death, but maternal survival is usually good

Burns in pregnancy
- Burns of >50% occurring in the second or third trimesters are associated with a high mortality rate

Management:
- Immediate delivery:
    - Maternal death is certain unless she is delivered and the fetal prognosis is not improved by waiting

23

Neonatal care

Neonatal resuscitation

Introduction

- Basic resuscitation of the newborn is a technique that all those involved in domiciliary obstetrics should be trained in and competent at performing, whilst those practising Immediate Care should be competent in performing advanced resuscitation of the newborn. This is becoming increasingly important with the run down in hospital based obstetric flying squads and their replacement by extended trained ambulance personnel supported by appropriately trained general practitioners

Incidence

- The number of newborn babies requiring resuscitation outside hospital is very small, but will probably increase in the United Kingdom, if the trend away from managed hospital obstetrics and towards more home confinement continues

Aetiology

- Babies born outside hospital fall into two groups:
    - Planned home confinements:
        - These are nearly all carefully selected beforehand and in particular the mothers are usually multiparous and have an uncomplicated previous obstetric history
        - The incidence of babies requiring resuscitation is very small in this group
    - Accidental pre-hospital delivery:
        - This usually occurs due to:
            - Failure or refusal to recognise pregnancy, or concealed pregnancy
            - Poor recognition of the beginning of the second stage of labour
            - Very rapid labour
            - Transport or geographical delay
        - The incidence of babies requiring resuscitation in this group is rather higher

Pathophysiology

The first breath

- The lungs actively secrete fluid in utero and at birth the baby's lungs are full of fluid
- The baby's first few breaths are vigorous so that the surface tension from the fluid is overcome. and the fluid is driven out of the alveoli and into the circulation, and the lungs begin to fill with air. Subsequent breaths do not normally need to be so forceful provided that there is sufficient surfactant

- Surfactant:
    - Surfactant helps to prevent the lungs from collapsing completely at the end of expiration, and reduces the inspiratory effort required for subsequent breaths
    - The ability of the fetus to secrete sufficient surfactant increases with increasing gestational maturity
    - Cold stress and acidosis reduce the amount of surfactant produced and increase the amount of respiratory effort required to breathe
- Blood flow through the lungs increases as the pulmonary capillaries open up and oxygenation improves
- The median time from delivery to the onset of spontaneous respiration is normally only 10 seconds
- If the newborn baby has never tried to breathe, it is more difficult to expand the lungs with air, as the lungs are still full of fluid, and more pressure than is usually necessary for normal ventilation will have to be applied initially to fill the alveoli "opening pressure". This is easier if the initial inflation/ventilation/inspiration is slightly prolonged
- If a baby stops breathing after having taken its first few breaths, less pressure will be required to ventilate it, than if it had never breathed

Circulatory changes

In the uterus
- Whilst the fetus is in the uterus, its heart pumps very little blood to the lungs because of:
    - The high resistance to blood flow of the pulmonary circulation
    - The much lower resistance to blood flow of the aorta and umbilical blood supply
- As a result of this most of the blood from the right ventricle is pumped via the pulmonary artery and the ductus arteriosus into the aorta

During delivery
- When the lungs expand with the first breath, the resistance to blood flow into the pulmonary circulation is reduced
- When the umbilical vessels are clamped or go into spasm, there is a rise in the resistance to blood flow into the aorta
- As a result blood is pumped from the right ventricle and from there into the rest of the pulmonary circulation, before returning to the left atrium via the pulmonary veins
- Soon after birth the ductus arteriosus and the foramen ovale (connecting the right and left sides of the heart at atrial level) close

Asphyxia

Primary apnoea
- Recent research suggests that if the neonate is suddenly severely deprived of oxygen at birth, it will stop trying to breathe. This results in:
    - A rapid rise in blood pressure, and a slowing of the heart rate, resulting in a reduced cardiac output
    - A rise in the peripheral vascular resistance
    - Production of catecholamines, vasopressin, angiotensin and other hormones
- These changes help to maintain blood flow to the vital organs (brain and heart) at the expense of all other organs including the lungs, where there is vasoconstriction
- This episode of apnoea continues for a variable length of time, after which deep agonal gasping (occurring about every 10-20 seconds) starts
- A neonate who is suffering from primary apnoea will probably recover with minimal help, and will tend, but not always, to look blue rather than pale
- The heart rate will improve when the airway is clear and air/oxygen enters the lungs. The skin will become pink after a gasp or two
- Administration of some drugs, including opiates and sedatives, to the mother, will tend to prolong the primary apnoeic phase

Terminal apnoea
- If the hypoxia continues:
  - The gasping will fade away and there is a second (terminal) apnoeic phase
  - The blood pressure begins to fall, the heart rate decreases further until there is asystole and death
- A neonate with primary apnoea will die unless actively resuscitated and will usually be:
  - Very pale rather than blue
  - Very floppy
- The neonate must be ventilated and will usually turn pink before taking its first spontaneous gasp

Note: 1. It may be difficult to tell whether a baby who doesn't breathe within a minute or two of birth is suffering from primary apnoea and is about to start gasping or is suffering from terminal apnoea having already passed through the gasping phase before birth. In each case resuscitation must not be delayed
     2. Hypoxia or acidosis results in:
- Narrowing of the pulmonary arterioles, which results in a further reduction in the blood supply to the lungs, and a further increase in hypoxia
- Reduced surfactant production and an increase in the inspiratory effort required to expand the lungs

Hypothermia
- If newborn babies are not kept warm and dry:
  - Their temperature will fall rapidly (10°C every 5 minutes) and they will become hypothermic, which in turn will result in hypoglycaemia, respiratory distress and acidosis

Procedure after the baby is born

Heat loss
- Immediately after birth:
  - Dry the infant, quickly, but thoroughly, using a warm towel
  - Having done this remove the now wet towel and replace it with a fresh warm dry towel

Assessment

Appearance
- Colour:
  - Ascertain, by examining the neonate's trunk, lips and tongue whether they appear to be centrally:
    - Pink
    - Cyanosed
    - Pale
- Tone:
  - Does the neonate appear to have good muscular tone or are they floppy

Breathing
- Observe:
  - The rate and quality of respirations
  - Whether there are any breathing problems, e.g. gasping, grunting

Circulation/heart rate
- Pulse
  - Asses the rate and quality by:
    - Listening to the apex beat with a stethoscope
    - Palpating the pulse at the base of the umbilical cord

Management
- The principle of management must be to prevent problems arising, and to recognise and treat those problems that do so as rapidly as possible
- Most healthy mature babies babies will usually breathe or cry within 90 seconds of delivery and have good muscle tone
- It is not usually necessary to suction the pharynx, and oxygen administration is not usually necessary
- Most neonates can be assigned to one of the categories below:

- **Breathing spontaneously *and* has a heart rate of >100 beats per minute *and* is centrally pink:**
    - Give the baby to the mother straight away
    - The baby will usually stay warm with skin to skin contact and may be put to the breast

- **Breathing inadequately *but* has a heart rate of >100 beats per minute *and* is centrally cyanosed:**
    - Wrap in a warm dry towel and put in a warm place, and attempt to dry
    - Drying the baby usually causes enough stimulation to induce effective breathing, but additional tactile stimulation may be necessary:
        - Gently flicking the soles of their feet
        - Rubbing the back for a few seconds
        - If this succeeds, subsequent gentle stimulation may help these infants to keep breathing
    - Administer supplementary oxygen
    - If there is no response, commence more active intervention (see below)

Oxygen
- Administer oxygen by face mask or funnel (if available), which should have perforations or a side vent to prevent a build-up of pressure

- **Breathing inadequately after stimulation *and* has a heart rate of <100 beats per minute *or* is pale:**
    - The baby needs urgent resuscitation:

Airway

Position
- Place the baby supine on a flat surface, with the head towards you
- Support the head in a neutral position with the jaw drawn forward to prevent the tongue obstructing the airway
- Maintain the neutral position by using a small pad under the shoulders
- Do *not* overextend or flex the head, which may result in kinking of the trachea and airway obstruction

- **If there is no meconium in the amniotic fluid:**
    - Look for respiratory efforts
    - Listen to the chest for breath sounds
    - If respiratory efforts are present and vigorous, but no breath sounds are audible; the airway may be obstructed:
        - Check the position of the baby and reposition the head if necessary
    - Gently suction the mouth and nostrils to remove any debris or mucus

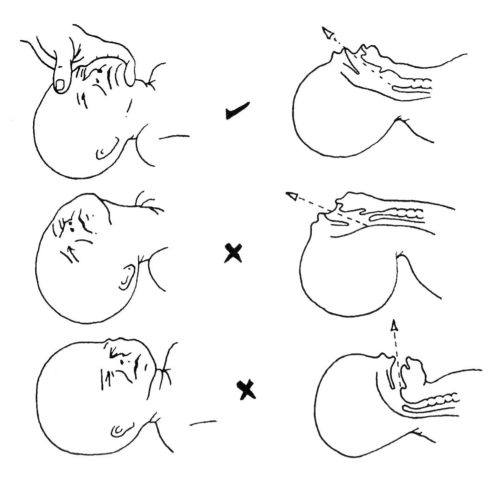

Figure 23-1 Positioning the neonate to maintain the airway

Suctioning
- Use a suction source with a negative pressure of less than 100 mmHg (the use of oral powered mucus extractors should be avoided, as congenital contamination with the human immunodeficiency virus (HIV) has been shown to occur)
- Catheter size: 10 or 8 FG (for pre-term neonates)
- Gently suck out the oropharynx by inserting a catheter no more than 5 cm
- Each attempt at suctioning should take no more than about 5 seconds

Note: Rough or deep suctioning may cause laryngeal spasm resulting in delay in the onset of spontaneous respiration or vagal stimulation resulting in bradycardia

- **If the airway is still obstructed:**
    - Consider insertion of an oropharyngeal airway

- If there is thick meconium in the airway:
    - Suction the mouth before delivery of the chest;
        - suction the mouth first and then the nose, trying to avoid making the baby gasp

Breathing

- **If respiratory efforts are shallow or slow:**
    - Count the heart rate over 10-15 seconds

- *If there is a regular heart rate of >100 beats per minute and no meconium is present:*
    - Stimulate the baby gently and administer oxygen, through a mask if the baby is cyanosed (the baby will usually start to breathe spontaneously)

- *If respirations do not improve within a further 20-30 seconds, and the heart rate is* **decreasing** *or if the baby remains* **cyanosed:**
    - Start lung inflations using a bag, valve and mask
    - Make certain that the chest wall moves with each inflation
    - Consider administration of Naloxone if the mother has recently received an opiate analgesic, but *only if the baby has become pink, with a good heart rate and is still not breathing*
    - If the heart rate continues to decrease over the next 30 seconds, in spite of adequate mask ventilation (by which time it will be about 2 minutes old), proceed to tracheal intubation

- **If respirations are absent or gasping, persistently shallow or irregular, or the heart rate is <100 beats per minute:**
    - Start lung inflations using a bag, valve and mask, and prepare to intubate

Circulation

Heart rate
- This is an important guide as to the need for, and response to resuscitation
- Check the heart rate by:
    - Auscultating or palpating the fetal heart over its apex
    - Palpating the base of the umbilical cord to check for an output
- If the heart rate is:
    - > 100 beats per minute; continue with the assessment
    - < 100 beats per minute and decreasing; commence or continue with positive pressure ventilation
    - < 60 beats per minute; commence or continue with positive pressure ventilation. Check technique and start external chest compressions

Note: The commonest cause of failure of the heart rate to improve is inadequate ventilation. Always check the adequacy of ventilation before starting external chest compressions

Colour
- Administer oxygen if the baby is centrally cyanosed
- Cyanosis may persist even after the baby develops an adequate heart rate and respiratory effort. This may be because the child has a congenital cardiac defect or be due to persisting pulmonary hypertension. Oxygen administration should be continued until the cause is ascertained (in hospital)
- Pallor may be evidence of asphyxia, anaemia or hypovolaemia

Positive pressure ventilation
- This may be achieved with a bag and mask or tracheal tube
- Both are techniques difficult to perform well and require skill and regular practice

Neonatal mask
- The mask should be soft, transparent and is usually circular
- It should cover the baby's mouth and nose
- It should be well fitting, so that when it is tightly applied it does not press on the eyes/overhang the chin

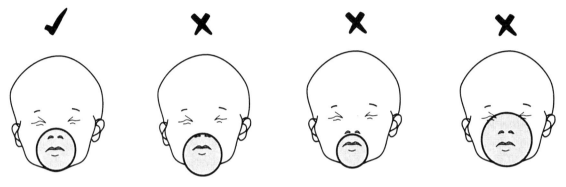

Figure 23-2 Position of mask

Lung inflation using a face mask

Method
  Airway
- Check for respiratory effort
- If this is present and perhaps vigorous, but doesn't result in chest expansion, there is probably airway obstruction

Clearing the airway
- Open the airway by slightly extending the neck
- Hold the chin gently forward using the finger on the mandible, being careful not to compress the soft tissues of the neck

Ventilation
- Hold the mask firmly in place
- Give intermittent ventilations by squeezing the bag gently with your fingertips, trying to maintain inflation times of 1-2 seconds for the five or six ventilations.

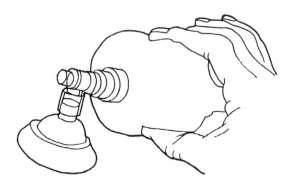

Figure 23-3 Gently squeeze the bag

- The initial inflation may require relatively high pressures (up to 30-40 mm H_2O) to overcome the initial opening pressure, but once this has occurred, a pressure of 20 mm H_2O is usually sufficient, to obtain adequate chest movement and ventilation by the fifth inflation
- If compression of the bag is too forceful, it may cause excessive pressure in spite of the pressure relief valve
- After five ventilations, check that the chest wall is moving satisfactorily, and then ventilate the lungs regularly at a rate of 30-40 ventilations per minute
    - Watch the chest rise and fall with each ventilation
- If synchronous chest movement does not occur:
    - Readjust the head position to ensure that the neck is adequately extended and the airway is not obstructed
    - Check that the mask makes an adequate seal
    - If necessary, clear the airway again by suctioning the mouth and nose
    - If in doubt gently insert an infant airway, making certain that it passes over the tongue to reach the pharynx
- If the lungs are particularly difficult to inflate and the chest does not move, increase the ventilation pressure to 40 mm H_2O

Oxygen
- Concentration: as high as possible
- Flow: 4-6 litres/minute

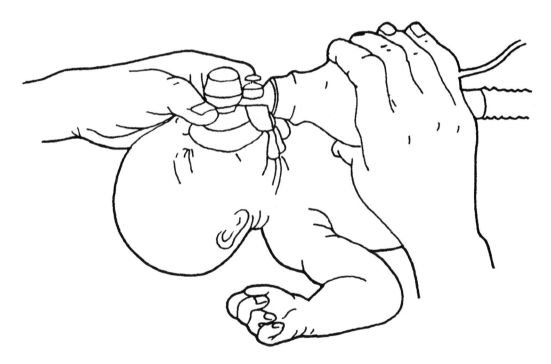

Figure 23-4 Holding the mask and squeezing the bag

- *If the heart rate is > 100 beats per minute and increasing, continue ventilating until spontaneous respiration is established*

    - Once the baby is being ventilated satisfactorily and the heart rate is adequate, reduce the ventilation pressure to 15-20 mm H_2O, provided adequate chest wall movement is occurring

- *If the heart rate is > 100 beats per minute and not increasing, proceed to intubate the baby*

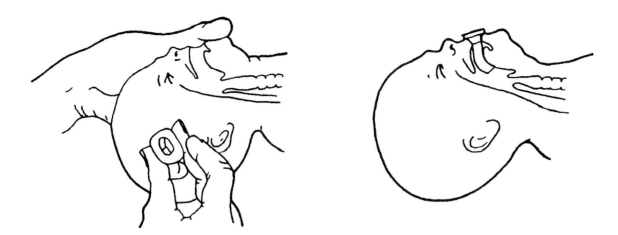

Figure 23-5 Insertion of a guedel airway

Tracheal intubation
- This usually requires a team of two in the pre-hospital situation:
    - The intubator
    - An assistant to pass over equipment as it is required, attach the ventilation bag when necessary and to monitor the baby's condition

Tracheal tube size
- This depends on the weight and gestation of the baby:

Tracheal tube sizes in neonates		
Size	Weight	Gestation
2.0-2.5	< 750 g	< 26 weeks
2.5-3.0	750-2000 g	26-34 weeks
3.0-3.5	> 2000g	34+ weeks

Figure 23-6 Tracheal tube sizes in neonates

Type of tube
- Plain uncuffed tubes are best (Coles tubes, which have a shoulder near the tip can cause glottic injury and are no longer recommended)
- A stylet may aid intubation, but it should be moulded to the same shape as the tube and should not protrude beyond the end of the tube

Laryngoscope
- A straight bladed laryngoscope is probably best for use in Immediate Care
- Blade size:
    - Small preterm baby: size 0
    - Term baby: size 1

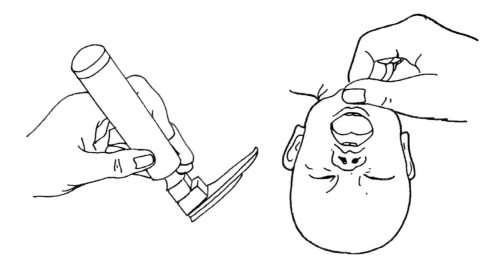

Figure 23-7 Neonatal intubation 1: Preparing to intubate

Method

- Place the baby on a flat surface, covered with a warm sheet or towel (if not already done)
- Position the baby, keeping the head in the midline, in a neutral position
- Before intubating, ventilate the baby several times with a bag and mask
- To intubate:
    - Gently insert a straight bladed laryngoscope into the mouth with the left hand, holding the lips apart with the fingers of the right hand
    - Guide the blade over the surface of the tongue, which is pushed to the left as the blade is advanced until the uvula is seen and continue until the epiglottis is visualised
    - The tip of the blade may be advanced by lifting the epiglottis gently

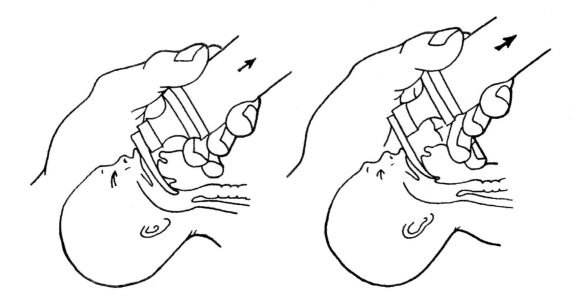

Figure 23-8 Neonatal intubation 2: Positioning the laryngoscope blade

- Use the laryngoscope blade to lift the tongue forward gently to view the larynx, by lifting the laryngoscope upwards and forwards in the direction of the handle (if the blade is inserted too far and enters the oesophagus, withdraw it gradually until the larynx is seen)

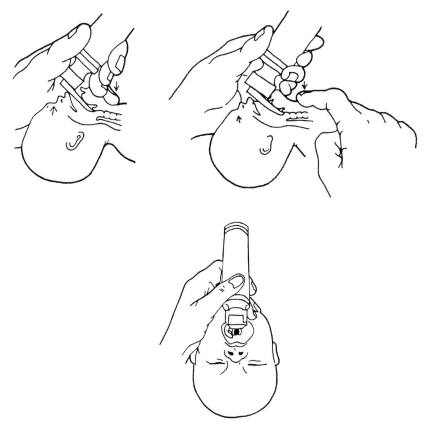

Figure 23-9 Neonatal intubation 3: Bringing the cords into view

- Clear the cords and posterior pharynx with a sucker
- Apply gentle pressure to the trachea with your fifth finger to bring the cords into view, ensuring that the trachea remains central
- Holding the tracheal tube in your right hand, pass it down from the right side of the mouth towards the larynx
- Insert the tip of the tube between the cords, and advance it until the mark is just above the cords
- Resting the right hand lightly on the baby's face, hold the tube firmly, and gently remove the laryngoscope (and stylet if one has been used)

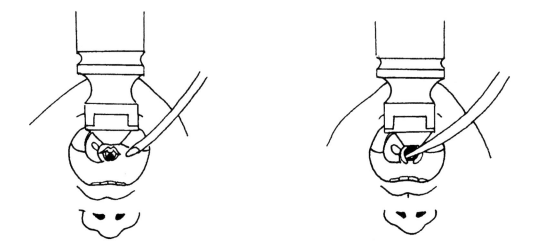

Figure 23-10 Neonatal intubation 4: Passing the tracheal tube

- Connect the oxygen tubing with blow-off valve set (at 345 kPa or 50 p.s.i.), to deliver 4-6 litres of oxygen per minute and connect it to a self inflating bag (usually 240 mL)
- Ventilate the baby five times at a rate of about 30 breaths per minute, then once the chest wall is moving adequately continue ventilating at a rate of 30-40 breaths per minute
- Watch the baby's chest for lung expansion, and monitor the pulse rate and colour.
- Auscultate the chest for breath sounds and check that air entry is equal
- Secure the tube with tape and check the position of the tube again
- Continue ventilation until the baby is breathing spontaneously
- Remove any secretions by suctioning down the tube
- Once the baby is breathing normally and has a good colour, normal pulse rate, good muscle tone and movement, allow it to breathe spontaneously through the tube, and if breathing is unobstructed, remove the tube during inspiration
- If ventilation has to be continued, secure the tracheal tube more securely prior to transportation

Problems
- Intubation should not take more than 30 seconds
    - If you are not successful within this time: withdraw the tube and ventilate the baby with a bag and mask before attempting intubation again
- If the baby remains cyanosed and the heart rate continues to decrease, consider the following:
    - If there are no breath sounds and no chest wall movement with inflation, the ventilation system has probably become disconnected:
        - Reconnect the system
    - If the heart rate is <60 beats/minute:
        - Administer external chest compressions followed by ventilation
    - If chest movement is poor with reduced breath sounds and abdominal distension after intubating; the tube is probably in the oesophagus:
        - Withdraw the tube and after ventilating the baby, try to intubate again
    - If breath sounds and chest movement are not symmetrical: the tracheal tube is probably in one of the main bronchi:
        - Withdraw the tube slowly, listening in the axilla for the restoration of equal air entry
    - If the baby's condition does not improve and chest movement remains inadequate:
        - Increase the inflation pressure

External chest compression
- Administer external chest compression if the baby has a bradycardia (<60 beats per minute), or the pulse rate is decreasing despite adequate ventilation or if the pulse is absent or is difficult to palpate. There is usually associated pallor
- The purpose of chest compressions in neonatal resuscitation is to deliver oxygenated blood to the coronary arteries to improve cardiac performance
- If successful, there should be an almost immediate improvement in the fetal heart rate
- Rate: about 120 compressions/minute with equal compression and relaxation times and a ratio of 3 compressions: 1 ventilation
- Check the spontaneous heart rate after 30 seconds:
    - If there is no response, in spite of good lung inflations and chest compressions; check the airway
- Continue with chest compressions, checking the spontaneous heart rate about every 2 minutes until:
    - The heart rate reaches 80 bpm and is increasing

Method 1 (preferred method)
- Grasp the baby's chest with both hands, placing the thumbs over the junction of the middle and lower third of the sternum
- Apply pressure to the sternum by pressing down with both thumbs, depressing it about 2-3 cms in a term baby

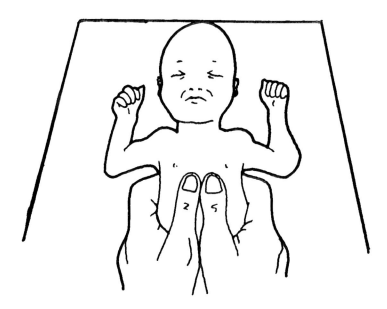

Figure 23-11 External chest compressions: method 1

Method 2 (less effective, but more commonly used as thumbs become fatigued quickly with method 1)
- Place two fingers 1-2 cm below a line joining the nipples *or* 1-2 cm above the xiphisternum
- One hand may support the back, while the other applies rhythmic sternal pressure

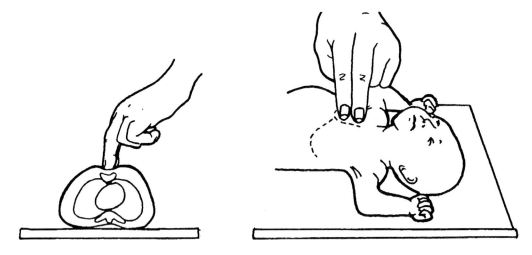

Figure 23-12 External chest compressions: method 2

Note: 1. During the relaxation phase, do not lift the fingers or thumbs off the chest
         2. Damage to the liver and other viscera, and fractured ribs may be caused:
             - If the finger or thumb positions are too low over the sternum or liver
             - If the compressions are too forceful

Co-ordination of inflations and chest compressions
- Following the initial ventilations, the ratio of ventilations to compressions should be 1:3

Naloxone (see chapter on Pain management)
- Considered naloxone if the baby's mother has had Pethidine or other opiates administered during labour
- The intramuscular route is preferred (as effective as the intravenous route, but the effect lasts longer)
- If naloxone is administered, remember to reassess the baby at regular intervals as the half life of opiates may exceed that of naloxone

Meconium
- If meconium is unexpectedly present as the head is delivered:
  - Suck out the mouth before delivery
- Dry and warm the baby
- Suck out the mouth and nose again
- Administer oxygen
- If the meconium was very thick, inspect the oropharynx and vocal cords under direct vision:
  - If meconium is present in small quantities in the trachea:
    - Intubate and apply suction
    - Continue to aspirate until the meconium is cleared, unless there is a bradycardia
    - If the tube becomes blocked, replace it rapidly with another

- *If the baby responds to resuscitation*
  - Transfer to hospital for admission to the neonatal unit

- *If the baby fails to respond to attempts at resuscitation*
  - Continue with resuscitation for at least 20 minutes
  - If the baby has a good pulse rate, but is not making any respiratory effort, continue with ventilation, and transfer to hospital for admission to the neonatal unit

Recording information
- Full details of the resuscitation should be kept, if possible without delaying the procedure, including:
  - The time taken from birth to the baby's first gasp and the onset of regular respiration and heart rate
  - The method of and response to resuscitation
  - Time of intubation and duration of ventilation

APGAR score
- The APGAR scoring system is a useful, commonly used method of assessing the condition of the baby at 1 and 5 minutes and gives information about the degree and severity of apnoea and the response to resuscitation
- Resuscitation should not be delayed to assess the score formally, but the condition of the baby noted mentally and recorded later

Apgar Score	0	1	3
Heart rate	Absent	< 100	> 100
Respiratory effort	Absent	Weak, or shallow cry	Good
Muscle tone	Limp	Some flexion	Active, well flexed
Reflex/ Irritability	None	Grimace	Cry
Colour	Pale/ Blue	Body pink Extremities blue	Pink

Figure 23-13 Apgar score

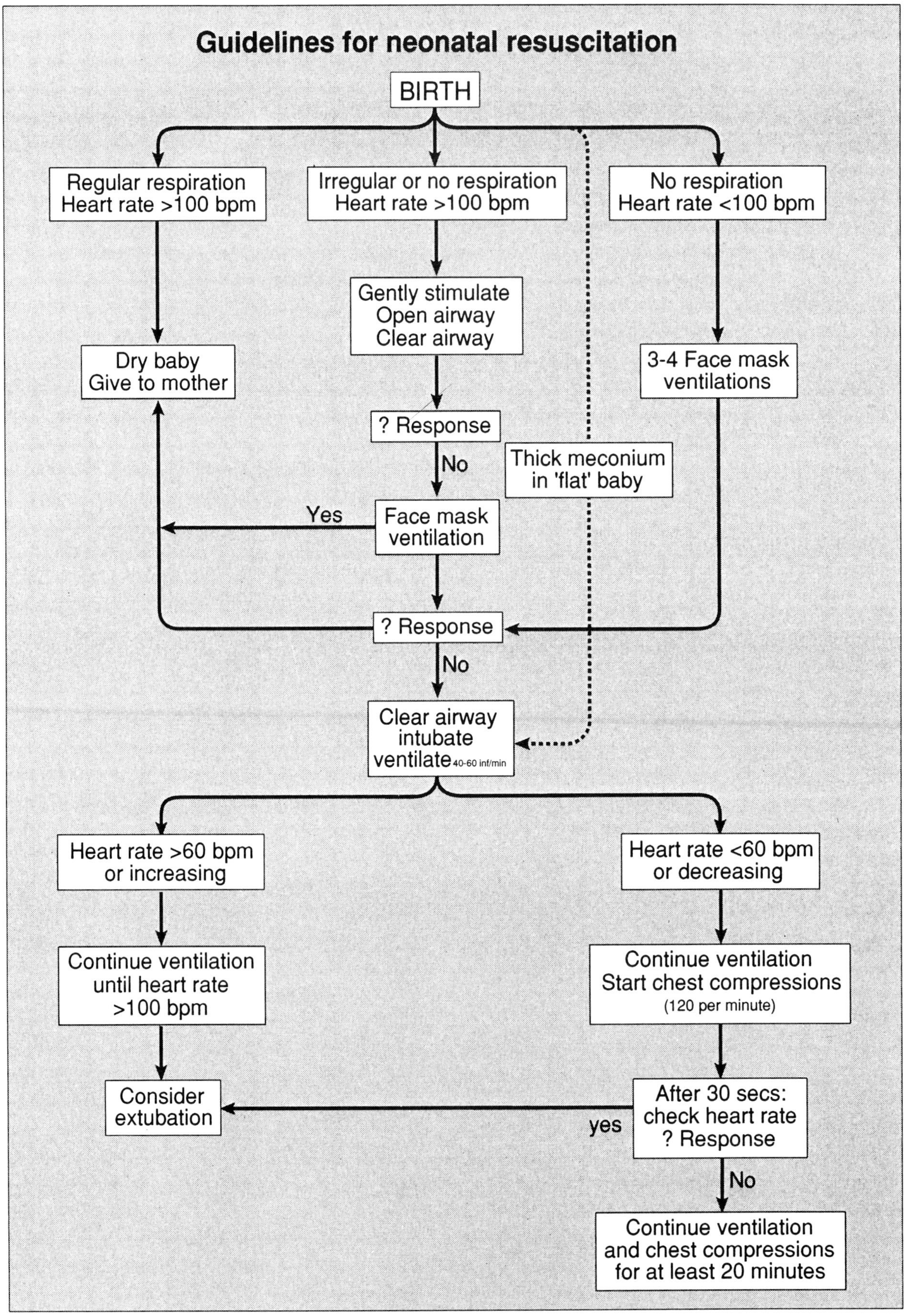

Guidelines for neonatal resuscitation

BIRTH

| Regular respiration Heart rate >100 bpm | Irregular or no respiration Heart rate >100 bpm | No respiration Heart rate <100 bpm |

Gently stimulate
Open airway
Clear airway

Dry baby
Give to mother

3-4 Face mask
ventilations

? Response

No

Thick meconium
in 'flat' baby

Yes — Face mask
ventilation

? Response

No

Clear airway
intubate
ventilate 40-60 inf/min

| Heart rate >60 bpm or increasing | Heart rate <60 bpm or decreasing |

Continue ventilation
until heart rate
>100 bpm

Continue ventilation
Start chest compressions
(120 per minute)

Consider
extubation

After 30 secs:
check heart rate
? Response

yes

No

Continue ventilation
and chest compressions
for at least 20 minutes

Figure 23-14 Algorithm for neonatal resuscitation
(copyright of the European Resuscitation Council, reproduced with permission)

24

Paediatric care

Paediatric resuscitation

Introduction

- Large numbers of fit and healthy children die every year as a result of trauma and a smaller, but nonetheless significant number die as a result of serious, but transient illnesses
- The importance of the efficient and effective practice of Immediate Care skills on children has been under-rated in the past, but this has now been recognised and the differences in the management of children and adults requiring Immediate Care defined, so that appropriate training and expertise can be developed for the benefit of these children

Definitions: An infant is a child under the age of one year
A child is aged between 1 and 8 years of age
Adolescents are children aged 8 years of age and over, and should still be treated as children, but may require different techniques for resuscitation

Life threatening problems in children

Age
- The type of problem encountered in children depends on their age:
    - Infants prior to toddling:
        - Mostly respiratory disease
        - Few accidents (including non-accidental injury)
    - Younger children (up to 8 years): liable to injury: adventurous and relatively oblivious of danger
        - Burns
        - RTAs
        - Ingestion of foreign bodies/dangerous chemicals
    - Older children/adolescents (8 years and over):
        - Accidents
        - Respiratory disease

Non-accidents/life threatening illness in children

Incidence
- Hypoxia due to upper airway obstruction (infection or foreign body, asthma and near drowning) is the commonest cause of cardiac arrest in infants and children

Aetiology
- Sudden infant death syndrome "SIDS"
- Gastroenteritis: hypovolaemic shock
- Congenital heart disease
- Septicaemia
- Laryngotracheal bronchitis
- Asthma
- Poisoning

Accidents/trauma in children

Incidence
- Accidents account for:
  - 11% of all deaths in children aged 28 days to 14 years
  - 32% of all deaths in children aged 5-14 years
- Trauma is:
  - The second most common cause of death in children aged 1-4 yrs (92/million population/annum)
  - The most common cause of death in children aged 5-14 yrs (86 per million population per annum)
- Accidents involving children account for one fifth of all emergency hospital admissions:
  - Slightly more boys are admitted to hospital than girls

Aetiology (age)
- 0-1 year: - Choking/suffocation
              - Burns
              - Drowning
              - Falls
- 1-4 years: - Road traffic accidents (as vehicle occupants)
              - Burns
              - Drowning
              - Falls
- 5-14 years: - Road traffic accidents (as vehicle occupants or pedestrians)
              - Bicycling accidents
              - Burns
              - Drowning

Types of injury/accident
- Burns/scalds (most common)
- Falls (next most common)
- Drowning
- Smoke inhalation
- Non accidental injury (NAI)
- Electric shock
- Poisoning/solvent abuse
- Road traffic accidents

Domestic accidents
- The 0-14 year age group accounts for 19% of all home accidents
- 72% occur in children between the ages of 1 month and 4 years
- The most dangerous rooms are:
  - The living room: 35%
  - The hall: 14%
  - The kitchen: 12%

Road traffic accidents
- Pedal cyclists: 26% of all pedal cycle accidents involve children
- Pedestrians: 17% of all pedestrian accidents occur in the 4-14 year age group
- Boys are injured in 70% of all RTAs involving children

Pathophysiology
- There are many differences between children and adults, in particular:

Anatomical differences between children and adults
- Greater relative surface area with less subcutaneous fat: greater heat loss
- Relatively large head for body size, with a protuberant occiput
- Shorter narrower airway:
    - Small oral cavity but a relatively large tongue which fills the oropharynx
    - Large angle of the jaw:
        - Infants: 140°
        - Adults: 120°
    - The epiglottis is more U-shaped than in adults
    - The larynx is conical and is situated further forward and higher up the neck in children:
        - The glottis is situated at the level of C3 in infants, C5-6 in adults
        - The cricoid ring is the narrowest part of the airway
        - Relatively little laryngeal swelling may result in airway obstruction
    - The trachea is relatively short:
        - Newborn: 4-5 cm
        - At 18 months: 7-8 cm
- Relatively small blood volume and small veins

Physiological differences between children and adults
- Small infants are obligatory nose breathers, because of the large tongue filling the oropharynx
- Children have a relatively high metabolic rate and a high oxygen consumption, with a reduced functional residual capacity and a high closing capacity resulting in a (physiological) right to left shunt
- In children, most breathing is diaphragmatic, and as children are unable to increase their tidal volume, they increase their respiratory rate in response to hypoxia
- Young children have soft ribs, which deform easily. If they breathe rapidly and deeply, e.g. in response to hypoxia, they develop intercostal muscle recession and use their accessory muscles (sternomastoids)
- The pulse rate increases in response to hypoxia and hypercapnia
- Relatively small volumes of blood or fluid loss can result in hypovolaemic shock due to the child's small total blood volume. Initial compensation, however is very effective and children tolerate fluid loss very well, before going into severe shock. Careful estimation of blood or fluid loss is therefore required, together with careful haemodynamic monitoring if over or under transfusion is to be avoided
- Liable to dehydration

Biochemistry
- Infants and small children are liable to hypoglycaemia due to their relatively small glycogen stores

Pharmacology
- Infants and children metabolise, distribute and react to drugs in a different way from adults, the difference depending on the drug

Pathophysiology

Cardiac arrest
- Usually occurs secondary to hypoxia/hypoxaemia
- The usual arrhythmia is asystole preceded by bradycardia

Trauma
- Because children are small, multisystem injury is common
- Major blunt injury usually results in thoracic and abdominal injury, often without bony injury (soft flexible bones)
- Penetrating injury is unusual
- Head injury is more common: children have a relatively large head
- Significant internal injury may occur in the absence of bony injury

Burns
- Relatively small burns may result in hypovolaemic shock

Normal values for vital signs in children at rest

Age	Heart rate (beats/minute)	Systolic blood Pressure (mmHg)	Respiratory rate (breaths/min)	Blood volume (mL/kg)
< 1 year	110-160	70-90	30-40	80-85
2-5 years	95-140	80-100	20-30	75-80
5-12 years	80-120	90-110	20-25	65-70
> 12 years	60-100	100-120	15-20	65-70

Figure 24-1 Normal values for the vital signs in children

PRACTICAL POINT: Systolic blood pressure in children = (age x2) + 80 mmHg)

Basic paediatric life support: care of the unconscious child

General management

- Follow the same basic guidelines as adults:
    - Ensure safety of rescuer and child
    - Assess and manage:
        - **Airway** (with cervical spine stabilisation in trauma)
        - **Breathing**
        - **Circulation** with haemorrhage control
        - **Disability** (neurological assessment and management)
        - **Exposure** (trauma only) with control of the environment

Assessment of the scene
- Ensure the safety of child and rescuer:
  - Look for out for any hazards, problems, etc.

Check the child's responsiveness
- Gently try to stimulate/awaken the child, and in a loud voice ask 'Are you all right?'

Note: Babies and anyone with a suspected cervical spine injury should *not* be shaken

- **If there is a response:**
  - Leave the child in the position in which they were found (provided that they are not in any further danger)
  - Keep warm as children are very prone to heat loss:
    - Use a woollen blanket, etc. with a warming device, e.g. a Hot pack, if appropriate, but beware of causing burns
  - Check their condition and get help if needed
  - Reassess regularly and monitor the pulse and respirations

- **If there is no response:**
  - Shout for help
  - Open the airway (see below)

Airway care
- Open the airway

Method
- If possible with the child in the position in which you found them, place your hand on the child's forehead and gently tilt the head:
  - Apply gentle neck extension, but be careful not to hyperextend it as this may kink the trachea and obstruct the airway
  - In small infants a support positioned under the shoulders may be helpful
- Lift the chin, with your finger tips under the tip of the mandible. Do not press on the soft tissue under the chin with your fingers as you may push the tongue into the airway, obstructing it
- If you have any difficulty, carefully turn the child onto their back, and open the airway as described above
- If an injury to the cervical spine is a possibility:
  - Do not apply head tilt, but try the jaw thrust method of opening the airway

Note: 1. Infants are obligatory nose breathers, and care should be taken to check and maintain the patency of the nasal passages
   2. Jaw thrust is nearly always successful in clearing the airway in children if head tilt, chin lift are not
   3. It may be necessary to try various positions before satisfactory airway control can be achieved

Breathing (ventilation)

- Check for airway patency by:
  - *Looking* for chest and abdominal movement
  - *Listening* for air movement
  - *Feeling* for the child's breath on your cheek or the back of your hand from their nose or mouth
- Look, listen and feel for evidence of breathing for up to 10 seconds before deciding that breathing is absent

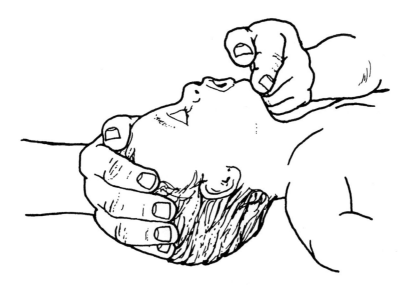

Figure 24-2 Airway maintenance: head tilt, chin lift

- **If the child is breathing:**
  - Turn the child onto their side
  - Check that the child is still breathing and that their ventilatory effort is normal by looking for normal chest expansion or abdominal movement
  - If there is intercostal recession, see-saw movement of the chest and abdomen (indicating residual airway obstruction) *or* flaring of the nares in small children

- **If the child is not breathing:**
  - Carefully remove any obvious airway obstruction
  - Give up to 5 expired air ventilations/effective rescue breaths, each of which makes the chest rise and fall

Expired air ventilation

Method

Infants
  - Hold the airway open:
    - Head tilt and chin lift
  - Take a deep breath and cover the infant's mouth and nose with your mouth, making certain that you have a good seal.
  - Blow out gently over 1-1½ seconds, watching to make certain that the infant's chest rises visibly, indicating lung expansion
  - Maintaining head tilt and chin lift, take your mouth away from the infant and watch for the chest to fall, indicating expiration as the air comes out
  - Repeat this sequence and administer up to five breaths (a minimum of 2 effective expired air ventilations/rescue breaths must be given)

  Note: If you have difficulty covering the infant's mouth and nose with your mouth, just cover the nose, and gently hold the mouth closed or seal it with your mouth

Children
- Hold the airway open:
    - Head tilt and chin lift
- Pinch the soft part of the nose closed with the index finger and thumb of the hand holding the forehead
- Open the mouth a little with the other hand, keeping the chin up
- Take a deep breath and cover the child's mouth with your mouth, making certain that you have a good seal
- Blow out gently over 1-1½ seconds, watching to make certain that the child's chest rises visibly, indicating lung expansion (when you stop blowing out)
- Maintaining head tilt and chin lift, take your mouth away from the child and watch for the chest to fall, indicating expiration as the air comes out
- Repeat this sequence and administer up to five breaths (a minimum of 2 effective expired air ventilations/rescue breaths must be given)

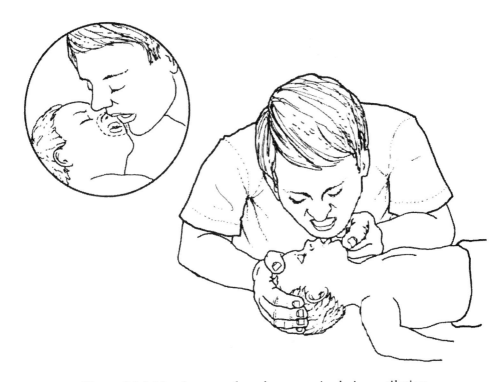

Figure 24-3 Mouth to mouth and nose expired air ventilation

- If the child requires ventilation only, adjust the rate to the size of the child:
    - Neonates: 20-30 breaths per minute
    - Children: 15-20 breaths per minute
    - Adolescents: 10-15 breaths per minute
- Volume:
    - This can be adjusted by watching the child's chest movement
- Any increase in ventilation should be achieved by raising the rate of delivery of expired air ventilations rather than the airway pressure and tidal volume, which can cause a pneumothorax
- Gastric distension:
    - This may occur resulting in splinting of the diaphragm
    - If gastric distension does occur, consider decompressing the stomach by applying manual pressure to the upper abdomen, with the child in the lateral position (beware of causing regurgitation and aspiration of gastric contents!)

- If you have difficulty achieving an effective breath, the airway may be obstructed:
    - Re-check the child's mouth and remove any obstruction
    - Re-check that there is adequate head tilt and chin lift, and that the neck is not over extended
    - Make up to five attempts to achieve 2 effective breaths
    - If still unsuccessful, manage as airway obstruction (see below)

Circulation

- **Look for signs of life or evidence of a circulation** (taking no more than 10 seconds to do so)
    - Look for any movement including swallowing or breathing (more than just an occasional gasp)
    - Check the pulse in a large artery:
        - Infants under one year old:
            - Feel for the brachial artery on the inner aspect of the upper arm
        - Children over one year old:
            - Feel for the carotid artery in the neck
        - Assess the volume, rate and rhythm
- If these pulses are absent, try the femoral or axillary pulses or monitor the apex beat

Note: 1. The right axillary artery is a common site for cardiac catheterisation, and operation scars should be looked for there (especially if there is an absent pulse)
2. Look for surgical scars in the chest or abdomen: may indicate congenital heart disease

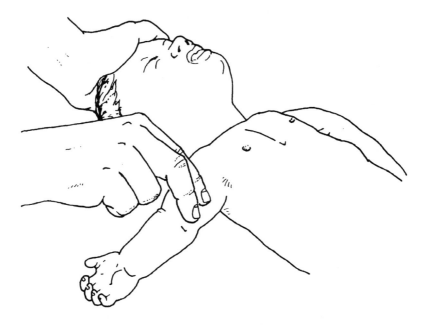

Figure 24-4 Monitoring the brachial pulse in an infant

- **If you are confident that you can detect signs of life or a pulse within 10 seconds**
    - Continue with expired air ventilations/rescue breathing, if necessary, until the child starts breathing effectively by itself
    - If the child remains unconscious:
        - Turn them onto their side (in the recovery position)

- **If there are no signs of life or a circulation, or if you are at all unsure**
  (or in infants, if the pulse is very slow - less than one beat per second/60 beats per minute)
    - Start chest compressions
    - Combine expired air ventilations/rescue breathing with chest compressions

External chest compression

Method

Infants
- Locate the sternum, and place the tips of two fingers, one finger's breadth below an imaginary line joining the infant's nipples
- Using the tips of two fingers, press down on the sternum and depress it about one third to one half of the depth of the infant's chest
- Release the pressure, then repeat chest compressions at a rate of about 100 compressions per minute (slightly less than 2 compressions per second)
- After 5 compressions:
    - Tilt the head, lift the chin and give 1 effective breath
- Place your fingers back on the sternum in the correct position and give 5 further chest compressions
- Continue giving chest compressions and expired air ventilations in a ratio of 5:1

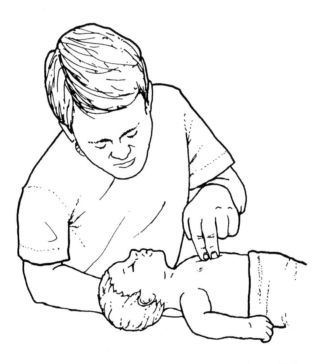

Figure 24-5 External chest compressions: Infants

Children
- Locate and place the heel of one hand over the lower half of the sternum, making certain that you do not compress the upper abdomen
- Lift the fingers to ensure that pressure is not applied over the child's ribs
- Position yourself vertically above the child's chest, and with your arms held straight, apply firm, but gentle downward pressure over the lower sternum and depress it about one third to one half of the depth of the child's chest
- Release the pressure, then repeat chest compressions at a rate of about 100 compressions per minute (slightly less than 2 compressions per second)
- After 5 compressions:
    - Tilt the head, lift the chin and give 1 effective breath
- Place your fingers back on the sternum in the correct position and give 5 further chest compressions
- Continue giving chest compressions and expired air ventilations in a ratio of 5:1

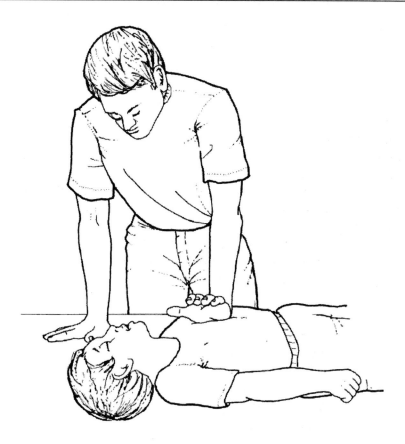

Figure 24-6 External chest compressions: Children

Children over 8 years old

- In children over the age of 8 years, it may be necessary to use the adult two handed method of chest compression to achieve an adequate depth of compression
- Locate the xiphisternal notch by running the index and middle fingers of one hand up the lower margins of the rib cage and find the point where the ribs join
- With your middle finger over the xiphisternum, place the tip of your index finger on the sternum above
- Place the heel of your other hand on the upper sternum, and slide it down towards the first hand until it touches the index finger. This should be the middle of the lower half of the sternum
- The heel of the first hand should then be placed on top of the other hand and the fingers interlocked, so that pressure is not applied over the ribs
- Lean well over the patient, so that your shoulders are positioned directly above the hands, with the arms held straight at the elbows
- Press down firmly and vertically on the sternum using just enough force to depress it 1½-2 inches (4-5 centimetres) without allowing your elbows to flex. The movement should be well controlled. Erratic or violent action is dangerous and may cause unnecessary injury to the patient
- Release the pressure, still keeping your hand on the patient, and repeat the procedure at a rate of approximately 100 compressions per minute
- Combine ventilations and chest compressions in a ratio of 15:2

Note: Compressions:
- Should be smooth.
- The compressive phase should last at least half the cycle

Ventilation:
- It is very important that adequate ventilation be achieved
- Flexibility:
  - Rescuer(s) should adapt his/their technique to achieve an adequate pulse and ventilation

- **Continue resuscitation until:**
  - The victim shows signs of life (spontaneous respiration, normal pulse)
  - Qualified help arrives
  - You become exhausted

When to go for help/assistance
- It is vital for rescuers to get help as soon as possible when a child collapses:
  - When more than one rescuer is available, one should start resuscitation, while another goes for help
  - If only one rescuer is present he should perform resuscitation for about **1 minute** before leaving the patient to go and get help. It may be possible to take infants or small children with you

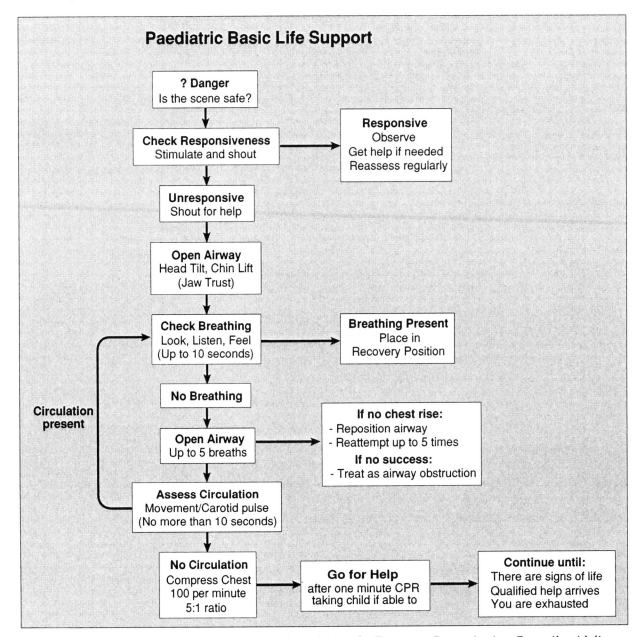

Figure 24-7 Paediatric Basic Life Support adapted from the European Resuscitation Council guidelines

Recovery position
- An unconscious child who has a clear airway, and is breathing spontaneously, should be turned on their side into the recovery position
- This prevents the tongue from falling backwards and obstructing the airway, and reduces the risk of inhalation of stomach contents
- There are a number of recovery positions, each of which have their own protagonists
- The important principles to be followed are:
    - The child should be in as near a true lateral position as possible, with the mouth dependent to allow free drainage of fluids from the mouth
    - The position should be stable. An infant may need to be supported by a small pillow or rolled up blanket placed behind their back to keep it in the correct position
    - A position that causes there to be any pressure on the chest, impairing breathing, should be avoided
    - It should be possible to turn the child onto their side, and then back again onto their back, easily and safely, especially if there is a possibility that they may have injured their cervical spine
    - The position should allow good access to the child for observing their general condition, and in particular should allow access to their airway

Airway obstruction
- Airway obstruction may be indicated by:
    - Inability to ventilate the child during basic life support (see above)
    - Increased respiratory effort
    - Choking or stridor (harsh high pitched inspiratory noise):
        - Usually due to an obstruction outside the thoracic cavity, i.e. in the larynx

Note: Expiratory noise (wheeze):
- Usually due to a fixed airway obstruction or a problem in the chest, e.g. asthma

Grunting (a noise at the end of expiration):
- Usually caused by a cardiac problem

Aetiology/management
- Tongue falling back into pharynx
    Aetiology:
    - Unconsciousness
    Management:
    - Elevate the jaw further and/or change the child's position (only use an airway in the deeply unconscious child)
- Foreign body ingestion
    Aetiology:
    - This may be blood, loose teeth, food, a toy or vomit
    Management:
    - Small objects: encourage to cough, suctioning
    - Large objects: *see management of choking (below)*
- Tissue swelling
    Aetiology:
    - Croup
    - Laryngotracheobronchitis (LTB)
    - Epiglottitis
    History:
    - This should be obtained from the parents, if possible, and may be useful in helping to distinguish between tissue swelling (infection), foreign body ingestion, asthma and other conditions
    Management: See chapter on Medical Emergencies

Foreign body ingestion/choking

Management
- If the child is breathing spontaneously, encourage them to clear the obstruction themself by coughing.
- Intervention is only necessary if these attempts are clearly unsuccessful and breathing is inadequate
- The technique used depends on the age of the child:
    - Try to use a technique which causes a sudden increase in pressure within the chest cavity (an artificial cough)

Finger sweeps
- This is *not recommended, except for removal of visible large objects* as it may cause:
    - Further impaction of the foreign body
    - Damage to the upper airway, with resultant oedema and sometimes haemorrhage, and may even precipitate acute laryngeal spasm

- **Administer 5 back blows:**

Back blows
- This should be attempted first

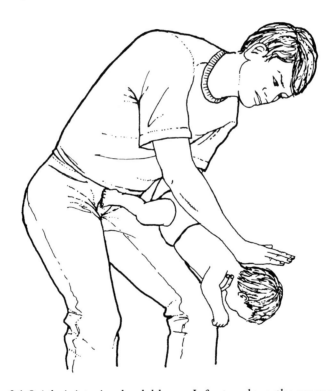

Figure 24-8 Administering back blows: Infants: along the rescuer's thigh

Method
- Position the child prone (face down), with the head lower than the trunk
- The method used depends on the child's size:
    - In infants this may be along the rescuer's thigh
    - In older children this may be across the rescuer's thighs/knees
- Deliver five firm blows to the middle of the back, between the shoulder blades initially

- **If this is unsuccessful, administer 5 chest thrusts:**

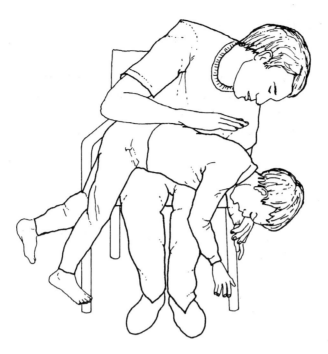

Figure 24-9 Administering back blows: Children: across rescuer's thighs/knees

Chest thrusts
- Turn the child into the supine position (lying on their back)
- The technique used is similar to that used for chest compressions:
  - Apply pressure at the same point on the sternum as for chest compressions, i.e. one finger's breadth below the nipple line
  - Chest thrusts should be sharper and more vigorous than chest compressions, and be performed at a rate of about 20 per minute

- **Check mouth**:
  - Check the mouth for a foreign body, which by then may have become visible, and extract it

- **Open airway**:
  - Open the airway using head tilt, chin lift (or jaw thrust)
  - Reassess breathing

- **If the child is breathing**:
  - Turn the child onto their side
  - Check that the child continues to breathe

- **If the child is not breathing**:
  - Administer up to 5 expired air ventilations, each of which makes the chest rise and fall
  - The airway may be apnoeic or the airway only partially cleared; in either case the rescuer may be able to achieve effective ventilation at this stage

- **If the airway remains obstructed, repeat the sequence:**

Infants
- Perform cycles of 5 back blows and chest thrusts
- Repeat the cycles until the airway is cleared or the child breathes spontaneously

Children
- Repeat the cycle as above, but substitute 5 abdominal thrusts for chest thrusts in alternate cycles

    Abdominal thrusts
    - Give five sharp abdominal thrusts upwards towards the diaphragm, taking care not to use excessive force
    - If the child is conscious; use the upright position
    - If the child is unconscious; lay them on their back with the heel of one hand placed in the middle the upper abdomen

- Alternate chest thrusts with abdominal thrusts in subsequent cycles

Note: Abdominal thrusts should not be performed on infants (under the age of one) as they may cause severe intra-abdominal injury including rupture of the liver and spleen

- **If there is still no improvement**:
    - Repeat the above cycle, but more forcibly
    - Consider advanced airways management (see below):
        - Laryngoscopy: (*only* for experts, as instrumentation may make a bad situation worse)
        - Cricothyrotomy
        - Ventilation

CAUTION: - If one foreign body is present, there may be another!

Tissue swelling

Management
- Steam or humidity may be beneficial, especially in croup
- Oxygen
- Consider nebulised budesonide or epinephrine
- If there is no improvement:
    - Administer expired air ventilation
    - Consider:
        - Laryngoscopy
        - Cricothyrotomy
- Treat the cause: See chapter on Medical Emergencies

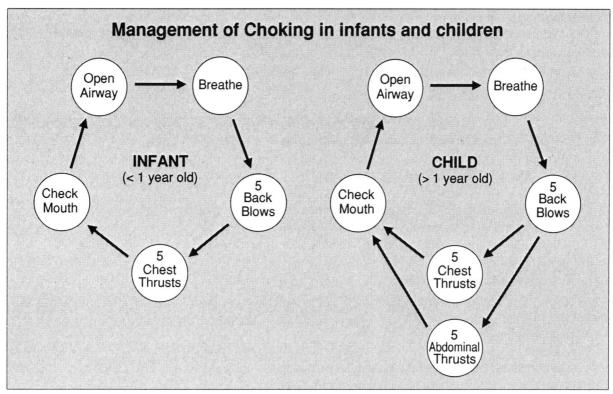

Figure 24-10 Algorithm for the management of choking in infants and children (copyright of the European Resuscitation Council, reproduced with permission)

Airway care

Oropharyngeal airway (Guedel)

Indications
- If the child is unconscious and has *no* gag reflex

Size
- 000-4 depending on the size of the child
- The length is best estimated by measuring the distance from the centre of the mouth to the angle of the jaw
- Too small an airway may not overcome the obstruction of the tongue and may force it backwards blocking the airway
- Too large an airway may damage the posterior pharyngeal wall when inserted

Insertion
- Insert the device by sliding it back over the tongue without rotating it

Complications
- If used inappropriately, it may precipitate choking, laryngospasm and vomiting

Nasopharyngeal airway
- Often a very useful and simple device to use in children
- Tolerated better than oropharyngeal airways in the conscious or semi-comatose child

Size
- The largest size which passes easily through the external nares

PRACTICAL POINT: A tracheal tube cut short, lubricated well, with a safety pin through the proximal end to prevent it slipping into the nose, makes a good substitute for a nasopharyngeal airway

Tracheal intubation in children
- This is the most reliable method of maintaining an adequate airway and ventilating infants and children
- As an approximate guide:
  - Tracheal tubes: *Size:* $\underline{\text{Age of child}} + 4$ mm   (*this gives a size 0.5 mm smaller than that*

    4*usually required for routine intubations*)

    Length: $\underline{\text{Age of child}} + 12$ cm

    2

  - Croup:
    - Use a smaller tracheal tube than usual (even so, intubation may be very difficult)
- Epiglottitis:
  - Intubation for epiglottitis should only be attempted by the experienced intubator in a hospital setting with all the necessary equipment available
  - In the pre-hospital situation; cricothyrotomy is to be preferred and may be life saving
- laryngoscopes:
  - A straight blade is used in children

Method: see chapter on Neonatal care
- After insertion:
  - Listen to the chest to ensure that air entry is adequate and equal on both sides and that the tube has not inadvertently entered the right main bronchus
  - Secure the tube and attachments firmly with tape

Tracheal tube sizes for children

Age	Internal diameter of T tube (mm)	Length (cm) Oral	Nasal	Suction catheter (FG)
Premature	2.5-3.0	11.0	13.5	6
Newborn-8 weeks	3.5	12.0	14.0	8
2-24 months	4.0	13.0	15.0	8
2 years	4.5	14.0	16.0	8
4 years	5.0	15.0	17.0	10
6 years	5.5	17.0	19.0	10
8 years	6.0	19.0	21.0	10
10 years	6.5	20.0	22.0	10
12 years	7.0	21.0	22.0	10
14 years	7.5	22.0	23.0	10
16 years	8.0	23.0	24.0	12

Figure 24-11 Tracheal tube sizes for children

Airway obstruction

Cricothyrotomy
- This is a difficult and dangerous technique in children
- It should be only considered in cases of severe upper airways obstruction by, e.g. foreign body maxillofacial trauma, severe laryngeal oedema, where all other methods have failed
- Needle cricothyrotomy (a 14G intravenous cannula is preferred)
- Difficult to perform in very small children and can result in permanent tracheal damage

Method: See chapter on Airway Care

Breathing (ventilation) care

Oxygen therapy
- Very important in children owing to their high oxygen consumption. Their physiological right to left shunt may be exacerbated by, e.g. thoracic injury or diaphragmatic splinting due to intra-abdominal injury
- Supplemental oxygen may be delivered by:
    - Facemask
    - Nasal cannulae (very useful for infants)
    - Tracheal tube

Ventilation
- If the child is not breathing, this must be achieved either by:
    - A resuscitation bag valve mask (preferably with an oropharyngeal or nasopharyngeal airway)
    - A resuscitation bag valve and tracheal tube

Masks
- Soft clear circular plastic masks are recommended

Resuscitation bags
- Sizes:
    - Infant: 250 mL
    - Child: 500 mL
    - Adult: 1600 mL
- Should:
    - Be self inflating
    - Have a pressure limiting valve (40 cms H_2O)
    - Have an oxygen filled reservoir fitted to increase the inspired oxygen concentration

Note: Automatic ventilators are *not* recommended for use with children

Circulation care
- Children with hypovolaemia or fluid loss require rapid active management

Incidence
- The commonest cause of shock in infants and children is hypovolaemia due to:
    - Haemorrhage
    - Diarrhoea and/or vomiting
    - Burns and peritonitis
- Other causes include septicaemia, anaphylaxis, cardiac problems, major chest injuries and poisoning

Aetiology
- Hypovolaemia occurs as a result of the loss of circulating blood volume from whatever cause

Pathophysiology
- What may be a relatively insignificant blood loss in an adult, may be highly significant in infants and children because of their smaller circulating blood volume
- The increased physiological reserve of children's circulation when compared to adults means that the vital signs may be only slightly abnormal in spite of significant blood loss
- In children, shock may be divided into three categories depending on its severity:

Compensated shock (Phase 1)
- The sympathetic reflexes maintain blood pressure and divert the blood supply to the essential organs
- The kidneys conserve water and salt and interstitial fluid is reabsorbed from the gastrointestinal tract
- The child may be pale, mildly agitated and tachycardic with a normal or slightly prolonged capillary refill time, but a normal systolic blood pressure and a normal or slightly raised diastolic blood pressure

Uncompensated shock (Phase 2)
- As the severity of shock increases, the compensatory mechanisms begin to fail, resulting in increasingly poor tissue perfusion in those tissues with a relatively poor blood supply
- The child will have a falling blood pressure, a prolonged capillary refill time, a tachycardia with pale cold extremeties, acidotic breathing, a reduced/absent urine output and a reduced level of consciousness
- In children this is a pre-terminal stage and must be managed very aggressively

Irreversible shock (Phase 3)
- In this phase irreversible vital organ failure has already occurred, and death will inevitably ensue in spite of adequate restoration of the circulation

Assessment
- Monitor the child's:
    - Heart rate and rhythm and the presence or absence of the peripheral pulses and their volume
    - Skin perfusion, capillary refill time, colour and mottling
    - Respiratory rate
    - Blood pressure ideally taken with a paediatric cuff with a width 2/3 length of child's upper arm
    - Mental state: AVPU, agitation, confusion, drowsiness
    - Temperature: taken with a rectal or axillary thermometer or thermocouple and blood glucose

PRACTICAL POINT: Except small infants an adult cuff, folded over, is sufficient for taking the blood pressure

Blood volume
- The circulating blood volume in infants and children is 80 mL/kg

Management

Intravenous cannulation in children
- Access to the circulation for administration of drugs and fluid replacement is difficult in children

Peripheral venous cannulation
- In practice, any visible vein may be cannulated
- The peripheral veins are likely to be shut down, although more central veins, such as the femoral and external jugular are often dilated and may be easier to cannulate
- If peripheral venous cannulation cannot be achieved within two or three minutes, another route for venous access needs to be established

Classification of hypovolaemic shock in children

	Compensated	Uncompensated	Pre-terminal (? irreversible)
Blood loss (%)	<25%	25-40%	>40%
Pulse rate	raised 10-20%	tachycardia >150/min	tachycardia/ bradycardia
Systolic BP	normal	normal or falling	plummeting
Pulse volume	normal/reduced	reduced +	reduced ++
Capillary refill	normal/increased	increased +	increased ++
Respiratory rate	tachypnoea +	tachypnoea ++	sighing respiration
Extremeties/skin	cool, pale	cold, mottled	cold, deathly pale
Mental state	mild agitation	lethargic, uncooperative	reacts only to pain or unresponsive

Figure 24-12 Classification of hypovolaemic shock in children

Central venous cannulation
- True central veins, i.e. the internal jugular and subclavian veins are probably the best routes for drug administration, although they are not of proven value in infants
- Central venous cannulation has the disadvantage that it is overly difficult to perform in children, and should not be performed by the inexperienced. In particular patient movement during chest compression makes central veins even more difficult to cannulate, and it can be difficult to differentiate between arteries and veins because of low arterial pressure and oxygen saturation. Accidental administration of calcium into a carotid or subclavian artery will have disastrous results. Central venous cannulation is therefore *not recommended* for use in the resuscitation of infants and children

Intraosseous infusion
- This is a useful route for drug and fluid administration
- For method, see chapter on Circulation care: shock

Intravenous infusion fluids
- Beware of over-transfusion and administer fluids sparingly, aiming to keep the systolic blood pressure 10-20 mmHg below normal, to prevent unnecessary further fluid loss, except in head injuries with probable raised intracranial pressure, when the systolic blood pressure should be maintained at normal or up to 15 mmHg above normal to maintain cerebral perfusion
- A careful record should be kept of the estimated blood loss and fluid transfused
- In hypovolaemic shock administer:
    - Crystalloid: 20 mL/kg, then:
    - Colloids: *Haemaccel®*, *Gelofusine®*, Hetastarch: 20 mL/kg
- In delayed resuscitation in infants administer 10% glucose, as their glycogen stores are easily depleted
- If possible all intravenous fluids should be warmed to body temperature prior to infusion

Disability (neurological state)

Assessment
- If the child is old enough and well enough to co-operate, the neurological status can be assessed using the AVPU scale
- Children change from being:
    - Happy/anxious
    - Miserable, crying: not too ill
    - Quiet, not interested in anything including parents: may be very ill
    - Restless: hypoxic
    - Exhausted: very ill (precedes respiratory arrest)

Management

Hypoglycaemia
- Take blood for later laboratory analysis
- Administer:
    - Oral glucose if the child is conscious and able to swallow
    - 0.5 g/kg dextrose (5 mL/kg of 10% dextrose). if the child is unconscious

Note: NEVER administer 50% dextrose to children as the hyperosmolar nature of the fluid may cause cerebral problems and even death

Fits
- Administer intravenous or rectal diazepam if fitting is prolonged

Exposure
- Removal of the child's clothing may be necessary to allow adequate physical examination and the execution of practical procedures
- Children and especially infants, lose heat very rapidly owing to their relatively large surface area, thin skin and lack of subcutaneous fat. A fall in body temperature results in a rise in oxygen consumption as compensatory metabolic processes start to provide an increase in heat production, peripheral vaso-constriction and a consequent lactic acidaemia
- It is very important therefore that if the ambient temperatures are low:
    - The child is not exposed unnecessarily before being put in the ambulance, which itself should be kept as warm as possible
    - The child should be kept warm, if exposure outside the ambulance is unavoidable, using:
        - Heat insulation
        - Warm or Hot packs *(being very careful not to burn the child)*
    - Keep the head covered, especially in infants/small children, as they lose a lot of heat from the head

Body weight estimation in children
- It can be extremely difficult to estimate an infant's or a child's weight in the Immediate Care situation, but the guides below may help. An alternative is to use the paediatric resuscitation chart (see below)
- Infants double their birth weight in 5 months and treble their birth weight in 1 year

Method:
- Between 1 and 9 years: (age in years + 4) x 2: (weight at 4 years: 16 kg)
- Between 7 and 12 years: age x 3: (weight at 10 years: 30 kg)

Note: Broselow® tape (colour coded), may be used to measure the length of the child and estimate the weight

Cardiac arrest in children

Incidence
- Primary cardiac or circulatory arrest is rare in children; the young heart is very resilient and will continue to beat for several minutes after respiratory arrest

Aetiology
- Bradycardia is a common response to hypoxia, and is best treated by maintaining adequate ventilation
- Restoration of alveolar ventilation with 100% oxygen usually improves cardiac output resulting in recovery
- Cardiac arrest in children usually only occurs after prolonged hypoxia due to an airway or breathing problem. It is associated with severe cerebral hypoxia and a very poor outcome; thus it is vital to recognise the warning signs, especially bradycardia, and act quickly to prevent hypoxic cardiac arrest

Note: Bradycardia with a rate <60 bpm should be treated as cardiac arrest in infants below the age of one year

Management
- As appropriate for the underlying cause

Advanced paediatric life support
- This is the use of aids in the management of the acutely ill child, and comes after Basic Life Support

Establish basic life support

Oxygenate, ventilate
- Provide positive pressure ventilation with a high inspired oxygen concentration

Attach a defibrillator or cardiac monitor
- Monitor the cardiac rhythm through the defibrillator pads/paddles, or monitoring electrodes placed in the conventional positions
- Paddle/pad size:
    - Select those which provide the best contact with the child's chest wall
- Paddle/pad position:
    - Infants:
        - On the front and back of the chest, just to the left of the midline
    - Children:
        - Place the defibrillator paddles/pads on the anterior chest wall; one just below the right clavicle and the other at the left anterior axillary line at about the level of the apex beat
        - If only large paddles are available; turn the child on its side, place the paddles on the front and back of the child and defibrillate through the chest

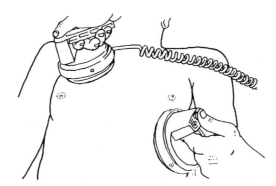

Figure 24-14 Defibrillation in children: paddle positions

Assess the cardiac rhythm (+ check for the pulse)
- Check the pulse:
    - Infants: brachial pulse in the inner aspect of the upper arm
    - Children: carotid pulse in the neck
- Take no more than 10 seconds
- Assess whether the rhythm is:
    - Non ventricular fibrillation or non ventricular tachycardia, ie. asystole, bradycardia and pulseless electrical activity
    - Ventricular fibrillation or ventricular tachycardia

Non VF/VT - Asystole, bradycardia and pulseless electrical activity (EMD)

Incidence
- Asystole/bradycardia: most common arrest arrhythmia in children
- Electromechanical dissociation (EMD): rare

Aetiology
- Asystole:
    - Usually occurs secondary to hypoxia, due to an airway or breathing problem
    - Bradycardia (= asystole): < 60 bpm for infants <1 year
- Electromechanical dissociation (4 Hs and 4 Ts):
    - Hypoxia   -   Tension pneumothorax
    - Hypovolaemia (commonest)   -   Toxic/therapeutic (e.g. drug overdosage)
    - Hypo/hyper-kalaemia   -   Thromboembolic
    - Hypothermia   -   (Cardiac) tamponade

Management
- Establish intravenous/intraosseous access
- Administer intravenous/intraosseous epinephrine: 10 µg/kg (0.1 mL/kg of 1:10,000 solution) *or* 10 x this dose via tracheal tube if intravenous/intraosseous access has not been established within 90 seconds
- Perform basic life support for about 3 minutes
- During basic life support/cardiopulmonary resuscitation:
    - Intubate and ventilate with 100% oxygen
- Reassess the cardiac rhythm, and if unsuccessful; repeat the cycle:
    - Administer epinephrine: 100 µg/kg (0.1 mL/kg of 1:1000 solution), followed by basic life/ cardiopulmonary resuscitation support for a further 3 minutes
- If unsuccessful; repeat the loop, administering fluids and alkalising agents if resuscitation is prolonged

Ventricular fibrillation

Incidence
- Uncommon in children, and is usually only seen as a terminal rhythm following cardiac arrest

Aetiology
- See 4Hs and 4 Ts above

Management
- Defibrillate with three defibrillation shocks:
    - 2 joules/kg initially, followed by:
    - 2 joules/kg, then increase to:
    - 4 joules/kg.
- Perform basic life support/cardiopulmonary resuscitation for about one minute

- During basic life support:
    - Intubate and ventilate with 100% oxygen
    - Establish intravenous/intraosseous access
    - Administer epinephrine: 10 μg/kg (= 0.1 mL/kg of 1:10,000)
- Defibrillate again, if you are unsuccessful:
    - 4 joules/kg; repeated up to twice (three times in all), if there is still no response
- If you are unsuccessful; perform CPR for about one minute, and repeat the loop, administering epinephrine: 100 μg/kg (= 0.1 mL/kg of 1:1000), every three minutes
- Consider the administration of sodium bicarbonate and/or an anti-arrhythmic
- Correct reversible causes

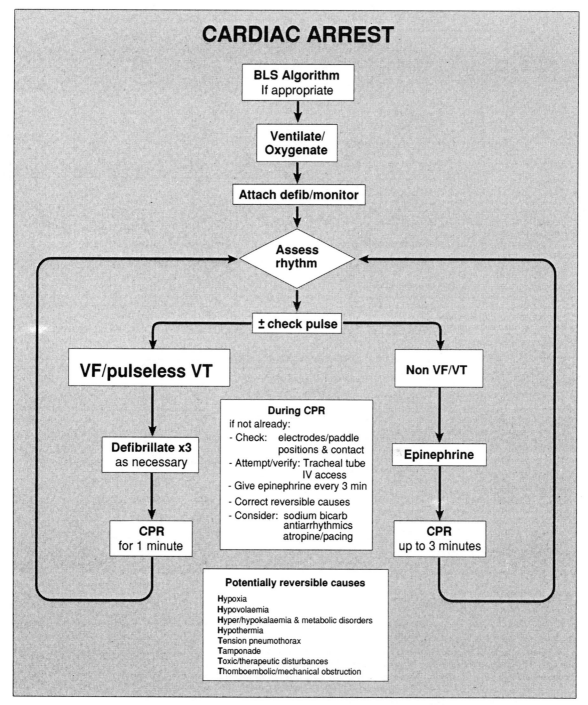

Figure 24-14 Advanced paediatric life support algorithm
(copyright of the European Resuscitation Council, reproduced with permission)

Paediatric Resuscitation Chart

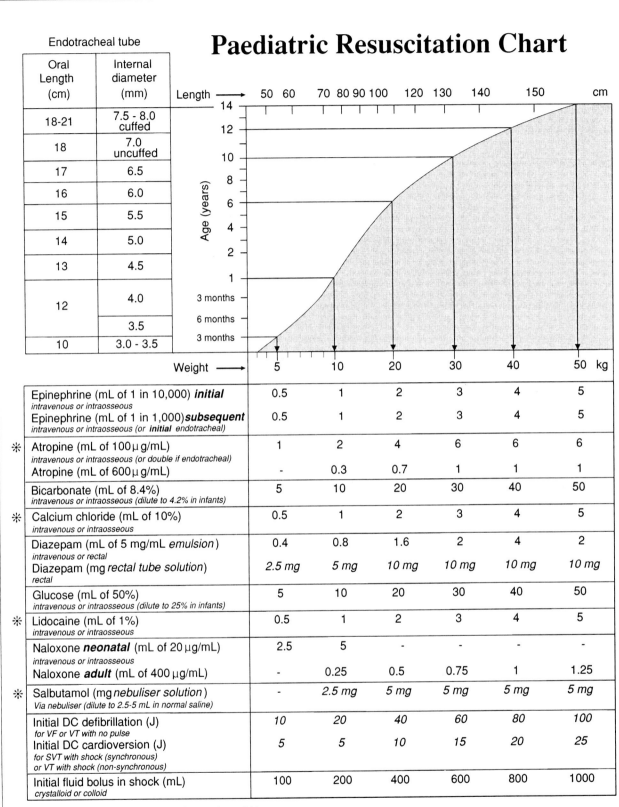

Endotracheal tube

Oral Length (cm)	Internal diameter (mm)
18-21	7.5 - 8.0 cuffed
18	7.0 uncuffed
17	6.5
16	6.0
15	5.5
14	5.0
13	4.5
12	4.0
	3.5
10	3.0 - 3.5

	5 kg	10	20	30	40	50 kg
Epinephrine (mL of 1 in 10,000) *initial* intravenous or intraosseous	0.5	1	2	3	4	5
Epinephrine (mL of 1 in 1,000) *subsequent* intravenous or intraosseous (or *initial* endotracheal)	0.5	1	2	3	4	5
✳ Atropine (mL of 100µg/mL) intravenous or intraosseous (or double if endotracheal)	1	2	4	6	6	6
Atropine (mL of 600µg/mL)	-	0.3	0.7	1	1	1
Bicarbonate (mL of 8.4%) intravenous or intraosseous (dilute to 4.2% in infants)	5	10	20	30	40	50
✳ Calcium chloride (mL of 10%) intravenous or intraosseous	0.5	1	2	3	4	5
Diazepam (mL of 5 mg/mL *emulsion*) intravenous or rectal	0.4	0.8	1.6	2	4	2
Diazepam (mg *rectal tube solution*) rectal	2.5 mg	5 mg	10 mg	10 mg	10 mg	10 mg
Glucose (mL of 50%) intravenous or intraosseous (dilute to 25% in infants)	5	10	20	30	40	50
✳ Lidocaine (mL of 1%) intravenous or intraosseous	0.5	1	2	3	4	5
Naloxone *neonatal* (mL of 20 µg/mL) intravenous or intraosseous	2.5	5	-	-	-	-
Naloxone *adult* (mL of 400 µg/mL)	-	0.25	0.5	0.75	1	1.25
✳ Salbutamol (mg *nebuliser solution*) Via nebuliser (dilute to 2.5-5 mL in normal saline)	-	2.5 mg	5 mg	5 mg	5 mg	5 mg
Initial DC defibrillation (J) for VF or VT with no pulse	10	20	40	60	80	100
Initial DC cardioversion (J) for SVT with shock (synchronous) or VT with shock (non-synchronous)	5	5	10	15	20	25
Initial fluid bolus in shock (mL) crystalloid or colloid	100	200	400	600	800	1000

✳ CAUTION! Non-standard drug concentrations may be available
Use **Atropine** 100 µg/mL or prepare by diluting 1 mg to 10 mL or 600 µg to 6 ml in normal saline
Note that 1 mL of **Calcium chloride** 10% is equivalent to 3 mL of **Calcium gluconate** 10%
Use **Lignocaine** (without adrenaline) 1% or give twice the volume of 0.5%. Give half the volume of 2% or dilute appropriately
Salbutamol may also be given by slow intravenous injection (5 µg/kg), but beware of the different concentrations available (e.g. 50 and 100 µg/mL)

Figure 24-15 Paediatric resuscitation drug dosage chart

Other cardiac drugs

- Lidocaine:
    - *Indication:* Ventricular arrhythmias
    - *Dosage:* 0.1 mL/kg of 1% (1 mg/kg), administered intravenously
            (This may be repeated after 5 minutes if necessary, followed by an infusion)
- Furosemide:
    - *Indication:* Cardiac failure
    - *Dosage:* 1-5 mg/kg administered intravenously

Drug administration in children
- When drugs are administered by the peripheral venous or intraosseous routes, they should be flushed through with 0.9% sodium chloride solution to help them to reach their site of action
- Access for drug administration may be difficult to achieve in children, and if intravenous or intraosseous access cannot be obtained within 90 seconds, then tracheal/endobronchial administration should be considered

Tracheal/endobronchial administration
- This route may be used for: epinephrine, lidocaine and atropine (*never* bicarbonate)
- It should only be used in the very early stages of resuscitation, as drug absorption may be unpredictable and unreliable for this route
- The dose should be double the intravenous dose (epinephrine ten times the intravenous dose), and the drug diluted in 2-3 mL of 0.9% sodium chloride solution
- After drug administration, the child should be hyperventilated (five inflations) to help distribution and absorption of the drug by the pulmonary vascular bed

Medical problems: life threatening illness in children

Heat loss in children

Pathophysiology
- Infants and young children can lose heat rapidly because of their relatively larger body surface, and may have difficulty generating enough heat to compensate for any heat loss. This is due to their relatively small glycogen stores and lack of body fat

Management
- Insulation:
    - Warm blankets, space blankets, cover the head
- Heat:
    - Hot water bottles, but beware of causing burns!
    - Prewarming intravenous fluids
- Energy:
    - Infusion of dextrose

Fits (see chapter on Medical emergencies)

Sudden infant death syndrome (SIDS)

Definition: The Sudden Infant Death Syndrome is the sudden death of any infant or young child (between the age of one week and two years), which is unexpected by history and in which a thorough necropsy (postmortem examination) fails to demonstrate an adequate cause of death

Incidence
- The incidence has been reduced by more than 50% following public education programmes encouraging mothers not to allow their babies to sleep in the prone position (sleeping on the side is also associated with an increased risk when compared with sleeping supine)
- Affects 1:500 children
- Age:
  - Most common cause of death in the first year of life
  - The majority of deaths occur between 4-20 weeks (peak incidence: 8-18 weeks), 80% of deaths occur before 8 months
  - Rare over the age of 1 year
- Responsible for:
  - >30% all cardiac arrests in children
  - 20% of all infant deaths in England and Wales

Aetiology
- At present the cause is unknown, but several mechanisms may be responsible
- Current research suggests that it may be due to a combination of:
  - Immature control of respiration and temperature (over wrapping and sleeping prone)
  - Carbon dioxide retention (sleeping prone on a soft mattress or loose bedding, especially duvets/quilts, which may slip over the baby's head)
  - A minor respiratory infection (pertussis has also been implicated)
  - A temporary defect in cardiac function (SIDS is associated with a longer than normal QT interval)
- Other factors include:
  - Intercurrent infection
  - Bottle feeding
  - Twins: especially if:
    - Delivered pre-term
    - Low birth weight
  - Male sex
  - Social and economic deprivation
  - Low birth weight, short gestation period and reduced birth length
  - Winter/cold weather (this trend has continued in spite of the general reduction in the incidence of SIDS)
  - Illegitimacy
  - Single parent family
  - Parents:
    - Who have smoked (risk increases with the number of smokers and the number of cigarettes smoked), or taken opiates or barbiturates
    - From ethnic minorities
  - Bed sharing, especially if a parent smokes
  - Sleeping on an old mattress, but not one covered totally by PVC
  - The incidence increases with ascending birth order and reduced birth interval

Management
- Basic/Advanced life support
- Treatment of the cause, if this is obvious

Trauma in children

- Children and adults react and respond to injury in very different ways both physically, physiologically and emotionally. Young children are unable to describe pain or localise symptoms, and if frightened tend to behave in an even younger way, sometimes even denying all symptoms. The parent/carer may be a valuable source of information and reassurance, provided that they are not themselves injured
- The way in which children are managed following injury should follow the same basic approach as adults

Primary survey

- Assessment of the:
    - Airway
    - Breathing
    - Circulation
    - Disability
    - Exposure with control of the environment

Primary management

- Resuscitation; care of the:
    - Airway with cervical spine stabilisation
    - Breathing
    - Circulation with control of haemorrhage

Airway and cervical spine

- The airway should be assessed following injury by:
    - Looking
    - Listening
    - Feeling
- A cervical spine injury should always be assumed unless it can be excluded from examining the mechanism of injury and the child
- Secure the airway:
    - Jaw thrust
    - Suction/removal of any foreign body
    - Oropharyngeal airway
    - Tracheal intubation
    - Surgical airway insertion (as a last resort)
- Stabilise the cervical spine (if the child is conscious this may require a lot of reassurance!):
    - Immobilise the cervical spine with in-line cervical stabilisation
    - Apply a semi-rigid cervical collar, shoulder pad, head blocks and tape down

Breathing

- Assess the adequacy of breathing:
    - The work of breathing;
        - Respiratory rate
        - Recession
        - Inspiratory (stridor) or expiratory (wheeze) noises
        - Grunting
        - Use of the accessory muscles
        - Flaring of the alae nasae
    - Effectiveness of breathing:
        - Breath sounds
        - Chest expansion
        - Abdominal excursion

- If breathing is inadequate:
    - Ventilate with a bag/mask and oxygen
    - Consider intubation
- If breath sound are unequal, consider:
    - Pneumothorax
    - Flail chest
    - Blocked main bronchus (? with misplaced tracheal tube)

Circulation
- Assess the:
    - Heart rate
    - Systolic blood pressure
    - Capillary refill
    - Skin colour
    - Temperature
    - Respiratory rate
    - Mental state
- All seriously injured children should have two wide bore cannulae inserted immediately, their haemodynamic state carefully monitored, and infusion commenced if there is any evidence of their decompensating, starting with:
    - Crystalloid 20 mL/kg, then:
    - Colloid 20 mL/kg
- If difficulty is experienced in obtaining intravenous access, intraosseous access should be obtained

Disability
- Assess the level of consciousness:
    - **A**   Alert
    - **V**   Responds to verbal stimuli
    - **P**   Responds to pain
    - **U**   Unresponsive
- Assess the pupil size and reactivity

Exposure
- Children lose body heat very quickly, so they should only be undressed if it is absolutely necessary to assess their injuries, and they should be covered up again as soon as possible, and kept warm

Secondary survey
- This follows the same order as in adults
- The secondary survey should only be performed on children, if it does not unduly delay their evacuation to hospital
    - Head
    - Face
    - Neck
    - Chest
    - Thorax
    - Abdomen
    - Pelvis
    - Spine
    - Extremities:
        - Upper limb
        - Lower limb

Secondary management
- This is done at the same time as problems are identified during the secondary survey

Pain relief
- If the child is in severe pain administer:
    - Morphine: 0.1-0.2 mg/kg, administered intravenously with care
    - Nitrous oxide/oxygen (*Entonox®, Nitronox®*):
        - Administered by mouthpiece rather than facemask (which children find frightening)
        - Contraindicated in chest injuries, especially pneumothorax, and base of skull fractures

Head injury in children

Incidence
- Head injury is the most common cause of death in children aged 1-15 years old, accounting for:
    - 15% of all deaths in this age group
    - 25% of deaths in children aged 5-15 years

Aetiology
- In children, the commonest cause of serious injury is road traffic accidents (pedestrians are the most vulnerable followed by pedal cyclists and then vehicle occupants), followed by falls
- In neonates child abuse is the commonest cause of serious injury

Pathophysiology
- As in adults, brain injury may occur as a result of the primary or secondary effects of injury:
    - Primary injury:
        - Cerebral laceration
        - Cerebral contusion
        - Dural sac tears
        - Diffuse axonal injury
    - Secondary injury:
        - Raised intracranial pressure resulting in reduced cerebral perfusion and cerebral ischaemia
        - Hypovolaemia and hypotension as a result of trauma resulting in cerebral ischaemia
        - Hypoxia caused by inadequate ventilation:pneumothorax
        - Hypoxia caused by airway obstruction
        - Hypoglycaemia
        - Vomiting and/or fitting
        - Hypothermia
        - Pyrexia

Intracranial pressure

Infants
- In infants, before the sutures have closed, the cranial volume can increase without causing the same problems that occur after they have fused. As a result large extradural and subdural bleeds may occur without causing a rise in intracranial pressure or neurological signs and symptoms, but may result in significant anaemia

Children
- The sutures between the bony plates making up a child's skull close between 12-18 months, after which the skull behaves like an adult's skull with a fixed volume
- In children cerebral oedema is the most common cause of raised intracranial pressure following a head injury

Scalp injury
- This may result in profuse bleeding with life threatening blood loss, aggravating any hypovolaemia, reducing blood pressure further and resulting in cerebral oedema and a further rise in intracranial pressure

Symptoms/signs
- The initial assessment of the head injured patient should follow the usual protocol, and should include:

Primary survey
- Airway with cervical spine stabilisation
- Breathing
- Circulation with control of haemorrhage
- Disability:
  - Assessment of the level of consciousness:
    A   Alert
    V   Responds to verbal stimuli
    P   Responds to pain
    U   Unresponsive
  - Assessment of the pupil size and reactivity
- Exposure

Primary survey and management
- The aim of the pre-hospital management of children with serious head injuries is the prevention of secondary brain injury by maintaining adequate oxygenation, ventilation and circulation, and by helping to avoid a rise in intracranial pressure
  - Airway management with cervical spine stabilisation
  - Breathing: ensure adequate ventilation
  - Circulation with control of haemorrhage
  - Disability
  - Exposure

Secondary survey
- Carefully examine the head:
  - Palpate the scalp for:
    - Bruises and lacerations
    - Depressed skull fractures
  - Look for evidence of base of skull fracture
    - CSF leak from the nose or ears
    - Racoon eyes
    - Battle's sign
- Assess the level of consciousness and responsiveness using the relevant coma scale
- Check the pupils for size and reactivity

Secondary management
- Intubate and ventilate any child with a significantly reduced level of consciousness
- Relieve pain:
  - Severe pain may result in an increase in intracranial pressure and may lead to misinterpretation of the level of consciousness
  - Morphine: 0.1-0.2 mg/kg, may be administered intravenously, and can be reversed if necessary with naloxone
  - Consider regional nerve blocks
- Fits should be controlled with diazepam

Glasgow coma scale		over 4 years		under 4 years	
Eye opening	Spontaneously		4	Spontaneously	4
	To verbal command		3	React to speech	3
	To pain		2	React to pain	2
	No response		1	No response	1
Best motor response	To verbal command:	Obeys	6	Spontaneous/obeys command	6
	To painful stimulus:	Localises pain	5	Localises pain	5
		Flexion/withdrawal	4	Withdrawal	4
		Flexion decorticate	3	Abnormal flexion (decorticate)	3
		Extension decerebrate	2	Abnormal extension (decerebrate)	2
		None	1	None	1
Best verbal response				*Crying*	*Interacts*
	Orientated/converses		5	Smiles	Yes, follows 5
	Disorientated/confused		4	Consolable	Inappropriate 4
	Inappropriate words		3	? Consolable	Moaning 3
	Incomprehensible sounds		2	Inconsolable	Irritable 2
	No response		1	No response	No response 1

Total   (3-15) _____   _____

Figure 24-16 Paediatric coma scale

Paediatric glasgow coma scale
- This is a version of the glasgow coma scale developed for use in children, however it is unproven, of variable value, and difficult to remember and apply in the pre-hospital setting

Chest injury in children
- Children who have suffered major trauma may have significant intrathoracic injuries, that can severely compromise respiration, and require immediate management during the primary survey

Incidence
- Chest injury is relatively common in children who have suffered major trauma

Aetiology
- Road traffic accident injuries are a major cause of thoracic trauma in children

Pathophysiology
- Children's thoracic cage is very flexible and the bones are rarely fractured, although the underlying organs may have suffered significant trauma
- Children who have been subjected to large transfers of kinetic energy may show very little evidence of this in the form of bruising, abrasions, etc.

Tension pneumothorax
- This is one of the most acute emergencies in the management of the severely injured child

Massive haemothorax
- This is relatively common in children who have suffered major trauma, because of the increased incidence of severe lung injury

Open pneumothorax
- Rarely seen in children

Flail chest
- This is a rare injury in children because of the elasticity of the child's thoracic cage
- When it does occur there is inevitably a greater degree of underlying soft tissue (lung) injury, which will result in even greater respiratory embarrassment

Cardiac tamponade
- May occur after both blunt and penetrating trauma

Pulmonary contusion
- This occurs relatively commonly in children because of the elasticity of the child's thoracic cage, resulting in an increase in the damage done to the underlying organs

Tracheal and bronchial rupture
- Often lethal

Great vessel injury
- Usually fatal

Ruptured diaphragm
- Usually occurs as a result of blunt abdominal trauma, usually on the left side

Symptoms/signs
- As in adults

Management
- As in adults

Abdominal injury in children

Incidence
- Abdominal injuries occur relatively commonly in children suffering from major trauma

Aetiology
- The majority of abdominal injuries in children are caused by blunt trauma, usually as a result of RTAs
- Blunt injury:
    - Hepatic and splenic rupture/laceration
- Deceleration/shearing injury:
    - Hepatic and splenic injury
    - Duodenal injury:
        - Rupture at the duodenojejunal flexure
        - Haematoma formation
- Straddling injury:
    - Urethral rupture

Pathophysiology
- The abdominal organs in children are very susceptible to injury because;
    - The abdominal wall is thin and provides little protection
    - The ribs are very elastic and provide little protection
    - The diaphragm is more horizontal than in adults, as a result of which the liver and spleen and liver are situated a bit lower and more anteriorly
    - The bladder is positioned more in the abdomen than in the pelvis and is more vulnerable to injury
- Abdominal injury may result in splinting of the diaphragm, causing impairment of ventilation

Symptoms/signs

Primary survey and management
- Initial assessment follows the usual protocol:
    - Airway management with cervical spine stabilisation
    - Breathing: ensure adequate ventilation
    - Circulation with control of haemorrhage:
        - If the child shows signs of shock and there is no obvious site of haemorrhage, consider an intra-abdominal cause
    - Disability
    - Exposure:
        - Consider exposure of the abdomen if an intra-abdominal injury is a possibility, and the shock appears not to be responding to fluid replacement

Secondary survey
- Examine the different parts of the child from top to toe in the usual sequence
- when examining the abdomen, look for:
    - Bruising:
        - This is highly significant as in children major abdominal injury may occur without any obvious external evidence
        - Children with obvious abdominal bruising have a high incidence of bowel perforation, especially if there is an associated injury of the lumbar spine
    - Lacerations
    - Penetrating wounds
    - Palpate the abdomen very gently, as it will make it harder for those who examine the child after you in hospital, if you cause any unnecessary pain

Pelvic injury in children

Incidence
- Pelvic fractures are relatively rare in children as the pelvis in children is relatively elastic, and the kinetic energy from a severe impact is usually transmitted to the intrapelvic organs, including the blood vessels resulting in their disruption and haemorrhage

Aetiology
- Pelvic fractures are usually caused by severe blunt injury, usually as a result of road traffic accidents

Pathophysiology
- Crush injuries of the pelvis causing pelvic disruption can result in life threatening hypovolaemic shock

Symptoms/signs
- Evidence of blunt pelvic/abdominal injury with signs of rapidly developing hypovolaemic shock

Management

Primary survey and management
- Initial assessment should follow the usual protocol:
    - Airway management with cervical spine stabilisation
    - Breathing: ensure adequate ventilation
    - Circulation with control of haemorrhage:
        - Rapid infusion of colloid and crystalloid with careful monitoring of the haemodynamic state
        - Stabilisation of the pelvis
    - Disability
    - Exposure

Extremity injury in children

Incidence
- Skeletal injury accounts for 10-15% of all injuries in children, 15% involving epiphyseal disruption
- Extremity trauma is unlikely to be immediately life-threatening in the child with multiple injuries, with the exception of massive open long bone fractures and traumatic amputations

Aetiology
- Injury in road traffic accidents is a major cause of serious extremity trauma

Pathophysiology
- Children's bones are more susceptible to injury than adults' bones because:
    - In children the bones are relatively elastic, resulting in greenstick and torus fractures caused when one or both cortices deform without actually fracturing. As a result the chances of fracture propagation is reduced in children and comminuted fractures are relatively rare
    - There are growth plates in children's bones, which are 2-5 times weaker than any other part of the paediatric skeleton, and are commonly involved in fractures
- In children, because their bones are more elastic, and thus less likely to fracture than adults' bones, the underlying structures may be significantly damaged without there being bony injury. This may lead to an underestimation of the severity of soft tissue injuries in children
- Massive, open, long bone fractures may result in life threatening blood loss, as open fractures may result in more blood loss than closed fractures because of the lack of tamponade from the surrounding tissues
- Partial amputations may result in more blood loss than complete amputations because completely severed blood vessels go into spasm, whereas partially severed blood vessels do not

Management
- It is vital to assess the child thoroughly and manage life-threatening problems first
- Unless extremity trauma is life-threatening, evaluation and management should be carried out during the secondary survey
- Remembered that:
    - Single, closed extremity trauma may sometimes rarely cause life-threatening hypovolaemia
    - Although multiple fractures may cause significant hypovolaemic shock, this is not usually an immediate life-threatening problem

Primary survey and management
- Initial assessment should follow the usual protocol:
    - Airway management with cervical spine stabilisation
    - Breathing: ensure adequate ventilation
    - Circulation with control of haemorrhage:
        - Open long bone fractures and partial traumatic amputations with rapidly developing hypovolaemic shock should be managed during the primary survey with an adequate intravenous infusion of colloid followed by crystalloid and splinting
    - Disability
    - Exposure

Secondary survey and management
- Examine the different parts of the child from top to toe in the usual sequence
- When examining the limbs expose them adequately, and look for any associated vascular or neurological injury:
    - Skin colour, temperature and neurological status
    - Peripheral pulses distal to a fracture
- Reduce and splint any fractures, especially if there is circulatory compromise, and re-check pulses, etc.
- Administer adequate analgesia

Severe haemorrhage in children

Incidence
- Uncommon in children

Aetiology
- Trauma

Pathophysiology
- Small children tolerate large volume blood loss very badly (see above)

Symptoms/signs
- Rapid weak pulse
- Monitor pulse rate, rhythm and volume in a large artery (see below)

Management
- Apply direct firm pressure over the bleeding point
- If there is evidence of the rapid development of hypovolaemic shock:
    - Put up intravenous infusions using two wide bore cannulae and infuse rapidly
    - Monitor the haemodynamic state continuously with the aim of keeping the systolic blood pressure 10-20 mmHg below normal so as not to increase blood loss
- If it is not possible to stop the haemorrhage; consider using a wide orthopaedic tourniquet, which should be placed as far distally as possible, and the time of its application recorded

Spinal injury in children

Incidence
- Spinal injuries are rare in children:
    - Cervical spine injuries account for 0.2% of all fractures/dislocations in children:
        - Injuries usually occur at or above the level of C2
        - Atlantoaxial rotary subluxation is the most common cervical spine injury, other injuries include odontoid epiphyseal separations and traumatic ligament disruptions
    - Thoracic and lumbar spine injuries account for <1% of all fractures/dislocations in children

Aetiology
- Spinal injuries occur most commonly in the child subjected to major trauma
- In children aged >10 years, sporting and recreational accidents account for over 40% of thoracic and lumbar spine injuries

Pathophysiology
- The spine is more flexible in children than adults as a result of which:
    - Impact energy is dissipated over a larger number of vertebrae
    - Fractures of more than one vertebra are relatively common
    - There may be spinal cord injury without obvious bony injury:
        - Occurs almost exclusively in children, especially under the age of 8 years
        - Affects the cervical spine more often than the thoracic or lumbar spine
    - The upper cervical vertebrae are the most flexible, as a result of which:
        - They are more likely to be damaged
        - The uppermost spinal cord is the most likely to be affected
- The most common mechanism of injury is hyperflexion resulting in compression of the anterior of the vertebrae and wedging

Symptoms/signs
- Torticollis after trauma indicates atlantoaxial rotary subluxation
- It is often very difficult to accurately assess the neurological status in children, as the result of which it is very important to assess the mechanism of injury and the most likely injuries sustained as a result

Management

Primary survey and management
- Initial assessment should follow the usual protocol:
    - Airway management with cervical spine stabilisation:
        - The cervical spine should always be immobilised if an examination of the mechanism of injury suggests a possible spinal injury
    - Breathing: ensure adequate ventilation
    - Circulation with control of haemorrhage:
    - Disability:
        - It is often very difficult to assess the neurological status in children, so all children who have suffered major trauma, and in whom an examination of the mechanism of injury suggests a possible spinal injury, should be immobilised on a spinal board
    - Exposure

Burns in children

Incidence
- Burns are a major cause of childhood mortality and morbidity:
    - In the UK, over 50 000 burnt and scalded children attend casualty departments each year, of whom over 5000 require admission, and nearly 100 die (about 5 from scalds)
    - 70% of severe burns occur in children less than 5 years old, most occurring in those aged 1-2 years
    - Boys are more likely to suffer from burns and major scalds

Aetiology
- Most fatal burns occur in house fires: smoke inhalation is the usual cause of death
- Most non-fatal burns involve clothing and are often associated with flammable liquids
- Scalds are usually caused by hot drinks, but may also be caused by hot cooking oil and hot bath water
- Burns are more likely to occur in households of low socioeconomic status, with family stress, poor housing conditions and over-crowding

Pathophysiology
- As adults, but children have a greater relative surface area than adults, so burns will have a greater systemic effect

Management
- As adults

Primary survey and management
- Airway management with cervical spine stabilisation
- Breathing: ensure adequate ventilation
- Circulation:
    - If the child has extensive burns:
        - Administer intravenous or intraosseous fluids
- Disability
- Exposure:
    - Assess the severity and degree of burns and dress them as appropriate
- Analgesia:
    - Provide the child with adequate analgesia

Electrical burns

Incidence
- One third of all victims of electrical injuries are children, of whom about 20% die as a result

Aetiology
- Over 90% involve generated electricity (rather than lightning strike)

Pathophysiology
- As adults

Management

Primary survey and management
- Airway management with cervical spine stabilisation, especially if the child is unconscious or has been thrown or fallen any distance
- Breathing: ensure adequate ventilation

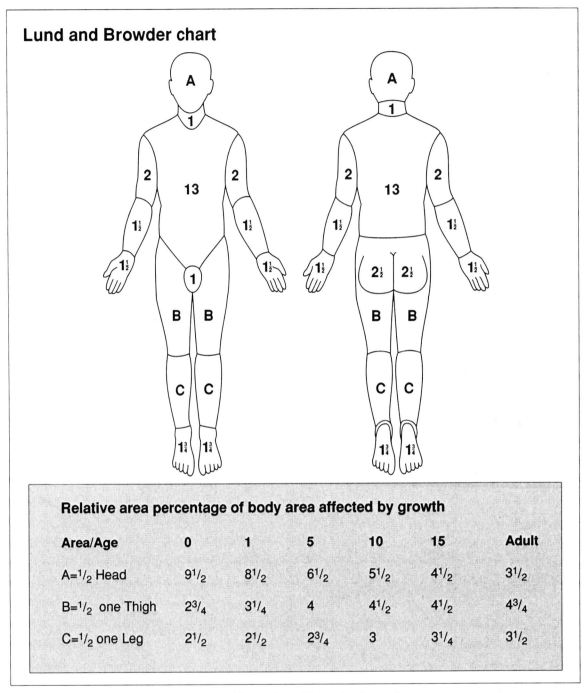

Lund and Browder chart

Relative area percentage of body area affected by growth

Area/Age	0	1	5	10	15	Adult
A=$\frac{1}{2}$ Head	$9\frac{1}{2}$	$8\frac{1}{2}$	$6\frac{1}{2}$	$5\frac{1}{2}$	$4\frac{1}{2}$	$3\frac{1}{2}$
B=$\frac{1}{2}$ one Thigh	$2\frac{3}{4}$	$3\frac{1}{4}$	4	$4\frac{1}{2}$	$4\frac{1}{2}$	$4\frac{3}{4}$
C=$\frac{1}{2}$ one Leg	$2\frac{1}{2}$	$2\frac{1}{2}$	$2\frac{3}{4}$	3	$3\frac{1}{4}$	$3\frac{1}{2}$

Figure 24-17 Lund and Browder burn chart

- Circulation:
    - Defibrillate immediately if the child has no pulse and is in VF
    - If the child has extensive burns:
        - Administer intravenous or intraosseous fluids
- Disability:
    - It is important to ascertain if there has been any significant nerve or muscle injury
- Exposure:
    - Assess the severity and degree of burns and dress them as appropriate
- Analgesia:
    - Provide the child with adequate analgesia

25

Care of the Elderly

Care of the elderly

Introduction
- Management of the elderly patient presents a unique problem in Immediate Care because of changes in their anatomy, physiology, pathophysiology and psychology brought about as a result of the ageing process, usually in combination with the effects of various illnesses and injuries, which themselves accelerate the ageing process
- The importance of recognising these differences is increasing as the number of elderly people in the population is increasing, both in absolute figures and as a percentage of the total population:
    - The number of people aged 100 and over rose from about 200 in 1951 to over 4000 in 1989
    - The number of pensioners is predicted to rise from 5.25 million in 1950 to about 10 million by the millennium, the greatest increase occurring in those aged 80 years and over, whose numbers are predicted to rise from 0.75 million to 2.5 million over the same period
- There is no precise definition of what is an elderly person, as some people age earlier than others, some may be affected by illness, which may cause premature ageing and immobility, and others not, and peoples' attitude to ageing may vary ranging from those who feel and behave as if they are young, to those who behave in a prematurely old fashion
- The Immediate Care practitioner should carefully evaluate the patient and if they appear to be elderly, manage them as such, and not base that judgement on age alone
- The Immediate Care practitioner needs to be aware that the elderly patient may be suffering from a multiplicity of inter-related problems, e.g. often an elderly patient may be injured as a result of a medical problem, e.g. a fall, as a result of a transient ischaemic attack, cardiac arrhythmia, postural hypotension, etc., which may cause a fractured hip and hypovolaemic shock, and hypothermia and pneumonia, if they are not found for some time

Incidence
- The elderly are more prone to injure themselves because of:
    - Reduced vision, e.g they are more likely to trip over objects, or not see sufficiently well to avoid an accident
    - Reduced hearing, which may prevent them from hearing well enough to avoid an accident or heed a shouted warning
    - Reduced ability to comprehend what may be about to happen and reduced ability to react rapidly enough to remove themselves quickly from a source of danger. This may be further aggravated by any drugs that the patient is taking
    - An increased tendency to fall over due to a combination of poor proprioreception, weak muscles and delayed reaction times

Aetiology
- Falls are the leading cause of mortality and morbidity in the elderly:
    - About 40% of elderly women and 20% of elderly men will give a history of a recent fall
    - The risk of falling increases with age rising from a 30% risk at the age of 65 to about 50% at the age of 80
- Road traffic accidents are the second most important cause of death in the elderly:
    - An elderly patient is five times more likely to be fatally injured in a road traffic accident than a younger patient, although excess speed is rarely a factor

Anatomy
- It may be difficult to distinguish between anatomical changes solely due to ageing and those due to pathological changes brought about by illness and injury. In practice most older people suffer from a combination of both these processes

Airway and respiratory system

Ageing

Upper airway
- With increasing age the older patient may suffer from dental caries, injury to the teeth and gum disease which may make the teeth vulnerable to trauma and may make it necessary for dentures or a bridge to be worn, which may itself be easily damaged, and become a foreign body likely to obstruct the airway or be aspirated
- The absence of some or all the teeth may alter the contour of the maxilla and mandible and may make it difficult to obtain a good seal for a mask for ventilating the patient
- The cartilage of the upper respiratory tract becomes more rigid making the soft palate less flexible and the larynx and tracheal cartilages more vulnerable to fracture

Lungs
- In older patients the thoracic cage becomes less flexible due to a combination of increasing rigidity of the ribs and stiffening of the joints, and there may be a reduction in muscle strength and tone
- The lung tissue may become less elastic

Cardiovascular system

Heart
- There will be some loss of strength of the myocardium, together with narrowing and stiffness of the coronary arteries due to atheroma, resulting in a reduction in coronary perfusion

Circulation
- There will be narrowing and stiffness of the arteries due to atheroma and plaque deposition, which may begin as early as late adolescence

Central nervous system

Brain
- With increasing age there will be general brain shrinkage with loss of neurones
- The circulation to the brain will be reduced due to narrowing of the arteries

Special senses
- In the eyes, vision may be impaired or reduced as a result of:
    - Macular degeneration
    - Cataract formation in the lens
    - Lens stiffening
- In the ears there may be otosclerosis

Musculoskeletal system

Bones
- Bones become more rigid and less flexible with ageing
- In post menopausal women and in some men. especially the less physically active, there is an increasing tendency to the development of osteoporosis, resulting in a thinning of the bones
- A reduction in height of the intervertebral discs may result in a reduction in height and an increase in stiffness of the spine
- Osteoarthritis of the spine may result in narrowing of the spinal canal

Joints
- With increasing age joints become stiffer, and some ankylose (become bony and rigid), e.g. the steromanubrial joint
- There may be degenerative disease resulting in joint stiffness, loose bodies. etc

Muscles
- With increasing age there is usually loss of muscle bulk and strength, especially if the person becomes less active

Physiology
- It may be difficult to distinguish between physiological changes solely due to ageing and those due to pathological changes brought about by illness and injury. In practice most older people suffer from a combination of both these processes

Airway and respiratory system
- Increasing rigidity of the thoracic cage and a reduction in the elasticity of the lungs results in a reduction in effective inspiratory lung volume, tidal volume and peak flow. To avoid a reduction in oxygenation, there may be a compensatory increase in respiratory rate

Cardiovascular system

Heart
- With increasing age there may be a reduction in heart rate, strength of myocardial contraction, stroke volume, compliance and efficiency of the cardiac valves, resulting in a reduction in cardiac output
- The blood pressure usually rises as the patient ages, the systolic pressure usually increasing more than the diastolic due to a reduction in the compliance of both arteries and veins. A further increase in arterial pressure occurs due to the need to overcome the increased resistance of arteries narrowed by plaque

Circulation
- Calcification of the arterial wall may make the arteries less able to respond to nervous and endocrine stimuli
- The result of the above is reduced circulation and tissue oxygenation making the ageing cardiovascular system less able to respond to trauma and sudden severe illness:
    - Acute myocardial infarction may be silent in that there may be either no pain or minimal pain, and the patient may simply present later with heart failure
    - The onset of hypovolaemic shock may appear to be delayed, resulting in a failure to compensate for blood volume depletion

Central nervous system

Brain
- Brain changes may result in impaired memory and concentration with depression
- The older brain is more vulnerable to hypoxia, and less able to compensate for and cope with the effects of injury and illness, resulting in confusion. This may be aggravated by poor vision and/or hearing; common causes are:
    - Hypoxia
    - Fluid loss; haemorrhage, dehydration
    - Head injury
    - Severe infection (the sudden onset of confusion may be the first indication of, e.g. pneumonia)
    - Diabetes mellitus with hypo- or hyperglycaemia
    - Liver and renal failure
    - Drugs
- As a result of confusion the elderly may:
    - Not realise what has happened to them or others with them in a trauma situation
    - React inappropriately to the death of others, e.g. they may appear to be callously unconcerned

Special senses
- There may be deafness and visual impairment with presbyopia

Peripheral and autonomic nervous system
- With increasing age there may be:
    - Reduced awareness of touch, temperature and pain, resulting in hypothermia, postural hypotension, falls, urinary incontinence and constipation
    - Impaired proprioception
    - Impaired control of posture and balance

Musculoskeletal system

Muscles
- The muscles become weaker with increasing age

Immune system
- Evidence of significant infection may be masked, e.g. classic evidence such as fever may be absent
- The older immune system is less efficient, in that it responds more slowly and less efficiently to infection, as a result of which the elderly are more vulnerable to sudden severe infection

Illness and disease
- Illnesses and disease may further reduce the ability of the body to respond to trauma and sudden illness

Airway and respiratory system
- There may be fibrosis and scarring of lung tissue from previous infection and inflammation effectively reducing the lung volume resulting in impaired lung expansion and ventilation, causing reduced blood oxygenation and increased carbon dioxide retention
- Lowered tissue oxygenation may make the body less able to cope with the sudden increase in energy demand that may occur as a result of trauma or severe illness

Cardiovascular system

Heart
- Hypertension may result in left ventricular hypertrophy to overcome the increased arterial vascular resistance; this results in an increased tendency to bleed profusely in trauma
- There may be severe narrowing and sometimes complete occlusion of some of the coronary arteries due to atheroma and plaque deposition, resulting in angina and myocardial infarction especially in the presence of reduced blood pressure, hypovolaemia and reduced SpO_2
- A previous myocardial infarction may result in an akinetic segment of heart muscle, which if large enough may form an aneurism of the heart wall, and result in impairment of the muscle pump of the heart and a relatively low blood pressure and tissue perfusion
- Impaired cardiac perfusion may also result in impairment of or damage to the cardiac conducting system resulting in various arrhythmias

Circulation
- There may be severe narrowing or evebn complete occlusion of some arteries due to atheroma and plaque deposition, resulting in impairment of the distal circulation. This may affect vital organs such as the brain and kidneys resulting in impaired function, and the limbs
- There may be peripheral vascular disease resulting in impairment of the peripheral circulation

Central nervous system

Brain
- Brain changes may result in severely impaired memory and concentration, and dementia

Peripheral and autonomic nervous system
- Diabetes mellitus may result in severe impairment of the peripheral and autonomic nervous systems, causing severe impairment of touch and proprioception

Musculoskeletal system

Bones
- Pathological osteoporosis may result in a flexion deformity (curvature) of the spine (kyphosis), and will make the person very liable to fractures which may occur as a result of only minimal force, e.g. a fracture of the hip occurring due to twisting the leg

Joints
- Arthritis will result in a reduction or even absence of the cartilage lining the joint, which together with bony deformity, may result in loss of movement and deformity, especially in the hips, knees and fingers

Muscles
- Diseases such as arthritis, and illnesses resulting in immobility, may result in severe loss of muscle bulk

Medication

- The elderly may take a large number of different drugs, both prescribed and non-prescribed for pre-existing medical problems
- They may not be taking these drugs correctly due to confusion or forgetfulness
- Some medication may alter or modify the patient's response to injury or sudden serious illness, and may interact with drugs administered by the pre-hospital practitioner to manage their acute problem
- Some drugs may interact with each other and cause further problems
- Anticoagulants will increase the tendency to bleed

Mechanism of injury

Airway and respiratory system

- The increased rigidity of the thoracic cage will make the elderly more prone to fractures of the ribs and sternum

Cardiovascular system

- Atheroma deposition may make arteries:
    - Less elastic making them more brittle and liable to shear injury, e.g. the bridging vessels supplying the brain, although paradoxically it may make some major vessels so stiff that they are less liable to shear injury, e.g. the arch of the aorta
    - Less able to constrict, if they are transected, resulting in an increase in haemorrhage

Central nervous system

Brain

- Brain changes may result in brain tissue becoming less elastic and therefore more likely to tear
- Cerebral artery atherosclerosis will make these vessels less flexible and vulnerable to deceleration/shear injury, resulting in an intracranial bleed, raised intracranial pressure and death
- Bridging veins may have to bridge a larger space than in the young due to brain shrinkage, increasing their vulnerability to excessive cerebral movement, resulting in an acute subdural haemorrhage
- Extradural haemorrhage is rare in the elderly due to the strongly adherent dura
- Chronic subdural haemorrhage is relatively common

Special senses

- Poor vision will result in an increased tendency to trip over objects and fall

Peripheral and autonomic nervous system

- Impaired proprioception may result in an increasing tendency to fall

Musculoskeletal system

Bones

- Old stiff bones are more likely to fracture than young supple ones, as a result of which multiple fracture are more common in the elderly
- Osteoporosis makes bones more liable to fracture if exposed to direct or indirect force, especially the hips, wrists and thoracic and lumbar vertebrae
- Osteoarthritis, loss of flexibility and narrowing of the spinal canal will make the spine and spinal cord more prone to injury

Joints

- Stiff joints are more vulnerable to injury than mobile ones
- Ankylosed joints are likely to 'fracture' through the affected joint

Muscles
- Weak muscles may result in immobility and tendency to have falls

Symptoms/signs

Approach
- Never treat the elderly as if they are small children or are mentally deficient:
  - Speak slowly and clearly but do not shout, unless the patient is obviously deaf
  - Introduce yourself
  - Only ask relevant questions
  - Explain what has happened to them (they may ask you repeatedly)
  - Be aware that any information they give you may not be 100% reliable, so try to ascertain how well orientated they are by first asking simple questions about their name, address and date of birth

Airway/breathing
- Elderly patients with a ventilation rate of less than 10 or more than 30 breaths per minute will not have a satisfactory minute volume and should be ventilated

Circulation
- Remember that a raised blood pressure is common in the elderly
- Measurement of the oxygen saturation from a peripheral digit may be unreliable due to poor tissue perfusion, and a more central site, e.g. the nose or ear is often better
- The capillary refill test may be unreliable in the elderly due to poor tissue perfusion

Disability
- The elderly patient is more likely to be confused, as a result of injury or illness, and it may be difficult to assess their neurological state

Exposure
- The older patient is more likely to become hypothermic, so unnecessary exposure should be avoided

Medical history
- Because of the high likelihood of elderly patients having a significant pre-existing medical problem and of being on some form of medication, it is even more important to obtain an accurate medical history

Management

Airway
- Leave well fitting dentures in place if a mask is going to be used for ventilation
- Handle the cervical spine with extra care as the elderly are more vulnerable both to fractures of the cervical spine and to damage of the spinal cord

Breathing
- Always administer oxygen
- Be extra careful to avoid damaging brittle teeth or dentures during tracheal intubation

Circulation
- There should be a lower threshold for putting up an intravenous infusion in the elderly, but infuse even more cautiously than usual, titrating infusion rate to the physical signs, to avoid either inadequate fluid replacement or fluid overload

26

The accident scene

The accident scene

Introduction

- Although almost every incident is unique, the procedures and guidelines to be followed are basically the same, and with experience should become instinctive
- It requires a lot of self discipline to adhere to guidelines and not to be distracted into doing either what others expect, or what your emotions tell you
- In particular, it is best to be relatively slow and sure, although a great deal of pressure may be put on you to do things either too quickly or not at all
- A few minutes doing things properly may save much time and even life, later on

Preparation

- Your **vehicle** should be:
    - Well prepared and maintained with:
        - Clean headlights
        - Regularly checked brakes, tyres, oil level, etc.
        - A full petrol tank
    - Highly visible: white or red, preferably with reflective strips and identifying panels
- Your **equipment** should be:
    - Well maintained, with expendable items replaced immediately after use (you never know when the next incident will be)
    - All drugs should be checked regularly for their expiry date
    - Stowed neatly, so that it is readily accessible for use, and easy for others to find. Similar boxes/ cases should be clearly labelled or colour coded according to their contents

PRACTICAL POINTS
- *It is advisable to have:*
    - *An arrangement with your local ambulance service/hospital for the replacement of medical gases*
    - *An arrangement with your local ambulance crews for the return of equipment after use.*
    - *An arrangement with your local Accident and Emergency Department and Ambulance Service for replacement of expendable or date expired items*
- *All drugs should have their expiry date clearly marked on the outside of their container*

Before setting off

- Ascertain the correct location of the incident before setting off, and try to work out a route to the incident in your mind, but do not waste too much time with this, as further directions are usually obtainable over the radio. The exception to this is motorways, when going the wrong way may result in many extra miles to travel
- Log in with the local ambulance service once you are on your way

Getting there
- Get there rapidly, but safely, and without hazarding or inconveniencing other road users
- Your **vehicle**:
    - Visible warning:
        - Green beacons: rotating light, strobe or light bar
            - This should be magnetic or permanently mounted, depending on the frequency of callout
        - Dipped headlights only should be used except in very heavy traffic, when rapid flashing of headlights may be permissible (a special unit can be fitted to your car for this purpose)
        - Fog lights should only be used in very poor visibility, i.e. fog, heavy rain
    - Audible warning devices/sirens:
        - Should only be used if prior permission has been obtained from the Police to do so
        - Twin tone horns/siren, may be mechanical or electric
        - These should be used with care as they can cause as many problems as they solve
    - Driving:
        - Do not take any unnecessary risks, and expect the unexpected
        - Driving training with your local traffic police is highly recommended
        - Always remember "*Safety fast*"

PRACTICAL POINT
- *The absence of oncoming traffic may mean that the road ahead is blocked, indicating a serious accident*

On arrival at the scene

Self protection

Protective identifying clothing
- Put on appropriate protective clothing preferably before setting off (especially if the accident/incident is on the motorway) or immediately on arriving at the scene
- It should be:
    - Protective, waterproof, warm, highly visible (fluorescent green/yellow)
    - Identifying with "DOCTOR" on the back and front
    - Chemical/fire resistant
    - Easy to clean
    - Allow you to "breathe"
    - Meet current regulations/standards for reflectivity/visibility.
- Consider: Helmet with a visor or protective goggles, jacket, tabard, gloves, over trousers, boots, etc.
- At night always wear a protective helmet with a head light, which will protect your head from unseen objects and the light will permit 'hands-free' operation

Note: Other items of equipment should include a personal ID card, torch, camera and mobile telephone

Hazards
- Do not expose yourself needlessly to any hazards, and look for those which may not be immediately obvious:
    - Oncoming traffic
    - Fire
    - Electricity
    - Dangerous chemicals/gases
    - Falling masonry
    - Strong water currents
    - Non-deployed airbags
    - Spilled fuels, battery acid and hydraulic fluids

Protecting the scene

Parking at the scene
- *Always park under police supervision.*
    - This should be as near to the incident as possible, so that you have all your equipment accessible but do not obstruct any ambulances or fire appliances
    - If necessary, particularly if you are the first on the scene, and there is poor visibility, park so as to protect the scene and minimise the chances of other vehicles colliding with any of the vehicles, etc. involved in the accident. Consider parking in the fend off position

The fend off position
- This is when a vehicle parks at an angle of about 45 degrees to the direction of travel
- It has the advantages that:
    - It makes a vehicle more visible to the oncoming traffic, as it displays a greater (side) area
    - If the parked vehicle is hit by another, it should tend to go in the direction in which its wheels are pointing, and not into the accident site
- The green beacon should be left on, and the hazard warning lights switched on
- If there is a danger of approaching vehicles not seeing the incident until too late and you are the first vehicle on scene, consider putting out a warning triangle, cones, etc.

PRACTICAL POINT
- *Leave the ignition keys in your vehicle, so that it can be moved if necessary*
- *Leave the engine running, so that you do not end up with a flat battery ("quitting" a vehicle, i.e. leaving it with the engine running, is permissible in these circumstances)*

Motorways
- These are particularly hazardous due to the high traffic density, and speed of vehicles, so special procedures have been agreed for the parking of emergency vehicles, using the ACECARD system (see diagram below)

Parking

Procedure:- Doctors attending an emergency on the motorway should:
- Put on protective clothing and safety helmets before proceeding to the incident or immediately on arrival
- Make sure of the location of the incident and access points onto the motorway
- En route, check the motorway marker posts against the distance from the incident
- Park the vehicle as follows:
- *Police first in attendance*
    - At most motorway incidents the Police will be in attendance before the arrival of the doctor, and will probably have placed "Police Accident" warning signs in position. Reflective cones and/or flashing lights may also be in use. A police vehicle should already have been parked 50 m on the approach side of the accident within the coned off area
    - The first doctor to arrive should park beyond the accident and first ambulance; leaving his green light and hazard warning flashers on
    - If an ambulance has not already arrived, he should leave room for an ambulance to park between the accident and his car
    - Reinforcing doctors should overtake the accident area and park 100 m beyond it on the hard shoulder displaying hazard lights but not green lights
    - If it is not possible to pass the accident area, the initial police vehicle in attendance will have stopped short of the accident, leaving enough space between itself and the accident for fire appliances, ambulances and doctors to park in

Motorway accidents: vehicle parking: either lane blocked

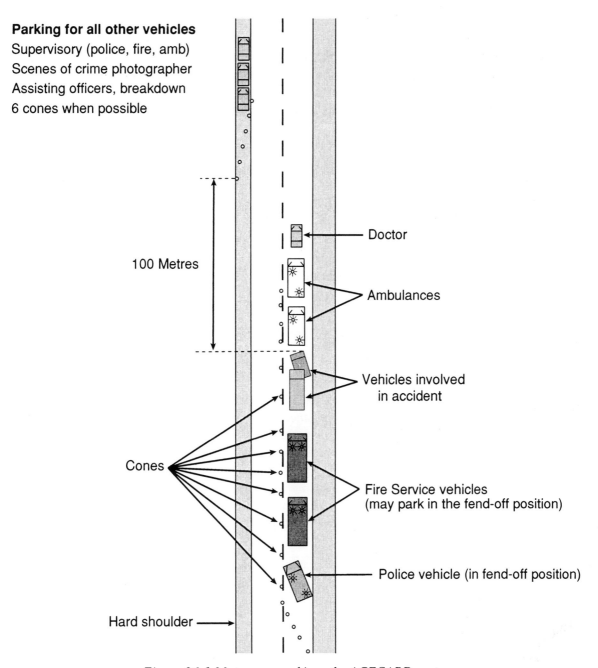

Parking for all other vehicles
Supervisory (police, fire, amb)
Scenes of crime photographer
Assisting officers, breakdown
6 cones when possible

100 Metres

Doctor

Ambulances

Vehicles involved
in accident

Cones

Fire Service vehicles
(may park in the fend-off position)

Police vehicle (in fend-off position)

Hard shoulder

Figure 26-1 Motorway parking: the ACECARD system

- *Doctor first in attendance*
    - Should he be the first to arrive, and part of the carriageway is still open, the first doctor should still park just beyond the incident
    - Immediately protect the scene by placing a warning triangle or reflective cones, flares and flashing lights if carried, at the rear of the accident site, i.e. nearest the oncoming traffic:
        - If possible, a warning triangle or a flare or flashing light should be positioned approximately 300 metres in advance of the accident. This should be on the hard shoulder if the accident is on the near side, and on the central reservation if the right hand lane is blocked
    - Vehicle lights, hazard warning lights and green beacons should be left on
    - Any reinforcing doctors should park in the positions as detailed previously

- *Liaison*
    - Where other services are in attendance, report to the officer in charge for information, and in particular liaise with the first ambulance crew or ambulance officer if he/she is in attendance

- *Leaving the scene*
    - When leaving the scene, switch off hazard warning lights and green beacons and drive off under police direction to enable safe merging with any passing traffic
    - Always be especially careful after attending an incident, as it is very easy to make errors at this stage, particularly if it has taken up a lot of time or energy or it has been difficult to deal with and you are tired

---

Guidelines for patient management at an accident

Initial scene assessment

Primary survey
- Initial triage of patients
- Initial patient assessment
- Initial patient management: resuscitation

Review of the scene/reading the wreckage
- Injury prediction

Secondary survey
- Secondary triage.
- Secondary patient assessment
- Secondary patient management
- Monitoring and recording the patient's condition

Monitoring
- Reassessment/review of management:
    - On the stretcher (with triage)
    - In the ambulance (with triage)
    - In transit

Figure 26-2 Guidelines for management of patients at an accident

Initial scene assessment

General principles
- Do not rush headlong into the incident towards those who are making the most noise, but inspect the scene carefully and methodically so as to get an overall picture
- This should be done rapidly without becoming over involved in the management of any individual casualties, except to carry out rapid life saving procedures

Specific points

Liaison
- Make contact as soon as possible with the ambulance crew in attendance
- Liaise with the senior ambulance, police, and fire officers present

The incident
- What has happened?
- What type of incident is it?

The casualties
- How many casualties are there?
- What kind of injuries do they have?
- How severely injured are they?
- Are they trapped?

Are there any hazards?
- Weather:
    - Cold, heat
    - Rain, sleet and snow
    - Wind, fog
- Dangerous chemicals (Hazchem code markings)
- Fire/explosion risk;
    - Petrol, gas
    - Explosives
- Unstable vehicles, buildings
- Electrocution from electricity power lines (see below)
- Non-deployed airbags

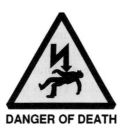

DANGER OF DEATH

Figure 26-3 High voltage danger warning sign

Electricity hazard
- All electricity, even 230 volt domestic supply can be lethal
- Touching electrical conductors or persons/objects in contact with them can be fatal
- Electricity can jump gaps (electricity may arc up to 10 metres from overhead power cables)
- Wearing rubber boots will not protect you
- Remember that trees, string, ropes, fences, crash barriers and water can all conduct electricity

Warning signs
- Towers and wooden poles carrying high voltage cables (more than 1000 volts) display a 'danger' warning sign. All electricity sub-stations are high voltage.
- Wooden poles without a danger sign are carrying low voltages (less than 1000 volts)
- *NEVER* assume that electrical equipment is dead, particularly fallen or broken wires/cables:
    - Electricity power supply companies normally restore the power supply following a short circuit after about 20-30 minutes, *without investigating the cause* (most are due to bird strike)
- It is therefore vital that the electricity power company is informed as soon as possible, to avoid the accidental electrocution of rescuers and rescued

Procedure
- Always keep at least 5 metres from a suspected live electrical conductor or anything touching it and await advice from the electricity power supply company
- If the electricity supply is less than 1000 volts, you may attempt to pull a live casualty clear with non-conductive gloves, or a dry wooden or other non-conducting pole

What is the geography?
- Are there any problems with access due to:
    - Ditches, ploughed fields
    - Water
    - Woods, trees
    - Buildings/building sites

Briefly examine the scene
- The road for:
    - Skid marks
    - Trail of wreckage, etc.
- Vehicle exteriors:
    - For deformity; which will give an idea of the collision/deceleration forces involved
- Vehicle interiors:
    - Is there any intrusion into and/or deformity of the passenger compartment
    - Have the seat belts been worn
    - Have airbags (if fitted) been deployed or not

Priorities in patient management
- Treat those patients who will die if not treated immediately, in particular:
    - The unconscious patient with an obstructed airway
    - The patient with a cardiac arrest, except possibly the elderly or those that have suffered major trauma and for whom the prospects of successful resuscitation are nil
    - Patient with severe haemorrhage from a major vessel
- Consider searching for ejected casualties and others whose presence may not be obvious initially especially in conditions of poor visibility, e.g. at night and in rough terrain, e.g. motorway ditches, embankments, hedges and in adjacent fields. This is best done by line searching (using a line of searchers who move forward together one step at a time)

Maximise medical/ambulance resources
- Use those doctors with the greatest expertise to treat those patients who most need those skills
- Identify ambulance personnel with special skills and make sure that they are used appropriately

Have other services been alerted?
- The Fire service:
    - Trapped patients
    - Dangerous chemicals/petrol or fire/fire risk
    - Illumination of the scene
    - Heavy lift, extra manpower

Medical/ambulance backup
- Are more doctors/ambulance personnel with extended skills needed?
- Is a surgical team required? (for field amputations)
- Is special medical equipment necessary?:
    - Pneumatic anti-shock garment (PASG)
    - Extrication devices
- Is helicopter evacuation required?:
    - Spinal injuries
    - Severe burns   } for rapid evacuation to a specialist unit
    - Injuries requiring immediate in-hospital management
- Are more ambulances required due to the number or severity of injuries of the casualties? (liaise with the ambulance crews (or ambulance officer if present))

The wreckage
- Do not interfere unnecessarily with any wreckage or debris from the accident site, which may be needed later by the police for forensic purposes

The dead
- Always insist that management of the living should take priority over confirming death
- Do not interfere with any dead casualties, but after confirming death in the presence of a police officer, leave them where they are until a police Scenes of Crimes Officer (SOCO) has arrived to examine the scene and take photographs
- It is advisable to note the date and time of confirmation of death, together with the name and number of the police officer dealing with the incident, for future reference, in case the coroner requires a statement
- Photographs of the deceased, taken with police permission, may also be useful

Triage
- Sort the casualties into various categories according to their needs for:
    - Immediate treatment
    - Special resources:
        - Experienced doctors
        - Extended trained ambulancepersons
        - Splints and other special medical equipment
    - Early evacuation
    - Evacuation to special (hospital) facilities
- If necessary label them according to their triage category, and be prepared to change their category according to any significant changes in their condition
- Triage should be dynamic, i.e. continuous and changeable

Primary survey and resuscitation (see chapter: Guidelines for Immediate Medical Care)

Guidelines
- This is the simultaneous assessment, identification and management of immediate life threatening problems, followed by an assessment of the potential for developing other serious life threatening problems or complications
- Airway with care of the cervical spine
- Breathing with control of ventilation
- Circulation with control of haemorrhage
- Disability; assessment of neurological function
- Exposure with control of the Environment

Reassessment of the scene/reading the wreckage (see below)
- If circumstances and the patient's condition permit, briefly reassess the scene in order to work out the likely mechanism of injury of your patient(s), before going back to the patient for the secondary survey:
    - Examine the scene
    - Examine the wreckage
    - Work out the mechanism of injury (you have already examined the patient)
    - Relate the two to each other
    - Do they correlate or might you expect injuries that you have not yet found?
    - If so look for them whilst doing the secondary survey

Reading the wreckage to determine the mechanism of injury in road traffic accidents

Introduction

- Examination of the accident scene for evidence as to why and how an accident occurred and for damage (wreckage) caused as a result of an accident may help the trained observer to predict the kind of injuries and problems that the casualty is likely to be be suffering from. These should be positively looked for, although they may not be obvious or even complained of initially. If there is no wreckage, for example when two bodies collide, then the severity of the injuries caused to one casualty are likely to be reciprocated by the other person involved in the impact

    Example: A common situation is one in which the driver of a vehicle anticipates the impending impact and produces endorphins to provide his own pain relief, enabling him to ignore his own pain and therefore injuries in the first few hours after injury. A notable historical example was the Marquis of Anglesey who had a leg shot off during the battle of Waterloo, but didn't realise it until the battle was over.

The Police, for forensic purposes, and the Road Research Laboratory, who carry out research into the causes of road traffic accidents and the mechanisms of injury, have a lot of experience in analysing the mechanism of injury from studying post-mortem reports and the wreckage from serious road traffic accidents

Examination of the accident scene

- How did the accident happen?:
    - What hit what? and what happened then?
    - What were the road conditions?
    - Assess:
        - The probable speed of impact
        - The forces involved (force = mass x acceleration), and their direction
- Why did the accident happen?:
    - Was the driver asleep?
    - Was alcohol involved?
    - Is the driver diabetic or epileptic?
    - Did the driver have a myocardial infarction?
    - Was there:
        - Too much speed?
        - A fault with one of the vehicles?
        - Adverse weather conditions?

Examination of the vehicle wreckage

- The type of impact:
    - Was it frontal, side, rear, or rollover, etc.
- Look for:
    - Deformity of the exterior of the vehicle:
        - Shortening of the front of the vehicle.
        - Rearward displacement of the wheels, doors and body panels
        - Buckling of the vehicle's floor or roof
        - The severity of the deformity can give a good idea as to the velocity of impact:
    - Intrusion into the passenger compartment:
        - Backwards displacement of the front wheel arch
        - Inwards displacement of the doors, roof and rarely the floor pan

- Deformity of the interior of the vehicle caused by the occupants, e.g. damage to the:
  - Windscreen (head)
  - Steering wheel (chest)
  - Front parcels shelf (knees), etc.
- The human body is softer than metal, and where there is major distortion of metal, it can be predicted that there will be even greater damage done to the human body involved
- Was a seat belt worn and did it lock?
- Was there any movement of objects inside the vehicle?:
  - Forward movement of seats
  - Unrestrained rear seat passengers
  - Loose luggage, etc.
- Examine a motor/pedal cyclist's helmet for signs of impact/damage

Evidence of high energy frontal impact
- Rearward displacement of wheels and body panels
- Deformity of the passenger compartment:
  - Buckling of the roof or floorpan
  - Rearward displacement of doors (making them difficult or impossible to open)
- Triggering of airbags (European specification airbags typically trigger at an impact speed of 18-20 mph, when crashing into a solid barrier)

Effects of severe frontal impact

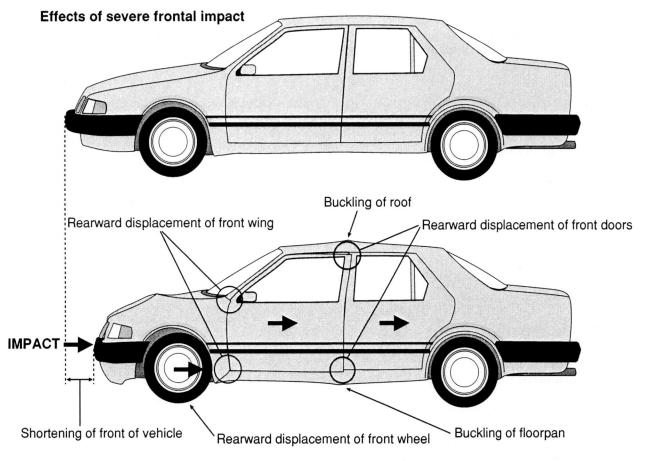

Figure 26-4 Effects of severe frontal impact

Examine the injury pattern of the casualty
- What are the apparent injuries? (look for pattern bruising)
- What forces acted on the victim, and how did they act?
- How rapid was any deceleration?
- Where was the force of the impact/energy transmitted to?
- What was compressed? (by cavitation or by secondary collision with internal organs)
- What injury producing movements were likely to have occurred as a result of ? (hyperflexion, hyperextension, excessive lateral flexion, etc.)
- What injuries are likely to occur as a result?

Injury prediction
- From consideration of all the above, and with a knowledge of the mechanisms of injury, it should be possible to predict the injuries that the patient is likely to be suffering from.
- In road traffic accidents, there are impacts involving:
    - The vehicle(s)
    - The patient(s)
    - The patient's internal organs.
- Determine the mechanism of injury:
    - How was the patient injured?
    - What forces were involved?
    - What injuries would you expect?
- Was deceleration rapid or gradual? (the more rapid the deceleration, the more serious the injuries are likely to be)
- Relate the mechanism of injury to the clinical findings

Secondary survey and management

Subjective interview

Objective examination

Head
- Scalp
- Neurological state
- Base of skull
- Face

Neck
Chest
- Chest wall and lungs
- Heart

Abdomen/pelvis
Extremities
- Upper limb
- Lower limb

Spine
- Back

Pain
- Analgesia

Medical history
- AMPLE

Monitoring/reassessment of the patient

Monitoring
- All the patient's vital sighns should be monitored at regular intervals:
  - Pulse
  - Blood pressure
  - Oximetry reading
  - Respiratory rate
  - Glasgow coma scale score

Trending
- Analysis of serial recordings of the patient's vital signs will give an early indication of any improvement or deterioration in their condition

Rescue of persons from vehicles fitted with airbags
- Airbags are being fitted to all new cars, and although only about 7% of all cars currently have airbags, this percentage will increase year on year until 2005, when it is estimated that about 80% of cars will have airbags fitted
- Whilst airbags undoubtedly save lives and help to prevent serious injury, they may cause some injuries, and are a major hazard for the rescue services if they are not deployed during an accident, as they may suddenly deploy and cause significant injury to the rescuers

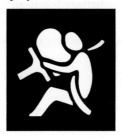

Figure 26-5 Airbag warning logo

Airbag deployment
- Airbags are fitted in the steering wheel boss (or front fascia in front of the front seat passenger), and an increasing number of cars are fitted with side impact airbags in the sides of the front seat back rest
- Airbags deploy immediately after a frontal/oblique frontal impact, due to a very rapid chemical reaction (controlled explosion) which produces a large volume of gas (and a loud bang) with a force of about 700 lbs/sq in at 200 mph (230 kph); this may have a stunning effect on the car occupants
- Airbags are designed to deploy:
  - In moderate to severe frontal impacts (within 20° of the mid-line or either side of the front of the vehicle) and are not designed to deploy in low speed frontal, rear end, or side impacts or in rollover accidents
  - When two electronic sensors simultaneously detect a deceleration in excess of the pre-set limits (in the UK and Europe, an impact of more than 18 mph). These sensors are:
    - A crash sensor which detects acceleration/deceleration
    - A safing sensor which detects deceleration only
- There are vents in the side or top seams of the airbag which allow the hot gases inside the bag to vent and allow the bag to deflate almost immediately after full inflation, thus releasing the driver or passenger
- Accidental airbag deployment may occur if:
  - The vehicle catches fire
  - Procedures performed by the rescue services generate sufficient voltage to trigger airbag inflation, e.g. cutting or pulling the steering column
- Airbag deployment is extremely loud and the vehicle occupants may appear stunned and deafened

Undeployed airbags
- Determine whether an airbag is fitted:
  - Vehicles fitted with a driver's airbag have the word AIRBAG, SIS or SRS on the steering wheel boss
  - Vehicles fitted with a front seat passenger's airbag have the word AIRBAG, SIS or SRS on the front fascia
  - Vehicles fitted with an airbag may have a label with the airbag symbol on the rear face of the appropriate door and on the VIN plate on the instrument panel
- All undeployed airbags should be treated as a potential hazard
- If an undeployed airbag is detected, a protection device should be used, e.g. a *Bag-Buster*^{TM}, which deflates the airbag as soon as it is triggered and prevents any particles from being released, before starting any rescue procedures
- Always carry out any procedures from the side of the vehicle and out of the potential path of the airbag, should it inflate unexpectedly
- Move the seat of the stabilised occupant as far backwards as possible or lower the back of the seat as far as possible
- Never position yourself, equipment or any other objects on or in front of a non-deployed airbag

Note: 1. Disconnecting the battery *will not* immobilise all airbag systems immediately, as there may be a residual energy reserve feature incorporated in the system, to enable the airbag to deploy in the event of battery failure. This has the energy to deploy the airbag for up to one minute after the ignition has been switched off or the battery has been disconnected
2. The steering column of a vehicle fitted with an airbag should *not* be cut or drilled. If in exceptional circumstances it is necessary to cut the steering column, the battery should be disconnected more than one minute beforehand
3. If the airbag is found to be punctured; *do not* touch any exposed chemicals
4. *Never* cut an airbag
5. Airbags will deploy spontaneously at high temperatures, e.g. if the vehicle catches fire

Deployed airbags
- The surface of a deployed airbag may be coated with a fine powdery residue, which is talcum powder or corn starch, used to lubricate the airbag as it deploys
- Some by-products of combustion may also be present. These are mainly sodium carbonates, but there may also be a very small amount of:
  - Sodium hydroxide, which can cause slight irritation of the skin and eyes
  - Sodium azide, which may cause hypotension, if it is accidentally absorbed through an open wound
- If gloves are not worn, the hands should be washed with soap and water after handling a deployed airbag
- Avoid getting any residue into the eyes or open wounds
- Be aware of the possibility of hot metal components under the airbag fabric, inside the steering wheel/front fascia
- Look positively for injuries that the patient may not yet be aware of, but you may suspect from your examination of the scene/vehicle

Entrapment

- Entrapment is a situation commonly encountered at the roadside but may also be a problem in industrial, recreational, aircraft, train, farming and domestic incidents
- Is usually but not always associated with significant injury
- In road traffic accidents entrapment is usually associated with extensive deformity of the vehicle, with intrusion into the passenger compartment
- There are usually problems with gaining access to the patient, both for assessing injuries, monitoring vital signs and treatment (initial resuscitation, followed by splinting, etc.)
- Almost always results in delay in full assessment and management of injuries, and evacuation to hospital may be delayed for several hours
- May result in prolonged exposure to hazards/hostile environment
- Special rescue equipment may be required to obtain the release of the casualty, and special medical equipment may be required for their actual removal, e.g. an extrication device
- Entrapment may be:
    - Relative
    - Absolute
    - Complicated

Relative entrapment

- This occurs when the casualty in unable to remove themself from the situation they are in after an accident, usually as a result of their injuries, which by themselves may not be very serious:
    - Unconsciousness will mean that a casualty is incapable of leaving the scene of their accident
    - A fractured ankle will prevent a casualty from descending/ascending a mountain after a fall
    - The pain and disability from a fractured humerus may prevent a casualty from leaving the vehicle in which they have been injured

Absolute entrapment

- Absolute entrapment occurs when the casualty is physically prevented from leaving the scene of their accident, because of modification to their environment as a result of what caused the accident, e.g.:
    - The casualty trapped in a vehicle due to deformity of the vehicle, resulting in interior intrusion, and/or seizing of the door locks
    - Collapse of a building, roof fall in a cave or mine may result in the casualty being physically trapped and unable to get out of where they are

Complicated entrapment

- Entrapment may be complicated or prolonged due to:
    - Impaction, when the casualty is trapped and physically restrained from moving
    - The patient's injuries, which may make extrication of the patient very difficult
    - Impalement
    - The need for amputation of a trapped part before the casualty can be released

Management of the trapped patient

- The management of the trapped patient should follow the usual guidelines, but in a slightly modified form because of the problems associated with lack of access for examination and management of the patient's injuries
- It may not be possible to examine and treat some parts of the patient until they have been released
- The aim of management is to:
    - Save life
    - Prevent and treat any complications
    - Extricate the patient rapidly, without causing any pain or aggravating/causing any injuries
- It should be remembered that the management of the trapped and injured patient is a team effort, everyone involved has their own special role and the more everybody works together as a cohesive unit, the greater the benefit will be for the patient. Ideally all potential members of the team should train together, so that they become familiar with each other's roles, equipment, strengths and weaknesses
- The whole entrapment situation is dynamic:
    - The cause of the patient's injuries may still be present and may continue to cause injury (unlike the patient in hospital, when the cause of injury has usually been removed)
- There may be more than one patient who is trapped and injured

Initial assessment of the scene

Primary survey and resuscitation
- Initial triage of patients
- Initial patient assessment/management: resuscitation

Reassessment of the scene/reading the wreckage

Secondary survey and management
- Secondary patient assessment/management
- Monitoring and recording the patient's condition
- Secondary triage

Overview of the scene

Monitoring
- Reassessment/review of management:
    - During extrication
    - On the stretcher
    - In the ambulance (with triage)
    - In transit

Assessment of the entrapment scene
- Scene assessment:
    - What is the cause of entrapment: why?
    - What is the method of entrapment: how?
- If trapped, is entrapment:
    - Relative? e.g. in the unconscious
    - Absolute? e.g. in the impacted casualty
- Are any special resources required to rescue the patient?

Primary survey and resuscitation in entrapment
- Identify the "time critical" patients (triage):
    - Those whose injuries and condition are such that they have priority for rapid extrication
- Determine the need for any additional medical support
- Liaise with the Fire Service especially over:
    - Safety and access to the patient during the extrication.
    - The release of trapped limbs, etc.
- Liaise with the ambulance service over:
    - The use of medical equipment
    - The method of patient removal, etc.

Airway
- Potential problems:
    - Access to the patient for:
        - Assessment
        - Management:
            - Cricothyrotomy
            - Intubation

Breathing
- Potential problems:
    - The position of the patient may inhibit breathing
    - Access to the patient for:
        - Assessment:
            - Monitoring the colour of the patient may be difficult due to poor lighting conditions.
        - Management:
            - Difficulty with carrying out practical procedures:
    - Oxygen may be contraindicated due to the risk of explosion
    - High ambient light levels may make it difficult to visualise the vocal cords for intubation

Circulation
- Potential problems:
    - The patient's position may impair their circulation
    - The environment, e.g.: cold:
        - May cause peripheral circulatory shutdown
        - May precipitate or aggravate shock
        - Intravenous fluids may freeze at very low temperatures (heat retaining cases and fluid warming devices may be necessary)
    - Access/adequate light for:
        - Assessing the patient (the capillary refill test is only reliable in relatively good light)
        - Management, e.g. setting up an intravenous infusion

Disability
- Potential problems:
    - Cerebral hypoxia resulting in confusion; consider:
        - Sedation, ventilation
        - This may also cause problems with extrication

Exposure with control of the environment
- This is not usually appropriate in the entrapment situation, except for:
    - Assessment of major injuries
    - Management of:
        - Life threatening injuries
        - Open injuries/lacerations requiring the application of dressings/protection
- Be careful not to let the patient get cold:
    - Cover them with blankets, etc.

Secondary survey and management in entrapment
- The full secondary survey is usually not possible until the patient has been removed from the place of entrapment to a "place of relative safety", usually an ambulance
- Depending on access, a modified secondary survey and management may be performed

Bony injury
- Potential special problems in the management of the trapped patient include difficulty with access for:
    - Assessment of:
        - Fractures
        - The peripheral pulses
    - Management:
        - Access for applying a splint:
            - Position
            - May not permit formal splint application
            - (Consider temporary splinting with: frac straps, bandages)

Analgesia/sedation
- Potential problems in administration of:
    - Nitrous oxide/oxygen gas mixture (*Entonox®, Nitronox®*):
        - Risk of fire
        - Room for the gas cylinder
    - Intravenous opiate ⎫
    - Intravenous midazolam ⎬ difficult intravenous access
    - Intravenous diazepam ⎭

Overview of the scene
- Stand back and review regularly:
    - The patient
    - The scene
    - The extrication process
- Review/repeat regularly

During extrication
- Anchor equipment securely, e.g. intravenous lines, splints
- Liaise closely with the ambulance crew and Ambulance Incident Officer (if present)
- Prepare:
    - The patient (for haemorrhage, pain)
    - For extrication:
        - Carrying sheet
        - Extrication device
    - The stretcher, e.g.: lay out a vacuum mattress, prepare traction splints

Assessment/management on the stretcher

- Take advantage of any open access to thoroughly reassess the patient if practicable, but be careful not to expose him/her unnecessarily or for too long to a hostile environment, e.g. the cold, wet or extreme heat
- Perform any procedures which may be difficult to perform in the confined space of an ambulance or helicopter, e.g. stabilisation or splinting
- Package/prepare the patient for loading making sure that all attached equipment is secure and accessible where necessary
- Liaise with the ambulance or helicopter crew to determine the most appropriate loading method and position of the patient in the ambulance or helicopter taking into account:
    - The patient's injuries, splinting, monitoring equipment, etc.
    - Any special characteristics of the ambulance's or helicopter's patient compartment

Assessment/management in the ambulance

- Reassessment of the patient prior to departure: take advantage of the stable platform, better lighting (if it is dark outside), and warm environment to thoroughly reassess the patient and perform any necessary practical procedures that it was not possible to perform whilst the patient was trapped:
    - *Primary survey and resuscitation*
        - Airway care:
            - Intubation
        - Breathing: ventilatory care
        - Circulation:
            - Further intravenous lines
            - Application of PASG
        - Disability
        - Exposure:
            - Remove all clothing to facilitate a full secondary survey
    - *Secondary survey and management*
- Triage: Identify the "time critical" patient ("scoop and run" vs "stay and stabilise")
- Select the hospital appropriate to the patient's injuries and medical condition according to local policies:
    - A hospital with a Burns Unit for those severely burnt
    - A hospital with a Neurosurgical Unit for head injuries
    - A major hospital for those with multiple serious injuries
- Determine any treatment required in transit
- Determine the need to travel yourself
- Determine the need for a police escort:
    - If traffic is heavy or the patient's condition is critical
- Brief the ambulance crew whether you are travelling with the patient or not

Note: In the case of motor/pedal cyclists, their crash hat/helmet should always be sent with them to hospital

- Keep the ambulance's doors closed to:
    - Conserve heat
    - Enable life saving procedures to be performed in private
    - Spare anxious relatives unnecessary distress
    - Keep all unnecessary personnel out

Assessment/management in transit

- Continuously monitor the patient's:
    - Airway
    - Breathing
    - Circulation
    - Dysfunction: neurological status
- Review the equipment in use and the patient positioning
- Radio the patient's clinical details to the hospital as necessary (according to local policies)
- Stop the ambulance if necessary to treat the patient:
    - To modify any splinting, etc.
    - To carry out defibrillation

Extrication

- If the patient is trapped they will need to be freed by the Fire and Rescue Service and then extricated
- This will involve teamwork from all involved

Routine extrication

- This is appropriate when there is no immediate risk to the life of the casualty
- In casualties with a suspected or possible spinal injury (if the patient has no other life threatening injuries, there is no need for rapid extrication):
    - An extrication device should be used and the patient extricated on a spinal board (an extrication device is significantly more effective than a spinal board alone in preventing rotation of the spine)

Urgent extrication

- This should be used when there is a risk to life, but access to the patient is limited
- In casualties with a suspected or possible spinal injury:
    - A spinal board should be used to facilitate, if possible/practicable, extrication through the rear of the vehicle, as the application of an extrication device is more time consuming and usually necessitates removal of the vehicle roof in most cases

Emergency extrication/Snatch rescue

- Emergency extrication should be used when there is an immediate major risk to life, e.g. risk of vehicle fire, or a serious airway or breathing problem
- In casualties with a suspected or possible spinal injury, the risk of aggravating the spinal injury should be weighed up against the risk of remaining in situ. In these circumstances:
    - Use of a spinal board with extrication through a side door is acceptable, using the "rapid extrication technique" in which the spine is immobilised using manual in-line stabilisation and the application of a semi-rigid collar before the patient is turned, and then slid out on the board

Special devices for patient extrication/transfer

For extrication

- Extrication device
- 'Scoop' chair
- Long spinal board, head blocks and body harness/straps
- 'Scoop' stretcher and straps

For a description of these devices, see chapter on Spinal injuries

Stretchers for carrying

- Ambulance trolley with canvas (and poles and spreader bars)
- Vacuum mattress (on ambulance trolley; for a description of this device, see chapter on Spinal injury)
- Neil Robertson stretcher
- Paragard stretcher

Neil Robertson stretcher

Description (for diagram; see chapter on Aeromedical evacuation)
- The stretcher is made of canvas with bamboo or wooden slats sewn into it longitudinally
- It has an upper set of short wings which fold around the thorax and a lower set of longer wings which may partially fold around the pelvis and legs
- Side straps to secure the wings around the body and legs, and immobilise the head, and rope handles at each end and on both sides
- The stretcher may be carried by the rope handles on each side, or lifted from the head end

Advantages
- Immobilises and splints the whole body
- Encloses and protects most of the body

Disadvantages
- Does not provide total immobilisation of the cervical spine
- May be difficult to apply if the casualty has had splints applied

Application
- Before use the device should be laid flat and folded out
- The casualty may be:
    - Transferred to the stretcher from a 'scoop' stretcher or carrying canvas with poles and spreader bars
    - Rolled onto the stretcher after the wings on one side have been rolled under the stretcher (similar to the long spinal board)
    - Slid onto the stretcher from the lower end
- Once the casualty is lying on the stretcher the wings are fasted around the body with straps, and the head secured with the head strap

CONCLUSION
- Useful for moving casualties through confined spaces (the Neil Robertson was originally developed for use in ships)

Paraguard stretcher

Description
- This is a relatively recent development of the Neil Robertson stretcher, which it resembles, but it is made from a reinforced plastic material with slats, and has a hinge in the middle, which allows it to be bent in the middle, even when holding a patient, to help it manoeuvre around obstacles, There is also a strap to secure the ankles
- The stretcher incorporates lifting/grab handles and approved lifting rings, so that it may be lifted by a helicopter winch

Application
- Before use the device should be laid flat and folded out and the hinge locked straight with the metal sleeves
- Lay the patient down on the stretcher (as above)
- Fold the upper and lower wings around the body and fasten their straps, and apply the head and ankle straps

CONCLUSION
- A usefully modernised version of the Neil Robertson stretcher, which has the added advantage of bending in the middle

Triage decision guidelines for hospital selection

1. *If:*
- The Glasgow coma scale score: <13
- The systolic blood pressure: <90 mmHg
- The respiratory rate: <10 or >29 breaths per minute
- The Triage Revised Trauma Score: <11

Then:
- Take the patient to a major hospital

2. *If not:*
- Assess the mechanism of injury, and the patient's actual injuries
- If the patient has:
    - A penetrating injury to the head, neck, chest, abdomen, pelvis or groin
    - Fractures of two or more proximal long bones
    - Burns totalling 15% or more, or burns to the face or burns involving the airway
    - A flail chest
    - Evidence of a high energy impact, e.g.:
        - Falls of 20 ft or more
        - An impact velocity of more than 20 mph
        - 20" deformity of front of vehicle or 30" if involving less than 2/3 of front of vehicle
        - Rearwards displacement of the front axle
        - 15" intrusion of the passenger compartment of the vehicle on the patient's side
        - Ejection of the patient
        - Vehicle rollover
        - Death of an occupant in the same car
        - A pedestrian hit at 20 mph or more by a car, or at more than 10 mph by a heavy vehicle, e.g. a lorry or bus

Then:
- Take the patient to a major hospital

3. *If not:*
- If:
    - The patient's age is <5 or >55 yrs
    or:
    - There is a known history of cardiac or respiratory disease, and moderate injury severity.

Then consider:
- Taking the patient to a major hospital

If in doubt take the patient to a major hospital

Reporting from the accident scene
- Reporting from the scene using report forms, printout from a patient monitoring device, photography, and any other relevant material will give the receiving doctor as much information as possible to help him determine how best to further treat and investigate the patient
- All doctors are taught, to a certain extent, to ignore what the other doctor has found and to examine the patient for themselves, but in Immediate Care they do so at their peril!

Report forms

Purpose
- To inform the receiving doctor of:
  - The patient's identity:
    - Name, address and date of birth
  - The type of accident:
    - RTA
    - Industrial
    - Domestic
    - Recreational
  - The history of the accident:
    - Alcohol?
    - Knocked out?
    - Vomited?
  - The mechanism of injury:
    - Driver/ front/rear seat passenger
    - Wearing/not wearing seat belt
    - Motorcyclist wearing/ not wearing helmet
    - Pedal cyclist, pedestrian, etc.
    - Details of the type of impact
  - The patient's suspected injuries
  - The patient's initial (baseline) condition:
    - Vital signs:
      - Glasgow coma scale
      - Trauma score
    - Changes in that condition (trends):
      - During extrication
      - In transit
      - In response to the treatment carried out
  - Treatment carried out since the time of injury:
    - Airway care:
      - Adjuncts used:
        - Airways.
        - Intubation
        - Oxygen
    - Breathing:
      - Ventilation
      - Chest drain
    - Circulation:
      - Intravenous infusion
    - Analgesia:
      - Nitrous oxide/oxygen gas mixture (*Entonox*®, *Nitronox*®), morphine
    - Splinting:
      - Spine, limb(s)

- The time intervals involved:
  - From first call (approximate time of accident) to first attendance
  - Duration of any entrapment
  - The time taken to stabilise the patient's condition.
  - The time spent in transit
- Any significant/relevant past medical history if available
- The patient's triage category:
  - Major incidents
- By whom the patient was examined and treated
- To help predict the likely patient outcome (trauma scoring)
- To act as a guide as to which hospital the patient should be sent and treatment priority (triage)
- For audit/research: for the ambulance service, Immediate Care doctors and the hospital
- To act as an aide memoire
- To act as a record for medico-legal purposes
- To be a training aid

Requirements

- Any report form should:
  - Provide all the above information
  - Be user friendly:
    - Easy to understand
    - Easy to carry, etc.
  - Be quick and easy to fill in:
    - Requiring the minimum of writing; with most questions answered by a tick
    - Should only contain space for observations and measurements which are readily obtainable in the field, e.g. pupil sizing is unreliable in the field where the lighting conditions can vary considerably, and so the terms: large, medium and small should be used
  - Have space for serial observations
  - Allow easy information retrieval:
    - Both clinical and research
  - Show uniformity:
    - Should use commonly understood terms and internationally agreed categories between ambulance services, Immediate Care schemes, and hospitals

Note: Consideration should be given as to whether any report form should be A4 size (or even A3 size), which is fairly large, but will show lots of information clearly or A5 size, which is more convenient and may fit into a pocket, but may be too small for all the information to be shown clearly

Patient Report Form

BASICS
BRITISH ASSOCIATION FOR IMMEDIATE CARE

INJURY ASSESSMENT?PRIORITY

Critical/Immediate	☐
Serious/Urgent	☐
Minor/Delayed	☐

CALLSIGN: Ambulance   **Dr.**

Date	Time Call		
Location	Arrival	Surname	Forename
	Depart	M/F d.o.b	Address
Hospital	Arrival	Vehicle No.	

ASSESSMENT ☐ RTA ☐ Work ☐ Home   ☐ Organised Sport   ☐ Leisure   ☐ Other (specify)

If RTA: ☐ Driver   ☐ Front/Rear Passenger   ☐ Pedestrian   ☐ Motorcyclist   ☐ Cyclist

Seatbelts? ☐ Yes ☐ No   ☐ Not known   Vomited? ☐ Yes ☐ No   Alcohol? ☐ Yes ☐ No   ☐ Not known

Crash helmet? ☐ Yes ☐ No   ☐ Not known   Ko'd? ☐ Yes ☐ No   Trapped? ☐ Yes ☐ No   How long?

PRIMARY SURVEY   Time:

Airway	☐ Clear	☐ Obstructed
C. Spine	☐ Normal	☐ Possible injury
Breathing	☐ Spontaneous	☐ Problem
Circulation/	☐ External	☐ Possible internal
Haemorrhage	☐ None/slight	☐ Moderate ☐ Severe
Disability	☐ Alert	Responds to ☐ Verbal stimuli ☐ Pain ☐ Unresponsive

Exposure/Injuries

C# Closed Fracture
O# Open Fracture
B Burn (shade area)   L Laceration
F Foreign body   A Abrasion
                            E Ecchymosis (bruising)

PRIMARY MANAGEMENT

Airway	☐ Oropharyngeal	☐ Nasal	☐ ET Tube
	☐ C/Thyrotomy	☐ Oxygen	☐ Suction
C. Spine	☐ C. Collar	☐ Ext Dev	☐ Long board
Breathing	☐ Ventilated	☐ Chest drain	

Circulation   Cannula size: Rt............   Lt..............

IV Fluids	Volume	Time
☐ H'manns/N. Saline _____		_____
☐ H'maccel/G'fusine _____		_____

SECONDARY MANAGEMENT

Analgesia ☐ N₂O/O₂   **Dose**   **Time**
Drugs   ☐ _____ _____ _____
(specify) ☐ _____ _____ _____

Splinting	☐ Frac Straps	☐ Traction: lbs/Kg_____
	☐ Box	☐ Other (specify)_____

SECONDARY SURVEY   Time: 1)   2)   3)

	1)	2)	3)
Respiratory Rate			
Oxygen Saturation (SpO₂)%			
Blood Pressure	-----	-----	-----
Pulse Rate			

Pupil reaction (✓ or X)   R ☐ ☐ ☐
                               L ☐ ☐ ☐

1 ○ Constricted   Size R [   ] [   ] [   ]
2 ○ Normal
3 ○ Dilated   Size L [   ] [   ] [   ]

Eye	Spontaneous	4	☐	☐	☐
Opening	To voice	3	☐	☐	☐
	To pain	2	☐	☐	☐
	None	1	☐	☐	☐
Best	Orientated	5	☐	☐	☐
Verbal	Confused	4	☐	☐	☐
Response	Inappropriate words	3	☐	☐	☐
	Incomprehensible	2	☐	☐	☐
	None	1	☐	☐	☐
Motor	Obeys commands	6	☐	☐	☐
Response	Localises pain	5	☐	☐	☐
	Withdrawal (pain)	4	☐	☐	☐
	Flexion (pain)	3	☐	☐	☐
	Extension (pain)	2	☐	☐	☐
	None	1	☐	☐	☐

COMA SCALE SCORE: 1)   2)   3)

COMMENTS

Signed	**Dr.**	**Nurse**
Crew		

© John Eaton/BASICS 1998

26-6 Patient report form

Procedure
- Any report form should be initiated by the first person attending the patient; ambulance personnel or Immediate Care doctor, be added to as necessary, especially if there are any serial observations, and go with the patient in the ambulance to the hospital casualty department, where they should be incorporated into the patient's notes
- Ideally there should be three copies; one each for the:
    - Ambulance service
    - Immediate Care doctor
    - Hospital

Coma Scale

introduction
- This was developed with the objective of indicating the patient's neurological injury and probable outcome following serious head trauma.

Glasgow coma scale

Eye opening	Spontaneously	4
	To verbal command	3
	To pain	2
	No response	1

Best motor response	To verbal command: Obeys	6
	To painful stimulus: Localises pain	5
	Flexion/withdrawal	4
	Flexion decorticate	3
	Extension decerebrate	2
	None	1

Best verbal response	Orientated/converses	5
	Disorientated/confused	4
	Inappropriate words	3
	Incomprehensible sounds	2
	Nil	1

Total   (3-15) _____

Figure 26-7 Glasgow coma scale

Trauma scoring

Introduction
- This is a method of measuring (scoring) the physiological state of the patient, in an effort to predict the outcome on a statistical basis
- It should be understood that as it is a statistical tool, it does not accurately estimate the outcome for a particular patient, but purely predicts the average outcome for a group of patients with similar scores
- It may be used for triaging patients at major incidents or to determine the appropriate hospital for any particular patient
- It can also be used as an evaluation tool, e.g. in statistical analysis
- To be of greatest value, it must use accurately obtained and recorded and repeatable measurements/ values, so as to reduce to the minimum any errors due to observer error or bias. If possible recording or measuring devices giving a clear readout and/or printout are to be preferred

Revised trauma score (RTS)
- The original trauma score was revised in 1987 to make scoring easier in the field, and to weigh it more in favour of the neurological state of the patient, using the Glasgow coma scale
- Capillary return and respiratory expansion, which are difficult to assess in the field, have been omitted
- A score below 4 for any variable indicates a survival rate of less than 90%
- A score below 6 indicates a survival rate of just over 45%
- Limitations of the revised trauma score include:
    - Patients with some severe injuries, e.g. long bone fractures, may have a normal score
    - It is unreliable if applied to paediatric casualties, so a paediatric trauma score has been developed

Note: A more sensitive trauma score is currently being developed using the addition of the SpO_2 reading

Revised trauma score		
Glasgow coma scale score	13-15	4
	9-12	3
	6-8	2
	4-5	1
	3	0
Systolic blood pressure	>90	4
	76-89	3
	50-75	2
	1-49	1
	0	0
Respiratory rate	10-29	4
	>29	3
	6-9	2
	1-5	1
	0	0
	Total score	**(0-12)**

Figure 26-8 Triage revised trauma score

Paediatric trauma score (PTS)

Introduction
- The paediatric trauma score is the paediatric counterpart of the triage revised trauma score
- It is rather more complicated and less easy to remember than the adult score. In particular, the weight can only be guessed, unless one of the parents knows it, and it is probably best reserved for use in the hospital, rather than the pre-hospital setting
- Skeletal injury is included because of its high incidence in children and its contribution to their mortality
- A score of greater than + 6 gives a predicted mortality rate of less than 1%
- A score of less than + 6 gives a predicted mortality rate of 25%

Paediatric trauma score

Weight	>44 lbs:20 kg	**+2**
	22-44 lbs:10-20 kg	**+1**
	<22 lbs:10 kg	**-1**
Airway	Normal	**+2**
	Oral/nasal airway	**+1**
	Intubated/tracheostomy	**-1**
Diastolic blood pressure	90 mmHg	**+2**
	50-90 mmHg	**+1**
	50 mmHg	**-1**
Level of consciousness	Completely awake	**+2**
	Drowsy, but rousable	**+1**
	Comatose/unconscious	**-1**
Open wound	None	**+2**
	Minor	**+1**
	Major or penetrating	**-1**
Fractures	None	**+2**
	Closed Fracture	**+1**
	Open or Multiple	**-1**
	Total score (-6 to+12)	

Figure 26-9 Paediatric trauma score

Problems with trauma scoring
- Trauma scoring lacks sensitivity
- There may not be enough time for the patient to deteriorate
- The patient may be hypertensive

Photography

Introduction
- This may play an important part in recording what has happened in an accident
- If possible the time, date (which may be recorded on the film by some cameras), and location where the pictures were taken should be recorded
- Can help with learning to read the wreckage

Legal and ethical aspects of photography and video recording
- There is no law of privacy in the UK and technically, taking a photograph of someone without their consent, is not an assault
- If photographs or video recordings are going to be used in lectures or for publication, it is permissible to record patients who require emergency treatment, but who cannot give consent. If the patient is capable of giving their consent, this should be obtained and the facts recorded in their clinical records. If the patient or a relative asks you to stop, you must do so
- Photographs and video recordinds should never be used or released for publication without first obtaining the consent of the injured or their relatives, or before the police have informed the next of kin
- Consideration should also be given to blanking out identifying marks, e.g. the number plates of vehicles facial characteristics of the patient, etc.
- If the photographs are only going to be used as part of the patient's clinical (medical) records, then the obtaining of their consent is probably implied
- Although not normally admissible as evidence, photographs may be requisitioned by the police, or asked for by the patient's solicitor
- In some areas, hospital photographers are prepared to go out to accidents, but need to be incorporated into the callout system, and to have personal and vehicle identification

Instant or Polaroid® photography
- This uses an automatic camera (autofocus, autoflash) which can produce instant pictures (Polaroid®) which can be sent with the patient to hospital
- Some cameras have the ability to "stamp" the date on the photograph
- In the near future digital cameras may be used, and the disc of the photographs from an accident sent with the patient to hospital to be downloaded onto a computer or printer in the Accident & Emergency department

Purpose
- To inform the receiving doctor of:
    - The mechanism of accident/injury
    - The forces involved:
        - Deformity of the exterior of the vehicle:
            - Deceleration
        - Deformity of the passenger compartment:
            - Prediction of injuries
    - Any special injuries:
        - Dislocations and fractures before and after reduction at the scene
        - Degloving injuries, etc. which are best not disturbed too often
    - Blood loss after haemorrhage
- They may also be:
    - A legal record of the above
    - Useful for helping the hospital staff, especially junior medical staff, to appreciate what the patient has been through and to help bridge the gap between pre-hospital and hospital care
- Ideally the camera should be robust and small enough to fit in a pocket or emergency medical case and should form part of the first response equipment

Method
- Pictures should be taken of:
    - The accident scene:
        - To give an idea of what happened when the accident occurred
    - The exterior of the vehicle:
        - To show any deformity of the vehicle, including any shortening, displacement of panels buckling of the floor pan, indentation of the roof, etc.
    - The interior of the vehicle
        - To show any intrusion into the passenger compartment, e.g. wheel arch, door panel
        - To show any deformity caused by impact with the occupants, e.g. steering wheel

Still photography
- This uses fully automatic compact cameras with autofocus, autoflash and a wide angle, zoom and close up (macro) facility. Those which can fit in a jacket pocket are to be preferred
- More bulky Single Lens Reflex cameras are probably best reserved for the professional photographer or when there is plenty of time
- Still photograpgs and slides can be useful as a teaching or learning medium, but to maximise their value, details of the injuries sustained by the patients, etc. should be kept
- In serious accidents involving the death or probable death of the injured, a police Scenes of Crime Officer (SOCO), is usually called in to photograph the scene to obtain forensic evidence as to the cause of injury or death, and can be a useful source of material

Video recording
- This requires bulky equipment and a professional camera operator to produce a professional result.
- It can be very useful as a training aid, and is being increasingly used by the Fire Service and Police Forces (also for forensic purposes)

Other aspects of recording
- Where possible, it is advisable to send with the patient to hospital any other items which may be useful to the receiving doctor
    - ECG recordings
    - Medication the patient may be taking
    - Poisons the patient may have ingested
    - Motor cyclist's helmet, etc.

27

The emergency services

The emergency services

Introduction

- The statutory emergency services are those services, whose responsibilities are laid down in law
- All those involved in pre-hospital emergency medical care, should consider themselves to be part of the emergency team, made up of all those members of the emergency services attending the incident, whose prime role is to treat the ill/injured as effectively as possible to save lives, reduce the effects of serious injury/illness, and stop any unnecessary suffering
- To do so they must integrate themselves into the team, realising that each member of the team is as important in his own way as any other, and each has his own area of specialist expertise and part to play
- To achieve this he must have an understanding of the roles of the other members of the team, together with some knowledge of their command structure, way of working and equipment, including its uses and limitations
- The team will need a leader, but this may not necessarily be the same person all the time provided that everybody in the team knows who it is, and recognises their authority. An example may be the motorway accident with a serious entrapment. The police will be in overall command and will direct all the other emergency services to an appropriate parking place. The fire service will usually be in control of the physical extrication process, but this may be under medical/ambulance direction if the patient's condition necessitates medical treatment before and during the extrication process. Once this is achieved the medical and ambulance services will manage the patient's treatment, before their eventual evacuation to hospital by the ambulance service. Each service will need continuous liaison with and assistance from each of the other services

The police

Role
- To preserve and safeguard life and protect property
- To uphold and enforce the law
- The prevention and detection of crime and the prosecution of offenders
- The enforcement of the road traffic law
- To control, co-ordinate and facilitate the work of the other emergency services
- To provide assistance for the other services moving to and from the scene of any incident
- To supply information to the press at major incidents and co-ordinate press releases from other agencies
- To establish and provide initial communications at the scene of any accident or incident
- To act on behalf of the coroner (or Procurator Fiscal in Scotland):
    - Investigate sudden or suspicious deaths
    - Arrange mortuary facilities, transport and custody of the deceased at major incidents
- To report the circumstances to the appropriate investigating authorities and facilitate their enquires

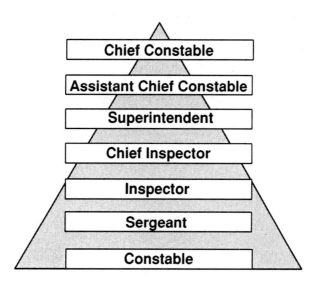

Figure 27-1 Rank structure of the Police Service

Command structure

- In each County or Metropolitan Area, there is a Police Force with its headquarters; each commanded by the Chief Constable, with his staff
- Attached to each headquarters is a Control Room and various specialist Departments:
  - Traffic
  - Scenes of Crime
  - Diving, etc.
- Each force is divided into Territorial Divisions, usually under the command of a Superintendent, with a senior staff of Chief Inspectors. Attached to each territorial division may be a number of specialist units, eg.:
  - Traffic
  - Community Service
- In most areas, the Division is further subdivided into Sub Divisions, under the command of a Chief Inspector or Inspector
- Each Territorial Division or Sub Division will include a number of Police Stations, usually under the command of a Chief Inspector or Inspector
- Each police station will usually be staffed by a number of shifts under the command of an Inspector or Sergeant

Note: 1. The (London) Metropolitan Police Force is commanded by a Commissioner, with a staff of Deputy Commissioners, Assistant Commissioners, Commanders and Chief Superintendents
2. In addition to County and Metropolitan Police Forces, there are a number of specialised Police Forces, which have a similar rank structure, e.g.:
   - British Transport Police
   - Royal Parks Police
   - Docks Police
   - Ministry of Defence Police
   - Military Police, RAF Police and Regulating Branch in the Royal Navy (have a military rank structure)

HM Coastguard

Role

- Similar to the police, but covering the coast and inshore waters
- Co-ordinate the other emergency services

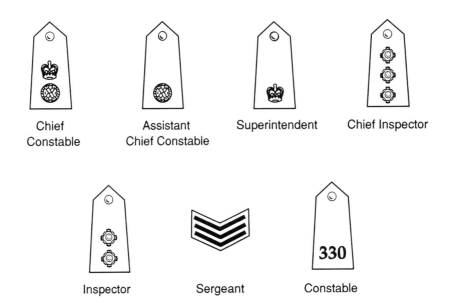

Figure 27-2 Rank identification: Police Service

The ambulance service

Role
-   To provide ambulance aid and where there are ambulance persons with advanced skills; paramedic ambulance aid to the seriously ill and injured
-   To provide appropriate transport to hospital for the seriously ill and injured, and to render ambulance aid en route
-   To provide appropriate transport to and from hospital for patients attending outpatient departments, day hospitals, physiotherapy departments, etc. and for non urgent admissions and discharges
-   Provide transport for inter-hospital transfers
-   To provide Health Service communications, logistical support and site management in close co-operation with the Police and Medical Incident Officers

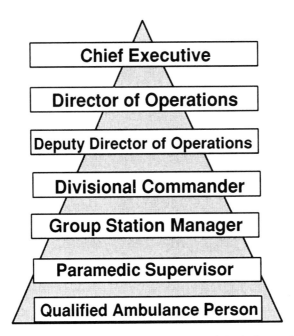

Figure 27-3 Rank structure of a typical Ambulance Service
NHS Trust (may vary)

Command structure

- In each National Health Service Region and Metropolitan Area, there was usually a Regional Chief Ambulance Officer, each County Ambulance Service in the Region being commanded by a Chief Ambulance Officer. Most of these have now become Ambulance Service NHS Trusts under the management of a Chief Executive
- Each Ambulance service has a Headquarters, usually situated adjacent to its control, which may also incorporate a training school, and is normally split up into three areas of activity:
    - Operations
    - Control and Communications
    - Support Services (Training, Fleet Transport)
- Services may be divided into Operational Divisions, which may be commanded by a Divisional Commander (Divisional Ambulance Officer)
- Each Ambulance Station or group of ambulance stations, depending on their size, is commanded by a Group Station Manager (Station Officer)
- Each small ambulance station may be supervised by a Paramedic Supervisor (Leading Ambulance Person)

Note: Each Ambulance Service is co-terminus with its Health Authority and its area may extend beyond the boundaries of the Police and Fire and Rescue Services within the County boundary, except in London where the London Ambulance Service covers two enlarged Health Regions and numerous Health Authorities

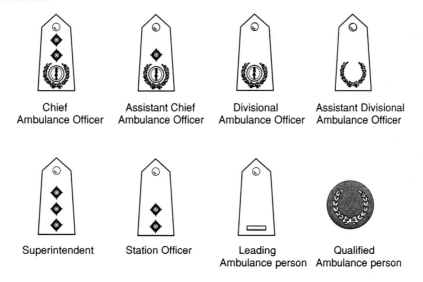

Figure 27-4 Rank identification: Ambulance Service

The fire and rescue service

Role

- To fight fires, protect life and property and advise on fire prevention
- To provide a rescue service for those trapped in road traffic, farming and industrial accidents or any other incident where people may become trapped
- To rescue patients from chemical incidents, and then deal with the chemicals themselves, rendering them harmless
- To monitor any radiation risk and rescue patients from radiation incidents
- To provide special equipment, e.g. Emergency lighting, pumping equipment, at incidents on request from the other emergency services
- To ensure safety at the scene of an incident and advise the other emergency services/agencies of any hazards

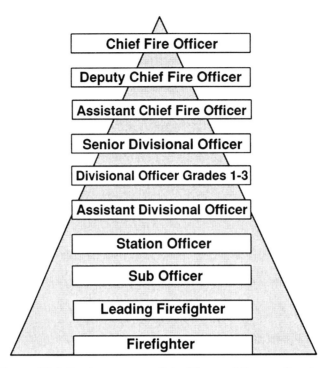

Figure 27-5 Rank structure of the Fire and Rescue Service

Command structure

- In each county or metropolitan area, there is a Fire and Rescue Service, commanded by a Chief Fire Officer, who has a Headquarters with an associated Central Control and a Headquarters staff
- The area in which the service operates is usually divided into Divisions, under the command of a Divisional Commander
- Each division will consist of a number of Stations, each under the command of a Station Officer
- In each Station there will be several Watches, which man the station in turn
- Each Watch is under the command of a Sub Officer, who has the assistance of a Leading Firefighter

PRACTICAL POINT: *It is often easier to identify firemen at an incident, by looking at their helmets. Officers above the rank of Sub Officer have white helmets, and below that rank yellow helmets. The greater the number and width of the black bands, the higher the rank*

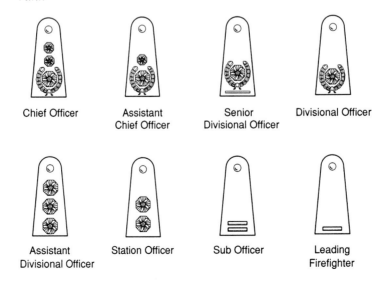

Figure 27-6 Rank identification: Fire and Rescue Service

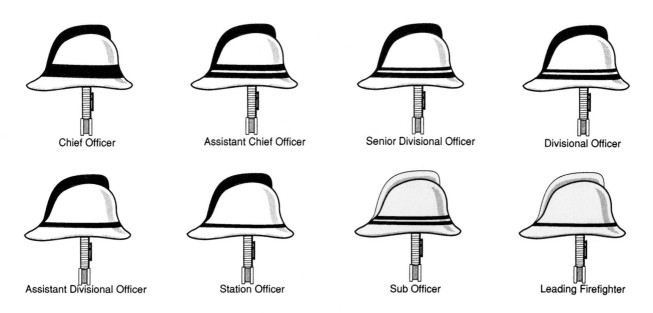

Figure 27-7 Rank identification: Fire Service helmets

Rural areas

-   In rural areas, where there is not enough work to justify employing full time firemen, Fire Services employ Retained Firemen, who have other full time jobs. They are alerted by long range radio pagers and proceed to the fire station, where the first to arrive form a crew and man the first fire engine/"Pump"

The medical services

Role

-   To prevent unnecessary death and suffering by providing assessment and medical treatment for the seriously ill or injured both out of hospital by General Medical Practitioners, and in hospital
-   General Practitioners have a legal duty as part of their terms of service to "give treatment which is immediately required owing to an accident or emergency" within their practice area
-   To confirm death

Note: Registered Medical Practitioners are the only people traditionally able to confirm death out of hospital

Organisation

-   The National Health Service in the United Kingdom is organised into "Providers" and "Purchasers"
-   In each NHS Region there are Health Emergency Planning Officers (HEPOs), to help plan and co-ordinate the Health Service response within that Region and with surrounding Regions
-   In each NHS Region, the providers are:
    -   Hospital Trusts, who hold contracts to provide hospital services
    -   Community Trusts, who have contracts to provide out of hospital services, except General Medical Services and General Dental Services
-   In each NHS Region, the purchasers are Unitary Health Authorities, who commission health care including General Medical (and Dental) Services and purchase it on behalf of the local population
-   All potential Receiving Hospitals are required to make provision to provide a Medical Incident Officer and a Mobile Medical Team, if requested to do so by the ambulance service. In the latest guidelines the ambulance service is advised not to nominate a Medical Incident Officer or ask for a Mobile Medical Team from any hospital receiving casualties from the incident, unless there is no alternative
-   In many areas there is now an agreement for the Ambulance Service to nominate the most appropriate doctor from a list of suitably trained senior doctors, including Consultants in Accident and Emergency Medicine and General Medical Practitioners, who are members of the local Immediate Care Scheme

Pre-hospital medical services

Doctors
- Out of hospital medical care is provided by General (Medical) Practitioners, who hold a contract with the local Health Authority
- In many areas, General Practitioners have developed a special interest in pre-hospital emergency medicine, and make themselves available to the Ambulance Service to assist in the medical management of sudden serious illness or severe injury in the community, as members of their local Immediate Care Scheme. The experience that they develop in emergency medicine and in working with the ambulance service, makes them particularly suitable for providing the medical input into Major Incidents

Ambulance Services
- Ambulance Services are usually a separate Health Service Trust which holds the contract from one or more Health Service Authorities to provide an Emergency Ambulance Service and, but not always, a non-emergency hospital patient transport service, within a specified area. In some areas this may be provided by another Ambulance Service or contractor

Relationships with ambulance crews
- Immediate Care doctors need to work very closely with their colleagues in the Ambulance Service:
    - Provide support
    - Advise
    - Supervise medical management
- Once in attendance, the doctor has legal and clinical responsibility for the purely medical management of the patient, regardless of who actually treats that patient

The local authorities

Role
- To maintain their own services and help those affected by the incident:
    - Local authorities have the task of obtaining additional manpower or specialised equipment and providing temporary accommodation, meals and other forms of relief to people in urgent need
- To co-ordinate the activity of the various organisations which support the emergency services and the the local authority including:
    - Health Authorities
    - Public and private utilities
    - The Armed services
    - Voluntary organisations, e.g. WRVS (Women's Royal Volunteer Service), British Red Cross
    - Adjacent local authorities

Organisation
- Local authorities are managed by a Chief Executive, who is responsible to a council of elected members
- There are a number of departments including:
    - Emergency planning:
        - Emergency planning officers (EPOs) who draw up contingency plans to cover a range of possible emergencies, from civil defence to peacetime disasters
    - Housing
    - Works, highways and structural engineering
    - Education and welfare

Inter-service co-ordination/co-operation
- There are usually dedicated land lines linking the central controls of each emergency service

28

Dangerous substances

Dangerous substances

Introduction
- The number, quantity and variety of dangerous substances transported by road, rail or in the air is steadily increasing and with it the risk of exposure and contamination following an accident
- The possibility of dangerous substances being involved should always be borne in mind when assessing the scene of any accident

Classification of dangerous substances
- The United Nations Committee of Experts on the Transport of Dangerous Goods has classified dangerous goods into nine groups, some of which have subgroups:
  - Class 1: explosives
  - Class 2; gases
  - Class 3: flammable liquids
  - Class 4: flammable solids
  - Class 5: oxidising and organic peroxides
  - Class 6: poisonous (toxic) and infectious substances
  - Class 7: radioactive substances
  - Class 8: corrosives
  - Class 9: miscellaneous dangerous substances

Labelling of dangerous substance containers

- The physical characteristics of a substance: colour, smell, etc., even if apparent, may not be sufficient to identify that substance or distinguish one substance from another
- The accurate labelling of the containers of dangerous substances is very important if accidental exposure/contamination and spillages are to be managed safely and effectively

United Nations number
- This is a four figure number, which is used worldwide, and is specific to each individual dangerous substance, so as to allow its rapid identification

Substance identification number
- This number is now used in the UK, as it includes some substances not covered by the UN list

United Nations warning label
- Recognised internationally and is included in most labelling systems
- It is a diamond shaped warning label indicating the primary hazard
- If there is more than one hazard, the diamond will show an exclamation mark

United Nations warning labels 1

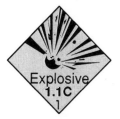

Class 1.1 - Mass explosion hazard

Class 1.2 - Projection hazard not mass explosion hazard

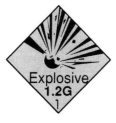

Class 1.4 Moderate explosion hazard

Class 1.6 Minor explosion hazard

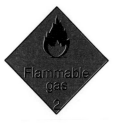

Class 2 - Flammable gas

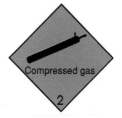

Class 2 - Non flammable compressed gas

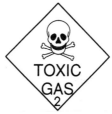

Class 2 - Toxic gas

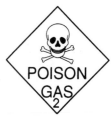

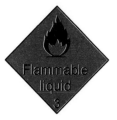

Class 3 - Flammable liquid

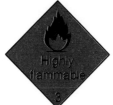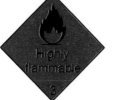

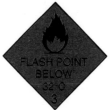

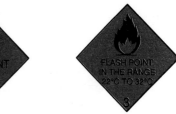

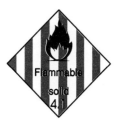

Class 4.1 - Flammable solid

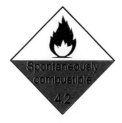

Class 4.2 - Spontaneously combustible substance

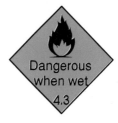

Class 4.3 - Dangerous when wet

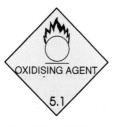

Class 5.1 - Oxidising substance

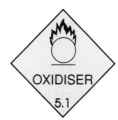

Class 5.1 - Oxidising substance

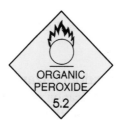

Class 5.2 - Organic peroxide

Figure 28-1 Examples of UN warning diamonds 1

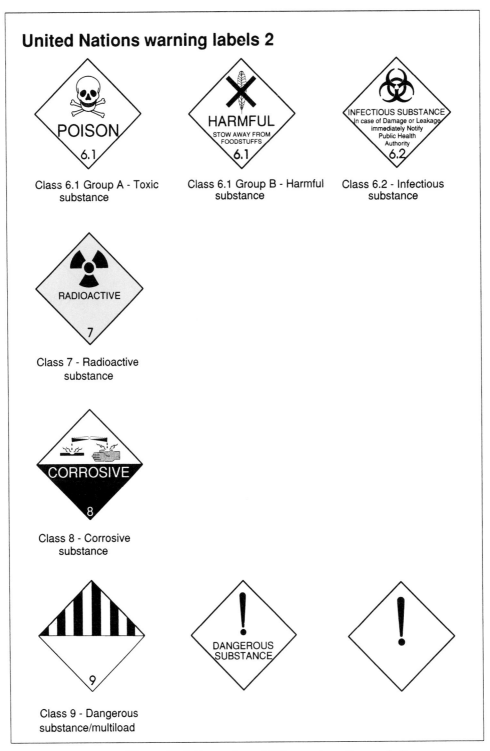

Figure 28-2 Examples of UN warning diamonds 2

Hazard warnings: United Kingdom hazard information system (UKHIS)/Hazchem label

- In order to provide rapid identification of individual dangerous chemicals, together with the hazard risk and method of dealing with them, all vehicles carrying prescribed dangerous substances in the UK are required to display warning labels on both sides and the rear
- In addition companies are obliged by law to inform the drivers of tankers of the significance of the warning panels and the load carried
- This labelling system will soon be replaced by the ADR labelling system (see below)

- The warning labels must give the following information:
    - Emergency action code, giving advice on how to control the chemical.
    - The United Nations identification number and name of the substance.
    - The United Nations hazard warning label.
    - The special advice telephone number.
    - The name and symbol/housemark of the manufacturer.

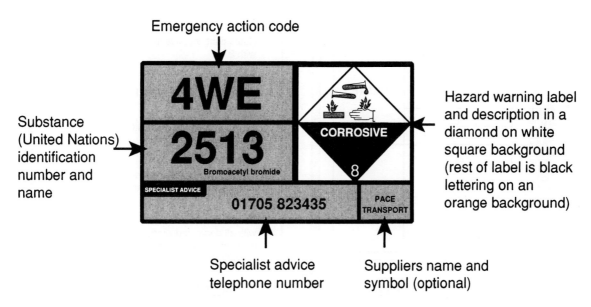

Figure 28-3 Example of a"UKHIS" board/Hazchem label

Specialist advice telephone number
- This is the 24 hour emergency telephone number of the supplier or manufacturer of the chemical

Emergency action code (formerly the Hazchem code)
- This gives the information necessary for the fire service to deal with the substance:
    - The recommended dispersal method:
        - Jets
        - Fog
        - Foam
        - Dry agent
    - The personal protection required
        - Full body protective clothing with breathing apparatus
        - Breathing apparatus plus protective gloves
    - The risk of explosion
    - The need for evacuation
    - The method of disposal:
        - May be diluted and washed down drains
        - Should be prevented from entering drains or water course

Hazchem card
- This is a small card designed for fire service use which details the management of chemical spillages
- Carried in all fire appliances and should also be carried by all Immediate Care doctors and ambulances

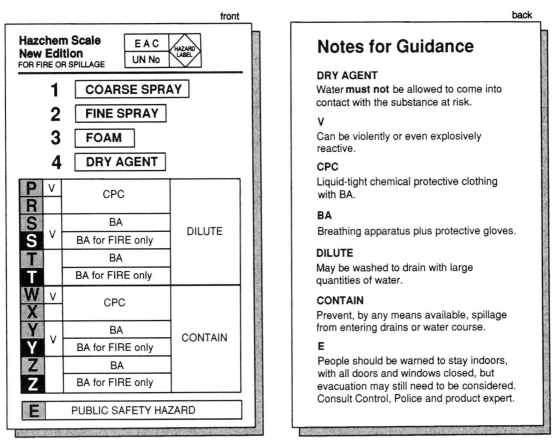

Figure 28-4 Hazchem card

CEFIC system of transport emergency cards (Road) - TREM card
- This is a system developed by the European Council of Chemical Manufacturers' Federation and is a manual of cards designed to give the emergency services information about dealing with hazardous chemicals, before expert advice can be obtained
- The cards are A4 sized and each gives the following information:
    - The correct British Standard chemical name of the substance
    - A description of the chemical's appearance and physical properties
    - The appropriate protection to be used
    - Advice on the immediate management of spillage or fire
    - The first aid management of contaminated casualties
- They are not always updated: always check that it is the correct one!
- It is usually kept in the nearside door pocket of the truck cab

ADR/CIM European Identification label
- This is a label displayed on the sides and rear of vehicles carrying hazardous substances to, from and on the European mainland and will shortly supersede the UKHIS board, bringing the UK into line with European practice
- It is in two parts:
    - The upper displays the Hazard Identification Number (HIN) or KemLer code (see below)
    - The lower part shows the Substance Identification (United Nations) Number
- United Nations hazard warning diamonds indicating from left to right the primary, secondary, and tertiary hazards (if appropriate) should be displayed together with the ADR label

RID identification label
- This is a similar labelling system to the ADR system, but used on railway wagons in Europe

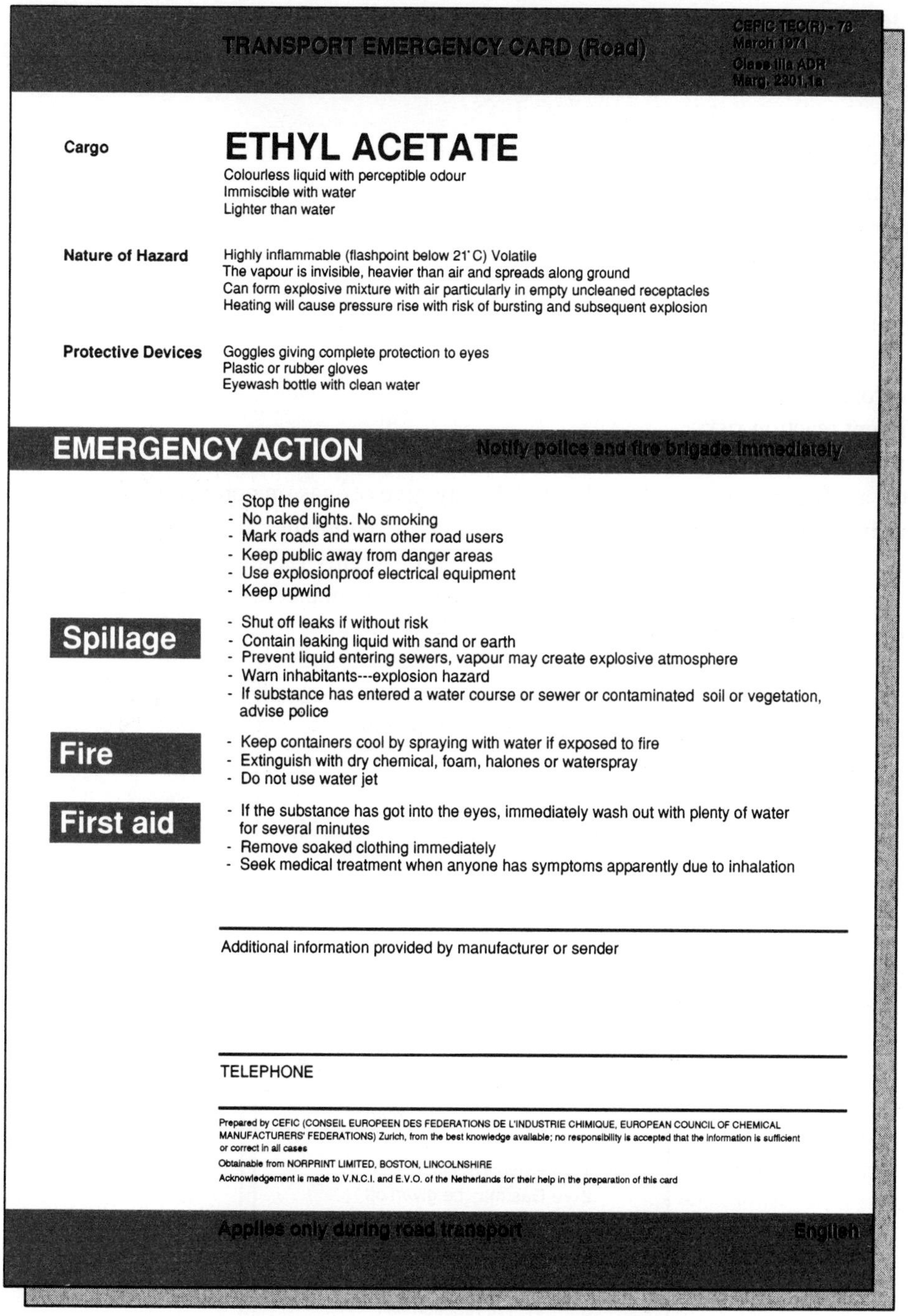

TRANSPORT EMERGENCY CARD (Road)

CEFIC TEC(R) - 78
March 1971
Classe IIIa ADR
Marg. 2301.1a

Cargo

ETHYL ACETATE

Colourless liquid with perceptible odour
Immiscible with water
Lighter than water

Nature of Hazard

Highly inflammable (flashpoint below 21°C) Volatile
The vapour is invisible, heavier than air and spreads along ground
Can form explosive mixture with air particularly in empty uncleaned receptacles
Heating will cause pressure rise with risk of bursting and subsequent explosion

Protective Devices

Goggles giving complete protection to eyes
Plastic or rubber gloves
Eyewash bottle with clean water

EMERGENCY ACTION   Notify police and fire brigade immediately

- Stop the engine
- No naked lights. No smoking
- Mark roads and warn other road users
- Keep public away from danger areas
- Use explosionproof electrical equipment
- Keep upwind

Spillage
- Shut off leaks if without risk
- Contain leaking liquid with sand or earth
- Prevent liquid entering sewers, vapour may create explosive atmosphere
- Warn inhabitants---explosion hazard
- If substance has entered a water course or sewer or contaminated soil or vegetation, advise police

Fire
- Keep containers cool by spraying with water if exposed to fire
- Extinguish with dry chemical, foam, halones or waterspray
- Do not use water jet

First aid
- If the substance has got into the eyes, immediately wash out with plenty of water for several minutes
- Remove soaked clothing immediately
- Seek medical treatment when anyone has symptoms apparently due to inhalation

Additional information provided by manufacturer or sender

TELEPHONE

Prepared by CEFIC (CONSEIL EUROPEEN DES FEDERATIONS DE L'INDUSTRIE CHIMIQUE, EUROPEAN COUNCIL OF CHEMICAL MANUFACTURERS' FEDERATIONS) Zurich, from the best knowledge available; no responsibility is accepted that the information is sufficient or correct in all cases
Obtainable from NORPRINT LIMITED, BOSTON, LINCOLNSHIRE
Acknowledgement is made to V.N.C.I. and E.V.O. of the Netherlands for their help in the preparation of this card

Applies only during road transport   English

Figure 28-5 Example of a TREM card

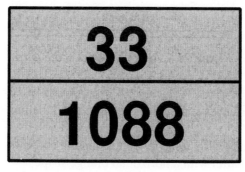

Figure 28-6 ADR/CIM "KemLer" board

The Hazard Identification Number (HIN) or Kemler code
- This is a numerical code using two or three digits which indicates the properties of the chemical
- The first digit indicates the classification of the primary hazard (see under Classification of dangerous substances)
- Second and third digits indicate any secondary hazard:
    - 0 No meaning
    - 1 Explosion risk
    - 2 Gas may be given off
    - 3 Inflammable risk
    - 5 Oxidising risk
    - 6 Toxic risk
    - 8 Corrosive risk
    - 9 Violent reaction risk
- An X in front of the first number indicates that the use of water is absolutely prohibited
- 22 indicates a refrigerated gas, 42 a solid which may give off gas on contact with water
- A repeated digit indicates an increased hazard, e.g. 3   flammable: flash point 21-100 °C
                                                      33   highly flammable: flash point <21 °C
                                                      333 spontaneously flammable

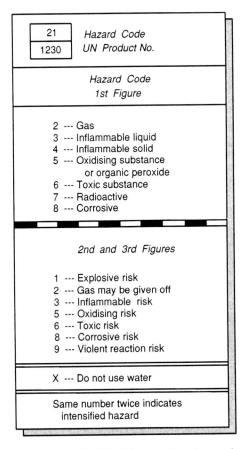

| 21 | Hazard Code |
| 1230 | UN Product No. |

Hazard Code
1st Figure

2 --- Gas
3 --- Inflammable liquid
4 --- Inflammable solid
5 --- Oxidising substance
        or organic peroxide
6 --- Toxic substance
7 --- Radioactive
8 --- Corrosive

2nd and 3rd Figures

1 --- Explosive risk
2 --- Gas may be given off
3 --- Inflammable risk
5 --- Oxidising risk
6 --- Toxic risk
8 --- Corrosive risk
9 --- Violent reaction risk

X --- Do not use water

Same number twice indicates
intensified hazard

Figure 28-7 ADR "Kemler" scale card

Labels on wagons
- Conveyors of dangerous substances sometimes use their own labelling system in addition that laid down in law
- The colour of a tank wagon may also assist in identifying the contents:
    - Liquefied gases: white barrel with a horizontal orange stripe
    - Highly flammable liquids: dove grey barrel with signal red sole bars

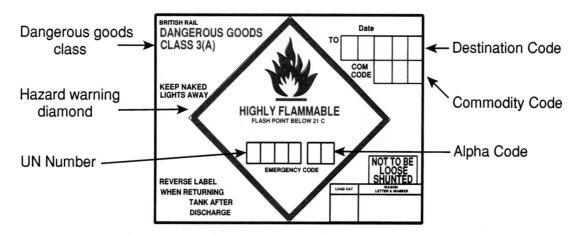

Figure 28-8 Example of a railway wagon label

Substances of low hazard
- The Chemical Industries Association has introduced a voluntary scheme, known as the "black and white marking scheme" for the marking of domestic tanker vehicles carrying substances of low hazard
- The panels are similar to the UKHIS panels, but:
    - The panels are only coloured black and white
    - There is no hazard warning diamond, but words of warning may appear in the same place
    - There is no substance identification number, but there is a description of the substance, e.g. chemical name

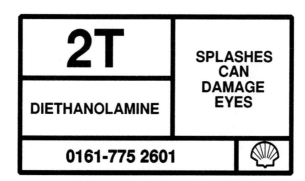

Figure 28-9 Example of a low hazard warning panel

Labels on packages
- The regulations for the labelling of hazardous goods carried or stored in packages are specified in the CHIP (Chemicals (Hazard Information and Packaging) Regulations)
- The label must include:
    - The full name of the substance, or the trade name if it is a mixture
    - One or two danger symbols and key words
    - Risk phrases
    - Safety phrases
    - The full name, address and telephone number of the manufacturer, importer, wholesaler or supplier
- If the package requires two danger symbols, the two labels should be attached so that they overlap at the middle edge. Twin labelling also indicates that the substance contained in it should not be mixed with other loads
- Packages may also have labels giving advice on their safe handling

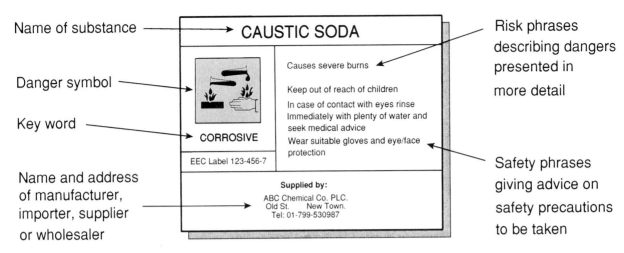

Name of substance

Danger symbol

Key word

Name and address of manufacturer, importer, supplier or wholesaler

Risk phrases describing dangers presented in more detail

Safety phrases giving advice on safety precautions to be taken

Figure 28-10 Label for dangerous goods in a package

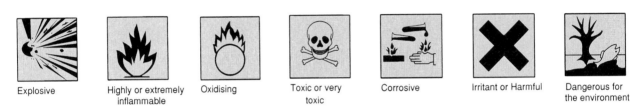

Explosive | Highly or extremely inflammable | Oxidising | Toxic or very toxic | Corrosive | Irritant or Harmful | Dangerous for the environment

Figure 28-11 Danger symbols for dangerous goods in a package (black lettering on an orange background)

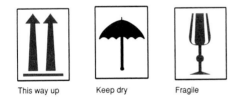

This way up | Keep dry | Fragile

Figure 28-12 Handling labels for packages

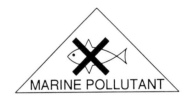

MARINE POLLUTANT

Figure 28-13 Label for marine pollutant

Management of chemical incidents

Principles

- It is the agreed responsibility of the Fire and Rescue Services to deal with the rescue and decontamination of contaminated casualties, which should be performed on-site
- In the UK, most Fire services have access to CHEMDATA, a computerised database, which gives advice on how to deal with most dangerous chemicals, and there is also the National Advice Centre, at the Atomic Energy Research Establishment Toxic and Hazardous Materials Group, at Harwell, which is prepared to provide 24 hour telephone assistance in identifying any chemical not in CHEMDATA
- If dangerous chemicals are involved in an incident, you should not risk your own safety to treat seriously contaminated casualties, as you may only add yourself to their number!
- Casualties should usually only be treated after they have first been rescued and if necessary decontaminated by the Fire Service
- Any personnel with a pre-existing skin condition or wounds involving breaches of the skin should not attend chemical incidents

Procedure

On arrival
- Inform ambulance control immediately if a chemical incident is suspected on arrival at the scene of an incident, and request the attendance of the Fire and Rescue Service, giving any details about the chemicals that may be immediately obvious
- Don protective clothing, if available, including overalls, boots, impervious gloves, "debris gloves" and eye protection

Initial assessment
- If you are the first to arrive, try to assess the wind direction if any gases are involved, and the flow of any liquids. Always approach the scene from upwind and uphill
- Advise anybody else in attendance to do likewise
- Perform life saving procedures during the initial assessment, provided this can be done without risking contaminating yourself
- If you are not completely protected, do not touch any chemical containers, etc., and if you are protected but contaminated do not touch anybody else especially any casualties, without first being decontaminated yourself
- If possible after identifying the chemicals involved, obtain details of the appropriate risk and immediate treatment indicated. Assess the number and severity of contamination of any casualties, and convey all this information to the Fire Service, Ambulance Service and Receiving Hospital immediately

PRACTICAL POINT: *All those involved in pre-hospital care should carry a copy of:*
- *"SUBSTANCES HAZARDOUS TO HEALTH: Emergency First Aid Guide"*
- *This gives the emergency treatment for most hazardous chemicals.*
- *Information about the management of contamination with chemicals not listed, can usually be obtained from the nearest Poisons Information Centre (see chapter on Poisoning)*

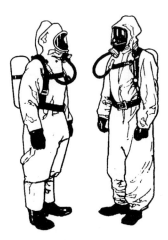

Figure 28-14 Examples of protective clothing

Chemical protective clothing
- There are two basic types of chemical protective clothing:
    - Chemical protective: a coveral suit with limited protection
    - Gas tight: very protective, vulcanised with an integral facemask, fireboots and gloves

PRACTICAL POINT: *Joint training in the use of both Breathing Apparatus (BA), and decontamination procedures should be developed with your local Fire and Rescue Service*

Breathing apparatus (BA)
- This is a pressurised air breathing system weighing 40-45 lbs and comprises:
    - A cylinder containing enough air for approximately 35 minutes of working time (depending on conditions), with a reserve of just under 10 minutes
    - An airtight face mask with a double reflex seal and an air demand valve
    - A harness to which the cylinder is attached incorporating:
        - A warning whistle indicating that there is just under 10 minutes of air left in the cylinder
        - A cylinder contents gauge
        - An inlet valve for a direct air supply (used during decontamination procedures, etc.)
        - A distress signal unit, which can only be reset using the safety tag. This tag records all the user details, e.g. time of start of use, state of the cylinder, etc., and is put on a control board, on which the movements of all personnel into the contaminated area, fireground, etc. are recorded

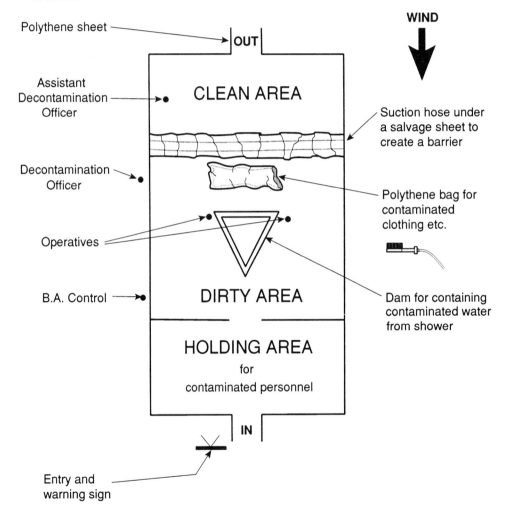

Figure 28-15 Typical layout of a decontamination zone

Decontamination
- The fire service will establish a decontamination area with a well defined entry and exit point, and control and perform the decontamination process
- Some industrial establishments may have their own facilities, with trained staff in attendance to assist the fire service
- If casualties are involved, they will usually be removed from the incident as rapidly as possible. In the case of noxious gases or smoke, removal to the fresh air may be all that is necessary, but for a few highly toxic and persistent chemicals, it may be necessary to decontaminate casualties at the scene

- In practice, stripping and washing the patients down with either water or soap and water is all that is required in most cases.
- Rarely, dry methods of cleaning: using intrinsically safe vacuum cleaners for dry powder contamination, or scraping, when tarry or viscous substances are involved, may be necessary
- Care must be exercised however, not to exacerbate any medical problems or injuries, and in particular shock. This can easily happen if the casualty is hosed down in the cold, and then not dried properly, which may result in him/her becoming hypothermic
- If the patient requires a stretcher, then they should be decontaminated on a "scoop stretcher". However care should be taken not to put undue stress on the stretcher, as it is not designed for carrying heavy casualties any distance
- In the case of female casualties, due account should be taken of their modesty, if circumstances and their condition permits. If available, female ambulance staff and firefighters should be provided
- If possible, at least one doctor should remain at the scene, until it is declared safe, to treat any member of the emergency services who may be injured or contaminated

Decontamination procedure
- The actual decontamination zone is usually divided into three areas:
    - Dirty:
        - This is where the initial decontamination is carried out, using wet or dry methods
        - Wet cleaning is carried out using a portable high pressure shower unit capable of delivering 2000 litres per minute for 3 minutes. This is capable of washing off nearly all known chemicals and the high rate of water delivery results in adequate dilution of any dangerous chemicals
        - The wearers' protective clothing will be decontaminated and removed in this area
    - Clean:
        - This is the area into which the cleaned personnel pass
    - Casualties:
        - Separate areas should be established for stretcher (P1 and P2) and ambulant (P3) casualties

Reducing the risk of contamination
- It is important that, all contamination is contained, and the risk of spread reduced to the minimum
- The fire service will seal contaminated clothing and property in polythene bags and labelled, and left at the scene, for disposal by a specialist contractor as arranged by the police
- All vehicles leaving the scene should if possible be made clean
- If patients are still contaminated, especially with volatile liquids:
    - They should be put feet first in plastic bags, leaving their heads clear, and if not contraindicated, given oxygen by oxygen mask
    - The ambulance should have all its windows opened, and the connecting door between the cab and patient area, closed
    - After use, each ambulance should be thoroughly decontaminated, before it re-enters service

Hospital decontamination
- The hospital should provide a suitable area for receiving the patient, with adequate ventilation and air extraction systems, together with showers and trolley baths for further decontamination
- In some cases further decontamination may be deemed necessary before severely contaminated casualties are allowed to enter the hospital

The contaminated dead
- The dead should be left where they lie after confirmation of death, so that forensic examination of the scene may take place, provided that to do so does not increase the risk of contamination for others.
- Following this they should be bagged up and labelled, before being decontaminated later during the forensic examination

Biological hazards

Introduction
- Contamination is caused by contact with pathogenic micro-organisms

Management
- The basic management principles are similar to those involving hazardous chemicals, and involves effective containment of the organisms or infected animals, incurring minimal unnecessary exposure to the hazard in the process

Radioactive contamination

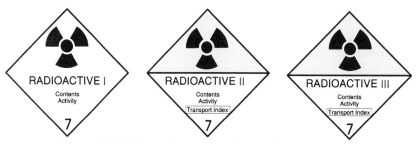

Figure 28-16 Hazard warnings for radioactive packages

Introduction
- There is an increasing use of radioactive substances (which give off radiation) in industry, research/ teaching and in medicine
- Large amounts of radioactive material are present in nuclear power stations, research laboratories and military establishments
- Nuclear materials are transported by road, rail, sea and in the air, as a result of which there is the potential for a nuclear incident almost anywhere. This should always be borne in mind whilst attending an accident, especially one involving a lorry, van, rail freight wagon or aircraft
- Sites where large amounts of nuclear materials are processed will have their own contingency plans, but the involvement of nuclear materials in a road, train, maritime or air accident may cause considerable concern and confusion, especially if members of the local emergency services are unaware of the procedures to be followed
- By law significantly radioactive materials have to be carried in extremely robust containers, which are designed to withstand a major impact without releasing any radioactive material, as a result of which any radiation emission is likely to be very small

Types of radiation

Alpha radiation
- In alpha radiation, small alpha particles are emitted, which:
    - Travel only a few millimetres in air
    - Will not penetrate materials such as clothing, dressings or a sheet of paper
    - May just penetrate skin, but are unlikely to cause any damage unless radiation occurs over a very long time
    - May cause damage to some sensitive internal organs if they are inspired or ingested
- Substances which emit alpha radiation include:
    - Uranium
    - Plutonium
    - Radon

Beta radiation
- In beta radiation, small negatively charged particles are emitted, which:
    - Travel only a few centimetres in air
    - Will not penetrate heavy clothing or metal, e.g. aluminium
    - May penetrate the skin and can damage the dermis and epidermis causing radiation burns, this is greatest if the substance emitting beta radiation is in direct contact with the skin, e.g. if clothing becomes contaminated with a beta emitting substance, it may cause radiation burns
    - If inspired or ingested may severely damage some internal organs, e.g. the thyroid gland
- Substances which emit beta radiation include:
    - Iodine
    - Tritium

Gamma radiation, neutrons and X-rays
- In gamma, neutron and X-ray radiation, particles are emitted which:
    - Travel many metres in air
    - Will penetrate most materials, except very dense materials, e.g. thick concrete, lead
    - Will penetrate body tissues, exchanging energy and causing cell damage as they go
- Substances which emit gamma, neutron and X-ray radiation include:
    - Caesium
    - Cobalt
    - Sources of industrial radiation

Safe contact time for Nuclear hazards

Category bar	at Zero Metres	at 1 metre	at 2 metres
I	20 hours	No restriction	No restriction
II	1 hour	20 hours	No restriction
III	3 minutes	1 hour	4 hours

Figure 28-17 Safe contact time for nuclear hazards

Types of radiation accident

Overexposure to penetrating radiation
- A patient who has been overexposed to radiation alone, is not radioactive and there is no risk at all to their medical rescuers

External contamination
- If the patient has been contaminated externally, there is a risk that they may still have the source of the contamination on their skin or clothes, and there is a risk of this contamination either being passed onto the skin or clothing of their medical rescuer, resulting in them being contaminated in turn and receiving penetrating radiation

Internal contamination
- If the patient has absorbed, ingested or inspired radioactive material, they are unlikely to be a hazard to their medical rescuers

Contaminated wound
- A patient's wound may become contaminated by radioactive material, in which case care must be exerted to avoid the radioactive material being spread any further

Protection
- Simple precautions will prevent the risk of spreading contamination, or of contaminating oneself:
    - Always assume that a casualty involved in an accident involving radioactivity, has been contaminated
    - Always wear a surgical face mask to prevent inspiring or ingesting radioactive material, and latex gloves to prevent contamination of the hands
    - Avoid disturbing the area any more than is absolutely necessary to prevent unnecessary spread of contaminated airborne particles
    - Cover all open wounds with a dressing to prevent wounds becoming contaminated, or contamination from wounds spreading further
    - Remove all the casualty's clothing if circumstances permit and seal them in a plastic bag, before wrapping the patient in a blanket or putting them in a contamination control envelope
    - Do not eat, drink or smoke, until you have been checked for contamination

Management
- The involvement of radioactive materials in an accident will usually be apparent from the labelling on a package, vehicle, container, etc.
- The usual procedure for management of the patient should be followed initially:
    - Assessment of the scene
    - Primary survey
    - Reassessment of the scene
    - Secondary survey
- The basic principles for managing patients contaminated by radioactive materials are broadly similar to those for chemical incidents with the exception that radioactivity cannot be detected or measured without special instruments
- Specific guidance on the management of such incidents is given in the document "National Arrangements for Incidents Involving Radioactivity" (NAIR)
- The objective of management of the patient who is contaminated with radioactive material is to remove the casualties from sources of high radioactivity and remove any other radioactive substances from the patient or their clothing. This can usually be achieved with soap and water

Evacuation
- In is very important to evacuate the patient to a hospital which is prepared to accept casualties contaminated by radioactivity, and to inform them well in advance that you will be sending them the casualty, so that they may make special preparations to receive him

29

Major incidents

Major incidents

Introduction

- Although major incidents may occur only rarely, their management is something with which all those involved in pre-hospital emergency medicine should be familiar, including Immediate Care doctors as they provide the initial medical response in many areas, and in those areas are usually the first doctors to arrive at the scene
- In some areas where there are Immediate Care Schemes, there are formal arrangements with the local ambulance service and hospitals for the scheme to provide not only the medical team, but also the Medical Incident Officer
- The procedures used should be considered to be an extension of those procedures commonly used at all incidents, except on a larger scale. Everyone is good at doing what they do often, and if major incidents are treated as being something special or different, there is the danger of there being even more confusion than is inevitable

Definitions

Major incident

- An unexpected event which overwhelms the normal resources of the unit be it Department, Hospital, Area or Region
- A major incident for one emergency service may not necessarily be a major incident for all the emergency services, but in most areas if one emergency service declares a major incident, the other emergency services automatically do the same
- There is almost inevitably initial chaos and confusion

Health circular: HC (90) 25 updated HSG (93) 24

- "A major incident arises when any occurrence presents a serious threat to the health of the community, disruption to the (health) service, or causes or is likely to cause such numbers of casualties as to require special arrangements by the health service"

Ambulance Officers Group 1992 (Section 2, Para. 2)

- "A major incident exists when......... the number and severity of *live* casualties requires special arrangements by the Health Service"

Emergency Planning in the NHS: EL (96) 79
- A Major Incident is 'any emergency that requires the implementation of special arrangements by one or more of the emergency services, the NHS or the local authority'
- For NHS purposes, a major incident is defined as 'Any occurrence which presents a major threat to the health of the community, disruption to the service, or causes (or is likely to cause) such numbers or types of casualties as to require special arrangements to be implemented by hospitals, ambulance services or health authorities'

Mass casualty situation
- A situation when the number and severity of injury of the casualties overwhelms the ambulance and medical resources available for their treatment

Multi casualty situation
- A situation when the number and severity of injury of the casualties is such that they can be managed by the ambulance and medical resources available for their treatment

Classification
- Major incidents may be classified in two different ways according to how they can be managed

Simple or compound
- Simple:
  - This is said to occur when the infrastructure i.e. roads, railways, communication systems and medical facilities including hospitals, surrounding the incident remains intact and can be used in the management of the incident and for the dispersal of casualties
- Compound:
  - Occurs in natural disasters and is when the infrastructure surrounding the incident is destroyed by the incident, resulting in:
    - Disruption to the inflow of resources required to manage the incident
    - Disruption to the outflow of the sick and injured
    - The non-availability of resources within the incident area

Compensated or uncompensated
- Compensated:
  - Occurs when the incident can be managed satisfactorily with the help of additional resources brought in to the scene, i.e. the supply of resources can cope with the demands put on them
- Uncompensated:
  - This occurs when the resources available for managing an incident are unable to cope adequately with the demands put on them. This happens in larger (mass casualty) or relatively isolated incidents, where there is a lack of local resources

Note: A multicasualty incident is an incident involving more than one casualty
A mass casualty incident is an incident involving a large number of casualties

Incidence
- Fortunately major incidents tend to occur relatively infrequently and by their very nature are usually unexpected
- Few health care professionals will experience more than one major incident, and most will not be involved in any major incidents throughout their entire careers

Aetiology
- Major incidents may be classified according to their aetiology into:

Natural
- Earthquake
- Volcanic activity
- Natural fire
- Storm including hurricane, tornado and waterspout
- Blizzard, snow and ice
- Flood
- Heatwave
- Famine
- Pestilence/disease:
    - Food poisoning, e.g. cholera, dysentery
    - Influenza
    - Rabies

Note: 1. One type of disaster is often followed by another, e.g. earthquake and storms often give rise to floods and fires
2. Most natural disasters will be followed by famine and an outbreak of disease, due to disruption of the supply of food and water, and disruption and contamination of the water supply and sanitation systems

Man-made
- Transport:
    - Road
    - Rail
    - Aviation
    - Maritime
- Industrial:
    - Construction
    - Mining
    - Chemical
    - Nuclear
- Crowd accidents, usually at large sporting events/mass gatherings
- Civil disorder/riots
- War and terrorist incidents

Note: Major fires may often occur as a result of man-made major incidents and may involve the release of highly toxic chemicals

Mass gatherings
- These are events, such as football matches and pop concerts where there are large numbers of people gathered together in a relatively small area, and where because of the nature of the event and the large numbers involved, there is the potential for a major incident
- They are unique in that the medical and ambulance resources already on site and available, should be adequate to deal with both the casualties which might usually be anticipated, and also manage any major incident that might arise until further resources arrive
- There should be a major incident plan, agreed by all the emergency services taking part

Preparation for a Major incident
- Adequate preparation is one of the key elements in the successful management of a major incident

Planning
- Every organisation involved in a major incident should have a major incident plan, which should be practised, reviewed and updated at regular intervals, with input from all the emergency services and relevant agencies
- The Department of Health in England has produced guidelines for the health services' response to a major incident which were included in HC (90)25, HSG (92)35 and Emergency Planning in the NHS: Health Services Arrangements for Dealing with Major Incidents: EL (96)79
- Planning the response to major incidents should be in accordance with the concept of "Integrated Emergency Management" (IEM), adopted by central and local government, the overall aim of which is to achieve maximum effectiveness by integrating the contributions made by a number of different agencies and authorities
- Plans should be produced which build on everyday procedures, so that most of those involved work in a way which is an extension of their usual role, rather than a new and different role
- The emphasis should be on producing a plan, which is sufficiently flexible to cope with a wide range of situations, which may increase in magnitude, duration, complexity or area and which may cross geographical and administrative boundaries
- Plans should integrate with those of the other emergency services, and be seamless across boundaries

Training
- This should include:
    - Theoretical instruction
    - Practical training, including:
        - Paper exercises
        - Tabletop exercises
        - Inter-service exercises

Equipment
- This should include:
    - Protective identifying clothing:
        - Jackets
        - Hard hats
        - Overtrousers
        - Stout waterproof and chemical resistant footwear
    - Communications equipment:
        - Hand-held radios
        - Cellular telephones
    - Recording equipment:
        - Notebook
        - Camera
        - Dictaphone
        - Casualty labelling system
    - Medical equipment:
        - This should be appropriate to the needs of the potential casualties (and is not required for those medical and ambulance personnel involved in the management of the incident)
        - Equipment used by immediate care doctors and Mobile Medical Teams should be compatible with that carried by the ambulance service
        - Equipment should be checked regularly and any perishable or limited-life items replaced
    - Reference material:
        - Telephone numbers of hospital, special resources, etc.

Major Incident management overview
- For the medical, ambulance and nursing services, this should be considered under the following headings:

Command and control
- To make the most effective and efficient use of all the personnel (resources) under their direction, commanders must have:
    - A thorough understanding of the way in which they work
    - Their differing strengths and weaknesses
    - The problems that they are having to face
    - Their requirements

Communications
- Good communication is the key to effective command and control and means not only an adequate exchange of information, but an understanding of that information by all parties concerned
- All personnel involved must be able to communicate effectively with:
    - Those directing them
    - Those working with them
    - Those working under their direction
- The senior doctor (Medical incident Officer) and other doctors with a command role need to be able to communicate with their counterparts in the other emergency services, especially the ambulance service, and with the Receiving Hospital(s)
- All medical personnel need to work closely with their counterparts in the Ambulance Service

Safety
- The safety of all those involved in a major incident needs to be considered, including:
    - Yourself
    - The incident scene
    - The casualties
    - Other rescuers

Assessment
- A rapid assessment of the overall incident is vital, if it is to be understood and managed effectively

Triage
- This is the rapid sorting of the casualties according to their need for rescue treatment and transportation
- Triage should be performed by doctors designated for that purpose, if available, or an experienced ambulance officer, using a recognised triage method

Treatment/management of the casualties
- This should be performed by teams of medical personnel, including ambulance service personnel, nursing staff and trained members of the voluntary aid societies, working under the direction of senior doctors

Transportation of casualties
- This is performed by the ambulance service after appropriate triaging and on-scene stabilisation according to patient needs
- Some patients may require special transport, e.g. the transport of spinal injuries by helicopter to a distant spinal unit
- Consideration should be given to dispatching patients directly to the hospital most appropriate to their needs, which may *not* be the nearest hospital, e.g. patients with burns to a burns unit, but this should be discussed with the hospital first, as they may be overwhelmed by a large number of casualties

Post incident

Debriefing
- After a major incident there should be a debriefing
- This should be done as soon as practical after the incident
- Each emergency service and unit within an emergency service will usually organise its own debriefing
- The following should be considered:
    - What actually happened?
    - What went right?
    - What went wrong?
    - What lessons have been learnt?
    - Could things have been organised better for a future event?
- Will help some of those emergency services personnel who have found the incident traumatic, come to terms with what happened, i.e. debriefing can be a kind of mass counselling
- Types of debrief:
    - *Hot debrief*:
        - At the scene prior to departure:
            - Informal
            - No formal minutes
            - Confirm that everyone is fit to go home; may identify those with early coping problems
            - Has the advantage that everything is fresh in the mind
    - *Single service/agency debrief*:
        - Formal
        - Minutes taken
    - *Multi-service/agency debrief*:
        - Involves senior members from each emergency service/agency involved
        - Formal
        - Minutes taken
        - May be used to produce a formal report/revisions of procedures

Documentation
- All medical personnel involved in an incident should write a brief summary of their actions and involvement at the incident, including times and decisions made.
- These reports should be given to the MIO for him to produce a summary, which should be disseminated widely to involved parties, in particular the Chief Executives of Ambulance Service Trusts, Health Authorities and receiving Hospital Trusts, identifying:
    - What went right
    - What went wrong
    - What could have been done better
    - Lessons learnt

Counselling
- Some rescuers as well as most survivors may need counselling
- Those medical and nursing staff with counselling skills, who have been involved in the same or similar incidents are probably the best people to do this

The emergency services in a major incident

- In general the priorities for all the emergency services are:
    - The preservation of life
    - The prevention of further loss of life and further injury
    - The relief of suffering
    - The protection of property
    - The protection of the environment
    - The restoration of normality
    - The investigation into the cause of the incident, including any criminal investigation

Information required

- The initial action required by the first emergency service to arrive at the scene of a major incident is to assess the scene without getting involved in the rescue operation, and to provide their control room with sufficient accurate information, for that emergency service and the other emergency services, when also given that information, to provide an appropriate and adequate response/attendance for the incident
- The information required is described by the pneumonics SAD CHALET or ETHANE:

S - Survey	C - Casualties	E - Exact location
A - Assess	H - Hazards	T - Type of incident
D - Disseminate	A - Access	H - Hazards?
	L - Location	A - Access
	E - Emergency services	N - Number of casualties
	T - Type of incident	E - Emergency services required/?extrication

Police

Scene management

- Any major incident is always treated initially as being the scene of a crime by the police, who will seek to establish early control over and access to and from the scene itself
- Controlling the scene may also help to:
    - Prevent escalation of the incident
    - Safeguard the public (evacuate the area if necessary)
    - Safeguard any property directly and indirectly involved in the incident
- Establish traffic and crowd control, both locally, and in the general area of the incident, by forming cordons. This may not be possible or practicable in the early stages of an incident, and assistance from others may be necessary in some circumstances;
    - There is usually an outer security cordon, manned by the police, and an inner evidential/safety cordon, which may be manned by the fire service and/or the police. There may also be a traffic cordon providing traffic diversions, etc.
    - Police officers may be sent through the scene, once an outer cordon has been established, to remove persons who have no real purpose being there. These may include members of the public comforting survivors and needs to be handled sensitively

Co-ordination of response

- The police have a coordinating and facilitating role at the scene of the incident and the surrounding area, except in the case of a fire, chemical or radiation incident, when the fire service, may have the lead role until that hazard is neutralised, and major aircraft accidents, when the Royal Air Force may have a coordinating role, especially when military aircraft are involved
- The police should plan and control:
    - Access/egress to the scene
    - Location of:
        - Incident Post, Ambulance Parking Area, Casualty Clearing Station, etc. (in consultation with the Ambulance Incident Officer)
- The police may provide the means of communication, if this is not otherwise available

Coordinating group
- The incident officers of the emergency services should:
    - Meet early at or near the scene
    - Meet regularly, at least every 2 hours
    - Share core information
    - Agree an action plan
    - Record key points
    - Produce minutes and circulate them
    - Retain documentary evidence of any meetings for subsequent inquiries, particularly a public inquiry
    - Plan media management

Liaison with other agencies
- There may be many other agencies, in addition to the emergency services, involved at a major incident, including:
    - Voluntary Aid Societies:
        - St John Ambulance, St Andrews Ambulance Association and the British Red Cross
        - WRVS
    - Borough and District Councils
    - Utility companies:
        - Gas, electricity and water companies
    - Transport companies:
        - Railtrack, and railway operating companies
        - British Airports Authority, airline companies and their handling agents
    - RAYNET; radio amateurs emergency network
    - Specialist international undertaking firms such as Kenyon Emergency Services and Global Partnership (DVI) Ltd, who have enormous experience of major disasters worldwide, and can provide teams for the forensic identification of the dead and their repatriation
    - The armed forces, especially the military (army)
- At a major incident the police may be responsible for notifying these other agencies, and initiating action to provide food, warmth, clothing, and shelter for those rendered homeless by the incident via the local Social Services Department
- The police have the lead role in coordinating the production of flexible emergency response plans by all the agencies likely to be involved in a major incident

Preservation of evidence
- The scene of any major incident is always initially treated as being the scene of a crime, and one of the purposes of placing a cordon around it and controlling access and egress, is to retain the integrity of any evidence that might be required in a subsequent enquiry

Media management
- Liaise with and control the media:
    - Provide good vantage points of the scene
    - Provide plenty of relevant information, updated at frequent regular intervals
    - Provide a press rendezvous point and establish a press centre
    - Provide access to a senior police officer

Other roles
- Other police roles may include:
    - Performing essential duties until the arrival of the specialist emergency service
    - Looking after VIPs visiting the scene

Casualty bureau
- The establishment of a casualty bureau is a core police function
- The casualty bureau is the central point for coordinating all information about the casualties (dead and surviving) from a major incident, and acts as the central contact and information point for all enquiries
- The casualty bureau is usually located in a relevant police headquarters, but often in a different location
- It carries out three functions:
    - Gathering information about all the people actually or potentially involved in the incident
    - Processing information about casualties
    - Providing authoritative information to relatives, friends, H.M. Coroner (Procurator Fiscal in Scotland), and the police senior investigating officer
- A public telephone number for enquiries is usually published via the media, as soon as the bureau opens
- Any incident involving members of the public. especially when there are known to be casualties, generates thousands of telephone calls from anxious relatives and friends, which will inevitably swamp local telephone switchboards and exchanges. The police service nationally has been considering the use of various information technology solutions to overcome this problem, including computer links with neighbouring forces to spread the workload

Investigation
- The police should carry out an investigation into the causes (including criminal) and management of the incident
- The police will act on behalf of the Coroner (Procurator Fiscal in Scotland):
    - Obtain confirmation of death and identification of the dead
    - Provide temporary mortuary facilities

Police Major Disaster Advisory Team
- A small team of senior police officers, who had had experience of managing a major incident, was established in 1993, to assist local police forces dealing with a major disaster by attending the scene with the purpose of giving experienced advice and support
- The skills of the team include:
    - Site clearance:
        - Cordoning and allocation of sectors using a grid system
        - Searching for bodies, body parts and property, and plotting and recording their position prior to packaging and labelling
    - Evacuation/relocation arrangements:
        - Ensuring the safe and rapid removal from the perceived danger of all those at risk, and their relocation (may be a complex procedure, especially if large numbers of people are involved)
        - Both procedures require close liaison with the local authority and emergency planning officer
    - Mortuary procedures:
        - All police forces and local authorities should identify suitable premises for use as temporary mortuaries in the event of a disaster resulting in the death of large numbers of persons
    - Antemortem (before death) inquiries and Casualty bureau
    - Identification procedures:
        - The object of these is to establish the identity of each of the deceased, by examining each potential identification against the evidence presented by post and antemortem teams, until all the victims have been identified
    - Liaison with relatives:
        - Obtaining antemortem data from the relatives to assist in the identification of the deceased
        - Assisting relatives throughout and after the incident with identification arrangements
    - Scene management: advisor to Tactical (Silver) Commander (see below)
    - Advising the senior investigating officer (SIO)
- The team may be called out by the chief officer of the police force involved with an incident, by contacting the National Emergency Procedures Unit, based at New Scotland Yard

Fire and rescue service
- Exert overall command and control of the incident in the case of fires, and chemical and nuclear incidents until the hazard is neutralized, when this role reverts to the police
- Save life and prevent escalation of the incident
- Neutralisation of hazards: fire, dangerous chemicals, radiation
- Rescue of the injured from immediate danger
- Release of the trapped including the dead
- Establish an inner safety cordon to control and supervise entry into the incident site
- Ensure the health and safety of all those entering the inner cordon of the incident site
- (May be a useful source of manpower once their primary role is accomplished)

Ambulance service
- Responsible for assessing the situation and mobilising and working with the medical services:
    - Immediately alert and mobilise the local Immediate Care Scheme doctors, where they are available
    - Select and alert the Receiving Hospital(s)
    - Provide transport for any hospital medical or surgical team
    - Provide on site and site to hospital communications
- Provide triage of, give ambulance aid to, and stabilise the injured, with medical supervision if appropriate
- Provide accommodation and extra medical equipment for the treatment of any casualties (many ambulance services can provide inflatable tents, in which casualties can be accommodated and treated)
- Transport the injured to the receiving hospitals, and provide inter-hospital transfers to specialist care facilities, e.g. for burns, spinal injury
- Provide transport home for those patients who are discharged early to make room for casualties from the major incident
- Has responsibility for the health and safety for all ambulance, medical and nursing personnel attending the incident
- Responsible for co-ordinating the activities of the Voluntary Aid Societies, and liaising with other organisations

Medical services
- Have legal responsibility for the medical treatment of the injured at the scene
- Provide medical triage, medical treatment and stabilisation of the injured, prior to their removal to hospital, by the ambulance service
- Provide confirmation of death
- Work in close unison with the ambulance service and receiving hospitals.
- Give advice on any occupational health matters or medical forensic aspects of the incident which may have a bearing on its overall management
- Provide medical support for the other emergency services if required

Hospital Mobile Medical and Surgical Teams
- In areas where there are no Immediate Care schemes, the medical input for pre-hospital medical care at Major Incidents should not be provided by a hospital likely to receive casualties
- The composition of the teams will usually depend on what is likely to be required of them
- The disadvantages of using Hospital Teams include:
    - Many have no experience in working in the field or with the ambulance service
    - The problem in the past was that if they were provided by the Receiving Hospital, they will deplete that hospital of medical and other staff, at the time when they will be required most for treating the injured as they arrive from the scene
- The advantages of using Hospital Teams include:
    - May be a valuable resource at a Casualty Clearing Station, if they are used to working together in the pre-hospital environment

Mobile Medical Team
- May be dispatched as soon as a Major Incident is declared by the Ambulance Service from a Listed, but non-Receiving hospital on request by the Ambulance Service or Medical Incident Officer

Mobile (Hospital) Medical Team

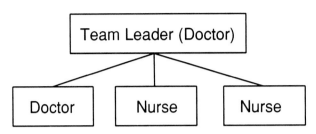

Figure 29-1 Composition of a Mobile Medical Team

Mobile Surgical Team
- May be requested to attend the scene on request by the Medical Incident Officer to perform surgical procedures, e.g. field amputations

Mobile Surgical Team

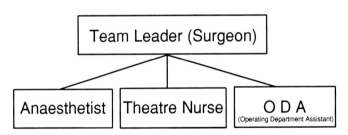

Figure 29-2 Composition of a Mobile Surgical Team

Pre-Hospital Medical teams
- Where there are doctors trained and experienced in Pre-Hospital Emergency Medicine (Immediate Medical Care), they should provide the medical personnel for the Medical Teams for Major Incidents, working as part of a team with members of the Ambulance Service

Pre-Hospital Medical Team

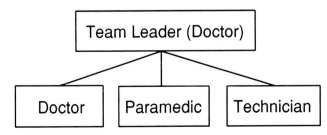

Figure 29-3 Composition of a Pre-Hospital Medical Team

Command and control

Introduction
- The proper command and control of all the personnel involved in a major incident is the key factor for the successful management of a major incident
- It will depend on all those involved in management knowing not only their own role, but also that of those subordinate to them, and a good knowledge of the working practices of the other services involved
- A personal knowledge and respect for the other managers involved will also be an advantage

Inter-service co-ordination
- The Police have overall responsibility for the coordination at any Major Incident, but should work very closely with each of the other emergency services
- The Police Incident Officer is the Police manager for an incident, but needs to work closely with and coordinate the work of the other emergency services through the Fire, Ambulance and Medical incident Officers as well as the senior representative of the local council and other agencies

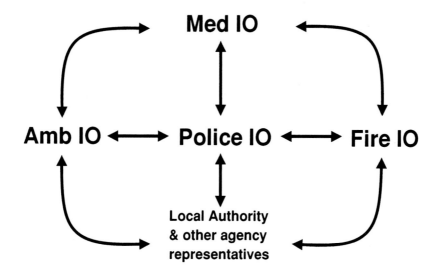

Figure 29-4 Relationship of Incident Officers to each other

Gold/silver/bronze system
- This is a system of status nomenclature for senior officers and Controls involved in the command and control of major incidents, and may be used by all the emergency services
- Its aim is to help identify the status, service and role of senior officers involved in the management of an incident principally for radio communications purposes
- In each emergency service, involved in a major incident, there is always only one officer of Gold status, and usually only one of Silver status, but there may be several of Bronze status
- The status (strategic/Gold, tactical/Silver or operational/Bronze) should be used as a prefix, followed by the service and role, e.g. Silver Ambulance Commander (Ambulance Incident Officer), Bronze Doctor Forward (Forward Medical Incident Officer)

Gold Control
- The major incident desk in control

Gold Commander
- The overall commander (**strategic**) of a service (usually the chief officer, chief executive or director)
- Usually based at the headquarters of a service, but may relocate if appropriate

Silver Control
- The on scene communications/incident control vehicle/room

Silver Commander
- The service's Incident Officer (**tactical**) at the scene

Bronze Commander
- The functional commanders/officers (**operational**) of a service at an incident with a management role

Gold, silver, bronze command

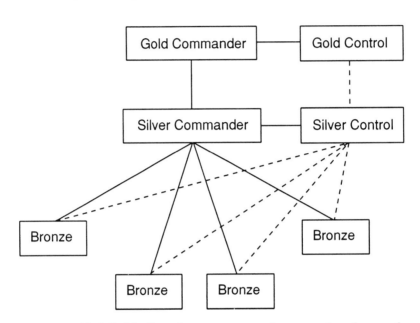

Figure 29-5 Gold, silver, bronze system of command and control

Ambulance service

Strategic/Gold Ambulance
- The Chief Ambulance Officer or nominated deputy

Strategic/Gold Ambulance Control
- The central Ambulance Control

Tactical/Silver Ambulance
- The Ambulance Incident Officer.

Tactical/Silver Ambulance Control
- The local Ambulance Control for the incident.

Operational/Bronze Ambulance Forward
- The Forward Ambulance Incident Officer

Operational/Bronze Ambulance Casualty Clearing/Treatment Officer
- The Ambulance Casualty Clearing Station/Treatment (area) Officer

Ambulance Command

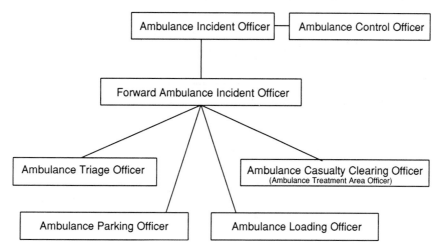

Figure 29-6 Ambulance command structure for a Major Incident

Medical services

Gold Doctor
- The senior doctor in Ambulance Control (Medical Coordinator)

Silver Doctor
- The Medical Incident Officer

Bronze Forward Doctor
- The Forward Medical Incident Officer/Senior Forward Doctor

Bronze Treatment Doctor
- The Medical Treatment (Area) Officer/Senior Treatment Area Doctor

Bronze Triage Doctor
- The Medical Triage Officer/Triage Doctor

Medical Command

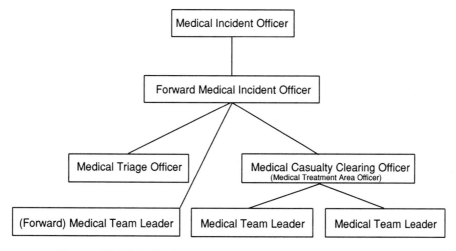

Figure 29-7 Medical command structure for a major incident

Organisation of the incident site
- The organisation of the incident site is the overall responsibility of the police
- The way in which the site is organised, has a direct bearing on how effectively the incident is managed
- It is vital to get the initial organisation correct, as once things begin to go wrong, there is virtually no chance of getting them sorted out correctly without bringing everything to a complete standstill
- It is therefore very important that all those involved have the same concepts about the way in which the site should be organised. To some extent this will involve having some idea of the working practices and procedures of the other emergency services as well as your own

Incident scene
- The actual location of the incident:
    - Wrecked vehicles
    - Aircraft
    - Train
    - Buildings
- May be spread over a very considerable area especially in aircraft, train accidents, etc. If so, it may have to be divided into sectors for management purposes
- As far as medical services are concerned, it is the area in which casualties both dead and alive remain following the incident

Outer (security) cordon
- This is a cordon set up around the whole incident (Controlled Area) and manned by the Police to:
    - Seal off the Controlled Area to prevent unauthorised personnel from entering the scene of a Major Incident
    - Monitor all those entering and leaving the scene; details of which will be kept in a log
- There will be Check Points at the entry and exit

Note: The police will also set up a traffic cordon around the incident to:
    - Prevent unauthorised vehicles approaching the scene
    - Direct authorised vehicles to the most appropriate place
    - Re-direct general traffic away from the scene

Emergency services rendezvous point/Marshalling area
- A predetermined area, usually manned by the police, where emergency service vehicles and personnel are assembled for logging and briefing prior to their being deployed forward to the scene of an incident
- Usually only found near special risk sites, e.g. airports, chemical complexes, nuclear sites, etc.

Incident control point
- A central point, readily identifiable, at which the Incident Officers and their emergency control vehicles are situated, and from which each service controls the response of their service to a land based incident.
- It is usually some distance from the actual incident scene, but ideally overlooking it
- In practice, the emergency control vehicles have to park a little distance apart to avoid mutual radio interference
- The police incident control vehicle should remain the only vehicle displaying a blue light between the inner and outer cordons. In some areas the fire and ambulance emergency control vehicles may also display flashing lights (red or red and white lights for the fire control point, and green or green and white for the ambulance and medical control point)

Incident Control Point

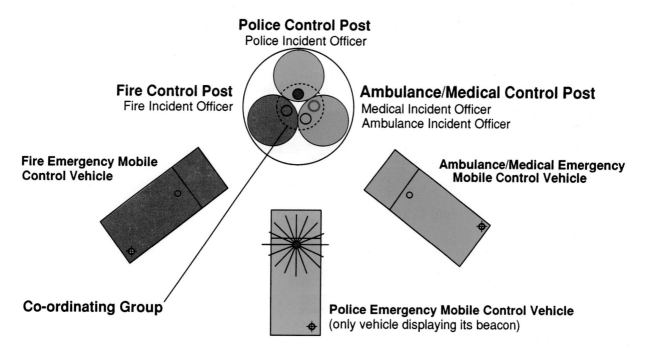

Figure 29-8 Incident Control Point and Control vehicles

Ambulance/medical control point
- An ambulance emergency mobile control vehicle providing an "on site" communications facility, which may be situated some distance from the incident scene, and may be identified by a green or green and white flashing light
- It provides a focal point for NHS/medical resources attending the incident

Inner (evidential/safety) cordon
- Surrounds the immediate site of the incident:
    - The Fire Service is in control within the inner cordon
    - Entry is controlled by the Police and/or Fire Service to:
        - Prevent unauthorised or unprotected personnel from entering the site of a major incident
        - Monitor all those entering and leaving the scene; details of which will be kept in a log
- The entry and exit will usually be at the same place

Triage Area
- This is a place of relative safety, close to or sometimes within the incident site, where the "triage sort" of the injured takes place

Casualty clearing station/Casualty treatment area
- A place of relative safety to which casualties are conveyed from the incident, and where assessment, triage, treatment and stabilisation is carried out by doctors and ambulance personnel working together under the joint direction of a senior doctor and the Ambulance Casualty Clearing Officer prior to their evacuation by ambulance

Ambulance (casualty) loading point
- An area, preferably of hard standing near the casualty clearing station, where casualties can be loaded into ambulances under the direction of the Ambulance Loading Officer, for transfer to hospital
- Some transfers may be effected by helicopter, necessitating that suitable landing arrangements be made

MAJOR INCIDENT ORGANISATION

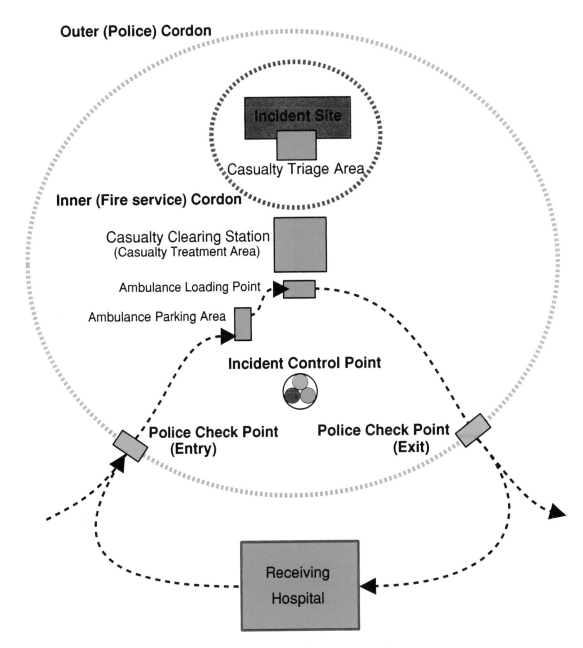

Figure 29-9 Major Incident site organisation

Ambulance parking area
- The area where ambulances are held prior to being called forward to load patients and is under the control of the Ambulance Parking Officer

Ambulance marshalling area
- Area to which ambulance resources (and staff) not immediately required at the scene, or being held for further use, can be directed to stand-by

Body holding area
- A place at or near the incident site where the deceased are collected together, once confirmed dead, under police supervision

Temporary mortuary
- A building, accessible from the disaster area, adapted for temporary use as a mortuary, to which the deceased will be taken from the scene for forensic medical/dental examination/identification purposes

Hospital organisation

Listed hospitals
- Hospitals listed by the Regional Health Authority as adequately equipped to receive casualties on a 24 hour basis and able to provide, when required, the Medical Incident Officer and/or a Mobile Medical Team(s)

Receiving hospital(s)
- The hospital(s) selected by the Ambulance Service (from those listed by the Regional Health Authority), to receive casualties in the event of any particular incident
- These are preferably Major Hospitals and are usually the nearest hospitals to which the first seriously injured casualties will be sent
- Hospitals to which the overflow of seriously injured casualties, and walking wounded may be sent are also designated Receiving Hospitals

Hospital mobile medical teams
- All Listed, but Non Receiving Hospitals near the scene should prepare a mobile medical team to be dispatched, on request only, from the Ambulance Service/Medical Incident Officer to provide on-site treatment

Note: In very rural or sparsely populated areas, the local District General Hospital may have to provide both a medical team and the Medical Incident Officer in the first instance. These should be relieved at the earliest opportunity by a medical team and/or Medical Incident Officer from another Listed Hospital or from the nearest Immediate Care Scheme

Hospital Coordination Centre
- This is the centre set up at a Receiving Hospital to manage the in-hospital response to the incident, and to collate for internal use, data concerning casualties received, their condition, bed states, theatres available; and to provide information to the Police Documentation Team as appropriate

Distribution of casualties
- Consideration should be given to casualties being conveyed to the hospital and facilities most appropriate to their needs, if the hospital is agreeable
- Ideally more than one hospital should always be involved so that there is an even distribution of patients between hospitals from the very start so that one hospital is not overstretched while another is idle

Senior site personnel

-   The precise nomenclature for the managers in each of the emergency services has been much debated and is constantly being reviewed. Because of this it may vary from one area to another and from one service to another. The titles given below are those used most commonly at present

Police Incident Officer

-   The senior police officer (tactical/silver) who assumes command of all police operations at the incident site, determines parameters set by gold command and establishes and maintains the police co-ordinating role of the emergency service response

Fire Incident Officer

-   The senior fire officer (tactical/silver) with overall responsibility for the management of the Fire Service at the incident site of a major incident

Ambulance Incident Officer

-   The senior ambulance officer (tactical/silver) with the overall responsibility for the work of the Ambulance Service at the scene of a major incident
-   He liaises closely with the Medical Incident Officer to ensure effective use of the medical and ambulance resources at the scene
-   He will also be responsible for the direction and control of the Voluntary Aid Societies' and Civil Aid input into the incident

Ambulance Senior Control Officer

-   The senior ambulance officer who has responsibility for providing and managing on site communications for all ambulance, medical and nursing officers at the incident and with ambulance control
-   He should usually remain in the ambulance/medical mobile control vehicle

Ambulance Forward Incident Officer

-   The senior ambulance officer (operational/bronze), in command of the ambulance resources at the scene or sector
-   He should work closely with the Forward Medical Incident officer

Ambulance (Primary) Triage Officer

-   The ambulance officer responsible together with the Medical Forward Triage Officer, for primary triage and labelling of casualties and organising their removal to the Casualty Clearing Station/Treatment Area

Ambulance Casualty Clearing (Station) Officer/Ambulance Treatment (Area) Officer

-   The ambulance officer in charge of ambulance resources in the casualty clearing station/treatment area
-   He should work closely with the Medical Casualty Clearing (Station) Officer/Treatment (Area) Officer to ensure the efficient throughput of casualties

Ambulance Loading (Area) Officer

-   The ambulance officer in charge of the ambulance loading at the casualty loading area. He is responsible for organising casualty movement in order of priority, with documentation, and for maintaining a supply of appropriate transportation

Ambulance Parking Officer

-   The ambulance officer in charge of the ambulances parked in the ambulance parking area

Ambulance Safety Officer

-   The ambulance officer who has responsibility of the safety of all ambulance, medical personnel within the inner cordon. He should liaise closely with safety officers from the other emergency services

Medical Incident Officer

- The senior doctor (tactical/silver), with overall responsibility, in close liaison with the Ambulance Incident Officer, for the medical resources at a major incident
- He should not be a member of any mobile medical team

Forward Medical Incident Officer/Senior Forward Doctor

- This may be the senior doctor (operational/bronze), in command of the medical resources at the incident scene
- He should work closely with the senior ambulance officer present, and report back to the medical incident officer
- He may be the leader of a medical team
- Should also deputise for the Medical Incident Officer as required

Medical (Primary) Triage Officer/Triage Doctor

- The senior doctor in charge of the initial (primary) triaging of the casualties, who determines and prioritises evacuation of the injured prior to their removal to the Casualty Clearing Station/treatment area
- He should work closely with the Ambulance (Primary) Triage Officer

Medical Casualty Clearing (Station)/Treatment (Area) Officer/Senior Treatment Area Doctor

- The senior doctor in charge of all the doctors working in the Casualty Clearing Station/medical treatment area
- He should work closely with the Ambulance Treatment Officer

Note: The Medical Incident Officer may also need several senior doctors to act as "gofers/fixers" (sector support doctors)

Local Authority Organisation

Survivor Reception Centre

- Secure area to which uninjured survivors can be taken for first aid, interview and documentation. This is normally short term accommodation

Rest Centre

- A building designated by the local authority for temporary longer term accommodation of evacuees

Senior personnel

CEPO (and EPO)

- County/Chief Emergency Planning Officer (and District Emergency Planning Officer) for the Local Authority

Local Authority Liaison Officer

- Officer designated by the local authority as the contact point for the emergency services

Welfare Co-ordination Team

- A team, normally coordinated by the local authority social services to look after the longer term welfare needs of those affected by a disaster. Teams may include social workers and representatives from the local authority, police, church, voluntary aid societies and the WRVS

Communications at Major Incidents

- Effective communication is the key to effective management, and is the area where there are most problems in major incident management, especially in the early stages
- The ambulance service will normally provide all communications for the Medical Incident Officer and medical teams.
- Strict radio discipline should be maintained at all times, but especially at major incidents, when air time is at a premium, and all messages kept brief and simple, so as to avoid misunderstandings and confusion
- The method of communication may vary according to the location, type of incident, and equipment available
- Off-site communications:
    - Ambulance service vehicles travelling to and from the incident:
        - Ambulance frequency/Emergency Reserve Channel (ERC)
    - Local immediate care scheme doctors:
        - Ambulance frequency/Emergency Reserve Channel (ERC)/immediate care scheme frequency
    - Adjacent ambulance services:
        - Telephone landline
    - Receiving hospitals:
        - Telephone landline
    - Other emergency centres, e.g. police, airport
        - Telephone landline
    - Health authority incident room:
        - Telephone landline
- On-site communications:
    - Between ambulance personnel and doctors:
        - Runner, VHF/UHF hand held radios
    - With ambulances:
        - VHF radio
    - Inter-service:
        - Runner, UHF hand held radios
    - With Receiving Hospitals via:
        - VHF radio on Ambulance frequency
        - Cellphones, although problems have been encountered due to media overusage blocking the system (see below)
        - British Telecom telephone (landline)
    - With ambulance control

Emergency reserve channel (ERC)

- This is a nation wide ambulance frequency (in England and Wales, but not in Scotland) which is usually only used during major incidents or major disasters
- It enables one ambulance service to communicate with vehicles from any other ambulance services that may be called in to assist it
- Many Immediate Care doctors also have radios on this frequency, with the permission of their local ambulance service

ACCOLC (Access overload control)

- This is a filtering system used on the Racal-Vodaphone cellular radio system
- It may be activated (usually by the police) at major incidents, and only allows access for those with prior authorization

Priority access

- A similar system to ACCOLC, but on the Cellnet cellular radio system

On Site communications (UHF)

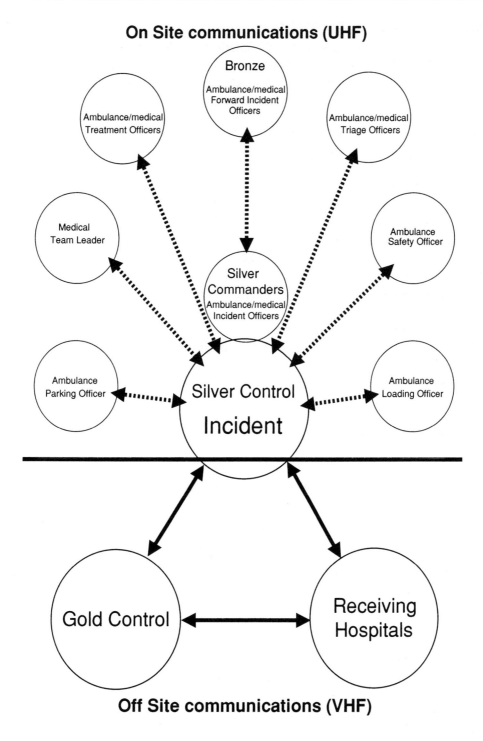

Off Site communications (VHF)

Figure 29-10 Ambulance/Medical Communications for a Major Incident

Safety at the scene of a major incident
- The fire service has overall responsibility for the safety of all those attending an incident, and will usually establish an inner safety cordon, and control entry though it, while the ambulance service has responsibility for the health and safety of all ambulance, medical and nursing personnel
- No rescuers should be needlessly exposed to any unnecessary risks, and become casualties themselves

Medical team
- The Medical Incident Officer should ensure that all members of the medical and nursing teams are not exposed unnecessarily to any hazards
- He should ensure the safety of:
    - The site itself
    - Those entering the site
    - Those working in the site
    - Arrange for the relief of the medical teams after about 4 hours into the incident
- Make certain that all medical and nursing personnel are wearing adequate approved identifying protective clothing, including hard helmets, jackets, overtrousers and stout footwear

Members of the other emergency services
- The Medical Incident Officer should be aware of the potential at a major incident for:
    - Exhaustion
    - Heat exhaustion
    - Hypothermia
    - Need for feeding
    - Minor injuries
    - Stress, etc.

Clothing/personal equipment for medical and nursing personnel
- This should be kept ready at all times, as major incidents are always unpredictable, and there is usually little or no time to prepare or assemble equipment ready for responding.
- Essential items include:
    - Fire-retardant overalls
    - An approved high visibility warm water and weatherproof jacket with the status of the wearer marked clearly on it
    - An approved hard hat with a helmet light, a protective visor or protective glasses, and the status of the wearer marked clearly on it.
    - Oil and acid resistant boots
    - Heavy duty and latex gloves
- Designated senior doctors should wear an approved green/white chequered tabard (provided by the ambulance service)
- Additional personal items should include:
    - An approved identity card
    - Notebook and waterproof pen/Dictaphone and spare tapes
    - Camera
    - Whistle
    - Money (for purchasing refreshments, etc.)
- Other useful items are:
    - Binoculars
    - Torch

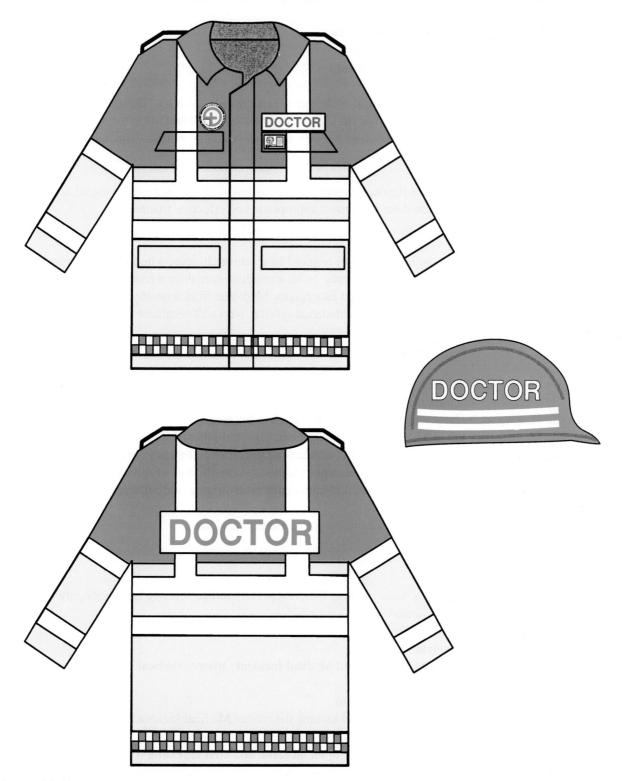

Figure 29-11 Doctor's jacket (top is fluorescent medical green, bottom fluorescent yellow) and green hard hat

Organisation of the medical services

The Medical Incident Officer (tactical/silver)

Definition (from EL (96)79): The senior doctor, with overall responsibility, in close liaison with the Ambulance Incident Officer, for the medical resources at the scene of the major incident. He should not be a member of any mobile medical team

Role
- He has overall responsibility for the deployment and management of the medical personnel at an incident to ensure that the injured have the most appropriate and effective treatment

Who ?
- The first doctor to arrive at the incident, until relieved by a senior clinician who has had appropriate training and/or experience in the role. This may be an immediate care doctor from the local Immediate Care scheme or a consultant in Accident and Emergency Medicine from a nearby hospital. Pools of potential MIOs are now organised by the ambulance service, who will nominate a MIO for the incident

Qualities
- Ideally he/she needs to:
    - Be known to and respected by the senior members of the other emergency services
    - Be disciplined and experienced in the role of medical management in Major Incidents
    - Be familiar with likely scenario for major incidents in his area
    - Be familiar with the organisation, role, equipment and requirements of Immediate Care and the attending medical teams, the ambulance service and the other emergency services
    - Be familiar with the organisation, role, requirements and capabilities of the surrounding hospitals, and location of any special facilities, e.g. burns unit, neurosurgical unit, thoracic unit and their admissions policies
    - Have the ability not to get involved in the treatment of individuals

Requirements
- He/she should:
    - Be readily identifiable, i.e. wear clothing (fluorescent tabard/hat), clearly labelled/highly visible
    - Have a runner, when indicated
    - Be able to communicate with:
        - Ambulance Incident Officer
        - Other senior doctors, e.g. Forward Medical Incident Officer, Medical Triage Officer

The first doctor at the scene of a major incident
- The first doctor to arrive at the scene should assume the role of Medical Incident Officer, unless or until relieved by a senior doctor who has been specially trained in the role
- If he is the first person to arrive at the scene of an incident, and after assessing it, decides that it is probably a major incident, he should discuss this with any other emergency services personnel present and then discuss/confirm this with Ambulance Control, before it is declared a major incident

Action
- He should assess the scene rapidly, without going too far away from his vehicle
- He must not treat any casualties
- He should give Ambulance Control the following information:
    - The exact location of the incident including a map reference or motorway marker post if possible.
    - A brief description of the general scene (e.g. type of incident, whether there is a fire, etc.)
    - The estimated number of casualties
    - If the other emergency services are already in attendance, and if not; whether they are required
    - The weather, road conditions and any dangers or hazards
    - Local accessibility
    - Estimate of number of ambulances and other doctors required

Assuming the role of Medical Incident Officer

Priorities/responsibilities
- Command and control of medical resources, working in close cooperation with the Ambulance Incident Officer
- Communication with medical/ambulance personnel and other Incident Officers
- Safety of the medical rescuers and the injured
- Assessment of the incident
- Triage of all those involved in the incident
- Treatment of those requiring immediate treatment
- Evacuation of the injured
- Press briefing
- Debriefing the medical resources post incident and helping to prepare any official report

Command and control
- On arriving at the scene, he should immediately:
    - Report to the Ambulance Emergency Control Vehicle
    - Locate and identify himself to the Ambulance Incident Officer (with whom he should stay at all times in order to ensure effective management of health service resources at the scene)
    - Don the Medical Incident Officer Tabard (if available)
    - Identify himself to and liaise with:
        - Police Incident Officer
        - Fire Incident Officer
    - Establish the Medical Control Point (this will be with the Ambulance Control Point) and take charge of all medical and nursing staff
- He should:
    - Appoint senior doctors to perform the following roles:
        - Forward Medical Incident Officer/Senior Forward Doctor
        - Medical Triage (area) Officer/Triage Doctor
        - Medical Treatment (area) Officer/Senior Treatment Area Doctor
        - Medical team leader(s) (in a large incident, there may need to be several medical teams)
    - Assess, together with the Ambulance Incident officer, the need for:
        - The continuance of, addition to or withdrawal of immediate care doctors/Mobile Medical Teams
        - The relief of the medical teams after about 4 hours into the incident or earlier if there are special circumstances, e.g. adverse environmental condition; high humidity, very cold weather
        - A continual medical presence until the whole incident has been closed down

- Be prepared (at the request of the Police) to provide doctors to identify human tissue and for the confirmation of death, once there are sufficient doctors to treat the injured
- Assess, together with the Ambulance Incident Officer, the need to activate additional Receiving Hospitals and the progressive release of activated Receiving Hospitals as the incident winds down
- Maintain a chronological log of all events
- Post incident:
    - Prepare a report for any inquiry, etc.
    - Organise:
        - The medical debriefing
        - Counselling for medical and nursing staff and members of the other emergency services

Communications
- He should ensure adequate communication between himself and other senior doctors with the ambulance service at all levels (preferably by radio)
- He should establish and maintain contact with the receiving hospital(s) to provide them with details and confirmation of the action plan, and provide them with situation reports with details of the:
    - Number of casualties and severity of their injuries.
    - The need for a Medical Team
    - Any special injuries requiring special facilities, e.g. burns
    - The need for a surgical team: for field amputation
    - Time of dispatch of casualties to the hospital, with as much relevant clinical information as possible (the Ambulance Incident Officer will arrange for the hospitals to be kept advised of incoming casualties; the Medical Incident Officer only has need to pass information or speak to the hospital in relation to those patients with special needs)
- He should be prepared to give a press interview, if requested by the Police Press Liaison Officer, and discuss and agree the contents of any statement with the Police and Ambulance Incident Officers

Safety
- Ensure that all doctors attending the incident have adequate protective/identifying clothing
- Determine (from the fire service) whether there are any potential or actual hazards
- Look after the health/safety of all nursing/medical personnel, and be aware of the possibility of potential problems, and watch other emergency services personnel for:
    - Exhaustion, heat exhaustion
    - Hypothermia
    - Feeding
    - Minor injuries, etc.

Note: The scene should be disturbed as little as possible so that post-accident forensic investigation into the cause of accident/mechanism of injury, etc. can be established

MAJOR INCIDENT ORGANISATION

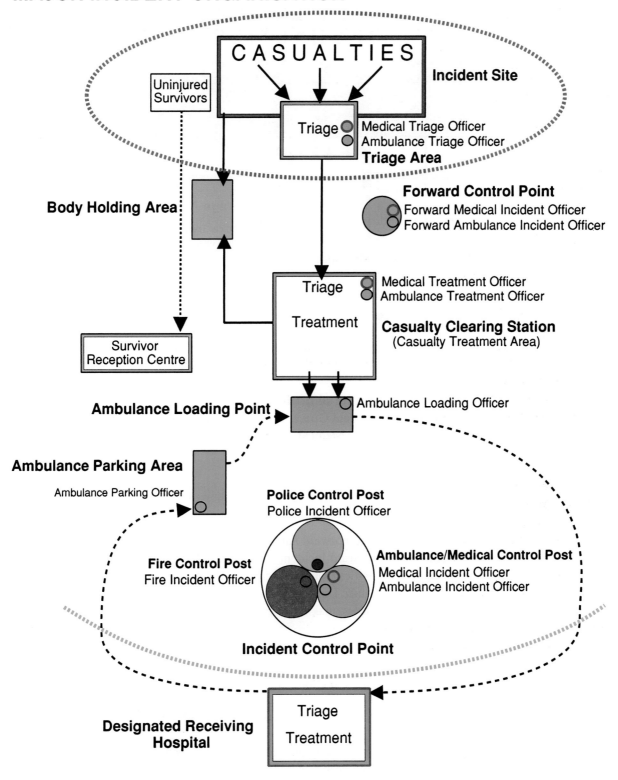

Figure 29-12 Medical and Ambulance Service organisation

Incident Site

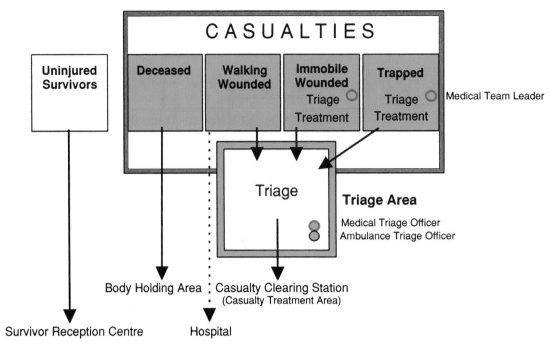

Figure 29-13 Organisation of the incident site

Forward medical incident officer (operational/bronze)
- Acts as the link between the Medical Incident Officer and those under him including the Medical Triage Officer, the Medical Treatment Officer and Medical Team Leaders
- Manages the medical resources at the incident site

Action

Command and control
- Liaise closely with the operational/bronze Forward Ambulance, Fire and Police Incident Officers
- After discussion with the Ambulance Forward Incident Officer and Medical Incident Officer:
    - Work out the lines of flow of casualties from the incident site (after initial triage) to the treatment areas and from there to the Ambulance Loading Point
    - Brief and deploy all medical resources, making certain that all medical personnel are fully briefed about the incident and their role
- Ensure that there is an adequate supply of medical equipment including standardised triage cards
- Consider:
    - The need for surgical teams for field amputations, etc.
    - The need for special medical resources/equipment
    - The use of paramedics/ambulance technicians (in consultation with the Forward Ambulance Incident Officer)
    - The possible use of nurses to escort severely injured patients to hospital
- Ensure that if minor injuries are treated on scene, that they are managed appropriately

Communications
- Ensure that there are adequate communications between all the senior doctors

Safety
- Ensure that the scene is safe before allowing medical personnel to enter the inner cordon

Assessment
- Assess the incident; reconnoitre the scene to ascertain:
    - The number and severity of casualties
    - If there are any trapped casualties
    - If there are any casualties with special injuries:
        - Burns
        - Spinal injuries
        - Those requiring field surgery
    - Any toxic risks and ascertain how to treat any contaminated casualties
- Determine the medical response required and agree his findings with the Ambulance Forward Incident Officer

Medical Triage Officer (operational/bronze)
- This is the senior doctor at the incident site who has responsibility for the initial triaging of the casualties
- He should work with the Ambulance Triage Officer
- Depending on the incident, and whether or not casualties are trapped, the initial triage may be performed at the site of the incident or in a triaging area near the incident
- He should ensure that the method of triaging and triage labelling system employed is uniform
- In consultation with the Forward Medical Incident Officer, the Ambulance Triage Officer and the Senior Fire Officer present, he may direct appropriate medical resources to those injured and requiring medical treatment in situ, e.g. those still trapped in any wreckage

Medical Casualty Clearing Station/casualty treatment officer (operational/bronze)
- This is the senior doctor in charge of all the medical treatment of casualties in the Casualty Clearing Station/Treatment Area(s), after they have arrived from the triage area/incident site
- He should work closely with the Ambulance Treatment Officer
- He may need to delegate senior doctors in charge of medical teams, Medical Team Leaders, if there is more than one Treatment Area
- He should ensure that there is an adequate supply of medical equipment for managing the care of the injured and identify the need for any special medical equipment or facilities, and convey his needs to the Medical Incident Officer

Action of all other doctors at a major incident
- On arrival at the incident:
    - Park under police supervision, switch off green light (this sequence may be reversed in special circumstances, e.g. at airports), leaving the keys in the ignition or deposit them at the Ambulance Control Vehicle
- Don adequate protective/identifying clothing, and always carry or show your identity card
- Log in with police (if the police are controlling entry into the Incident Site)
- Make certain that you have sufficient appropriate equipment with you (it is unlikely that you will be able to go back to get any more equipment)
- Report to the Medical Incident Officer/Ambulance Control Vehicle
- Carry out the instructions of senior doctors in a disciplined manner
- Do not give press interviews without permission from both the Police and Medical Incident Officers

Casualty Clearing Station
(Casualty Treatment Area)

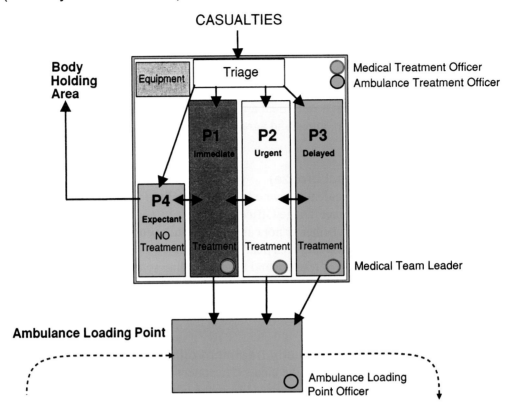

Figure 29-14 Organisation of the Casualty Clearing Station/Casualty Treatment Area

Medical Coordinator (Gold Doctor)
- In some areas there are arrangements for bringing a senior doctor into Ambulance Control
- His role is to act as the link between the Designated Hospital and the Medical Incident Officer, thus freeing the Medical Incident Officer for his main role as the senior medical manager at the incident
- He may also assist in prioritising the rest of the routine ambulance work

Action
- He should:
    - Report to Ambulance Control as soon as possible after a Major Incident has been declared
    - Remain in Ambulance Control throughout the incident, or until relieved by another doctor approved for the role
    - Try to match patients, especially those with special needs, with suitable available bed space, within a reasonable distance from the incident
    - Liaise with the Medical Incident Officer, who should keep him constantly appraised of the requirements of the patients at the incident
    - Have a good knowledge of the capabilities of all the medical facilities in his area
    - Liaise with the County and Regional Emergency Planning Officers
- He may need to remain in Control for some time after all patients have been cleared from the scene of a major incident to facilitate the secondary transfer of some patients from the Designated Receiving Hospital to specialised facilities

Triage

Definition: Triage is the sorting of casualties into different categories according to the severity of their injuries for the purpose of prioritising evacuation and treatment

- In the mass casualty situation, the objective must be to do the most good for the greatest number of casualties
- In the simple compensated major incident, the objective must also be to ensure that the right casualties reach the right hospital within the right time
- In many cases the early removal from the scene of the uninjured and walking wounded removes a source of distraction and allows the rescuers to give their undivided attention to the more seriously injured.
- Once they have been triaged, casualties should be reassessed and re-triaged if necessary, at regular intervals

Triage Categories

	Trauma score						Expected (untreated) % survival
Red	1-10	Priority 1	P1	Critical	Immediate	T1	10%
Yellow	11	Priority 2	P2	Serious	Urgent	T2	30%
Green	12	Priority 3	P3	Minor	Delayed	T3	60%
Blue	0				Expectant	T4	none
White (black lettering)				Dead	Deceased	T0	
(Police label is light blue with black lettering)							

Figure 29-15 Triage categories

First (Immediate) priority
- Those casualties requiring life saving procedures

Second (Urgent) priority
- Those casualties requiring surgical intervention within 4-6 hours

Third (Delayed) priority
- Those with minor injuries (the walking wounded) who do require urgent treatment

Expectant casualties
- This category is only used in the mass casualty or battlefield situation
- Are those severely injured casualties who are unlikely to survive even if treated aggressively, but would require a greater than appropriate medical resource in the process, thus depriving potential survivors of treatment

Uninjured survivors
- It is thought that these should also be included in the categories of casualties, as they too will require special handling and treatment, e.g. counselling
- The police may need them for identification and documentation purposes and as witnesses of the event
- They should be coralled and directed to the Survivor Reception Centre

The dead
- A new numbered blue label has been produced by the police service for labelling the dead. The Association of Chief Police Officers (ACPO) has recommended its use to all police forces, and advised them to make the label available to ambulance and fire services for use at major incidents

Types of triage

Self triage
- Walking wounded:
  - These will tend to walk away from the site of the incident and in many civilian incidents may present first at the nearest casualty department or even to casualty departments some considerable way from the incident, as they know that the nearest hospital will be more than busy!
- Crawling wounded:
  - Will try to get away from incident in any way they can
- Severely injured/trapped wounded:
  - Those unable to get away from the incident either because they are physically trapped, or as a result of their injuries

Note: Some seriously injured patients may attempt to get away and later collapse some distance from the scene of the incident

Medical triage
- Categorization according to the medical condition/injuries/Triage Revised Trauma Score of the injured.
- It should always be performed by the most senior and experienced person available

Triage Methods
- Triaging begins at the incident scene and should take place continuously and in greater depth as the patient passes down the evacuation line

Triage sieve/primary triage
- This is the rapid initial triage performed at the Incident scene, before any casualties are treated
- The initial assessment of the scene should be followed by a sweep of the casualties which should include a brief assessment of each casualty
- This should be a rapid assessment of their airway, breathing and circulation, and appropriate labelling
- Only rapid life saving procedures should be performed at this stage e.g., clearing the airway, arresting life threatening haemorrhage
- Those patients requiring special resources, e.g. the trapped and seriously burnt should also be identified
- By its nature this initial triage, which may be performed by first aiders or members of the emergency services who lack specialised medical knowledge, will only be rough, but any errors made at this stage can probably be corrected as the casualties move down the evacuation chain

Triage Sort/secondary triage
- A more selective triage process performed at the Casualty Clearing Station/Treatment Area and later at the:
  - Casualty Loading point
  - A & E Department.
- At any other time as indicated by a change in the patient's condition

TRIAGE LABELLING

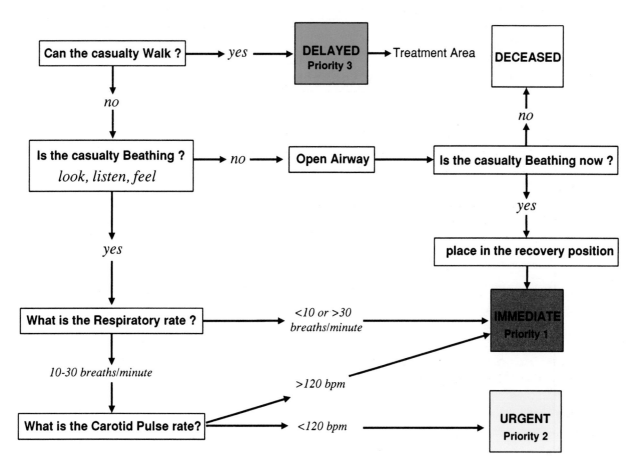

Figure 29-16 Triage sieve labelling scheme

Triage labelling
-   This is a simple system of casualty labelling according to the patient's triage category
-   Unfortunately, currently there is no universally accepted triage system or even method of labelling

Triage labelling requirements
-   Any labelling system should:
    -   Be highly visible:
        -   Colours are often difficult to distinguish in poor visibility; the category description should also be clearly shown
    -   Be robust, waterproof and easy to write on
    -   Be easy to attach to the patient and difficult to remove
    -   Allow a change in the triage category of a casualty in either direction
    -   Allow a casualty's details to be filled in rapidly
    -   Have space for serial observations
    -   Allow trauma scoring, if circumstances permit
    -   Be uniform for all those involved at any single incident

CASUALTY NUMBER
GMAS 0000000

CASUALTY ASSESSMENT MODULE

PRIMARY SURVEY			Time:	
Airway	☐ Clear		☐ Obstructed	
C. Spine	☐ Normal		☐ Possible injury	
Breathing	☐ Spontaneous		☐ Problem	
Circulation/	☐ External		☐ Possible internal	
Haemorrhage	☐ None/slight		☐ Moderate ☐ Severe	
Disability	☐ Alert	Responds to	☐ Verbal stimuli ☐ **P**ain ☐ **U**nresponsive	

Exposure/Injuries

C# Closed Fracture
O# Open Fracture   L Laceration
B Burn (shade area)   A Abrasion
F Foreign body   E Ecchymosis (bruising)

PRIMARY MANAGEMENT

Airway	☐ Oropharyngeal	☐ Nasal	☐ ET Tube
	☐ C/Thyrotomy	☐ Oxygen	☐ Suction
C. Spine	☐ C. Collar	☐ Ext Dev	☐ Long board
Breathing	☐ Ventilated	☐ Chest drain	

Circulation	Cannula size:	Rt.............	Lt.............
	IV Fluids	**Volume**	**Time**
	☐ H'manns/N. Saline	_____	_____
	☐ H'maccel/G'fusine	_____	_____

SECONDARY MANAGEMENT

Analgesia	☐ N₂O/O₂	**Dose**	**Time**
Drugs	☐ _____	_____	_____
(specify)	☐ _____	_____	_____

Splinting	☐ Frac Straps	☐ Traction: lbs/Kg_____
	☐ Box	☐ Other (specify) _____

SECONDARY SURVEY Time:

Respiratory Rate	
Oxygen Saturation (SpO₂)%	
Blood Pressure	_____
Pulse Rate	

Eye Opening	Spontaneous	4 ☐
	To voice	3 ☐
	To pain	2 ☐
	None	1 ☐

Best Verbal Response	Orientated	5 ☐
	Confused	4 ☐
	Inappropriate words	3 ☐
	Incomprehensible	2 ☐
	None	1 ☐

Motor Response	Obeys commands	6 ☐
	Localises pain	5 ☐
	Withdrawal (pain)	4 ☐
	Flexion (pain)	3 ☐
	Extension (pain)	2 ☐
	None	1 ☐

Pupils	React	R ☐
	(✓or X)	L ☐

1 ∘ Constricted   Size R [   ]
2 ○ Normal
3 ○ Dilated   Size L [   ]

TRAUMA SCORE:	
COMMENTS	

Signed
Status:

Figure 29-17 Triage card: Casualty assessment module

The dead
- It is important that the dead should be clearly labelled as soon as circumstances permit. This will prevent personnel from being diverted from resuscitating the living by other members of the emergency services who are unsure if the resuscitation should be attempted
- If possible, bodies should never be disturbed more than necessary to confirm death, and *always* be left in situ for later photography by the police, for forensic purposes, and eventual removal to the temporary mortuary facilities, so that valuable information about the accident is not destroyed

Confirmation of death
- In the UK, it is generally accepted that the only person who can legally confirm death out of hospital, is a registered medical practitioner
- Death should be confirmed in the presence of a police officer, who represents Her Majesty's Coroner in England and Wales, and the Procurator Fiscal in Scotland, with the relevant details recorded on the patient's triage label, and the new numbered blue police label, recommended by ACPO, if it is available

Method
- In a Major Incident, the initial classification of a casualty as dead will usually occur during the triage sieve. However, it may not be possible to carry out the full procedure to confirm death, with a police officer, due to the lack of policemen at the Incident Scene. If this is the case, a triage label should be attached to the casualty, and the full procedure carried out later when more personnel are available
- For practical purposes, it is usually sufficient to classify a casualty as dead, if they do not breathe, after the airway is opened, initially. The doctor confirming death however should carry out a more complete examination, including the presence of apnoea, an absent pulse/heartbeat, and fixed dilated pupils
- The job of confirming death will usually be delegated to a specific doctor by the Medical Incident Officer. The nominated doctor should go round the incident scene with a delegated police officer completing the procedure, and filling in the triage label and the blue police label, if it is available

Note: The dead should be covered with a blanket, salvage sheet or whatever else is available, so that they are out of sight of the press and public, especially any survivors (who may need to be kept forcibly away)

Body Holding Area
- The best position for this should be considered early on in the incident
- In some areas there may be a pre-designated site, e.g. a hanger, empty factory or school
- A dead body should *only* be moved initially if it is;
    - Necessary to obtain access to living casualties lying underneath them
    - In danger of being destroyed by fire, chemicals etc.
- If it is necessary to move a dead body, its position should be carefully recorded (ideally photographed)

Temporary Mortuary
- This should be set up if the nearest mortuary is any distance from the incident site
- The local authority in conjunction with the police will locate pre-designated sites in each area, usually a sheltered dry place, out of sight of the public and the media in, e.g. a school, village hall, or barn
- It will be used by the Coroner's Officer (or Procurator Fiscal's Officer in Scotland) and pathologists for the initial post-mortem examinations to determine the cause of death and for identifying the deceased

DEAD

Death Pronounced:

Time: Date:

Name of Doctor:

Signature:

Witnessed by PC:

Number:

Name:

Figure 29-18 Triage card: The dead

Identifying the dead
- The Police have the responsibility for identifying the dead and also for informing the next of kin
- In the case of foreign nationals, the Police also have the responsibility for informing the deceased's Consulate, High Commission or Embassy of the death of one of their nationals under the Vienna Convention on Consular Relations as directed by the Foreign Office
- Unfortunately in many Major Incidents, the deceased may not be easy recognise, because of severe deformity or dismemberment caused by an impact, fire, or explosion, and the separation of bodies from their clothing and personal effects
- The Police may set up a Casualty Bureau, which will have the job of collating all the information about casualties from known passenger lists, and lists of those thought or known to be involved from relatives and friends. This is then reconciled with the known position of the deceased immediately after the incident and from their clothing, personal effects and dental records
- It is therefore very important that no items or human material is removed from the scene of an incident unnecessarily, so that they can be photographed in situ and then bagged up and labelled, before being sent for forensic examination
- In air crashes, the Emergency Procedures Information Centre (EPIC), at Heathrow Airport, staffed by British Airways staff, will also collect information working closely with the Police and HM Coroner, if it is contracted to the airline involved in the accident

The media
- A Major Incident is of great interest to the media and they will attempt to obtain as much information as early as possible for their public
- Some will be less scrupulous than others, and may go to any lengths to obtain an exclusive story
- The initial response will probably be from the local media; press, radio and television, and will usually be followed by the national and international media
- The speed of the response of the television and radio media, in particular, and the sophistication of their communications equipment often compares very favourably with that of the emergency services
- Media attention will usually be directed at the scene and also to any hospitals to which the injured may be conveyed

Requirements
- Photographic opportunities, especially good vantage point of the scene
- A supply of accurate information, updated at regular frequent intervals
- A media rendezvous point or press centre
- Interviews with/access to key personnel, especially a senior police officer
- Access to witnesses, casualties, survivors, relatives, and any 'hero' or 'villain' stories. They will also want to know if any criminal proceedings are contemplated, and how soon the local community will return to relative normality

Management
- Managed correctly the press may be an asset:
    - Give notice of disrupted services/road closures
    - Advise the public to stay away
    - Appeal for witnesses
    - Appeal to key medical staff to go to their place of work urgently
    - Appeal for blood donors
- If allowed uncontrolled access to the scene, they may:
    - Obstruct and distract the emergency services away from their prime role of saving lives and safeguarding property
    - Destroy or remove forensic evidence as to the cause of the incident
    - Subject the survivors to unreasonable and inappropriate pressure and impinge on their dignity.
- If over restricted, they may force entry to the site

Media Liaison Point
- All media should be directed to this
- It should be reasonably close to the scene, but outside the outer security cordon

Access to the scene
- Media access to the scene itself should be restricted, but not unreasonably so
- May be allowed at the discretion of the Police Incident Officer, who should authorise passes to be issued to those allowed access
- Often, it is only practical to allow a small number of individuals access for security and safety reasons. In this case the media should be allowed to choose representatives from each type of medium - known as a *Media Pool,* to enter the scene

Parking
- Consideration should be given as to where the media should park their vehicles, so that access for the emergency services is not compromised

Overflying
- Rules must be established early for overflying to take aerial photographs (air exclusion zone)
- The noise and downwash from helicopters may seriously impair the work of the emergency services.

Facilities
- A Media Liaison Officer should be appointed as soon as possible by the police and should provide the press with updated information in the form of statements and press conferences at regular specified times
- Consideration should be given to establishing a media centre, especially in extended incidents

Information
- Interviews should be avoided (refer the enquirer politely but firmly to the Press Officer)
- Statements to the press should only be given by the Ambulance or Medical Incident Officer, but only after first agreeing the contents with the Police Press Officer, other Incident Officers, and the site owners, where appropriate, so that there is no contradiction or conflict to be exploited
- Any statement should be brief and factual
- Avoid giving opinions
- Do not give details of any individual casualties

30

Aeromedical evacuation

Aeromedical evacuation

Introduction

- All personnel involved in the management of Major Incidents require some understanding of aeromedical problems as there is an increasing tendency to use helicopters in primary evacuation of some patients, especially those with burns or a spinal injury

Rotary wing aircraft: helicopters

Uses
- To *deliver* medical and ambulance personnel very rapidly to the scene for:
    - Patients suspected of having very severe or multiple injuries, requiring immediate life saving treatment
    - Incidents in:
        - Remote or inaccessible places
        - Metropolitan areas, where traffic congestion may make road transport very slow
    - Incidents at sea
- For *primary evacuation* of casualties especially for:
    - Major disasters
    - Patients with very severe or multiple injuries
    - Patients with special injuries, e.g. burns, spinal injuries to appropriate specialist medical facilities
    - Remote places:
        - Scarce ambulance resources
        - Long travelling distances
        - Rough terrain
    - Inaccessible places
    - Metropolitan areas
    - Maritime accidents
- For *secondary evacuation*:
    - Hospital to hospital direct short haul transfer:
        - Often used for:
            - Spinal injuries
            - Severe burns

Helicopter types

- They may be:
    - Civilian:
        - Usually a small helicopter with some provision for transporting casualties
    - Police:
        - A small helicopter, which may be owned or chartered by the police
        - Its prime role is traffic control/surveillance, with some provision for carrying casualties
    - Ambulance service:
        - Small helicopter. Often chartered and specially adapted for ambulance use
    - Military:
        - Usually Royal Navy or Royal Air Force
        - This is usually a large helicopter, whose primary role is Search and Rescue, or troop or cargo transportation
        - They have provision for transporting casualties, but there is little sound insulation so they tend to be particularly noisy

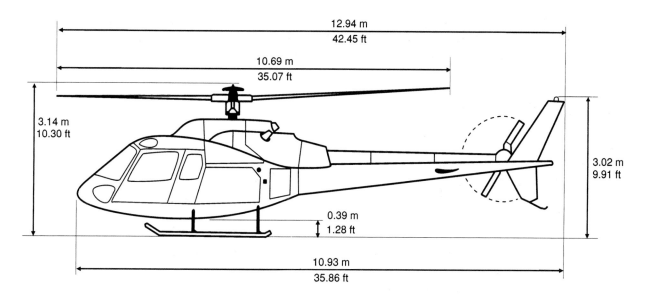

Figure 30-1 The main dimensions of the AS 355 helicopter

Advantages

Access

- Helicopters do not require an airfield or landing strip on which to land
- They have:
    - The ability to land in relatively small spaces
    - The ability to land on rough ground if equipped with skids (on soft ground, the rotors may have to be kept going to provide enough lift to prevent the helicopter from sinking in)
    - A winching facility (military and coastguard helicopters only) which can be used to lift up a stretcher from places only accessible from the air:
        - Very rough terrain
        - Cliffs

PRACTICAL POINT: Military helicopters usually have their winch and cargo doors on the port (left) side
Civilian helicopters and aircraft usually have their cargo doors on the starboard (right)

Speed
- Helicopters are relatively fast compared to road transport
- Can travel in a straight line

Range
- Their range is:
    - Wessex/MBB 105: 300 miles
    - Sea King/Dauphin 2: 600 miles

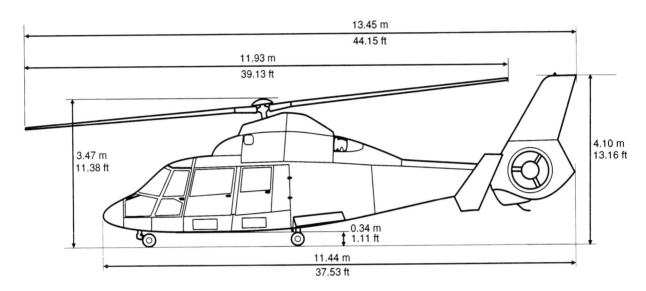

Figure 30-2 The main dimensions of the SA 365 Dauphin helicopter

Disadvantages

Cost
- Helicopters are very expensive to operate

Range
- Have a relatively short range of action compared to fixed wing aircraft

Static
- The static generated by the aircraft may have to be earthed, and this may cause problems, especially during winching (size dependent and occurs with the Sea King, but not the Wessex)

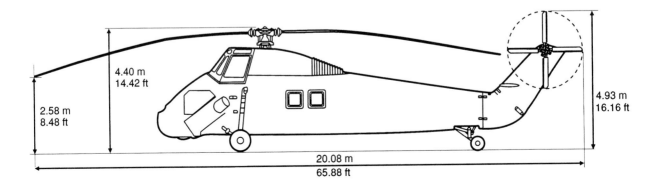

Figure 30-3 The main dimensions of the Wessex helicopter

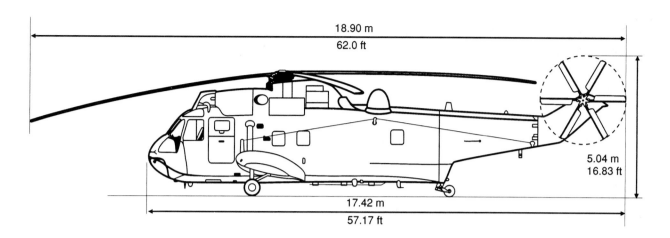

Figure 30-4 The main dimensions of the Sea King helicopter

Rotor blades
- These can be very dangerous for those on the ground, especially if it is sloping
- All those approaching a helicopter should do so cautiously and under the direct control and guidance of the pilot
- May generate considerable downdraught, which can be unpleasant for those on the ground. All loose items should be secured

Stokes litter

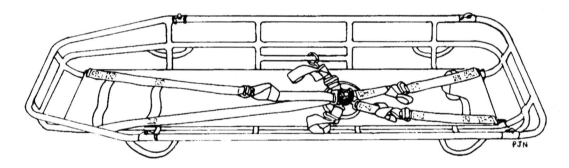

Neil Robertson stretcher

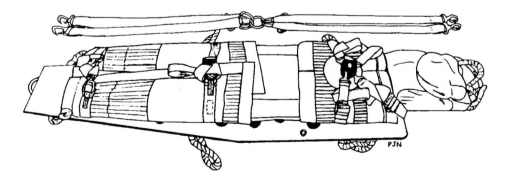

Figure 30-5 Devices in which patients can be winched/carried in helicopters

The high levels of noise
- Cabin levels 80-115 dBA (pain >140 dBA):
- This may be uncomfortable, and can necessitate the use of ear defenders for all (this includes the patient, even if he is unconscious)
- Causes difficulty with communication:
    - Necessitates the use of hand signs/headphones

Vibration
- This may be quite unpleasant

Flicker
- This occurs when the rotor blades interrupt the light from a strong light source, causing it to appear to flicker
- It may:
    - Cause vertigo, which may be uncomfortable.
    - Induce epileptiform fits (rarely)

Wind chill/cold
- This may precipitate hypothermia and aggravate shock:
    - Consider using an insulating (space) blanket

Other problems
- There also may be problems with:
    - Compatibility of equipment:
        - Different voltage, etc.
    - Interference with the aircraft's avionics:
        - LEDs.
        - Defibrillator discharge (in practice, this does not appear to be the problem that it might seem to be in theory)
    - Lack of space

Helicopter landing site

Site selection
- The site should be clear of all tall obstacles (25 metres or over):
    - Trees, buildings, pylons
- The actual landing spot should be firm and at least 15 metres in diameter
- The maximum slope should be no more than 12%

Helicopter landing site preparation
- Clear an area 100 metres in diameter
- Remove or secure all loose material which may be either blown about causing injury or sucked into the engine air intake:
    - Paper debris
    - Stones
    - Medical equipment
    - Leaves and loose branches
- Keep the area clear of any crowds and animals
- Indicate the wind direction using smoke if possible
- Mark out the intended landing place with "*Day-glo*" or similar markers, if available

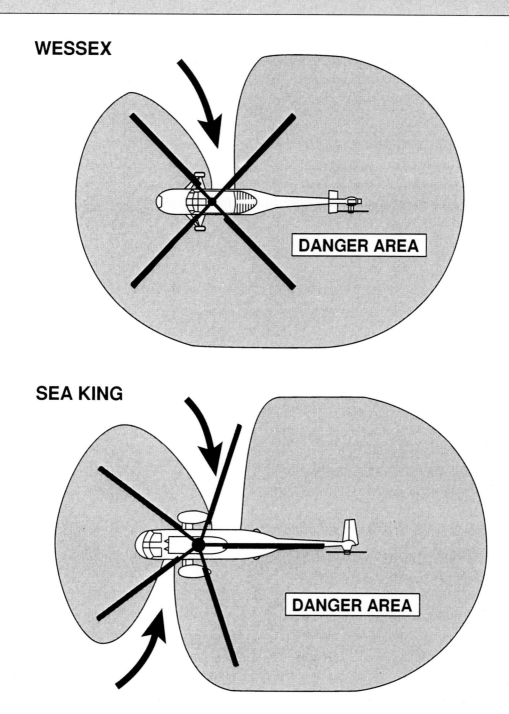

Figure 30-6 Helicopter entry points and danger zones

Landing helicopters
- Most helicopter pilots are skilled and practised in unaided landings, and do not usually require any assistance
- If the selected site is particularly difficult for any reason guidance may helpful:
    - Guide the helicopter in by standing or kneeling well beyond the edge of the 15 metre landing spot, with your back to the wind and with both arms raised

Approaching helicopters
- Only approach a helicopter, when you have been directed to do so by a crew member, ideally the pilot.
- If the blades of a helicopter are rotating, approach it in a crouched position, to avoid being blown over.
- Never go near a rotating tail rotor

In the helicopter
- Patients must have a secure harness fastening them to the stretcher
- All medical equipment must be made secure:
    - Fixation of the endotracheal tube
    - Intravenous lines
- Make sure that you are prepared for all likely medical emergencies:
    - Make sure that there is enough room around the patient
    - Prepare and place equipment ready to use
    - Establish intravenous access, if you have not already done so
- Prepare yourself for a possible emergency evacuation of the helicopter

Fixed wing aircraft

Uses
- Fixed wing aircraft are usually only used for the secondary transfer or evacuation of patients over relatively long distances

Types
- The aircraft may be:
    - Piston or jet engined
    - Pressurised or unpressurised
- The flights may be:
    - Long, medium or short haul
    - By air ambulance or scheduled flight

Advantages
- May be extremely rapid, and the only practical method of long distance patient transport

Selection of which type of aircraft ?
- This depends on:
    - What is available
    - The finance/insurance that is available
    - The airport facilities:
        - The length of the runway
        - The time that the airport is open
    - The time to be spent in transit:
        - The risk to the patient is directly proportional to the length of time spent travelling
    - Any compromise between range versus speed, and altitude, e.g. cabin pressurisation for open skull fractures, pneumothorax and diving dysbarism
    - Whether a stop-over is necessary:
    - Consider the risk of unnecessary exposure of the aircraft crew and other passengers to any endemic health problems in the pick up country
    - Limits on the crew's flying time
    - Whether pressurisation is necessary:
        - This depends on the aircraft's altitude

- Whether there is a problem with:
    - Hypoxia:
        - Hypoxia is exacerbated by increasing height, as the atmospheric pressure decreases, the partial pressure of oxygen and oxygen concentration also decreases
        - ? Therapeutic oxygen supply needed/available, e.g. for patient with:
            - Cardiac failure
            - Myocardial ischaemia
            - Severe anaemia
            - Respiratory disease
            - Cerebral artery insufficiency
- The reduced ambient temperature
- Decompression/high flying (low pressure):
    - This should be avoided:
        - In patients with abnormal gas containing cavities whether traumatic, therapeutic/ investigative
        - Following recent diving:
            - Within 12 hours of "no-stop" diving (<10 metres)
            - Within 24 hours of "stop" diving (>10 metres)
        - In patients suffering from any diving related disease of recent onset
- Dehydration:
    - This is worse on long flights, due to the low humidity of the aircraft's air conditioned cabin air
- The risk of "Jet lag":
    - This is the disturbance of circadian rhythms, which is caused by transmeridian flight, i.e. crossing time zones. This is far worse after eastward flights compared with westward flights
    - It does not occur when travelling along time, i.e. from North to South or vice versa
- Poor lighting and lack of adequate space in all types of aircraft
- Drug schedules:
    - There may be problems due to changes in time
    - It is probably best to maintain these on the departure zone time until arrival at the final destination
- The different voltage used in the aircraft (28 volt DC)
    - This may cause problems (non functioning) of some essential medical equipment:
        - Monitors
        - Infusion pumps, etc.
- There are special regulations regarding the importation and carriage of "Dangerous cargo":
    - Relevant items are oxygen, mercury, aerosols and flammable materials
- There is a legal requirement to have a Home Office Licence for the importation and reimportation of "Controlled Drugs"

Planning

- Road ambulance liaison:
    - The collection of the patient from the point of arrival
- Medico-legal:
    - Obtain permission from the treating doctor abroad for the transfer
- Make certain that the UK destination is adequate for the patient's needs, and that there will not be any need for a further transfer within the UK
- If repatriation is for the insurer's economic reasons, make sure that:
    - The patient gives their consent
    - There is no increased medical risk to the patient in the transfer
    - The medical care in the UK is as good, if not better, than that abroad

Problems
- Getting enough accurate information about the patient:
    - Language/translation:
        - From medical foreign language into foreign language into English into medical English
        - The doctors/officials in the foreign country may be economical with the truth in order to expedite transfer of the patient

Information required
- Ideally all this information should be obtained before setting off to collect the patient, although invariably not all of it is
- The name, age, sex, religion and home address of the patient
- The name, address and telephone number of the patient's general practitioner, and hospital consultant
- The patient's destination:
    - Hospital, nursing home, etc.
    - It is always advisable to check that there is actually a bed available for the patient
- The patient's height, size, weight:
    - Can he/she fit in the aircraft?
- The diagnosis, treatment carried out, and the time intervals involved
- Details of any special requirements both medical and nursing care:
    - Diet
    - Suctioning
    - Intravenous fluids, etc.
    - Monitoring
    - Splinting
- The available facilities in the hospitals involved in the patient's care, both in the foreign country and the UK (if appropriate)
- The experience and expertise of the hospital staff in the foreign country, and accompanying the patient to and in the aircraft
- The drugs used and to be used:
    - Names
    - Doses
    - Times given

In the aircraft
- Patients must have a secure harness fastening them to the stretcher
- All medical equipment must be made secure:
    - Fixation of the tracheal tube
    - Intravenous lines
- Make sure that you are prepared for all likely medical emergencies:
    - Make sure that there is enough room around the patient
    - Prepare and place equipment ready to use
    - Establish intravenous access, if you have not already done so
- Prepare yourself for a possible emergency evacuation of the aircraft

31

Radio communications

Radio communications

Introduction
- Effective communication is the key to the command and control of resources at Major Incidents
- An understanding of the most appropriate method of communication, and the best way to use it is also very important
- The ambulance service has responsibility for Health Service communications in the UK

Radio communication
- The efficiency of radio communication is dependent on correct procedures being followed and accurate information being given to Control, which will enable the correct decisions to be made about the provision of resources at its disposal and to manage them effectively

Organisation

Control
- This is the central radio, usually in a fixed place, which manages the radio network
- There is usually a control console which is connected to the transmitter and receiver by a landline
- The transmitter and receiver are situated adjacent to the radio mast near the top of which is the aerial to which they are connected, and which receives and transmits the radio signals
- At Major Incidents, each emergency service usually has a mobile control, carried in a mobile control vehicle, which manages the local radio network for that service

Mobile radios
- These are small radio sets which incorporate both a transmitter and a receiver, connected to an aerial
- They may be:
    - Vehicle mounted: usually permanently fixed in the vehicle, possibly with hands-free operation
    - Transportable: portable, with good range, but rather heavy and bulky, and may be used in-vehicle
    - Hand held (portable): usually lightweight, but with a limited range

Radio frequencies

Bands
- There are three radio frequency bands used in the United Kingdom by the statutory ambulance services, Immediate Care schemes, voluntary aid societies and motor sport organisations:
    - Low band AM: 77-88 MHz (voluntary aid societies, motor sport organisations)
    - High band FM: 165-174 MHz (statutory ambulance services, Immediate Care schemes, voluntary aid societies and motor sport organisations)
    - UHF: various (statutory ambulance services for short range communications)

Modulation
- Radio waves may be modulated in two ways:
  - FM: frequency modulation
  - AM: amplitude modulation
- A radio using one kind of modulation cannot usually communicate satisfactorily with a radio using the other kind of modulation

Radio reception
- Radio waves travel in straight lines, although they can be reflected off some of the layers of the upper atmosphere, or off some buildings

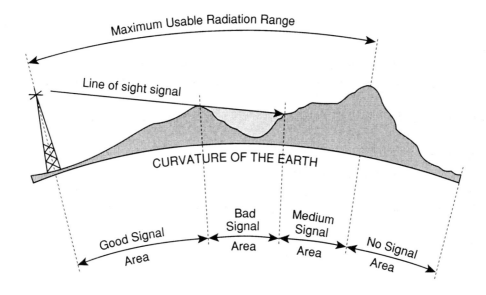

Figure 31-1 Radio reception

Transmitter range
- Radio has a limited range
- Radio reception is always best from a high unobstructed location
- If a mobile cannot receive (hear) Control (which usually has a higher powered transmitter and better aerial siting than mobiles), then it is unlikely that Control will be able to receive the mobile
- If radio reception is poor, e.g. at the limit of the range, or in a radio black spot, the mobile should move to a more favourable location (usually higher up, or on the opposite side of a hill), before attempting to transmit

Interference
- Transmission and reception can be upset by weather: thunderstorms, heavy rain, etc.

Radio black-spots/shadows (areas of poor radio reception)
- Can be caused either by the terrain, tall buildings, steel cladding, etc.

Methods of transmission

Single frequency simplex
- This is where both the base station and the mobiles transmit and receive on the same frequency
- This means that all the radios in a system can hear transmissions from all the other radios
- Used by the voluntary aid societies, in motor sport, and by ambulance services UHF (short range communications)

Advantages
- Useful when mobiles need to be able to communicate directly with each other

Disadvantages
- If two mobiles transmit at once, they will cause mutual interference "heterodyne"
- Two mobiles can engage the whole system and make it difficult for Control to exercise control

CONCLUSION
- Suitable for systems covering a relatively small area, when mobiles are involved in the same incident or event and need to be able to communicate directly with each other, but radio discipline needs to be strictly enforced. May also be useful in schemes with very few mobiles covering large areas, which are unlikely to interfere with each other

Two frequency simplex (semi-duplex)
- The base station transmits on one frequency, and the mobiles transmit on another adjacent frequency
- This means that all mobiles can receive the base station, but only the base station can receive transmissions from the mobiles (which cannot usually receive transmissions from each other):
    - Base: transmits on frequency A and receives on frequency B
    - Mobiles: transmit on frequency B and receive on frequency A
- Used by ambulance services and Immediate Care schemes

Advantages
- Easier for Control to exercise control
- Useful when a base station controls a large number of mobiles, and there is usually no need for mobiles to be able to transmit to and receive each other

Disadvantages
- Occupies two channels
- Mobiles cannot listen to each other (and learn what is going on), unless Control switches on talkthrough

CONCLUSION
- The system of choice for large systems covering large geographical areas

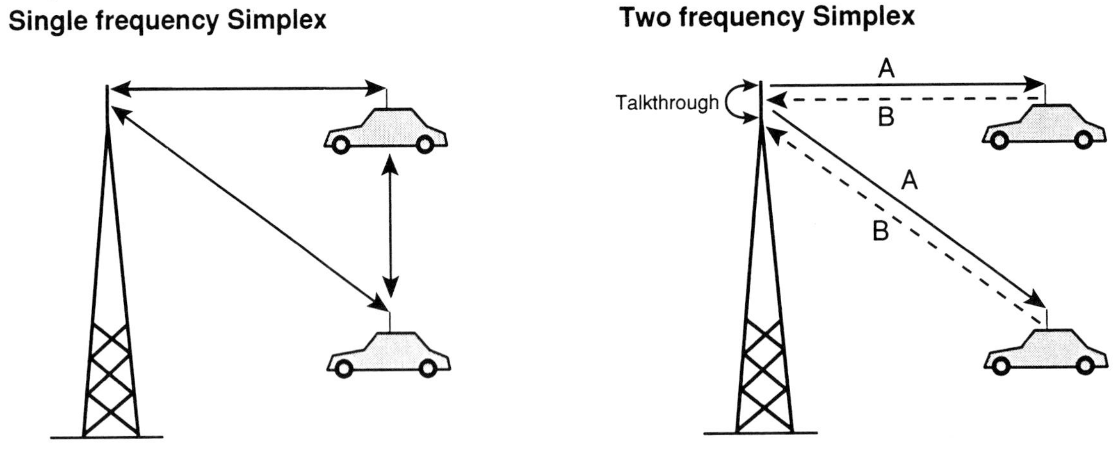

Single frequency Simplex   **Two frequency Simplex**

Figure 31-2 Single and two frequency simplex

Two frequency duplex
- The use of a two frequency system, in which both the transmitter and receiver can both operate simultaneously (like a telephone)
- Electronically complicated
- Used in Cellular radio

Facilities

Talkthrough
- A facility used in two frequency simplex, which enables the base station to re-transmit everything that it receives
- Enables mobiles to hear all transmissions, and for one mobile to communicate with another
- May be switched by the base station console, and may also be switchable by mobiles using a tone control system (see below)

Encoders/decoders
- These encode or decode a series of audio tones (usually three or five), which can be used to selectively 'page' (the radio will emit a bleep similar to a pager) and 'open up' a radio from a stand-by (dormant) state (when they are switched on, but their loud speaker is muted)
- The sequence of tones may also be used to activate a pager on the same radio system, so that when a mobile is paged, not only will the radio open up, but the pager will go off at the same time
- Useful:
    - When a channel or frequency has to be shared with other users, and mobiles do not want to have to listen to irrelevant transmissions
    - When used in conjunction with a pager, for alerting a radio operator who may not be close to the radio

Sub-audio tone
- This is an inaudible tone (unique to a particular system), which is transmitted simultaneously with any speech. The receiving radio will only 'open up' and switch on its speaker, when it receives this tone. The radio will revert to a 'closed down' state with its speaker muted as soon as it ceases to receive the sub-audio tone
- Its purpose is to only open up radios when there is a transmission on their radio system and is useful when a channel or frequency has to be shared with other users, and mobiles do not want to have to listen to irrelevant transmissions

Squelch
- A control found on older sets, which reduces the amount of receiver interference, but at the same time increases the threshold/strength of signal required for the radio to receive a transmission

Callsigns

Fixed stations
- Fixed stations are usually called 'Control' or 'Base', with a prefix indicating the name of the service, e.g. Essam Control (Essex Ambulance Control), SWAG Base (Saffron Walden Accident Group Base)

Mobiles and portables
- Mobiles and portables are usually given letter names of the the NATO phonetic alphabet or numbers of the NATO figure pronunciation (see below). This may be:
    - Preceded by a prefix indicating the name of the service, e.g. Essam 181 (Essex Ambulance Service mobile 181)
    - Preceded or followed by an indication of the status of the mobile, e.g. Medic SWAG 01 (Doctor 01 from the Saffron Walden Accident Group), Essam 181 Papa (Essex Ambulance Service mobile 181 with a paramedic on board)
    - Callsigns usually belong to an emergency vehicle, rather than to members of its crew
    - Doctors and officers in the emergency services usually have their own individual callsigns

Note: Full callsigns should always be used when starting and closing any exchange of messages

Radio procedure

Introduction
- Correct Control, vehicle and individual 'callsigns' must be used at all times and *never* the names of control operators, vehicle crews or doctors
- Messages should be spoken in a way that will ensure the receiver has full understanding of them
- The three characteristics of a good radio message are:
    - Clarity:
        - Pronounce words distinctly and slowly
    - Accuracy:
        - In the situation where communications are difficult, or the pronunciation of words, names or numbers is difficult and liable to cause uncertainty in the mind of the receiver, the word or name should be spelt out using the NATO phonetic alphabet or in the case of numbers use the NATO figure pronunciation (see below)
    - Brevity:
        - Messages must be as brief as possible, using well recognised abbreviations and codes
- The following factors are therefore important:
    - Rhythm;
        - This should be steady
    - Rate:
        - Slightly slower than normal speed of talking is 40-60 words per minute
    - Volume:
        - keep your mouth close to the microphone and speak across it
        - Do not shout or whisper
    - Pitch
        - The pitch of the female voice is considered best for radio communications. Gruff voiced men should try to raise the pitch of their voice and avoid muttering
- Never use obscene language or swear words over the air. This is an offence under the Radiotelephone Licensing Regulations, and offenders may be prosecuted

Proper use of radio
- Radios should be switched on the moment the vehicle becomes mobile
- Remember, only one mobile or radio user can use the radio frequency or channel at one time and that messages of a non-urgent nature could be blocking another mobile's urgent call for assistance
- Always try to be as polite and friendly as possible, but do not take up any unnecessary airtime

Preliminary call
- This is a transmission to ensure that communications are possible before air space is wasted in passing a message which cannot for one reason or another be received
- It is essential to stop and think before passing a radio message - plan it, and until you get enough experience, try to write it down on paper to prevent confusion (if circumstances permit)
- Before transmission, make sure that the channel is clear:
    - Always listen before transmitting. If you are not certain if the channel is in use, ask briefly
    - Operators should *never* attempt to call Control when another transmission is in progress, except in life threatening emergencies, when the call should be prefixed 'Safety', 'Priority' or 'Priority Urgent' (in motor sport)
- After this, call once only; using full call signs, and always give your own call sign after that of the station you are calling
- When an individual or a mobile initiates the call to Control, the following procedure should be used:
    - Control 'call sign' (this is usually repeated once), followed by the doctor's or vehicle's 'call sign'

Example:
    Mobile: *"Essam Control, Essam Control, Medic 01,* over"
    Control: *"Medic 01, Essam Control,* go ahead, over"

Messages
- Each message should end with 'over'

Example:
    Mobile: "Good morning Essam, responding to your call to an RTA on the M11, *over*"
    Control: "Good morning to you Medic 01, we have a report of persons trapped, *over*"

Acknowledgements
- Every message must be acknowledged, otherwise the calling station may think the exchange is incomplete and may continue to keep the channel clear of other users
- Important or complicated messages may be repeated by the receiving station to indicate that they have got the message correct

Example:
    Control: "Can you proceed to marker post Alpha Bravo 201 please, over"
    Mobile: "Roger, *Marker post Alpha Bravo 201,* over"

Closing
- At the end of a message or series of messages, stations may end with either the words:
  - 'Standing by' indicating that they will continue to monitor that radio frequency *or*
  - 'Out' indicating that they do not expect any further communications
- It is usually the prerogative of Control to indicate that the exchange is over

Example:
    Mobile: "I am leaving the scene and will RTB, over"
    Control: "Roger, Medic 01, Control *out*"

Locations
- When giving a location, reference should be made to distances, cross roads, road junction numbers, and well known buildings along with the area location

Corrections
- 'Wrong' or 'Correction' should be used to indicate that a mistake has been made

Example:
    Control: "Good morning, Medic 01, please can you proceed to a collapse in Saffron Walden, on the B1184, *wrong* the B1183 outside the Eight Bells, over"

Long messages
- In general all messages should take up no more than about 30 seconds
- Long, complicated or important messages should be split up into sequential sentences to ensure accuracy and allow others to interrupt if they have a more urgent message:
  - Only one sentence should be transmitted at a time, and the next sentence only transmitted after acknowledgement that the preceding sentence has been received and understood

NATO phonetic alphabet
- Different accents and methods of pronunciation, and the fact that radio transmission may distort some sounds, makes it easy for some sounds to be confused
- In this alphabet, each letter has an unmistakable sound
- Used to spell out difficult or important words or letters

A	ALPHA	*AL-FAR*		N	NOVEMBER	*NO-VEM-BER*
B	BRAVO	*BRA-VOH*		O	OSCAR	*OSS-CAH*
C	CHARLIE	*CHAR-LEE*		P	PAPA	*PAH-PAH*
D	DELTA	*DELL-TAH*		Q	QUEBEC	*KEY-BECK*
E	ECHO	*ECK-OH*		R	ROMEO	*ROM-ME-OH*
F	FOXTROT	*FOX-TROT*		S	SIERRA	*SEE-AIR-AH*
G	GOLF	*GOLF*		T	TANGO	*TANG-GO*
H	HOTEL	*HO-TELL*		U	UNIFORM	*YOU-NEE-FORM*
I	INDIA	*IN-DEE-AH*		V	VICTOR	*VIK-TAH*
J	JULIET	*JEW-LEE-ETT*		W	WHISKEY	*WISS-KEY*
K	KILO	*KEY-LOH*		X	X-RAY	*ECKS-RAY*
L	LIMA	*LEE-MAH*		Y	YANKEE	*YANG-KEY*
M	MIKE	*MIKE*		Z	ZULU	*ZOO-LOO*

Numeral pronunciation
- This is a method of pronunciation for numerals, similar to the NATO phonetic alphabet for letters

1	*WUN*		6	*SIX*
2	*TOO*		7	*SEV-EN*
3	*THUREE*		8	*ATE*
4	*FOUR*		9	*NINER*
5	*FIYIV*		0	*ZERO*

Radio check
- When using a radio for the first time or after moving to a fresh location, it should be checked to make certain that the radio is functioning properly and that it can receive the base station and other radios on the network

Signal strength
- This is used when checking signal strength and radio reception with another radio:
  1. Unreadable
  2. Very noisy and barely readable
  3. Noisy but readable
  4. Good, but slightly noisy
  5. Loud and clear (OK)

- The following may be used as a simpler alternative, but is not commonly used in the ambulance service:
  - OK
  - Difficult
  - Broken
  - Unworkable
  - Nothing Heard

Example:
>   Mobile: "ESSAM control, this is MEDIC SWAG 01, *radio check* please, over"
>   Control: "Roger MEDIC SWAG 01, *I read you strength 3*, over"

Kilo code

- This is a code system which is used by some ambulance services, but there is little uniformity between different services
- It is used to save air time and prevent confidential information being understood by outsiders

Example: Kilo

1	Death unconfirmed by a doctor
2	Death confirmed by a doctor
3	Overdose not seen by a doctor
4	Overdose seen by a doctor
5	Myocardial infarction
6	Unconscious patient
7	Abortion
8	Psychiatric patient
9	AIDS patient
10	Terminally ill patient

Common abbreviations/expressions used in radio communications

Acknowledge	Indicate that you have received my message
ETA	Estimated time of arrival
ETD	Estimated time of departure
Go ahead	Usually used after a 'wait' period.
OK	All right, correct
Over	Used at the end of each message, apart from the final one
Priority!	Should prefix an urgent life saving message (only to be used in exceptional circumstances)
Repeat	Repeat your message
Roger	Message understood
RTB	Return to base
Safety!	Should prefix an urgent safety message
Say again	Repeat your message
Send	Transmit your message
Stand by!	Wait!

Standing by   Used at the completion of an exchange of messages, indicating that the radio is expecting further transmissions and will remain 'opened up'

Wait   Indicates that you are unable to reply immediately (within 5 seconds). It is normally followed by an indication of time, e.g. "wait one (minute)"

Wait out   I am not in a position to reply; I will contact you later

32

Psychiatric emergencies

Psychiatric emergencies

Psychiatric emergencies

Definition: A psychiatric emergency is a situation in which the patient exhibits psychological distress which exceeds the ability of that individual, their carers or society to cope with it, and which may pose a possible risk to the patient or others

Incidence
- Psychiatric emergencies are common in areas of social deprivation, poor housing, and ethnic minorities

Aetiology
- Causes include:
    - Psychoses
    - Depression and mania
    - Anxiety
    - Dementia
    - Alcohol and drug abuse
- May be precipitated by:
    - Social difficulties:
        - Financial problems
        - Lack of food, warmth and shelter
    - Breakdown in relationships:
        - Family
        - Society
    - Physical illness
  - Medication
  - Alcohol, illegal drugs and substance abuse

Assessment
- In order to obtain a useful history it is necessary to:
    - Engage the patient
    - Take a rapid selective history from all those available

History of current problem
- This should be obtained from family, neighbours, work colleagues, friends
- History of current problems
    - Sudden onset
    - Gradual onset
- Previous medical history

- Previous psychiatric history:
    - Depression
    - Psychotic illnesses
    - Drug and substance abuse
- Current prescribed medicines
- Current alcohol, illegal drug and substance abuse
- Domestic circumstances

Mental state assessment
- Appearance and behaviour
- Speech (coherence) and content
- Thoughts and beliefs expressed
- Overall state of mind (mood) and whether it it is congruent with the content of the thoughts
- Observable abnormal perceptions and expressed experiences
- Assessment of the level of consciousness and orientation in time, space and person
- Short-term memory and concentration
- Insight into their problems by the patient
- Suicidal intent

Physical examination
- This should be performed as rapidly as possible, especially where the history and mental state assessment indicate that there might be a causative physical problem:
    - Hypoglycaemia
    - Infection
    - Cardiac failure
    - Myxoedema
    - Uraemia
    - Delirium tremens
    - Subdural haematoma
- Breath odour may indicate:
    - Alcohol
    - Ketones
    - Solvent abuse
- Recent skin puncture marks and scarring over veins used may indicate drug abuse

Psychosis
- In psychosis the patient has a disorder of thought and behaviour with delusions and hallucinations
- The acutely ill psychotic patient may be a danger to themselves, their family and the public

Incidence
- An acute psychosis is one of the commonest causes of an acute psychiatric emergency

Aetiology
- Causes include:
    - Schizophrenia;
        - Affects about 1: 100 people during their lifetime
        - Many patients are also depressed; about 10% of schizophrenics commit suicide
        - The onset is usually in the late teens in men and slightly later for women
    - Hypomania
        - Affects about 8: 1,000 people during their lifetime
    - Psychotic depression

Symptoms/signs

Delusions
- A delusion is a firmly held belief, which has no foundation in reality, often based on spurious and inappropriate evidence, in spite of any logical arguments or evidence to the contrary
- The delusions may be:
    - Paranoid;
        - That they are being persecuted/pursued by others often the police or people in authority
        - That others are listening to their thoughts and/or sending them coded or secret messages via the television, radio or newspaper
    - Grandiose:
        - That they are for example God, Jesus, Napoleon, and that they have a some special role to perform

Hallucinations
- A hallucination is the perception of receiving a sensory stimulus in the absence of any actual stimulus
- The sensory stimulus appears totally real, but often frightening/threatening to the patient, e.g.:
    - Hearing voices or noises which are not present
    - Seeing things which are not visible to others
    - Tasting special flavours
    - Being sexually stimulated by non-existent beings
- In many cases the patient will offer a delusional explanation for their hallucination, e.g.
    - That the voices are transmitted down the electric cable, or come from the radio/television, etc.

Psychotic depression
- Underactivity
- Lack of concentration
- Social withdrawal
- Emotional emptiness with inability to experience pleasure
- Poverty of speech and thought
- Poor response to traditional medication

Overactivity
- Restlessness
- Over talkative

Psychotic behaviour
- Many patents suffering from an acute psychosis, may appear threatening or dangerous to others, but are only so on very rare occasions, with the exception of a very small minority
- Warning signs of possible impending violent behaviour include:
    - A previous history of violence
    - Immediate recent violent behaviour
    - The patient's appearance and behaviour
    - Intoxication with drugs and/or alcohol
    - The content of any delusional thoughts

Management
- Try to gain the confidence of the patient
- Gently, calmly, patiently and confidently listen to the patient and persuade them that they need help. Often the patient will accept that they need medical assistance, as they commonly find their hallucinations frightening and unpleasant

- Avoid:
    - Questioning the validity of their beliefs and do not threaten or provoke the patient in any way
    - Inappropriate force
    - Verbal aggression
    - Confining the patient in an enclosed environment as this will often make them worse
- Never expose yourself to unnecessary danger, and always have a prepared avenue for escape
- Consider oral or intravenous sedation with:
    - Chlorpromazine
    - Haloperidol
    - Droperidol

Depression and mania

- Depression is the most common cause of suicide

Depression

Incidence

- Depression severe enough to warrant medical treatment affects 5-10% of the population at any one time
- 10% of depressed patients commit suicide

Symptoms/signs

- Depression is a persistent and debilitating mood disorder characterised by:
    - Sadness and low mood sustained for at least two weeks
    - The inability to derive pleasure from any activity (anhedonism)
    - Poor self-esteem and hopelessness
    - Lethargy, lack of motivation, poor concentration and lack of drive
    - Suicidal ideas
- Other common symptoms include:
    - Sleep disturbance often with poor or unrewarding/unrefreshing sleep, or prolonged sleep
    - Loss of or increased libido
    - Loss of appetite, resulting in dehydration and exhaustion, or sometimes increased appetite
    - Anxiety
    - Self neglect

Hypomania, bipolar affective disorder, manic depressive illness

Incidence

- The lifetime risk of developing hypomania is about 0.5%

Symptoms/signs

- In hypomania the patient's mood will swing from episodes of severe depression and lethargy to episodes of mania, characterised by:
    - Elation
    - Over-activity with increased speed of thought and excessive expansive speech
    - Grandiose delusions of their self-importance or over-confidence in their own abilities
    - Over-spending, often extravagantly
    - Sexual excess or disinhibition
    - Hallucinations which may reinforce their beliefs
    - Lack of sleep, food and water intake
    - Neglect of their appearance or dressing up in inappropriate extrovert manner
- When severely depressed the patient may develop a manic stupor in which they appear mute and motionless, although fully conscious

Management
- Patients suffering from depression are rarely dangerous to others, except when they are determined to commit suicide, and take others with them (family, loved ones, or enemies, who they perceive as being responsible for their condition)
- Admit as an emergency psychiatric admission
- Sedate (rarely necessary)

Anxiety disorder
- Anxiety disorders include:
    - Anxiety states/panic attacks (attacks of severe anxiety with an overpowering fear of severe physical illness, dying, being trapped, or the wish to escape)
    - Phobias
    - Obsessive compulsive disorder

Incidence
- Anxiety disorders rarely by themselves cause an acute psychiatric emergency, but anxiety is a common feature of many other psychiatric illnesses, including depression and alcohol abuse, and will increase the patient's distress

Symptoms/signs
- Emotional:
    - Fearfulness
    - Irritability
    - poor concentration
    - Restlessness
    - Sensitivity to noise
- Physical (due to sympathetic overactivity):
    - Dry mouth
    - Tachycardia
    - Hyperventilation
    - Churning stomach

Management
- Massive and repeated reassurance
- Treatment of hyperventilation if present
- Sedation with:
    - Diazepam
    - Lorazepam (a short acting benzodiazepine suitable for the treatment of panic attacks)

Personality disorder
- This is a broad term which encompasses many diagnosis ranging from inadequate personality to hysterical personality, etc.
- Patients suffering from personality disorder are amongst the most difficult to assess, as:
    - They may appear to be impatient, demanding, attention seeking, manipulative, hysterical, inadequate and hostile and it may be difficult to engage with them
    - They may antagonise and alienate the health care professional with whom they come into contact
    - There have been a number of previous unsuccessful suicide attempts, which have not been life-threatening
- However patients with personality disorder have a significant risk of developing other psychiatric disorders, e.g. depression, and with it the risk of suicide, which may be missed
- If a patient who appears to be suffering from personality disorder expresses suicidal intent, 'cries for help', they should be assessed thoroughly and in the same way as any other 'at risk' psychiatric patient

Physical causes of psychiatric illness

Incidence
- Acute toxic confusion state/delirium is relatively common in the elderly

Aetiology
- There are many physical causes of acute psychiatric illness, including:
    - Hypoglycaemia
    - Infection
    - Cardiac failure
    - Myxoedema
    - Uraemia
    - Delirium tremens
    - Subdural haematoma
    - Senile dementia

Symptoms/signs
- Impaired consciousness with:
    - Drowsiness
    - Poor concentration
    - A lack of lucidity
- Increased arousal with
    - Fearfulness
    - Acute anxiety
- Delusions and hallucinations
- Disorientation in time, space and person

Risk factors for suicide
- A past or present history of significant depressive illness, schizophrenia or eating disorder
- Personality disorder
- A family history of suicide
- Single status and social isolation
- Unemployment
- Problem drinking
- Previous attempts at self-harm
- Recent bereavement
- Older age

Alcohol, Illegal drug and substance abuse

- All those involved in pre-hospital care will increasingly be involved in caring for patients suffering from drug and substance abuse, which in itself has a high incidence of acute physical morbidity and more rarely mortality, and may be associated with acute injury or illness

Incidence

- Confusion and psychosis caused by drug and alcohol abuse is a common cause of psychiatric emergency
- The range of problems requiring immediate medical care may include:
    - Acute intoxication
    - Acute behavioural disturbances
    - The secondary effects of trauma and severe infection
- The abuser may be using more than one drug, often of doubtful purity and strength
- The Immediate Care practitioner should always be aware of the possibility of illegal drugs and substances being involved, and the patient and their companions questioned appropriately, especially if:
    - They show an inappropriate response to their circumstances or any other behavioural disturbance
    - They are noted to have injection marks
    - Syringes, powders, or tablets are found amongst their personal effects

Alcohol abuse

Ethanol (ethyl alcohol) abuse: acute alocoholic intoxication

- Widely available as a beverage, but is also an important constituent of cosmetics, aftershave, hair tonic, antiseptics, mouth washes, dishwasher detergents and glass cleaners, as well as being commonly used in industry as a solvent

Incidence

- Acute poisoning is common in adults, but may also occur in children either accidentally or deliberately
- Recent alcohol consumption is a factor in 10% of all road traffic accidents: resulting in 800 deaths and 22,000 casualties annually in the UK
- Drunken drivers account for 1/3 of all fatal RTAs (2/3 of all fatal RTAs between 10 pm and 4 am)
- One third of drivers in injury accidents fail the breath test

Aetiology

- Acute alcohol poisoning is an uncommon cause of death by itself, unless exceptionally large quantities are consumed, and when fatalities occur, aspiration of gastric contents is an important factor
- Alcohol ingestion may predispose the patient to other life threatening conditions especially major trauma
- Every year people die because their condition is presumed to be due to alcohol, rather than the real cause, e.g. head injury
- The patient may have taken drugs as well as alcohol, the effects of which may often be potentiated by it
- In adults severe ethanol intoxication will follow the consumption of 300-500 mL of a strong spirit, e.g. whisky, gin, vodka, which may be fatal if the recovery period is not supervised adequately

Pathophysiology

Absorption
- Alcohol is absorbed rapidly through the mucosa of the stomach and small intestine. The rate of alcohol absorption may be reduced by the presence of food in the stomach, and in heavy smokers, and is partly determined by genetic factors
- Peak blood ethanol concentrations usually occur within 30-90 minutes of ingestion
- Moderate amounts of ethanol may be metabolised before absorption by gastric alcohol dehydrogenase, so that not all the ethanol enters the circulation. This enzyme is present in lower quantities in women and alcoholics of both sexes, resulting in higher ethanol absorption

Metabolism
- About 95% of ingested alcohol is oxidised to acetaldehyde and acetone, and the remainder is excreted unchanged in the urine, and to a lesser extent in the breath
- In young children, who have not eaten for 8-12 hours, ingestion of even modest amounts of alcohol may result in permanent neurological damage as a result of the ensuing hypoglycaemia

Action
- Ethanol is a CNS depressant, which in small doses depresses the cortical inhibitory centres resulting initially in disinhibition (inebriation), and in larger doses cortical and medullary depression
- Vomiting whilst unconscious can be a problem
- Causes vasodilation especially of cutaneous vessels, resulting in increased heat loss and may precipitate hypothermia and hypotension
- Ethanol ingestion causes inhibition of hepatic gluconeogenesis resulting in hypoglycaemia, especially in children or after fasting, exercise or chronic malnutrition. In these circumstances, alcohol induced hypoglycaemia typically occurs within 6-36 hours of ingestion of a moderate or large amount of alcohol
- Heavy drinking may precipitate acute cardiac arrhythmias, whether heart disease is present or not
- Lactic acidosis (which is usually only mild) is an uncommon but potentially serious complication of acute ethanol poisoning and occurs especially in patients with severe liver disease, pancreatitis or sepsis
- Alcoholics who have regularly consumed large amounts of alcohol may develop an alcoholic ketoacidosis, caused by a combination of dehydration, glucopenia, increased lipolysis and ketogenesis. An ethanol-free interval with nausea and vomiting usually precedes the onset of ketoacidosis and ethanol may not be found in the blood

Symptoms/signs
- History of alcohol ingestion
- Smell of alcohol on breath (unreliable as a guide of the blood alcohol level)
- Nausea, vomiting due to alcoholic gastritis
- Hypoglycaemia, convulsions (especially in children)
- Impaired neurological state:

Blood ethanol concentration. (mg/l)

<500	Talkativeness, subjective feeling of wellbeing
500-1000	Inebriation:
	- Slurred speech
	- Emotional instability with irrational behaviour and aggression
	- Poor coordination
	- Loss of sensory perception
	- Drowsiness
1000-3000	Intoxication
	- Loss of sensory perception
	- Lack of coordination, and ataxia with an unsteady gait
	- Blurred or double vision, nystagmus
	- Flushed, warm skin
	- Hypotension, tachycardia
	- Coma
	- Convulsions
>5000	Very severe intoxication
	- Coma
	- Hyporeflexia
	- hypothermia
	- Respiratory depression
	- Poor airway protection with loss of gag reflex and risk of aspiration of vomit

Note: Even if the patient's breath smells strongly of alcohol; other causes of impaired consciousness should be positively looked for:
- Head injury
- Hypoglycaemia
- Physical illness, etc.

Management
- Induce emesis/gastric emptying with airway protection
- Care of the unconscious patient, especially the airway, as vomiting may occur and the patient may have a reduced gag reflex and respiratory drive
- Full examination to exclude other cause for the patient's condition
- If the patient is confused and violent, sedation should be considered, e.g. with diazepam
- Respiratory depression, cardiac arrhythmias and shock should be treated appropriately
- Blood glucose monitoring and intravenous/oral glucose if indicated

Acute alcohol withdrawal

Aetiology
- Only found in alcoholics
- Usually comes on within 24-72 hours of the last drink, but may be delayed for up to 10 days
- Has a high mortality

Symptoms/signs
- History and signs of alcoholism
- The severity of the withdrawal reaction is related to the amount and duration of alcohol intake, but there is considerable variation in symptoms from one individual to another and even from one episode to another in the same individual
- The withdrawal reaction is characterised by sympathetic nervous system overactivity:
    - Sweating, tachycardia, hypertension and tremor
- The clinical features may be partially related to or occur as a result of very high glucocorticoid levels

Minor withdrawal
- May occur within a few hours of the blood ethanol concentrations suddenly falling or reducing to zero
- Full recovery usually occurs within 24-72 hours
- Apprehension, weakness, faintness, sweating and irritability
- Catecholamine induced hypertension, insomnia and (often coarse and irregular) tremors

Intermediate withdrawal
- Hallucinations ("delirium tremens");
    - Occur in less than 5% of patients, usually within 48 hours of ceasing alcohol ingestion
    - Auditory and/or visual hallucinations, which are often, but not always threatening or unpleasant, e.g. spiders, snakes, hedgehogs, etc.
    - Individuals are usually able to describe the nature of their hallucinations, and are aware that they are not real
- Withdrawal fits:
    - These occur in up to 2% of patients, usually within 12-24 hours of ceasing alcohol ingestion, but may be delayed for up to 72 hours
    - Are usually of the uncomplicated grand mal type, and are few in number, although status epilepticus may rarely occur
- Cardiac arrhythmias:
    - Uncommon, and are probably caused by an underlying metabolic disorder

Major withdrawal
- Occurs in about 5% of patients, usually within 3 days of ceasing alcohol ingestion, and may last from 3-7 days
- It is characterised by:
    - Severe agitation
    - Confusion
    - Delusions
    - Gross tremulousness
    - Tachycardia
    - Excessive sweating
- The patient becomes completely disorientated and experiences visual and sometimes auditory hallucinations, which are often associated with extreme fear and apprehension, leading to aggressive, destructive and suicidal behaviour
- The mortality is about 1%, provided that there is adequate medical supervision, and death is usually associated with cardiovascular collapse or concurrent infection

Management
- Reassurance and sedation:
    - Oral benzodiazepine, e.g. diazepam
- Circulatory support
    - Intravenous infusion of crystalloid
- Treatment of fits:
    - Intravenous diazepam/midazolam
- Hallucinations and delirium:
    - Intramuscular haloperidol (*Serenace®*) 2.5-10 mg, every 4-8 hours depending on response, up to a maximum of 60 mg

Note: Alcoholics are also at risk from other acute problems, e.g. haematemesis

Methyl alcohol (methanol, wood alcohol) abuse

Incidence
- Accidental poisoning is relatively common in the desperate and poor alcoholic, who uses it as a substitute for ethyl alcohol, resulting in chronic poisoning

Aetiology
- Found in paints, paint thinners, paint removers, varnishes and antifreeze
- Usually only toxic when ingested

Pathophysiology
- Can cause a profound metabolic acidosis
- Methanol is metabolised to formic acid, which cannot be further metabolised by the body and is toxic to retinal ganglion cells, commonly causing blindness

Symptoms/signs
- Alcoholic odour
- Nausea, vomiting, dizziness and headache
- Visual blurring, or other visual disturbance (may occur after the signs of intoxication have subsided)
- Drowsiness and coma
- Tachypnoea with deep respirations
- Hypotension and shock

Management
- Consider induction of emesis with airway protection
- Oxygen
- Circulatory support:
    - Intravenous infusion of crystalloid
    - If the patient shows signs of a metabolic acidosis:
        - Consider administration of 50 mL 8.4% bicarbonate intravenously.
- Cardiac monitoring
- Give one measure of whisky every hour (ethanol selectively impairs the metabolism of methanol to formic acid and thus promotes its excretion unaltered)

Heroin and opiate abuse
- Drugs made from the milky fluid that seeps out of the cut surface of unripe seed capsules of the opium poppy *Papaver somniferum*

Heroin
- Heroin is the most commonly abused opiate

Known as:
- 'smack', 'junk','H', 'skag'

Description
- Available as a grey, pink, brown or white powder, which can be dissolved in water and injected, sniffed, or smoked

Action
- Cerebral depression
- Peripheral vasodilation
- Constipation
- Many heroin addicts will contract hepatitis B or C, or AIDS due to sharing needles with other addicts
- Induce a feeling of total relaxation and detachment from pain and anxiety
- Makes the user drowsy, happy, warm and content, and appears to relieve pain, stress and discomfort
- Causes both physical and psychological dependence in weeks to months
- First time users may experience nausea and vomiting
- Prolonged use may cause:
    - Anorexia and malnutrition
    - Amenorrhoea
    - Constipation
    - Reduced immunity
- Withdrawal:
    - Occurs within 4-12 hours of ceasing to use the drug, peaks at 48 hours and abates after about a week. Insomnia and craving may last for weeks
    - Results in muscle aches and spasms, tremor, sweating and chills, restlessness, sneezing and yawning
- Overdosage results in:
    - Unconsciousness and coma
    - Respiratory depression eventually resulting in death

Symptoms/signs
- Euphoria, drowsiness/impaired consciousness
- Constricted pupils
- Respiratory depression
- Needle marks and abscesses on hands arms, legs and feet, with blood stains on clothing and bedding

- Look for:
    - Wraps of paper
    - Syringes and needles
    - Blackened tinfoil
    - Tourniquet (belt, tie, string)
    - Bent spoons, spent matches, bottle caps

Management
- Basic Life Support
- Oxygen
- Circulatory support with an intravenous infusion
- Consider use of activated charcoal if the opioid has been ingested
- **Naloxone** (400 µg/mL: 1/2 mL amps) may be used both as a diagnostic and as a therapeutic agent:

Dosage: 0.8-2.0 mg given as an intravenous bolus

- Reversal of symptoms should begin within about 1 minute, but beware of "recovery" followed by further collapse (for more information: see chapter on Pain management)
- A partial response indicates that a further dose should be administered, although the patient may also have ingested other central nervous system depressants, e.g. alcohol, or a benzodiazepine, or may already have suffered a degree of hypoxic cerebral damage, resulting in dilated pupils
- The initial dose of naloxone may need to be repeated, as naloxone has a short half life

Note: Although naloxone administration may precipitate a withdrawal reaction in a heroin addict, this should *not* be considered to be a contraindication to its use

Morphine abuse
- The fatal dose may be as little as 100mg

Methadone abuse
- This is a synthetic opiate, which is prescribed to help patients withdraw from heroin usage, but is abused by many addicts
- It is designed to be taken orally, but may also be injected intravenously
- It has a half life of about 15 hours, which delays the onset of withdrawal symptoms

Volatile substance abuse: glues and solvent abuse
- Commonly used by school children, especially teenage males, often as a group activity
- Results in over 100 deaths per year

Description
- Glues and solvent used include industrial and household products, containing volatile substances, including acetone, chloroform, ether, toluene, that can be sniffed.
- The substances most frequently abused may be classified into:
    - Fuel gases:
        - Butane gas lighter fuel (butane is also used as the propellant in 'ozone friendly' sprays
        - Paraffin hydrocarbon lighter fluid
        - Petrol vapour
        - Propane

- Solvents:
    - Trichloroethane (typewriter correction fluid)
    - Trichloroethylene
    - Bromochlorodifluoromethane (fire extinguishers)
    - Butylnitrite (also used as a room deodoriser)
    - Paint and paint stripper
    - Nail varnish and nail varnish removers
- Glues (account for 20% of deaths):
    - Toluene
- Aerosols which use CFCs (usually halon) as the propellant (account for 20% of deaths):
    - Polishes
    - Hair lacquer

Administration
- Solvents are usually put on a piece of cloth, which is held near the nose for inhalation ('huffing')
- Adhesives are emptied into a plastic bag, the opening of which is gathered together and held over the nose and mouth and inhaled ('bagging')
- Some users increase the effect by inhaling inside a plastic bag, placed over the head, and sniff until they lose consciousness
- Fuel gases and aerosols are sprayed directly into the mouth

Action
- Volatile solvents cause the rapid onset of intoxication similar to that produced by alcohol, including:
    - Initial excitement with a feeling of wellbeing, euphoria, disinhibition and exhilaration
    - Auditory and visual hallucinations which may be frightening
    - Dizziness and ataxia with nausea, vomiting, flushing and increased salivation
    - Sneezing and coughing due to mild irritation of the mucous membranes of the nasal and respiratory tracts
- Increasing exposure causes:
    - Progressive impairment of consciousness with mental confusion and loss of self control
    - Ataxia, dysarthria, and nystagmus
    - Unconsciousness, coma and occasionally fits
- Heavy or long term use may cause:
    - Permanent brain, renal and hepatic damage
    - Cardiotoxicity (may be cause of death)
- Regular use causes psychological dependence
- Suffocation or unconsciousness may occur from the fumes or putting the head inside a plastic bag

Symptoms/signs
- Rash around the nose/mouth
- Stomach cramps
- Drunken behaviour with aggression and uncoordinated movements
- Conjunctivitis
- Look for:
    - Empty tubes or cans
    - Plastic bags with traces of glue in them
    - Strong chemical smell
    - Traces of substance on clothing

Management
- Airway care if the patient is unconscious
- Oxygen
- Sedation with diazepam if the patient is rowdy or in a state of panic

Sedative abuse
- These include:

Benzodiazepine abuse (also see above):
- Widely as a drug of abuse, especially temazepam and diazepam

Known as:
- 'Tranx', benzos', 'eggs', 'jellies'

Description
- Available as tablets and capsules (temazepam)
- Temazepam in particular is often abused; it is available in capsules, the contents of which are dissolved and then injected intravenously

Action
- Lessen alertness, and may lower the inhibitions, resulting in aggression
- Psychological addiction is common in long term abusers
- Withdrawal may cause confusion, irritability and anxiety, and the inability to cope generally

Symptoms/signs
- Drowsiness
- Slurred speech and ataxia
- Partial ptosis and nystagmus
- Coma
- Mild hypoxia and respiratory depression

Management (see chapter on Poisoning and Overdosage)

Barbiturate abuse (also see above)
- Amylobarbitone (*Amytal*®), barbitone, butobarbitone (*Soneryl*®), pentobarbitone (*Nembutal*®), phenobarbitone, quinalbarbitone (*Seconal*®), sodium amylobarbitone (*Sodium Amytal*®)

Known as:
- 'Barbs', 'downers', 'blues', 'reds', 'sekkies"

Description
- Most are supplied in powdered form and are sold in coloured capsules, and are often consumed with alcohol.
- Some abusers dissolve the contents of the capsules for intravenous injection
- Some injecting addicts will contract hepatitis B or C, or AIDS due to sharing needles with other addicts

Action
- Sedating, causing drowsiness, ataxia, and dysarthria
- Heavy or prolonged use may cause:
    - Irritability, nervousness, twitching, delirium and convulsions
    - Insomnia
    - Hypotension
    - Nausea and vomiting
- Rapid withdrawal in an addict may result in sudden death
- Regular use results in physical and emotional dependence

Symptoms/signs
- Flushed appearance
- Slurred speech
- Staggering/unsteady gait
- Drowsiness, stupor
- Vomiting

- Look for:
    - Tablets or capsules of various colours
    - White powder
    - Needles and syringes

Management
- Basic Life Support, oxygen
- Intubation and ventilation in the deeply unconscious patient

Cannabis
- Widely used as a social drug

Known as:
- 'Dope', 'blow', 'wacky backy', 'grass', 'shit', 'ganja'

Description
- Produced from the Indian hemp plant, *Cannabis sativa,* which is found worldwide, and contains several active constituents, known as tetrahydrocannabinols
- May be used as:
    - Hash/hashish:
        - Cannabis resin scraped from the plant and compressed into dark brown blocks, and usually mixed with tobacco
    - 'Grass', 'pot', 'dope', 'marijuana':
        - Dried, chopped, cannabis leaves which are mixed with tobacco, rolled into a cigarette and smoked, or eaten or brewed into tea
    - Concentrated oil
        - Smoked or taken orally
- Psychologically but not physically addictive
- May rarely be brewed up into a kind of tea and injected

Action
- If smoked, the symptoms start within 10-20 minutes and last for up to three hours
- If ingested, the symptoms take up to 2 hours to begin, and last up to 6 hours
- Helps people to relax and become disinhibited
- Enhances sensory perception, especially colour and sound
- Co-ordination is impaired with delayed reaction times
- May also cause:
    - Hallucinations
    - Anxiety and panic
- Prolonged use may result in:
    - Permanent psychological changes
    - Lung damage caused by regular smoking
- Accidental ingestion by children may result in coma with dilated pupils, hypotonia, and hyporeflexia
- Cannabis may also be brewed into a kind of tea and injected, when it may rapidly cause:
    - Nausea, vomiting, abdominal pain, and watery diarrhoea, accompanied by rigors, fever, hypotension and shock

Symptoms/signs
- Impaired co-ordination
- Red eyes, with dilated pupils
- Tachycardia
- Disinhibition with irrelevant giggling, etc.
- Look for:
    - Butt ends of hand-rolled cigarettes ('joints')
    - Strong smell of burning leaves
    - Large cigarette papers

Management
- None is usually necessary when cannabis has been smoked or ingested
- If the patient is unconscious: care of the airway
- Panic reactions:
    - Reassurance
    - Sedate with diazepam
- Intravenous cannabis
    - Circulatory support with an intravenous infusion of crystalloid

Hallucinogenic drug abuse

LSD (lysergic acid diethylamide)
- Widely available

Known as:
- 'Acid'

Description
- A white powder or colourless, odourless liquid, it is usually mixed with other substances and formed into very small tablets or capsules, or supplied in sugar cubes or impregnated paper squares, and taken orally after food and swallowed

Action
- Produces pleasant hallucinations, including auditory and visual, and a feeling of being outside the body, which may occur for several months after the initial trip without any recent drug exposure
- Onset of effects occurs about one hour after ingestion and lasts for up to twelve hours
- It may also cause unpleasant hallucinations leading to depression, dizziness, panic/extreme agitation leading to violence, and bad flashbacks (more likely if the user is anxious or in unfamiliar surroundings)
- Long term use may result in a sense of unreality and permanent personality disorder
- Death may result from accidents or violence whilst under the influence of this drug

Symptoms/signs
- Detection may be difficult
- Perceptual changes, especially auditory and visual
- Illusions and hallucinations
- Paranoid delusions
- Confusion, agitation, wild excitement and unmanageability
- Dilated pupils, piloerection, tachycardia and hypertension (after large doses)

Management
- Physical restraint may be necessary to prevent the patient from injuring himself or those trying to manage him
- Reassurance and sedation with chlorpromazine (50-100 mg administered intravenously) is usually adequate
- If the patient is unconscious; care of the airway, etc.

'Magic mushrooms'
- See chapter on Poisoning and overdosage under 'plants and fungi'

Stimulant abuse

Cocaine
- Cocaine is used medically as a local anaesthetic
- Becoming more popular as a drug of abuse

Known as:
- 'Snow', 'rock', 'base'

Description
- A crystalline white powder produced from the leaves of the coca bush grown mainly in Peru, Bolivia, and Columbia
- It may be sniffed, smoked or more rarely injected (sometimes mixed with heroin)
- Causes psychological dependence

Action
- Cocaine blocks the reuptake of the neurotransmitters norepinephrine, serotonin and dopamine in the brain resulting in a stimulant effect producing feelings of euphoria, wellbeing, indifference to pain and tiredness, anaesthesia, and illusions of physical and mental strength
- These effects tend to peak quickly, and lessen rapidly. The drug then has to be taken more often to maintain the 'high'
- Cocaine also has a local anaesthetic effect, which in overdosage may cause arrhythmias and myocardial depression, resulting in a fall in cardiac output and eventually death
- Other effects include:
    - Dry mouth
    - Anorexia
- Long term use results in:
    - Hyperexcitability, loss of libido and impotence
    - Nausea, insomnia, weight loss, paranoia, loss of sense of smell (anosmia)
    - Pruritus
    - Sniffing may cause damage to the nasal mucous membranes, which can be very painful
- Some cocaine addicts will contract hepatitis B or C, or AIDS due to sharing needles with other addicts

Symptoms/signs
- Increased alertness and excitation
- Euphoria
- Increased respiratory rate, increased temperature
- Tachycardia and raised blood pressure
- Dilated pupils
- Fits
- Look for:
    - Folds of paper
    - Syringes and needles
    - Handbag mirror and razor blade
    - Straw for sniffing or snorting

Management
- There is no direct antidote for cocaine toxicity, but it is now accepted that high dose intravenous diazepam effectively antagonises the central stimulant and hypertensive effects of cocaine, and should be administered immediately
- Treat cardiac arrhythmias with β-blockers, e.g. atenolol

Crack cocaine

Description
- Cocaine which has been chemically treated so that it can be smoked using a water pipe

Action
- The initial high is followed by unpleasant after-effects which encourage compulsive use and lead to dependence
- Highly addictive
- May cause respiratory depression and is cardiotoxic
- Smoking crack causes black sputum, chest pain and lung damage

Symptoms/signs
- Extreme euphoria with loss of self control
- Agitation and aggressive behaviour with dilated pupils
- Look for:
    - Paper wraps
    - Small plastic bags
    - Water pipes or tubing

Management
- As cocaine

Amphetamine abuse
- Amphetamines are widely used as stimulants
- Include dexamphetamine (*Dexedrine*®), and amphetamine-like drugs including methylphenidate (*Ritalin*®), and diethylpropion (*Tenuate Dospan*®)

Known as:
- 'Speed', 'uppers', 'sulphate', 'sulph', 'whiz', 'amph'

Description
- A powder or tablet that can be eaten, smoked with tobacco, mixed with water and injected, or sniffed

Action
- Stimulant, giving an initial feeling of having extra energy and confidence, excitement, staying power and reduced need for sleep
- Increasing use is required to maintain the same effect
- Physically addictive
- The initial effects are followed by a feeling of anxiety, irritability, paranoia, disturbed sleep, and loss of appetite, and are followed by depression and hunger
- High doses may produce panic attacks, delirium, hallucinations, and hypertension and tachycardia resulting in cardiac damage and cerebrovascular accidents
- Withdrawal may result in severe depression, dysphoria, fatigue and lethargy
- Prolonged use may result in immunosuppression
- Some amphetamine addicts will contract hepatitis B or C, or AIDS due to sharing needles

Symptoms/signs
- Abundant energy, talkative, excitable and confident with anorexia and insomnia
- Jerky movements and a dry mouth
- Confusion, changing moods, aggressive behaviour
- Long term heavy use may result in:
    - Exhaustion and paranoid toxic psychoses
- Needle marks
- Look for:
    - Folded wraps of paper
    - Powder or tablets
    - Syringes and needles

Management
  - Treat hypertension and cardiac arrhythmias with β-blockers, e.g. atenolol

Ecstacy (MDMA)
  - Ecstacy has recently been associated with several highly publicised deaths in young people due to cardiac arrhythmias and malignant hyperthermia
  - Used as a dance drug at parties and 'raves'

Known as:
  - 'E', 'dennis the menace', 'rhubarb and custard', 'new yorker', 'love droves', 'disco burgers', 'phase 4', 'adam', 'fantasy'

Description
  - Several drugs are marketed as ecstasy, including the original ecstasy MDMA, (3, 4-methylene-dioxymethylamphetamine), MDA (3, 4-methylene-dioxyamphetamine), MDEA (3, 4-methylene-dioxyethamphetamine) and MBDB (3, 4-methylene-benzodioxolbutanamine)
  - They are hallucinogenic semisynthetic amphetamines
  - Comes as tablets or differently coloured capsules

Action
  - A stimulant, it makes people very sociable, and gives them extra energy. Once this wears off they may feel depressed and low. It may also affect co-ordination
  - There are two ways in which death may result from ecstasy ingestion:
    - Early:
      - Excessive fluid intake compounded by failure of renal water excretion, due to inappropriate secretion of antidiuretic hormone, may cause hyponatraemia and result in fatal cardiac arrhythmias
    - Late:
      - If taken in a hot atmosphere, e.g. at a rave, ecstasy use can have an effect on muscles resulting in malignant hyperthermia with severe heatstroke and death
  - Some deaths may occur after exposure to doses which have previously well tolerated, and may be due to an idiosyncratic reaction resulting in direct brain injury
  - Taken in large amounts ecstasy may cause anxiety, confusion and paranoia
  - Prolonged use can result in hepatic damage; regular users may develop insomnia, and girls may develop menorrhagia

Symptoms/signs
  - Polydipsia, thirst
  - Abundant energy
  - Increased colour perception
  - Enhanced empathy
  - Look for:
    - Excess drinking
    - Tablets of varying colours
  - Hyperthermia with a core temperature of 39-42°C:
    - Collapse or fits
    - Dilated pupils
    - Sweating (although in severe cases this may have ceased)
    - A marked sinus tachycardia (140-160 bpm) and hypotension

Management
  - Basic Life Support, oxygen
  - Hyperthermia (this is an acute life threatening condition):
    - Administer an infusion of 1 litre of N-Saline immediately
    - If this brings down the pulse rate and raises the blood pressure; administer a further 1 litre
  - Convulsions/fits: administer intravenous diazepam

The Mental Health Act 1983 (or Mental Health (Scotland) Act 1984)

- If a patient who needs admitting to hospital as a psychiatric emergency refuses, then they may be detained under a section of the 1983 Mental Health Act
- Indications for admitting a patient as a psychiatric emergency include some or all of the following:
    - Where they are at risk of harming themselves
    - Where there is a risk that they will harm others
    - Where they are at risk of severe self-neglect or are unable to make rational decisions about their treatment because of psychiatric illness

Section 2 (Section 24 in Scotland): admission for assessment

- A Section 2 lasts up to 28 days (24-72 hours, extendable to 28 days in Scotland) and allows for a patient to be removed to hospital for assessment
- Section 2 is usually used when the diagnosis is uncertain or the patient does not have a previous known history of mental illness

Section 3 (Sections 18 in Scotland): admission for treatment

- Section 3 lasts up to six months and can be renewed
- It is used for admitting a patient with a past psychiatric history when the diagnosis is already known
- In Scotland, the application must be approved by a Sheriff

Section 4 (Section 24 in Scotland): admission for assessment as an emergency

- This lasts up to 72 hours, and is useful when there is a risk of the patient absconding or becoming violent before a second doctor can arrive (it requires one doctor and an approved social worker for completion)
- A section 4 should be converted to a section 2 or 3 as soon as possible by an approved doctor

Section 135 (Section 117-118 in Scotland): gaining access

- This may be used when it is not possible to gain access to the patient's home to complete an assessment
- A warrant must be issued by a magistrate
- A section 135 warrant is normally obtained by the social worker, who should arrange for the patient's general practitioner and a psychiatrist to be present, so that a section 2 or 3 section can be completed after access has been gained

Section 136: removal from a public place to a place of safety

- This may used by the police to remove the patient to a place of safety, e.g. a police station

Method

- The process for detaining a patient under Sections 2 and 3, are similar and require input from:
    - Two doctors, who have to examine the patient together or separately to assess the patient's physical and mental health, make a diagnosis and decide whether admission to hospital is indicated:
        - One doctor should have prior knowledge of the patient (ideally the patient's own GP)
        - The other doctor, usually a psychiatrist, should be approved under section 12 (2) of the Mental Health Act (1983) as having experience in diagnosis or treatment of mental disorder
        - If the patient's own GP is unable to attend a second Section 12(2) doctor may be used instead
    - An approved social worker, or rarely the patient's nearest relative, who applies for the section. Their principal role is to explore whether there is any viable and safe alternative to detention, taking into account the social circumstances of the patient and the wishes of their family
    - A manager at the designated hospital who receives the patient
- For a Section 3 application:
    - Additional information needs to be provided about the patient's mental state
    - If the nearest relative objects, the application cannot proceed
- Once the medical recommendation forms have been completed, they are passed to the approved social worker for activation

Notes

33

Counselling accident and disaster victims

Counselling disaster and accident victims

Introduction

- Those involved with Immediate Care should be aware of the need for counselling for all those involved in incidents resulting in serious physical or emotional trauma, because they may be involved both as a sufferer and in the treatment of sufferers
- It is now well recognised that the best counsellors are not only those trained in counselling, but also those who were themselves involved in the actual or similar events, and as such, those involved in Immediate Care who are not affected, may have a unique and very special role
- Counselling should not be thrust unthinkingly on all those involved in horrific events, but there should be an understanding that they may require help and if so should not feel embarrassed or awkward about seeking it
- Many of those involved in Immediate Care may already give themselves and their colleagues a kind of counselling, by discussing the event with their colleagues or others involved in it, or even by holding informal or formal debriefing sessions, at which feelings can be vented in a non threatening and non judgemental environment
- It should be remembered that even the experts may be upset by "the Big One"

Post-traumatic stress disorder (PTSD)

- This is an adjustment disorder occurring as a result of an exceptional mental or physical stress, not normally experienced by most people

Incidence

- 40-70% of all those directly involved in a disaster, experience symptoms during the following month
- 20% may experience chronic levels of anxiety for more than 2 years
- Long term effects (lasting up to 5 years) are possibly most common in those involved in fires or explosion at sea
- Up to 70% of rescuers may be affected
- Associated with an increase in physical and psychiatric illness and accidental and non-accidental death

Aetiology

- The causative event does not have to be a major disaster, but may be a particularly traumatic event including:
    - Serious injury accidents
    - Torture
    - Rape, attempted rape or sexual abuse
    - Assault
    - Accidental killing of others
    - Witnessed death of a child or spouse
    - Difficult childbirth
- Those at risk may also include:
    - Battle shocked soldiers
    - Hijack victims
    - Concentration camp survivors
    - Hostages
- Disasters which expose their victims to a prolonged risk of death or mutilation are more likely to result in severe and prolonged effects
- It is not only the victims themselves that may suffer from this condition, but also their friends, relatives, and emergency services personnel and rescue workers
- Community workers and members of the voluntary agency involved in the care of the survivors of a disaster may also be at risk
- Emergency services personnel are more likely to suffer from PTSD if:
    - They are unable to do anything active to help the survivors
    - There are gruesome tasks involving multiple deaths, mutilated bodies or the deaths of young children
    - There is poor organisation and management of the disaster with a lack of command and control, and explanation of their tasks, leading to frustration over lives than cannot be saved, equipment failure, delays and overwhelming demands being made on them
- Those involved in a near miss situation (i.e. those who but for some accident of fate would have been a victim) may also be affected

Pathopsychology

- *PTSD affects normal individuals; it is the event which is abnormal/exceptional*
- The traumatic event is by definition, one which is distressing for all those involved with it, and in particular gives them feelings of acute fear, terror, and usually a sense of helplessness, and impotence
- Characteristics of the disaster, the rescue operation and the sufferer may all affect the degree of stress experienced
- Psychopathic personalities may to a certain extent be protected
- Head injury with retrograde amnesia seems to protect patients from the condition
- Some of the effects may be worse in those who are uninjured and in those involved in the near miss situation, who may have feelings of guilt about having survived
- Those most at risk include:
    - The unemployed
    - Those from lower socioeconomic class
    - Those from large families
    - The divorced and those with little support
    - Females
    - The young, especially children (including those born from victims shortly after the disaster)
    - The elderly (because of their reluctance to ask for help)

- Severity:
    - Those with a predisposition for pre-morbid depressive or neurotic traits are more likely to be affected and probably also more severely affected than those without such personality traits
    - Repeated similar stress may increase the severity
    - The severity is likely to be increased if the stressor is caused by another person

Prognosis
- The overall prognosis is:
    - Good if treatment is early and specific
    - Poor if symptoms and treatment are each delayed more than 6 months

Symptoms
- The onset of symptoms may be delayed by up to 6 months after the event (many patients will avoid seeking medical help in an effort to avoid anything to do with their experience)
- Symptoms must have been present for at least 1 month before the diagnosis can be made

Presenting symptoms
- May include:
    - *History of:*
        - Anxiety
        - Depression
        - Exhaustion
        - Poor concentration
        - Marital problems
        - Palpitations
        - Irritability
        - Sudden outbursts of anger
        - Alcohol or drug abuse
    - *Appears:*
        - Apathetic
        - Withdrawn

Diagnosis

DSM-IV diagnostic criteria
- As PTSD was originally an American Psychiatric Association Diagnostic and Statistical Manual, Fourth Edition (DSM-IV) diagnosis, this is the system most commonly used to make the diagnosis
- The DSM-IV diagnostic criteria for 309.81 post traumatic stress disorder are:

    A. Exposure to a traumatic event in which both of the following were present:
    - The person experienced, witnessed or was confronted with an event(s) that involved actual or threatened death, serious injury or a threat to physical integrity
    - The Person's response involved intense fear, helplessness or horror

    B. The event is persistently re-experienced in one (or more) of the following ways:
    - Recurrent and intrusive distressing recollections of the event, including images, thoughts or perceptions

        Note: In young children, repetitive play may occur in which themes or aspects of the traumatic event are expressed

- Recurrent distressing dreams of the event (repetition syndrome)

   Note: In children, there may be frightening dreams without recognisable content

- Acting or feeling as if the traumatic event was reoccurring (this includes a sense of reliving the experience, illusions, hallucinations and dissociative flashbacks, including those that occur on awakening or when intoxicated)

   Note: In young children, trauma specific re-enactment may occur

- Intense psychological distress at exposure to internal or external cues that symbolise or resemble an aspect of the traumatic event

C. Persistent avoidance of stimuli associated with the traumatic event and numbing of general responsiveness (not present before) with depressive symptomatology and suicidal thoughts as indicated by three (or more) of the following:
   - Efforts to avoid thoughts, feelings or conversations associated with the traumatic event
   - Efforts to avoid activities, places or people that arouse recollections of the traumatic event
   - Inability to recall an important aspect of the traumatic event
   - Markedly reduced interest or participation in significant activities
   - Feeling of detachment or estrangement from others (who have not experienced the same trauma)
   - Restricted range of affection (e.g. unable to have loving feelings)
   - Sense of a foreshortened future (e.g. does not expect to have a career, marriage, children or a normal life span)

D. Persistent symptoms of increased arousal (not present before the traumatic event), as indicated by two (or more) of the following:
   - Difficulty in falling or staying asleep
   - Irritability or outbursts of anger
   - Difficulty in concentrating
   - Hypervigilance
   - Exaggerated startle response (excitability)

E. The duration of the disturbance is more than one month

F. The disturbance causes clinically significant distress or impairment in social, occupational or other important areas of functioning

International Classification of Diseases, ICD-10. diagnostic criteria
- PTSD is also recognised as a separate diagnostic category in the latest revision of the International Classification of Diseases, ICD-10. The diagnostic criteria, which are less specific than DSM-IV, are:

Essential
   - Onset within six months of a traumatic event of exceptional severity
   - Repetitive intrusive recollection or re-enactment of the event in memories, daytime imagery or dreams
Not essential
   - Emotional detachment, numbing of feeling and avoidance
   - Autonomic disturbances
   - Mood disorder
   - Behavioural abnormalities

Management

- Although a wide range of treatment methods have been used for PTSD, there is no specific treatment
- In general, the treatment of PTSD is based on:
    - The provision of support, preferably in groups, helps the victim to understand that he is not alone (the key is talking about and sharing the experience)
    - The prevention of avoidance behaviour, and encouragement and support for patients to face any situations about which they have become phobic
- The treatment of PTSD may depend on the presentation:
    - Acute onset
    - Delayed onset (after six months):
        - May be associated with significant depression requiring concurrent pharmacological treatment
    - Chronic:
        - The longer treatment is delayed, the harder it is to manage successfully

Primary intervention

- Immediately following a disaster, victims may experience:
    - Confusion
    - Fear
    - Shock
    - Disorientation
    - Feelings of being overwhelmed
    - Anger
- They have a basic need for:
    - Comfort
    - Reassurance:
        - Good communication conveying rapid accurate information about:
            - What has happened to their fellows
            - What has happened to them
            - What is still happening/going to happen, e.g. operations, discharge from hospital
    - Protection
    - Security
    - To be reunited with their natural group:
        - Friends, relatives, co-workers
- Early psychological intervention may have several advantages:
    - Personal experience of the disaster and its immediate aftermath may increase credibility (as may experience of similar disasters)
    - Allows the professional to be seen and regarded as part of the team, rather than as a distant and possibly threatening figure to whom the victim is referred later
    - Assists in the forming of a special relationship (bonding) between victim and helper
    - May facilitate psychological triage:
        - Identifies those most at risk of developing problems later
- Immediate treatment of any sleep disturbance with a benzodiazepine may be beneficial, but should be of limited duration, to minimise the risk of dependence

Secondary intervention

- This should be started once the basic threat to survival has ended and basic needs met
- Should generally only be in response to symptoms

Specific techniques
- Individual or group counselling/critical stress debriefing (possibly best):
- Desensitisation
- Learning relaxation techniques/anxiety management
- Psychotherapy
- Tricyclic antidepressants (may also improve sleep quality and prevent nightmares)
- Eye movement desensitisation and reprocessing (EMDR)

Individual or group counselling/critical stress debriefing
- Eases the expression of feelings
- Helps in the understanding of reactions and methods of coping
- Informs the victims what they may expect of themselves
- Identifies specific problems and suggests realistic solutions
- Inspires hope for the future
- Allows identification of positive achievements and progress
- Must help the patient to take a realistic and unbiased view of what has happened to them and prevent them from seeing themself as a "permanent victim" for the rest of his life

Critical incident stress debriefing (CISD)
- Should take place 48-72 hours post incident, and after any operational debriefing
- The aim should be to:
    - Review the helper's role
    - Ease the expression of feelings
    - Explore particular problems and their solutions
    - Identify positive gains
    - Explore the consequences of disengagement
    - Identify those at risk
- Confidentiality is essential

Method
- Begin by reporting factual information
- Then lead on to more delicate issues such as their psychological and emotional reactions following the incident
- Debriefing should be conducted in a thoroughly professional manner, and should be considered a natural extension of the normal procedure following a disaster
- Discussion should be encouraged to be as honest and open as possible, which will require a constructive and non-judgemental attitude on the part of the group leader and other senior personnel
- Debriefing will be most effective if sessions are organised in naturally occurring groups, which encourages camaraderie, rather than a group of individuals who have little in common
- Males may get very angry due to the build up of emotions which they are unable to express to other males. Females are usually better at expressing their feelings and feel less vulnerable doing so
- The violence with which feelings may be expressed can be very frightening for others

Note: Successful debriefing makes demands on the group leader; he/she should have:
    - Some personal knowledge of the specific disaster and its effects
    - A knowledge of the psychological reaction to trauma and of group dynamics

Taped imaginative exposure
- The victim is asked to write a script and then make an audio tape of their experiences, and to play it back to themselves twice daily
- After two weeks while the victim should make a revised and more detailed recording (dealing with the real issues) and to continue listening to it
- This process may enable the casualty to separate their memories from the triggers which spark off their most painful and violent emotions, and allows them to ventilate their feelings

Note: Compliance with treatment may be a problem in PTSD and some victims may go to any length to avoid memories of the incident

Eye movement desensitisation and reprocessing
- This is a new technique used for the treatment of flashbacks

34

Organisation of immediate medical care

Organisation of immediate medical care

Liaison
- For any Immediate Care scheme to be effective, there must be good liaison with:
  - Ambulance Service
  - Police
  - Fire Service
  - Local A & E Departments
  - Other local immediate care schemes

Equipment
- The equipment used in or by a scheme depends on:
  - The funds available:
    - In general, equipment must give value for money, and when setting up a scheme it is best to provide relatively basic equipment initially, and then slowly add to it as the doctor's experience grows
  - The equipment carried by the local Ambulance Service. It may be either:
    - Additional
    - Complementary
    - Should always be compatible
  - The experience and training of the doctors involved
  - The physical size of the doctor's car
    - It should be realised that there is a limit as to how much can be squeezed into the average car boot, and some items which are bulky and may be used only on rare occasions are probably best issued to the busier and more experienced doctors
  - Although given to an individual doctor for his personal use, the equipment should continue to be the property of the scheme
  - The actual choice of equipment is discussed in another section (see below)

Identity cards
- It is essential for all doctors to carry identity cards (obtainable from BASICS headquarters):
  - The card identifies the holder as being a BASICS doctor. Especially at major incidents, there may be large numbers of doctors volunteering their services. These may include imposters and doctors inexperienced and untrained in Immediate Care. The police and ambulance services need to identify the genuine doctors who are going to be useful to them
  - In addition, if there is any element of security risk, the police will only allow doctors who are either known to them or who have identification into the scene
  - There is a register of all BASICS ID card holders, held at a central point. At some time in the future, this will be contactable on a 24 hour basis for verification purposes

Green beacons

The Law
-   The relevant regulations are contained in "The Road Vehicles Lighting Regulations 1984, Statutory Instrument number 812", which state that:
    -   Any vehicle being used by a Registered Medical Practitioner for the purposes of an emergency may display one or more green lamps
    -   Each green lamp or warning beacon is a device capable of emitting a flashing or rotating beam of light throughout 360 degrees in the horizontal plane
    -   Only those people entitled to use a green beacon may in fact have one fitted to their vehicle, whether or not it is in working order
    -   Each beacon must be visible at a reasonable distance from the vehicle, be mounted not less than 1200 mm above the ground and must flash at a rate between 60 and 240 equal times per minute
    -   Although not specified in this legislation, no vehicle may use bulbs in their headlights or beacons exceeding 55 watts

Twin tone horns/sirens
-   At present there is no facility in law for doctors to use either twin tone horns or sirens, or for anybody to legally give them permission
-   Many doctors, however, use these devices with the unwritten "permission" of their local Chief Constable, on the understanding that if the privilege is ever abused, it would result in action being taken against them

Training
-   The value of proper training in Immediate Care should not be underestimated. Although it shares a lot of common ground with several other disciplines, especially anaesthetics, accident and emergency medicine, and orthopaedics, it really is a discipline in its own right and has some subject matter that is unique
-   Because it is such a practical subject, like many other branches of medicine, it is difficult to learn by theory alone. By its very nature, and unlike many other disciplines, there is usually little time for much thought and so those involved in Immediate Care have to learn to get it right automatically. Such automatism can only be developed by constant practice, and working to guidelines

Training on the job
-   The best way to train for Immediate Care is to do it. However it is important to remember that every incident is unique, and should be treated as part of the learning process

Audit/follow up
-   If possible every casualty, other than those with minor injuries, should be followed up in hospital to find out what their actual injuries were, and to try to evaluate the benefit of the Immediate Care that was given, and to see if anything else could have been done, or if it was, whether it might not have been done better or differently
-   A log book should be used to record the results, which can be audited later

Debriefing
-   If possible most incidents should be discussed afterwards in an honest constructive and critical way with the other members of the emergency team present, especially ambulance personel, as this will help everyone understand each other's roles, and so improve the treatment for the one person who really counts: the patient. This must be tackled delicately initially, as it is very easy for one's motives to be misunderstood before good relationships are established
-   May act as a mutual counselling session following particularly horrific accidents/incidents

Theoretical training

- The value of theoretical training should not be underestimated, although Immediate Care is such a practical subject. For the experienced doctor it may be particularly useful for describing recent advances in Immediate Care

Practical training

- Practical training is particularly useful for procedures, such as intubation, intravenous cannulation, cricothyrotomy and insertion of chest drains, which may only be carried out infrequently on live patients, and where a special technique is necessary
- It is also invaluable for practising Basic and Advanced Life Support including recognition of arrhythmias, defibrillation and administration of cardiac drugs, using mannikins
- Any doctor who is issued with a defibrillator should be trained and certified in Advanced Life Support
- The value of joint training, especially with the ambulance service and possibly the fire service (in extrication) should be not underestimated and will not only improve technical skills and the understanding of each other's roles, but will also help develop a team approach

Hepatitis B/HIV disease

Introduction

- The prevalence of HIV is growing rapidly in the UK, whilst that of Hepatitis B is relatively static, averaging about 1000 reported cases per year
- So far as is known, no member of the emergency services has yet been contaminated or infected with either virus in the course of their duties, but the potential for being infected is a very real one
- The overall risk for occupational percutaneous exposure to HIV blood in a health care environment is about 3 per 1000 injuries, whilst that for Hepatitis is very much greater. The risk from saliva is very low

Pathophysiology

- Both the viruses responsible for Hepatitis B and HIV disease can be found in the body fluids of infected individuals, although so far only blood contamination has resulted in infection
- Infection usually enters the body through a defect in the dermis, e.g. a scratch or minor laceration, or through the mucous membranes. Such minor injuries are often sustained by emergency services personnel at an incident site, from broken glass, sharp metal, etc.
- Many studies have shown that there is no evidence of risk where contaminated blood is in contact with intact skin

Contamination

- High risk of contamination situations include:
  - Percutaneous injury from needles, surgical instruments, bone fragments
  - Exposure of broken skin due to abrasions, lacerations and eczema
  - Exposure of mucous membranes, including the eye, to contaminated blood or body fluids
- Low risk situations include contact with low risk materials including urine, vomit, saliva or faeces

Needlestick injury
- Needlestick injuries which carry a relatively high risk of transmission of HIV and hepatitis include:
  - Those resulting in deeply penetrating injury
  - Those caused by hollow bore needles, which may hold a reservoir of blood
  - Those caused by needles which are visibly blood stained or have been in an artery or vein
  - Those caused by needles which have been used on patients terminally ill with AIDS or hepatitis

Hepatitis B immunisation
- All those involved in Immediate Care be vaccinated against Hepatitis B, and their status checked at regular intervals (every 3-5 years)
- Vaccination is effective in preventing infection in individuals who produce antibodies. Ten to fifteen percent of those over 40 years of age do not respond, with a smaller proportion in younger people
- The vaccination course consists of the initial dose, followed 1 month later by another, and a third 6 months after the first. The response to immunisation should be checked 2-4 months later, and a booster dose given if the individual has a low response
- Non-responders should consider Hepatitis B immunoglobulin (HBIG) administration if exposure occurs

Protection/Prevention of contamination
- All those involved in Immediate Care should wear latex protective gloves to protect themselves from contamination with infected blood
- Many doctors, prefer not to wear gloves as they feel that it makes delicate manipulation of instruments difficult. In these circumstances the hands should be washed thoroughly after dealing with the incident, especially if there are any minor lacerations or eczema
- All sharps should be put in a sharps safety bin or container at the earliest opportunity. Most ambulance services equip their ambulances with these, and Immediate Care doctors are also advised to carry them
- Ideally a small sharps bin should be carried in the same equipment container as your emergency drug and intravenous fluid administration kit, so that any sharps can be put in the bin immediately after use

Management of contamination
- Immediately after contamination:
    - Wash the contaminated wound with water or saline
    - Encourage the contaminated wound to bleed
    - Cover the wound with a waterproof dressing
- If the source patient or blood is known to be or strongly suspected to be HIV or Hepatitis positive, or is at high risk of being HIV or Hepatititis B positive; contact the nearest available senior doctor on call for Infectious Diseases immediately

Hepatitis B
- Those contaminated with blood or body fluids thought to be infected with Hepatitis B should be given anti-Hepatitis B immunoglobulin (HBIG), which provides passive immunity, immediately, together with immunisation, if they have not previously been immunised

HIV
- The risk of acquiring HIV may be reduced following high risk exposure if zidovudine is taken prophylactically as soon as possible (preferably within one hour) following occupational exposure (post exposure prophylaxis: PEP) to body fluids from HIV positive patients
- PEP is not necessary following low risk exposure

Cleaning and disinfection

Cleaning
- All reusable medical equipment should be thoroughly cleaned with warm soapy water whilst wearing rubber household gloves, before attempting to disinfect or sterilise it
- Disposable equipment should not be reused
- Equipment which is reusable and likely to become contaminated includes laryngoscopes, pulse oximeter probes, stethoscopes, ventilation equipment (excluding tracheal tubes, etc.)

Disinfection
- This should be done with a fresh aqueous solution of bleach or dichloroisocyanurate (*Milton*®)

Tetanus immunisation

Introduction

- Tetanus is an acute disease, with an appreciable mortality. Tetanus spores are found in the soil and may be introduced into the body during injury, especially puncture wounds; but also through burns and trivial and often unnoticed scratches and abrasions
- By the very nature of their work, everyone involved in Immediate Care is at risk of being infected
- The staff of casualty units should be aware of the risk of tetanus contamination in any patients under their care and advise and treat them as necessary

Note:-   In patients under 6 years of age, substitute DPT (absorbed diptheria, pertussis and tetanus) for TT
- Patients with impaired immunity may not respond to the vaccine and may require additional TIG

Guidelines for the administration of tetanus toxoid (TT) and adsorbed tetanus human immunoglobulin (TIG)

Immunisation status	Wound type	Recommendations
Unimmunised or incompletely immunised	Low risk	One dose of TT followed by complete immunisation (Second dose 4 weeks later; third dose at 4-6 months) *Note:* - In order to maintain satisfactory protection a reinforcing dose should be given 10 years after the initial dose and again 10 years later - Reinforcing doses at less than 10 year intervals are *not recommended*, since they have been shown to be unnecessary and can result in considerable local reactions
	Tetanus prone: When the wound/burn is neglected for more than 6 hours. If there is a puncture wound, evidence of sepsis, direct contact with soil, or there is a significant amount of devitalised tissue	One dose of TT plus 250 u TIG (500 u if more than 24 hr since injury or there is a high risk of contamination) followed by a complete course of immunisation. The remaiming two injections should be given at *monthly* intervals *Note:* - Use separate syringes and limbs as sites of injection for TT & TIG
Full first course + booster within preceding 10 years	Low risk	No vaccine necessary
	Tetanus prone	If there is a high risk of tetanus, e.g. after contamination with manure: one dose of adsorbed vaccine
	Neglected more than 24 hours	One dose TT plus 250-500 u TIG administered at a different site
Last of 3 dose course *or*	Low risk	One dose TT
Booster more than 10 years previously	Tetanus prone	One dose TT plus 250-500 u TIG administered at a different site

Figure 33-1 Guidelines for administration of tetanus toxoid and absorbed tetanus human immunoglobulin

Callout policies

Selective callout
- Doctors are only called out to incidents which have either been assessed by an ambulance crew at the scene, or when persons are known either to be trapped or seriously injured

Advantages:
- Doctors are only called out when they are known to be needed
- Extended trained ambulance persons/paramedics may be able to cope adequately on many occasions

Disadvantages:
- In rural areas, it may take the ambulance a considerable time to get to the incident. Even if there are seriously injured patients, who need Immediate Care, it may not make sense for the ambulance to wait for a doctor, who may have to travel a similar distance to the ambulance, especially if the hospital is not that far away
- There will nearly always be a delay before the doctor reaches the scene. It is now accepted that the earlier Immediate Care begins, the more effective it will be
- Doctors may only be called out rarely, and gain little experience. "We are all only good at doing what we do often; and there is no substitute for repeated experience". A small number of callouts tends to lead to poor doctor morale and loss of enthusiasm, poor working relationships and poor discipline

CONCLUSION: - The method of choice for urban areas, where both the ambulances, doctors and hospitals are near the incident, and little time is spent in transit

Non-selective callout
- Doctors are called to every incident regardless of the initial assessment, except for obvious trivia

Advantages:
- Doctors reach the scene early, so that immediate treatment begins early
- Doctors attend many incidents, and even if their presence may not be strictly necessary in a considerable percentage of calls, they gain considerable experience and expertise in Immediate Care
- On some occasions doctors may save ambulance time by either deciding that a patient does not require treatment or in the case of casualties with minor injuries only, divert the ambulance to their surgery or local cottage hospital for treatment
- Doctors also develop a close working relationship with the ambulance crews, so that when there is a major incident, they all work together as a team
- A large number of successful callouts leads to good doctor morale and good discipline
- Doctor callout becomes a routine for ambulance control, so time is not wasted deciding whether or not a doctor is required

Disadvantages
- On some occasions, the callout may be a waste of doctor time, although, even if their attendance is not strictly necessary, it is very seldom ever a complete waste of time
- Doctor callout may take up ambulance control time, which can be at a premium

CONCLUSION
- The callout method of choice for rural areas

Limited selective callout
- This is when the control officer has a list of priorities and decides from the incoming information from the public, whether or not a doctor is required
- It is really a variation of selective callout and suffers from the same disadvantages, as well as the fact that the initial information from the public is often inaccurate
- It could however be developed using flow diagrams and carefully applied criteria to a very satisfactory callout system, especially for medical emergencies (see below)

Criteria based dispatch (CBD)
- This is a computer aided system, in which the control officer interrogates the initial informant with a set of questions based on flow diagrams, provided by the computer, which then decides the priority of the call and the appropriate response, including whether or not a physician should be dispatched
- Several systems, based on those developed for use in the USA, are currently being piloted by selected UK ambulance services

Advantages
- Such a system may be most useful for evaluating the appropriate response to medical emergencies, which are relatively easy to assess, and are more likely to occur in the domestic environment with ready telephone and patient access for patient reassessment

Disadvantages
- In trauma cases, the initial assessment of minor versus life threatening trauma is often more difficult than for medical cases, because for example there is often limited access to the patient
- The majority of accidents occur outside the home, making telephone access more difficult, the nearest telephone may be some distance from the incident, which makes it difficult to provide accurate information in response to interrogation
- Current systems do not take into account the average response time to an incident or distance to the nearest appropriate medical facility, both factors which are of vital import, when assessing the level of response, including whether or not dispatching a doctor is appropriate

CONCLUSION
- Criteria based dispatch is an exciting new development, which will require careful evaluation and subsequent modification, and should be used as an aid to dispatch, together with local knowledge, to determine the appropriate level of response

Automatic vehicle location (AVL)
- This is a satellite based system used for determining the precise location of ambulances and other emergency vehicles, including BASICs doctors in some areas, so that the nearest appropriate vehicle is dispatched

Commitment of doctors

Introduction
- Whether an Immediate Care Scheme uses an on call rota, a continuous on call commitment, or a mixture of the two, it will depend on the personal preferences of the participating doctors

Rota
- The on call commitment is shared between several doctors, usually partners in the same practice

Advantage:
- There is nearly always a doctor available in each area

Disadvantages:
- No one doctor really gets enough experience to be good at Immediate Care, and it is rare to find that all doctors in a partnership are equally enthusiastic about practising Immediate Care
- It is usually too expensive to equip all the doctors in one area to a high standard

Continuous
- Every doctor is on call continuously, except when he is either out of the area, or not available for personal reasons

Advantage:
- In each area there are one or two doctors who get a lot of experience, have high morale and discipline and can be equipped to a high standard

Disadvantage:
- It can be a very considerable commitment for a doctor to be on call continuously, and can put a strain on personal and professional relationships

CONCLUSION: - If possible a small number of highly committed and highly professional doctors who attend a relatively large number of incidents, is desirable to provide a professional service, but may be an unrealistic ideal in some areas

Medico-legal aspects of immediate care

Negligence
- At present the practice of Immediate Care is considered a normal part of hospital and general practice, and there have been no cases of doctors being sued for medical negligence. However, with an increasingly litigation minded population, the time may come when doctors are at risk of being sued
- A registered medical practitioner is expected to provide "appropriate and prompt action upon evidence suggesting the existence of a condition requiring urgent medical intervention"
- GPs are expected as part of their terms of service to provide emergency treatment to any person who requires it within their practice area. A practitioner with special skills in resuscitation, who offers assistance, takes on a duty of care, and must exercise it within the constraints imposed by the prevailing circumstances
- Having taken on the duty of care to a patient, a doctor is expected to provide a reasonable standard of treatment. "A doctor is not negligent, if he is acting in accordance with a practice accepted as proper by a responsible body of medical men skilled in that particular art, merely because there is a body of such opinion, that takes a contrary view"
- It is advisable for all doctors actively involved in Immediate Care to make sure that they are trained and competent in its practice. Training should include proper instruction, supervised practice and self audit.
- Records should be made and retained, as they would be for any other branch of medicine
- It should be remembered that once he has seen a patient, that doctor becomes legally responsible for the medical management of that patient, until the patient is handed over into the care of another doctor. He may also be considered legally responsible for the actions of any ambulance persons present, who may be considered to be working under his direction as far as the actual medical management of the patient is concerned

Police statements (Section 9 statements)

Introduction
- The Immediate Care practitioner may be asked by the police to provide them with a statement, as a result of attending an accident or incident
- The statement may be required for:
    - The Coroner when there has been a death, which he needs to investigate
    - The purposes of a criminal investigation
- The circumstances for this may include:
    - When there has been a sudden death, and the doctor is asked to confirm death
    - When someone has been killed in an accident, e.g. a road traffic accident, industrial accident, and the doctor is asked to confirm death
    - When there has been an assault, one of the parties to which has been treated by the doctor
    - Where a crime has been committed, which has been observed by the doctor

Format

Paper
- Most police forces have headed statement paper with continuation sheets, plain for typewritten statements, lined for handwritten statements
- Handwritten statements should be submitted only in an emergency (lawyers may delight in questioning the the clarity of a doctor's handwriting)
- A word processor with a spell-check facility may be used and ensures that the statement can be read through to check for errors and sense before a corrected version is printed out
- Any amendments to a handwritten or typed statement should be initialled
- Some police forces have pre-prepared statements for doctors to complete and sign after confirming death at a road traffic accident
- It is advisable to keep a copy of the statement for future reference

Content
- Statements are designed to be read by lay people, and should be written in plain English, avoiding medical terms if possible; where there is no alternative it is a good idea to provide a simple explanation of what the medical term means in brackets, e.g. periorbital haematoma (black eye)

Layout
- A statement should include the following:
    - Name
    - Address
    - Age of witness (if over 21, just state 'over 21')
    - Occupation of witness:
    - Preamble as below:
        - " Who states: This statement, consisting of .... page (s), signed by me, is true to the best of my knowledge and belief and I make it knowing that if it is tendered in evidence I shall be liable to prosecution if I have wilfully stated in it anything which I know to be false or do not believe to be true".
        Dated the .... day of .... 199 ....

        (Signed) ....

    - In addition to the first signature, the bottom of each sheet should be signed immediately below the last paragraph in the right hand corner (so that no further information can be added later)

- Then follows the statement. Each subsequent page must be headed as follows:
  - Continued statement of .... Sheet No ....
- If the statement is typed out it should be set out in paragraphs
- If the statement is hand written, there should be continuous text with no paragraphs (so that no further information can be added later)
- The first paragraph should contain the writer's:
  - Relevant qualifications
  - Current appointment
  - Experience relevant to the case
- The next paragraph should provide:
  - An explanation as to how the writer became involved in the case, e.g. as an Immediate Care Scheme doctor called out by the ambulance service
  - The date and time of the callout (this may be obtained from ambulance control, if necessary)
  - The time of arrival and of examining the patient
  - The location of the incident, e.g. name and location of road, precise room in house
  - The name, age, date of birth and address of the patient (the patient's name should always be written in capital letters, wherever it appears)
  - A description of the vehicles involved, including manufacture, colour and index number

Note: In some accidents/incidents, the precise identity of a casualty may not be known at the time. In this case it is probably best to record the name and telephone number of the police "Officer Dealing" with the case, and contact him the following day

  - The following paragraph may include:
    - The results of examining the patient
    - Details of any treatment carried out
    - Details of any other persons present, e.g. ambulance crew
    - The time of confirmation of death, and the name, rank and serial number of the police officer present at that time
  - If *Polaroid*® photographs are taken for forensic purposes, you should:
    - Add the patient's name, date and your signature to the paper strip on the back of the photo.
    - Record the fact in your statement
  - It is usually best not to express an opinion about the cause of the accident or cause of death, unless you are very sure of all the facts, and are happy to appear in court to be cross questioned!

Essex Police

Witness Statement

Statement of: Dr Christopher John Eaton

Ageof Witness (if over 21, state 'over 21'): Over 21   Occupation: Medical Practitioner

Address: 2 Borough Lane, Saffron Walden, Essex CB11 4AF   Tel. No. 01799-524224

Who states: This statement, consisting of one page, signed by me, is true to the best of my knowledge and belief and I make it knowing that if it is tendered in evidence I shall be liable to prosecution if I have wilfully stated in it anything which I know to be false or do not believe to be true.

Dated the   23 rd   day of   August   1998

(Signed)   J Eaton

I am a fully Registered and qualified medical practitioner, having obtained the degrees of Bachelor of Medicine and Bachelor of Surgery of the University of London, and being a Licentiate of the Royal College of Surgeons of Physicians of London, and a Member of the Royal College of Surgeons of England. I also hold the Diploma in Immediate Medical Care of the Royal College of Surgeons of Edinburgh, and have been certified proficient in Advanced Cardiac Life Support and Advanced Trauma Life Support. At present I am engaged in General Practice in the Saffron Walden area, where I have been since 1978.

At approximately 14.30pm on Tuesday18 August 1998, I was called to attend a serious road traffic accident by Essex Ambulance control in my capacity as a member of MEDICS (The Mid Essex Immediate Care Scheme), on the M.11 Motorway, North-bound near the Strethall Road Bridge, by marker post 6662A.

On arriving at the scene, I found a white Ford Scorpio motor car Index No: H268 LTF, near which was the body of a male, who I now know to be that of JOHN THOMAS, of 16 The Willows, Great Chesterford, Essex CB10 1ZL. On examination he had no spontaneous pulse or respiration, and I confirmed him deceased at 14.43pm in the presence of P.C. 1580 Smith.

(Signed)   J Eaton

Figure 33-2 A specimen statement

35

Immediate medical care equipment

Immediate medical care equipment

Introduction
- This is a very brief and basic list of the various types of equipment used in Immediate Care, together with some of the manufacturers. It is by no means exhaustive, and the omission of a product does not mean that it is not recommended
- There may be positive advantages in using equipment from a common manufacturer, which may facilitate interchange of equipment or parts of equipment, e.g. ECG chest leads
- It is easy to get carried away by new and increasingly complex equipment. The value of any new item of equipment is unproven, and there needs to be careful pre-hospital and hospital evaluation of its role in Immediate Care before purchase
- If new equipment is introduced, then to be used effectively, there needs to be instruction in its use not only for the ambulance service, but also for Immediate Care doctors and possibly even the fire service, so that all the members of the team are familiar with its use and applications

Key: * - Basic Equipment: suitable for most doctors
     ** - More Advanced Equipment: more expensive and probably best reserved for doctors who are called out a lot, are trained and competent in its use and are more experienced

Radio equipment
- Radiopagers:
    - Commercial:
      - Cellular
    - VHF
- Hand portables:
    - UHF:
        - Short range, only used for on-site communication
    - VHF:
        - Long range, but there may be problems with "shadowing"
    - Cellular
- Car radios:
    - UHF:
        - Usually only used as a relay in conjunction with a link to a VHF radio
        - VHF with selective calling, status reporting, etc.
    - Cellular

Vehicle equipment

Green beacons
- Light source may be either:
    - Quartz Halogen bulb with:
        - Rotating reflector
        - Stroboscopic tube
        - * Single light
    - ** Multiple lights often a pair of rotating lights with a forward facing strobe
    - ** Bar light
- Mounting:
    - * Magnetic:
        - May fall off due to buffeting at high speeds
        - Dashboard mounted
    - ** Permanent:
        - Bolt on
        - Gutter mounting
        - Integrated into the vehicle's light clusters/radiator grille

Audible warning devices/sirens
- * Air operated (pneumatic):
    - Cheap, need maintaining
    - Not so loud
- ** Electronic:
    - Expensive, but very audible

Safety equipment
- * Hazard warning triange
- * Reflective strips
- * Compressed gas warning triangle
- * Spray-on disinfectant

Protective identifying clothing
- * High visibility jacket which meet the BSI standard for visibility and is fire retardant
- * High visibility tabard
- ** High visibility over trousers
- * Green protective helmet with visor and headlight
- * Heavy duty boots (preferably steel capped)
- * Gloves:
    - * Latex
    - ** Heavy duty rubber: debris gloves
- ** Protective goggles
- ** Fire-resistant suit (usually a "Proban" coated overall)
- ** Chemical-resistant overall suits (to BASICS specification or from the *Germa*® clothing range)

Rescue equipment
- * Shears/scissors
- * *SOS*® rescue device
- ** Seat belt cutter

Patient management equipment

Airway management device
- * Lubricating jelly and gauze swabs
- * Stethoscope
- * Oropharyngeal Airways:
    - Guedel sizes 000-4
- Nasopharyngeal airways:
    - * Latex.
    - ** Linder balloon
- ** Modified Oesophageal Airways:
    - Pharyngeal Tracheal Lumen Airway
    - Combi tube
    - Laryngeal Mask Airway
- Cricothyrotomy devices:
    - * Large intravenous cannula: 12-16 G
    - ** Mini Trach II
    - ** Quicktrach
- **Small tracheostomy tube: 5
- * Tracheal introducers:
    - Gum elastic bougie (facilitates intubation)
    - Malleable plastic introducer
- Suction:
    - * Hand operated
    - * Foot operated
    - ** Oxygen driven from ventilator
    - ** Electric/battery operated

Ventilation management devices
- * Pocket Mask Professional with oxygen inlet and strap
- * Bag and mask with an oxygen reservoir and additional paediatric mask
- * Oxygen cylinder with multiflow ability and high concentration mask (?plus recharging device)
- ** Ventilators
- ** Chest drainage kits
- * Laryngoscopes:
    - Penlon (plastic)
    - Plastic with interchangeable blades
    - Metal with adult and paediatric blades (may have bulb or fibre optic illumination)
- Asherman chest seal

Circulation care devices
- ** *Cardiopump®*
- * Wide bore cannulae: 12, 14, 16 G
- ** With dilator for very rapid infusion
- ** Intraosseous needles
- * Giving sets
- ** IV Push - Pressure Infusor
- * Elbow splint: ArmLok
- ** Wrist splint
- * Tourniquet:
    - * For phlebotomy
    - ** For haemorrhage control

- - * 3-Way tap
- - * Fluid warmers:
    - - Reusable hot pack
    - - Infupack
    - - Hot sack
- - ** Pneumatic Anti Shock Garment: *Gladiator*®
- - * Hooks for drips:
    - - Butcher's
    - - Magnetic

Splints for the management of fractures
- - * Triangular bandages
- - * Wide crepe bandages
- - * Cervical spine:
    - - Stifneck Select
    - - Ambu Perfit Ace
    - - Necloc
    - - Hines
- - * Femur: Traction splints:
    - - Pneumatic (bicycle pump):
        - - Donway splint
    - - Spring tension:
        - - Sager
    - - Locked winder:
        - - Conway Trac 3
    - - Winder and ratchet:
        - - Hare (latest versions as Conway)
    - - Light weight portable:
        - - Kendrick
- - * Limb splints:
    - - Box: adult and paediatric
    - - Frac straps
    - - Sam splints
- - ** Spencer splints (upper and lower limb)

Burns
- - * Burns dressings
- - * Kling film

Extrication devices **
- - KED
- - RED
- - Fallon
- - ED 2000

Equipment for medical emergencies
- - ** Defibrillators
- - * Nebulisers
- - * Blood glucometer
- - * Peak flow meter: *Mini Wright*®

Drugs for use in Immediate Care
- Prefilled syringes, e.g. the IMS *Min-I-Jet*® system are prefered for use in Immediate Care, because they are easy to assemble and use in an emergency

Miscellaneous
- Dedicated drugs case with syringes and needles or injection; 21G (green) and 23 G (blue)
- Ampoule opener
- Disposable sharps box

Cardiovascular system

Diuretics
- Furosemide:
    - 10 mg/mL in 2, 5 mL ampoules
    - 10 mg/mL in 25 mL prefilled syringe (IMS)

Antiarrhythmic drugs
- Lidocaine:
    - 10 mg/mL, 10 mL prefilled syringe (IMS)
    - 20 mg/mL, 5 mL prefillled syringe (IMS, Xylocard)
- Atropine:
    - 100μg/mL, 10, 20, 30 mL prefilled syringe (IMS)
    - 300 μg/mL, 10 mL prefilled syringe (Aurum)
- Bretylium: 50 mg/mL, 10 mL ampoules or prefilled syringe (IMS)
- Calcium chloride: 1g/10 mL (10%) prefilled syringe (IMS)
- Adenosine: 3 mg/mL, 2 mL ampoules

Nitrates
- Glyceryl trinitrate spray
- *Suscard*® buccal 1, 2, 3, 5 mg

Sympathomimetics
- Epinephrine: 10 mL 1:10,000 prefilled syringe (IMS)

Anti-coagulants
- *Hepsal*® (should be stored in a refrigerator)

Antiplatelet drugs
- Aspirin 75, 300 mg tablets

Thrombolytics
- Anistreplase 30 unit vial with 5 mL water for reconstitution (should be stored in a refrigerator)

Intravenous infusion fluids
- Crystalloid:
    - Hartmann's solution
    - N-Saline intravenous infusion, 500, 1000 mL packs
- Colloids:
    - *Haemaccel*®
    - *Gelofusine*®
- Buffering solution:
    - Sodium bicarbonate: 50 mL 8.4% prefilled syringe (IMS)

Respiratory system

Bronchodilators
- β_2 adrenergic agonists:
    - Salbutamol nebules: 2.5/5 mg
    - Terbulaline respules: 2.5 mg/mL in 2 mL
- Adrenoceptor stimulants:
    - Epinephrine: 1 mL 1:1000 prefilled syringe (IMS)
- Anticholinergic:
    - Ipratropium bromide: nebuliser solution: 0.25 %
- Methylxanthene:
    - Aminophylline: 250 mg/10 mL

Steroids
- Hydrocortisone: 100 mg/mL ampoules
- Prenisolone: tabs 5 mg

Antihistamines
- Chlorpheniramine: injection 10 mg/mL

Central nervous system

Analgesics
- Opiates:
    - Diamorphine 5, 10, 30 100, 500 mg ampoules (should be administered with an anti-emetic, e.g. metoclopramide 5 mg/mL, 2 mL ampoules)
    - Nalbuphine: 10 mg/mL, 1, 2 ml ampoules
- Opiate antagonist: naloxone: 20, 400 µg/ml, 1 mL ampoules
- Gases: nitrous oxide/oxygen
- Non steroidal anti-inflammatory: diclofenac: 25 mg/mL, 3 mL ampoules

Anaesthetics/sedating agents
- Diazepam:
    - Intravenous injection: 5 mg/mL 2mL
    - Rectal tubes: *Stesolid*®: 2 mg, 4 mg/mL 2.5 mL
- Midazolam: 10 mg/2 mL/5mL
- Ketamine: 10 mg/mL, 20 mL vial, 50 mg/mL, 10 mL vial, 100 mg/mL, 5 mL vial
- Propofol: 10 mg/mL, 20 mL ampoooules
- Etomidate: 2mg/mL, 10 mL ampoules
- Flumazenil: 100 µg/mL, 5 mL ampoules

Infections: antibiotics

Penicillin
- Benzyl penicillin injection: 600 mg vial

Chloramphenicol
- Chloramphenicol injection: 300 mg,1 g, 1.2 g vials

Endocrine system
- Diabetes, treatment of hypoglycaemia:
    - Glucose: 50 mL 50% prefilled syringe (IMS)
    - Glucagon: 1, 10 mg vial with diluent

Obstetrics/gynaecology

Oxytocics
- Ergometrine: 500 µg/mL, 1 mL amoules
- Syntometrine (ergometrine 500 µg, oxytocin 5 units/mL) 1 mL ampoules

Skin disinfectant/cleanser
- Povidone iodine dry spray (*Betadine*®)

Monitoring equipment
- * Stethoscope preferably with amplification
- * Pen torch
- * Sphygmomanometers:
    - Aneroid
    - Audio
- ** Pulse oximeter
- * Disposable end tidal CO_2 detector
- * Ear thermometer
- ** Multi measurement devices:
    - Non invasive BP
    - ECG
    - Oximetry
    - Temperature
    - Capnography

Equipment containers
- Preferably lightweight and easily portable:
    - Rigid
    - Soft

Recording information/reporting
- * BASICS report forms
- * BASICS triage labels
- ** Cameras: still, instant, polaroid
- * *Broselow*® paediatric tape

Miscellaneous equipment
- Lighting:
    - * Flood/spotlight:
        - Hand held
        - Magnetic
- Space blankets:
    - * Single use
    - ** Heavy duty
- Labels for identifying contents of equipment cases
- Book: Substances Hazardous to Health: Emergency First Aid Guide

Bibliography

Books: Title	Author	Publisher	Date
ABCs from the BMJ		BMJ Publishing Group	
ABC of Antenatal Care *Third Edition*	Chamberlain		1997
ABC of Atrial Fibrillation	Lip		1996
ABC of Emergency Radiology	Edited: Nicholson & Driscoll		1995
ABC of Diabetes *Fourth Edition*	Watkins		1998
ABC of Major Trauma *Second Edition*	Edited: Skinner et al		1996
ABC of Mental Health	Edited: Davies & Craig		1998
ABC of Resuscitation: *Third Edition*	Edited: Evans et al		1996
ABC of Spinal Cord Injury: *Third Edition*	Grundy & Swain		1996
ABC if Sports Medicine	Edited: McLatchie		1995
Accident & Emergency Diagnosis & Management	Brown	Butterworth Heinemann	1996
Accidents & Emergencies *Second edition*	Kirby	Castle House	1991
Accidents & Emergencies *Sixth Edition*	Bache & Hardy	Oxford Universiy Press	1994
ACLS Manual		American Heart Assoc	1989
Acute Medicine *Second Edition*	Sprigings	Blackwell Science	1995
Advanced Life Support Course Manual *Third Edition*	Edited: Handley	Resuscitation Council (UK)	1998
Advanced Paediatric Life Support *Second Edition*	Advanced Life Support Gp.	BMJ Publishing Group	1997
Advanced Trauma Life Support *Sixth Edition*	American Coll of Surg		1997
Acute Poisoning *Second Edition*	Proudfoot	Butterworth Heinemann	1993
Aeromedical Transportation	Martin & Rodenberg	Ashgate	1997
Basic Rescue and Emergency Care	American Academy of Orthopaedic Surgeons		1990
British National Formulary *Number 35 (March 1998)*		British Medical Assoc & Pharmaceutical Soc of GB	1998
Cambridge Textbook of Accident & Emergency Medicine	Editors: Skinner et al	Cambridge University Press	1997
Care of the Acutely Ill & Injured	Edited: Wilson & Marsden	John Wiley	1989
Clinical Forensic Medicine	Edited: McLay	Pinter	1990
Common Obstetric Emergencies	Gibb	Butterworth Heineman	1991
Current Emergency Diagnosis & Treatment	Edited: Ho and Saunders	Appleton & Lange	1990
Disasters: Current Planning and Recent Experience	Walsh	Edward Arnold	1989
The ECG Made Easy *Fifth Edition*	Hampton	Churchill Livingstone	1997
The ECG in Practice *Second Edition*	Hampton	Churchill Livingstone	1997
Emergency Care	Edited: Greaves et al	WB Saunders	1997
Emergency Care and Transportation of the Sick and Injured: *Fifth Edition*	Edited: Heckman	American Academy of Orthopaedic Surgeons	1992
Emergencies in the Home	Various	BMJ Publishing Group	1990
Essentials of Sports Medicine *Third Edition*	McLatchie	Churchill Livingstone	1993
Guide to Major Incident Planning	Edited: Hines & Robertson	BASICS	1986
Guide to the Misuse of Drugs Act 1971 and the Misuse of Drugs Regulations	Department of Health	1989	
Handbook of Immediate Care	Greaves et al	W B Saunders	1995
The High Altitude Medicine Handbook	Pollard & Murdoch	Radcliffe Medical Press	1997
Immunisation against Infectious Diseases *1996 Edition*	Dept of Health	HMSO	1992
Lecture Notes on Accident & Emergency Medicine	Yates & Redmond	Blackwell	1985
The Management of Acute Pain	Park and Fulton	Oxford University Press	1992
Major Incident Medical Management and Support	Advanced Life Support Gp	BMJ Publishing Group	1995
Management of Disasters and their Aftermath	Wallace, Rowles, Colton	BMJ Publishing Group	1994
Medicine for Disasters	Edited: Baskett & Weller	John Wright	1988
The New Police Surgeon	Edited: Burges	Hutchinson	1978
Outline of Fractures	Adams & Hamblen	Churchill Livingstone	1992

Oxford Handbooks of Emergency Medicine	Editors: Illingworth et al	Oxford University Press	
Accidents and Emergencies in Children *Second Edition*	Morton & Phillips		1996
The Management of Wounds and Burns	Wardrope & Smith		1992
Cardiopulmonary Resuscitation	Skinner & Vincent		1993
The Management of Head injuries	Currie		1993
Anaesthesia and Analgesia	Illingworth & Simpson		1994
Maxillo and Dental Emergencies	Hawkesford & Banks		1994
Emergencies in Obstetrics and Gynaecology	Stevens & Kenney		1994
The Management of Major Trauma *Second Edition*	Robertson & Redmond		1994
Environmental Medical Emergencies	Steedman		1994
Psychiatric Emergencies	Merson & Baldwin		1995
History Taking, Examination, and Record Keeping in Emergency Medicine	Guly		1996
Acute Medical emergencies	Guly & Richardson		1996
Pre-Hospital Trauma Life Support *Third Edition*	PHTLS Committee of the National Assocn. of EMT	Mosby-Year Book Inc	1994
Principles and Practice Series	Editors: Hahn & Adams	BMJ Publishing Group	
Capnography	O'Flaherty		1994
Pulse Oximetry	Moyle		1994
Rescue Emergency Care	Edited: Easton	Heinemann	1977
Resuscitation of Babies at Birth	Royal College of Paediatrics and Child Health UK	BMJ Publishing Group	1997
Resuscitation Handbook *Second Edition*	Baskett	Lippincott/Gower	1993
RTA: Persons Trapped	Watson	Greenwade	1991
Simpsons Forensic Medicine *Tenth Edition*	Knight	Edward Arnold	1991
Substances Hazardous to Health: Emergency First Aid Guide	Edited: Houston	Croner Publications Ltd	1994
Trauma Care	Edited: Driscoll & Skinner	BMJ Publishing Group	1998
Trauma: Pathogenesis & Treatment	Edited: Westaby	Heinemann	1989
Trauma Resuscitation; The Team Approach	Driscoll et al	Macmillan	1993
What to do in a Paediatric Emergency	Higginson et al	BMJ Publishing Group	1996
Yearbooks of Emergency Medicine	Wagner	Mosby-Year Book Inc	1992/3/4/5/6/7

Journals

The British Medical Journal
Care of the Critically Ill
European Journal of Emergency Medicine
Injury: The British Journal of Accident Surgery
Journal of Accident & Emergency Medicine
Journal of the British Association for Immediate Care
Journal of Clinical Forensic Medicine
Pre-Hospital Immediate Care
Resuscitation: Official Journal of the European Resuscitation Council

The above list is is by no means exhaustive, but reading most of the above should give the reader a very good grounding in the ever developing art and science of Immediate Care

Index

Notes